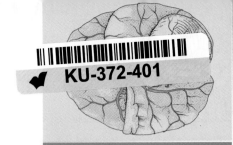

BARR'S
The Human
Nervous System
AN ANATOMICAL VIEWPOINT

NINTH EDITION

John A. Kiernan, MB, ChB, PhD, DSc
Professor
Department of Anatomy and Cell Biology
The University of Western Ontario
London, Canada

 Wolters Kluwer | Lippincott Williams & Wilkins
Health
Philadelphia • Baltimore • New York • London
Buenos Aires • Hong Kong • Sydney • Tokyo

Acquisitions Editor: Crystal Taylor
Developmental Editor: Kathleen H. Scogna
Managing Editor: Jessica Heise
Marketing Manager: Valerie Sanders
Production Editor: John Larkin
Creative Director: Doug Smock
Compositor: Maryland Composition

Ninth Edition

Copyright © 2009, 2005 Lippincott Williams & Wilkins, a Wolters Kluwer business.

351 West Camden Street
Baltimore, MD 21201

530 Walnut Street
Philadelphia, PA 19106

Printed in China

The publisher is not responsible (as a matter of product liability, negligence, or otherwise) for any injury resulting from any material contained herein. This publication contains information relating to general principles of medical care that should not be construed as specific instructions for individual patients. Manufacturers' product information and package inserts should be reviewed for current information, including contraindications, dosages, and precautions.

The publishers have made every effort to trace the copyright holders for borrowed material. If they have inadvertently overlooked any, they will be pleased to make the necessary arrangements at the first opportunity.

To purchase additional copies of this book, call our customer service department at (800) 638-3030 or fax orders to (301) 223-2320. International customers should call (301) 223-2330.

Visit Lippincott Williams & Wilkins on the Internet: http://www.lww.com. Lippincott Williams & Wilkins customer service representatives are available from 8:30 am to 6:00 pm, EST.

Library of Congress Cataloging-in-Publication Data
Kiernan, J. A. (John Alan)
 Barr's the human nervous system : an anatomical viewpoint / John A. Kiernan. — 9th ed.
  p. ; cm.
 Includes bibliographical references and index.
 ISBN 1605473960
 ISBN 9781605473963
 1. Neuroanatomy. I. Barr, Murray Llewellyn, 1908-1995. II. Title. III. Title: Human nervous system.
 [DNLM: 1. Nervous System—anatomy & histology. WL 101 K47b 2009]
 QM451.B27 2009
 611.8–dc22
                    2008014726

Preface to the Ninth Edition

Murray Llewellyn Barr (1908–1995) obtained his medical degree in 1933 from the University of Western Ontario in London, Canada, and after a few years in practice, he entered the Department of Anatomy at the same institution. He studied and taught neuroanatomy there until 1978. This period of service was interrupted by the Second World War, when he served in the Medical Branch of the Royal Canadian Air Force. In 1949, the direction of Barr's research changed abruptly from neurohistology to cytogenetics. With Ewart G. ("Mike") Bertram, who was then a graduate student, he had observed an intranuclear inclusion in neurons of female animals. This was the sex chromatin, now widely known as the *Barr body*; its discovery was an early landmark in the science of human cytogenetics. For this and his later work in the field, Murray Barr received more than 30 awards and honors, including the Kennedy Foundation International Award in Mental Retardation, Fellowship of the Royal Society of London, the Order of Canada, and seven honorary doctorates.

Although Barr's research career was largely concerned with the cytological diagnosis of inherited diseases, he continued to teach neuroanatomy. The first edition of this book, published in 1972, was one of the first medium-sized texts in its field. It was written to make life easier for those approaching neuroscience for the first time, especially medical students and those in the allied health sciences. This objective has not changed, although a greater variety of students now study the subject. Advances in the science necessitated much revision over the years, and the book became larger with successive editions. With the Eighth Edition, this trend was reversed, resulting in a somewhat smaller book. The illustrations were enhanced, however, with more extensive use of colors.

New to This Edition

In this Ninth Edition, the improvement and changing of illustrations has continued, and nearly all are now colored. The text and recommended readings have, of course, also been updated. Readers of this edition have access to the publisher's Web site—www.lww.thepoint.com—which includes a variety of additional materials. These include labeled and unlabeled versions of all the illustrations for instructors, sample exam questions and clinical cases, an extended glossary, and biographical information about researchers and physicians whose names are associated with anatomy, physiology, and diseases of the nervous system. ThePoint also carries expanded versions of some chapters. A marginal icon in the printed book indicates subjects for which additional material is available online.

Acknowledgments

An important feature in the production of the Ninth Edition has been the publisher's extensive use of external reviewers. I'd like to thank Robert Cambridge, Erica Grimm, Vaishnav Krishnan, Anna Likhacheva, Sidney L. Palmer, PhD, James Pinckney II, and Maria Thomadaki, DC. The book is undoubtedly much improved as a result of their recommendations and comments, for which I thank them. It is a pleasure to acknowledge also the helpful advice given by present and former colleagues during the writing of this and the five preceding editions: Drs. J. Ronald Doucette, Jonathan Hore, Kost Elisevich, Brian A. Flumerfelt, Elias B. Gammal, Alan W. Hrycyshyn, Arthur J. Hudson, Peeyush K. Lala, Peter Merrifield, D.G. Montemurro, David M. Pelz, N. Rajakumar, David Ramsay, A.

Jon Stoessl, Shannon Venance, Tutis Vilis, and Chris Watling. I appreciate also the numerous insightful comments of Professor Ronan O'Rahilly (Villars-sur-Glâne, Switzerland), especially on matters of embryology and terminology.

The artwork for the first seven editions of the book was prepared by local artists (Margaret Corrin, Louise Gadbois, Jeannie Ross, Nancy Somerville) supervised by the authors. For this edition, all the illustrations were prepared in electronic form by the publisher's art department, Jennifer Clements and artist Kim Battista, working from older artwork and from my sketches. Among other staff at Lippincott Williams & Wilkins, Crystal Taylor arranged the reviewing and the contract for the Ninth Edition, and Kathleen Scogna, Jessica Heise, and John Larkin presided over production of the book. I thank them all for their contributions.

J. A. KIERNAN
London, Canada

Contents

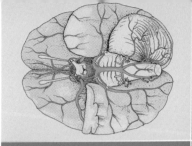

PART I

Introduction and Neurohistology

Chapter 1

DEVELOPMENT, COMPOSITION, AND EVOLUTION OF THE NERVOUS SYSTEM

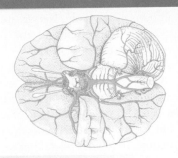

Important Facts

- The nervous system is derived from the ectoderm of the embryo.
- The central nervous system is formed from the neural tube, and the peripheral nervous system is formed from the neural crest.
- The first cells to differentiate in the nervous system are neurons, which are specialized for communication. They are followed by supporting cells known as neuroglia (or simply glia).
- Abnormal development of the brain or spinal cord can result from faulty closure of the neural tube or failed development of the overlying bone and skin.
- Obstruction of the flow of cerebrospinal fluid within or out of the cavities of the brain results in fluid accumulation known as hydrocephalus.
- The major divisions of the central nervous system are present from the 4th week after fertilization. They are the spinal cord, medulla, pons, midbrain, diencephalon, and cerebral hemispheres. The cerebellum appears later, as an outgrowth of the brain stem.
- Within normal limits, the size of the brain does not correlate with intelligence.

All living organisms respond to chemical and physical stimuli. The response may be a movement, or it may be the expulsion of biosynthetic products from cells. These receptive, motor, and secretory functions are combined in a single cell in both unicellular organisms and the simplest multicellular animals, the sponges. In all other groups of animals, cells are able to communicate, so that the reception of a stimulus by one cell may result in motile or secretory activity of other cells. Specialized cells known as **neurons** or nerve cells exist to transfer information rapidly from one part of an animal's body to another. All the neurons of an organism, together with their supporting cells, constitute a **nervous system**.

To carry out its communicative function, a neuron exhibits two different but coupled activities. They are **conduction** of a signal from one part of the cell to another and **synaptic transmission**, which is communication between adjacent cells. An **impulse**, also called an **action potential**, is a wave of electrical depolarization that is propagated within the surface membrane of the neuron. A stimulus applied to one part of the neuron initiates an impulse that travels to all other parts of the cell. Neurons commonly have long cytoplasmic processes, known as **neurites**, that end in close apposition to the surfaces of other cells. The ends of the neurites are called **synaptic terminals**, and the cell-to-cell contacts they make are known as **synapses**. The neurites in higher animals usually are specialized to form **dendrites** and **axons**, which typically conduct toward and away from the cell body, respectively. Most axons are ensheathed in **myelin**, which is a lipid-rich material composed of tightly packed membranous layers. The arrival of an impulse at a terminal triggers synaptic transmission. This event normally involves the release of a chemical compound from the neuronal cytoplasm, which evokes some type of response in the postsynaptic cell. At some synapses, the two cells are electrically coupled. Another type of neuron exists that discharges its chemical products into the circulating blood, thereby influencing distant parts of the body. Neurons of the latter type, known as neurosecretory cells, are functionally related to endocrine gland cells.

The **central nervous system** (CNS) consists of the brain and spinal cord and is protected by the cranium and the vertebral column. Bundles of axons called **nerves** connect the CNS with all parts of the body. Nerves are the most conspicuous components of the **peripheral nervous system**. The cell bodies of neurons in the CNS are in regions known as **gray matter**. A compact aggregation of gray matter is called a **nucleus**, not to be confused with the nucleus of a cell. Regions of CNS tissue that contain axons but not neuronal cell bodies are called **white matter**. In the peripheral nervous system, neuronal cell bodies occur in nodular structures called **ganglia** (singular: **ganglion**). This word is also used (commonly but wrongly) for certain nuclei in the CNS.

Development of the Nervous System

The neurons and other cells of the nervous system develop from the dorsal **ectoderm** of the early embryo. The ectoderm is the layer that also becomes the epidermis, which covers the surface of the body. The first indication of the future nervous system is the neuroectoderm, consisting of the **neural plate**, which appears in the dorsal midline of the embryo at the 16th day after fertilization. The cells of the neural plate become taller than those of the ordinary ectoderm. This change is induced by the underlying mesodermal cells. The neural plate grows rapidly, and in 2 days, it becomes a **neural groove** with a **neural fold** along each side.

A note on times and ages. In clinical practice, pregnancy is timed from the 1st day of the last menstrual period, about 14 days before fertilization. The age of an embryo is stated from the known or estimated time of fertilization. When it is 8 weeks old and all the organs are formed, an embryo is renamed a fetus. The embryonic period is divided into 23 Carnegie stages, based on anatomical development. The neural folds appear at stage 8, when the embryo is 1.0 to 1.5 mm long.

NEURAL TUBE, CREST, AND PLACODES

By the end of the 3rd week (stage 10), the neural folds have begun to fuse with one another, thereby converting the neural groove into a **neural tube** (Fig. 1-1). This transformation begins in the middle (in what will eventually be

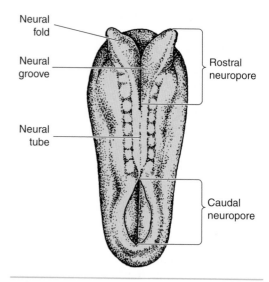

FIGURE 1-1   Dorsal view of a human embryo about 22 days after fertilization. Closure of the neural tube is in progress.

the cervical segments of the spinal cord) and proceeds rostrally and caudally. The openings at each end (the rostral and caudal **neuropores**) close at about the 24th and 27th days, respectively (stages 11 and 12). The neural tube is the forerunner of the brain and spinal cord. The cells lining the tube constitute the **neuroepithelium**, which will give rise to all the neurons and most of the other cells in the CNS.

Neuroectodermal cells that are not incorporated into the tube form **neural crests**, which run dorsolaterally along each side of the neural tube. From the neural crests are derived the dorsal root ganglia of spinal nerves, some of the neurons in sensory ganglia of cranial nerves, autonomic ganglia, the nonneuronal cells (neuroglia) of peripheral nerves, and secretory cells of the adrenal medulla. Thus, the cells of the neural crest are notable for their extensive migrations. Many of them even differentiate into cells of nonneural tissue, including the melanocytes of the skin; the calcitonin-secreting cells of the thyroid gland; cells in the carotid and aortic bodies; odontoblasts of teeth; and some of the bones, muscles, and other structures of mesenchymal origin in the head. The connective tissue cells in nerves and ganglia are derived from the local mesoderm.

Some peripheral nervous elements are derived from **placodes**, which are thickened regions of the ectoderm of the head's surface. Thus, the olfactory neurosensory cells, the sensory cells and associated ganglia of the inner ear, and some of the neurons in the sensory ganglia of cranial nerves are derived from placodes. Some cells of the olfactory placode migrate into the rostral end of the neural tube and become intrinsic neurons of the CNS.

PRODUCTION OF NEURONS AND NEUROGLIA

The first populations of cells produced in the neural tube are **neurons**. (The old term *neuroblasts* is inappropriate for these cells because after they are formed, they do not divide again.) Most of the neurons are produced between the 4th and 20th weeks. The young neurons migrate, grow cytoplasmic processes, and form synaptic connections with other neurons.

The number of neurons formed in the neural tube exceeds the number in the adult brain and spinal cord. Large numbers of neurons die in the normal course of development. This occurrence, known as **cell death** or **apoptosis**, is seen in many embryonic systems throughout the animal kingdom. In invertebrates, the cell death is genetically programmed. Experimental studies carried out by Hamburger in the 1930s showed that in vertebrates, the cells that died were those that failed to make synaptic connections. In some animals, new neurons are generated throughout life in some parts of the brain, from pluripotent precursor cells. Quantitative histochemical studies have provided no evidence of such activity in the adult human brain.

The neurons in sensory ganglia derived from the neural crest send neurites into peripheral nerves and into the neural tube. By the 8th week of intrauterine life, the centrally directed neurites have extensive synaptic connections with neurons in the spinal cord. The number and complexity of synapses continue to increase until well after birth, as does the generation of neuroglial cells.

Neuroglia, more commonly called **glia**, comprises the cells of the nervous system that are not neurons. The structures and functions of different glial cell types are dealt with in Chapter 2.

The first glial cells, known as radial glia, develop alongside the first neurons, having cytoplasmic processes that extend from the lumen to the outside surface of the neural tube. The processes of radial glia guide the migration of the young neurons. Most astrocytes and oligodendrocytes, however, are generated from the neuroepithelium during the fetal period. Mature glial cells are visible with classical staining methods by 19 weeks, but some can be detected by immunohistochemical techniques as early as 7 weeks. Microglial cells arise from hemopoietic tissue and enter the brain and spinal cord by passing through the walls of blood vessels.

In the peripheral nervous system, neurons (in sensory and autonomic ganglia) and glial cells (satellite cells in ganglia and Schwann cells in nerves) are derived from the neural crest.

FORMATION OF THE BRAIN AND SPINAL CORD

Even before the closure of the neural folds, the neural plate is conspicuously larger at the rostral end of the embryo, and irregularities corresponding to the major divisions of the developing **brain** are already visible. The remainder of the neural tube becomes the **spinal cord**. The site of closure of the caudal neuropore corresponds to the upper lumbar segments of the cord. Further caudally, the spinal cord is formed by "secondary neurulation," which is the coalescence of a chain of vesicles that becomes continuous with the lumen of the neural tube about 3 weeks after the closure of the caudal neuropore. The vesicles are derived from the **caudal eminence**, a mass of pluripotent cells located dorsal to the developing coccyx.

As described conventionally, three major divisions of the brain appear at the end of the 4th week: the **prosencephalon** (forebrain), **mesencephalon** (midbrain), and **rhombencephalon** (hindbrain). During the 5th week, secondary swellings develop in the prosencephalon and rhombencephalon, so that the number of major parts becomes five: the **telencephalon**, **diencephalon**, **mesencephalon**, **metencephalon**, and **myelencephalon** (Fig. 1-2). The same words are used for the corresponding parts of the adult human brain. (In the chick embryo, a favorite subject for embryological investigation, the swellings in the embryonic brain are known as "brain vesicles," a term that should not be used in human anatomy.) The early embryonic CNS is also divisible longitudinally into smaller segments known as **neuromeres**. The neuromeres become

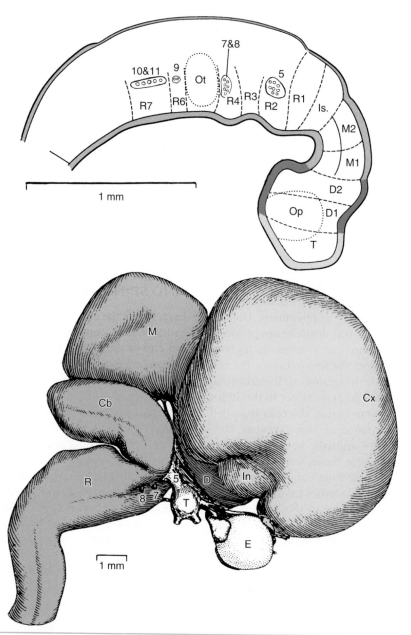

FIGURE 1-2   Major parts of the brain in human embryo at 4 weeks (above, a midline section) and fetus at 8 weeks (below, reconstucted from serial sections). Color scheme: Telencephalon (forebrain), yellow; diencephalon, blue; mesencephalon (midbrain), orange; rhombencephalon (hindbrain, composed of medulla, pons, and cerebellum), gray. In the embryo, some neuromeres are indicated for the telencephalon (T), diencephalon (D1, D2), mesencephalon (M1, M2), isthmus (Is), and rhombencephalon (**R1** to **R7**). The levels of the optic (**Op**) and otic (**Ot**) vesicles, which are lateral to the neural tube, are indicated. (These vesicles will become the lens and inner ear, respectively.) In the fetus: Cb, cerebellum; Cx, cerebral cortex; D, diencephalon; E, eye; In, insula; M, mesencephalon; R, rhombencephalon; T, trigeminal ganglion; 5, sensory root of trigeminal nerve; 7, 8, rootlets of facial and vestibulocochlear nerves. (Modified from O'Rahilly R, Müller F. *The Embryonic Human Brain. An Atlas of Developmental Stages*, 3rd ed. Hoboken, NJ: Wiley-Liss, 2006.)

indistinguishable as the complex structure of the brain develops, but segmental organization of the spinal cord persists throughout life.

As cellular proliferation and differentiation proceed in the neural tube, a longitudinal groove called the **sulcus limitans** appears along the inner aspect of each lateral wall. The sulcus demarcates a dorsal **alar plate** from a ventral **basal plate**; they acquire afferent and efferent connections, respectively, and are present from the rostral end of the mesencephalon to the caudal end of the spinal cord. Responding to an inductive effect of the nearby notochord (which marks the position of future vertebrae), the basal plates of the left and right sides become separated by a thin **floor plate**. Some of the basal plate cells differentiate into motor neurons, with axons that grow out into the developing muscles. The growing axons of neurons of the sensory ganglia enter the alar plate.

FURTHER DEVELOPMENT OF THE BRAIN

As the parts of the brain differentiate and grow, some of the formal embryological names are replaced by others for common usage (Table 1-1). The myelencephalon becomes the **medulla oblongata**, and the metencephalon develops into the **pons** and **cerebellum**. The mesencephalon of the mature brain usually is called the **midbrain**. The names *diencephalon* and *telencephalon* are retained because of the diverse nature of their derivatives. A large mass of gray matter, the **thalamus**, develops in the diencephalon. Adjacent regions are known as the **epithalamus**, **hypothalamus**, and **subthalamus**, each with distinctive structural and functional characteristics. The left and right halves of the telencephalon are known as the **cerebral hemispheres**. These undergo the greatest development in the human brain, in respect both to other regions and to the brains of other animals. The telencephalon includes the olfactory system, the corpus striatum (a mass of gray matter with motor functions), an extensive surface layer of gray matter known as the cortex or pallium, and a medullary center of white matter.

The lumen of the neural tube becomes the **ventricular system**. A **lateral ventricle** develops in each cerebral hemisphere. The **third ventricle** is in the diencephalon, and the **fourth ventricle** is bounded by the medulla, pons, and cerebellum. The third and fourth ventricles are connected by a narrow channel, the **cerebral aqueduct**, through the midbrain. The lumen also remains narrow in the caudal part of the medulla and throughout the spinal cord, where it becomes the **central canal**.

Flexures in the neural tube help to accommodate the initially cylindrical brain in what will eventually be a round head. The first to form are the cervical flexure at the junction of the rhombencephalon with the spinal cord and the mesencephalic flexure at the level of the midbrain. The pontine flexure in the metencephalon soon follows. These flexures in the brain (Fig. 1-3) ensure that the optical axes of the eyes (which connect with the prosencephalon) are at right angles to the axis of the vertebral column. This necessary feature of the erect posture of humans contrasts with the posture of quadrupedal animals, in which there is no abrupt bend at the junction of the midbrain with the forebrain.

TABLE I-I Development of the Brain

	Embryonic Brain Major Division	Mature Brain Subdivision
Rhombencephalon	Myelencephalon	Medulla oblongata
	Metencephalon	Pons and cerebellum
Mesencephalon	Mesencephalon	Midbrain, consisting of tectum and cerebral peduncles
Prosencephalon	Diencephalon	Thalamus, epithalamus, hypothalamus, and subthalamus
	Telencephalon	Cerebral hemispheres, each containing olfactory system, corpus striatum, cerebral cortex, and white matter

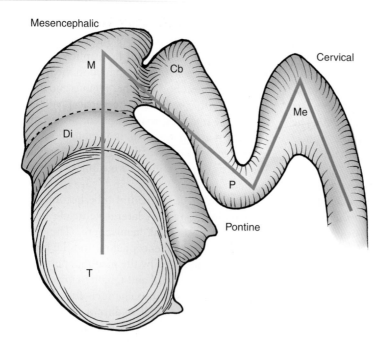

Mesencephalic

M

Cb

Cervical

Me

Di

P

Pontine

T

FIGURE 1-3 Embryonic brain at 7 weeks (stage 20) showing the three flexures in the approximate form of the letter M. The major divisions of the brain are colored: telencephalon **(T)**, yellow; diencephalon **(Di)**, blue; midbrain **(M)**, orange; rhombencephalon, gray; comprising medulla **(Me)**, pons **(P)**, and cerebellum **(Cb)**. (Modified from O'Rahilly R, Müller F. *The Embryonic Human Brain. An Atlas of Developmental Stages,* 3rd ed. Hoboken, NJ: Wiley-Liss, 2006:221.)

Development of the Meninges

The membranous coverings of the brain and spinal cord first appear in the 4th week as a single mesodermally derived **primary** (or primitive) **meninx**. Fluid-filled spaces appear within the primary meninx 1 week later, and subsequent differentiation leads to formation of the three layers that constitute the meninges: the **pia mater**, closest to the nervous tissue; the **arachnoid**; and the **dura mater**, which lines the cranial cavity and spinal canal. The **subarachnoid space**, which contains **cerebrospinal fluid** (CSF), is between the inner two meningeal layers.

Summary of Main Regions of the Central Nervous System

Certain features of the main regions are now briefly reviewed, by way of introduction and to provide a first acquaintance with some neuroanatomical terms. *Before proceeding to later chapters, the student should know the meanings of all the words used in the following eight*

paragraphs. There is a glossary at the end of the book. The major divisions of the adult brain are shown in Figure 1-4.

SPINAL CORD

The spinal cord is the least differentiated component of the CNS. The segmental nature of the spinal cord is reflected in a series of paired spinal nerves, each of which is attached to the cord by a dorsal sensory root and a ventral motor root. The central **gray matter**, in which neuronal cell bodies are located, has a roughly H-shaped outline in transverse section. **White matter**, which consists of myelinated axons running longitudinally, occupies the periphery of the cord. The spinal gray matter includes neuronal connections that provide for spinal reflexes. The white matter contains axons that convey sensory data to the brain and others that conduct impulses, typically of motor significance, from the brain to the spinal cord.

MEDULLA OBLONGATA

The fiber tracts of the spinal cord are continued in the medulla, which also contains clusters of neurons called **nuclei**. The most prominent of these, the inferior olivary nuclei, send fibers to the cerebellum through the inferior cerebellar

Abnormal Development of the Nervous System

ANENCEPHALY AND SPINA BIFIDA

Congenital malformations of the CNS include those that result from failure of the neural tube to close normally. Developmental failure occurs also in associated bone and skin. In **anencephaly,** the neural folds do not fuse at the rostral end of the developing neural tube, so that the forebrain, cranial vault, and much of the scalp are missing. The abnormal brain (the brain stem and, sometimes, the diencephalon) is exposed to the exterior. Anencephaly occurs once in about 1,000 births and is incompatible with sustained life. The equivalent condition at the caudal end of the CNS is **myeloschisis** (cleft spinal cord), in which there is extensive exposure of nonfunctional nervous tissue in the lumbosacral region. Sometimes these two conditions coexist in the same baby.

Myeloschisis is the severest form of **spina bifida**. In less severe types, the spinal cord and its adjacent connective tissue ensheathment (the leptomeninges; see Chapter 26) are intact, but the overlying mesodermal derivatives are not. In **meningomyelocele**, the dura mater, vertebral arches, and skin are missing, and a visible protrusion contains either the caudal part of the spinal cord or its associated nerve roots. If

the neural elements remain in the vertebral canal, the lump at the surface is a **meningocele**, a cyst containing CSF. These types of spina bifida can be corrected surgically, but permanent paralysis or weakness of the lower limbs often persists. **Spina bifida occulta** is a common condition in which the dura and skin remain intact but one or more bony vertebral arches fail to develop. Usually there are no symptoms other than a dimple, a tuft of hair, or some other minor irregularity of the overlying skin.

HYDROCEPHALUS

Cerebrospinal fluid accumulates in the ventricles of the brain if its normal flow is obstructed (see Chapter 26). Nervous tissue is destroyed by the pressure, and the head can become greatly enlarged. Causes include **stenosis of the cerebral aqueduct** in the midbrain and the **Chiari malformation**, in which the medulla and part of the cerebellum are located in the upper cervical spinal canal rather than in the skull. This abnormal anatomy can obstruct the flow of CSF out of the ventricular system, resulting in **internal hydrocephalus**. Spina bifida is also present in many infants with Chiari malformation. Internal hydrocephalus is treated by installing an alternative pathway for drainage of the ventricular system of the brain.

peduncles, which attach the cerebellum to the medulla oblongata. Of the smaller nuclei, some are components of cranial nerves.

PONS

The pons consists of two distinct parts. The dorsal portion or **tegmentum** has features shared with the rest of the brain stem. Therefore, it includes ascending and descending tracts, together with some nuclei of cranial nerves. The ventral portion or **basal pons** is special to this part of the brain stem. Its function is to provide for extensive connections between the cortex of a cerebral hemisphere and that of the contralateral cerebellar hemisphere. These connections contribute to maximal efficiency of motor activities. A pair of middle cerebellar peduncles attaches the cerebellum to the pons.

MIDBRAIN

Similar to other parts of the brain stem, the midbrain contains ascending and descending pathways, together with nuclei for two cranial nerves. A dorsal region, the roof or **tectum**, is concerned principally with the visual and auditory systems. The midbrain also includes two prominent nuclei, the **red nucleus** and the **substantia nigra**, which are concerned with motor control. The cerebellum is attached to the midbrain by the superior cerebellar peduncles.

CEREBELLUM

The cerebellum is especially large in the human brain. Receiving data from most of the sensory systems and the cerebral cortex, the cerebellum eventually influences motor neurons that

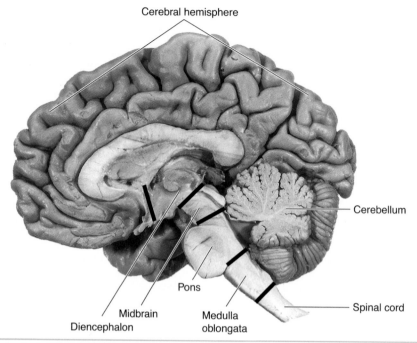

Cerebral hemisphere

Cerebellum

Pons

Spinal cord

Midbrain

Medulla
oblongata

Diencephalon

FIGURE 1-4   Regions of the mature central nervous system, as seen in sagittal section. (Photograph courtesy of Dr. D. G. Montemurro.)

supply the skeletal musculature. The functions of the cerebellum are to produce changes in muscle tone in relation to equilibrium, locomotion, and posture and to coordinate the timing, force, and extent of contraction of muscles being used for skilled movements. The cerebellum operates at a subconscious level.

DIENCEPHALON

The diencephalon forms the central core of the **cerebrum**. The largest component of the diencephalon, the **thalamus**, consists of several regions or nuclei, some of which receive data from sensory systems and project to sensory areas of the cerebral cortex. Part of the thalamus has connections with cortical areas that are concerned with complex mental processes. Other regions participate in neural circuits related to emotions, and certain thalamic nuclei are incorporated into pathways from the cerebellum and corpus striatum to motor areas of the cerebral cortex. The **epithalamus** includes small tracts and nuclei, together with the **pineal gland**, an endocrine organ. The **hypothalamus** has an important controlling influence over

the sympathetic and parasympathetic systems, which supply internal organs, exocrine glands, and blood vessels. In addition, neurosecretory cells in the hypothalamus synthesize hormones that enter the bloodstream. Some act on the kidneys and other organs; others influence the hormonal output of the anterior lobe of the pituitary gland through a special portal system of blood vessels. Some of the neurosecretory cells in the hypothalamus and in the immediately adjacent part of the telencephalon are derived from the olfactory placode, not from the epithelium of the neural tube. These neurons contain and secrete a polypeptide known as gonadotrophin-releasing hormone (GnRH). They migrate along the **terminal nerve** into the forebrain. The terminal nerve is a tiny cranial nerve (sometimes given number zero) rostral to the olfactory nerves. The **subthalamus** includes sensory tracts that proceed to the thalamus, axons that originate in the cerebellum and corpus striatum, and the **subthalamic nucleus**, which has motor functions. The **retina** is a derivative of the diencephalon; therefore, the optic nerve and the visual system are intimately related to this part of the brain.

TELENCEPHALON (CEREBRAL HEMISPHERES)

The telencephalon includes the cerebral cortex, corpus striatum, and cerebral white matter. The **cerebral cortex** is much folded, with ridges (**gyri**) separated by grooves (**sulci**). Major sulci separate the **frontal, parietal, occipital,** and **temporal lobes** of the cerebral hemisphere, which are named after the overlying bones of the skull. Different modalities of sensation and motor functions are represented in distinct areas of the cortex, and there are also large expanses of association cortex, in which the highest levels of neural function take place, including those inherent in intellectual activity.

The **corpus striatum** is a large mass of gray matter with motor functions situated near the base of each hemisphere. It consists of the **caudate** and **lentiform nuclei,** which are parts of a system known as the **basal ganglia,** discussed in Chapters 12 and 23. The **cerebral white matter** (medullary center) consists of fibers that connect cortical areas of the same hemisphere, fibers that cross the midline (most are in a large commissure known as the **corpus callosum**) to connect cortical areas of the two hemispheres, and fibers that pass in both directions between cortex and subcortical parts of the CNS. Fibers of the last category converge to form the compact **internal capsule** in the region of the thalamus and corpus striatum.

Size of the Human Brain

At birth, the average brain weighs about 400 g. Further increase in size is attributable to continuing formation of synaptic connections, production of neuroglial cells, and thickening of the myelin sheaths around axons. The most rapid growth of the brain occurs in utero and during the first 20 postnatal weeks. By age 3 years, the average weight (1,200 g) of the brain is almost that of an adult, although slow growth continues until age 18 years. After age 50 years, there is a slow decline in brain size. This decrease in size does not lead to intellectual deterioration unless there is considerable atrophy caused by disease.

The weight of the mature brain varies with age and stature. The normal range in adult men is 1,100 to 1,700 g (mean, 1,360 g). The lower figures for adult women (1,050–1,550 g; mean, 1,275 g) are mainly attributable to the smaller stature of women compared with men. There is no evidence of a relation between brain weight, within normal limits, and a person's level of intelligence.

Suggested Reading

Campbell K, Gotz M. Radial glia: multi-purpose cells for vertebrate brain development. *Trends Neurosci* 2002;25:235–238.

Del Bigio MR. Proliferative status of cells in the human dentate gyrus. *Microsc Res Tech* 1999;45:353–368.

Doucette R. Transitional zone of the first cranial nerve. *J Comp Neurol* 1991;312:451–466.

Hill M. UNSW Embryology. Ver. 6.1. An educational resource for learning concepts in embryological development. Available online at http://embryology.med.unsw.edu.au.

Jessen KR, Richardson WD, eds. *Glial Cell Development: Basic Principles and Clinical Relevance,* 2nd ed. Oxford: Oxford University Press, 2001.

Konstantinidou AD, Silos-Santiago I, Flaris N, et al. Development of the primary afferent projection in human spinal cord. *J Comp Neurol* 1995;354:1–12.

Lemire RJ, Loeser JD, Leech RW, et al. *Normal and Abnormal Development of the Human Nervous System.* Hagerstown, MD: Harper & Row, 1975.

Miller RH. Oligodendrocyte origins. *Trends Neurosci* 1996;19:92–96.

Müller F, O'Rahilly R. The timing and sequence of appearance of neuromeres and their derivatives in staged human embryos. *Acta Anat* 1997;158:83–99.

O'Rahilly R, Müller F. Minireview: initial development of the human nervous system. *Teratology* 1999;60:39–41.

O'Rahilly R, Müller F. Two sites of fusion of the neural folds and the two neuropores in the human embryo. *Teratology* 2002;65:162–170.

O'Rahilly R, Müller F. *The Embryonic Human Brain. An Atlas of Developmental Stages,* 3rd ed. New York: Wiley-Liss, 2006.

O'Rahilly R, Müller F. Significant features in the early prenatal development of the human brain. *Ann Anat* 2008;190:105–118.

Webb JF, Noden DM. Ectodermal placodes: contributions to the development of the vertebrate head. *Am Zool* 1993;33:434–447.

Weiss S, Dunne C, Hewson J, et al. Multipotent CNS stem cells are present in the adult mammalian spinal cord and ventricular neuraxis. *J Neurosci* 1996;16:7599–7609.

Zecevic N, Chen Y, Filipovic R. Contributions of cortical subventricular zone to the development of the human cerebral cortex. *J Comp Neurol* 2005;491:109–122.

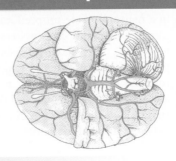

Chapter 2

CELLS OF THE NERVOUS SYSTEM

Important Facts

- Neurons are cells specialized for rapid communication. Most of the cytoplasm of a neuron is in long processes, the neurites (dendrites and axon, which conduct signals toward and away from the cell body, respectively).
- In the central nervous system (CNS), neuronal cell bodies and dendrites occur in gray matter. White matter consists largely of axons, most of which have myelin sheaths that serve to increase the velocity of conduction.
- A neuronal surface membrane has a resting potential of −70 mV, maintained by the sodium pump. This is reversed to +40 mV in an axon during the passage of an action potential.
- The fastest signals, known as impulses or action potentials, are carried in the surface membrane of the axon. There is rapid (saltatory) conduction in myelinated axons because the ion channels in the axolemma are confined to the nodes.
- The surface membrane of the perikaryon and dendrites does not conduct impulses. Potential changes move more slowly and are graded. An action potential is initiated when the region of the axonal hillock is depolarized to a threshold level.
- Neurons communicate with one another at synapses. Chemical transmitters released by axonal terminals evoke changes in the membrane of the postsynaptic cell, which may be either stimulated or inhibited. The effect depends on the transmitter and the type of receptor molecule in the postsynaptic membrane.
- Local reductions of membrane potential (excitatory postsynaptic potentials or depolarizations) add together and may result in initiation of action potentials. Hyperpolarization (inhibitory postsynaptic potentials) reduces the likelihood of initiation of an impulse.
- Proteins and other substances are transported within axons at different speeds and in both directions.
- Much of the cytoplasm of a neuron is removed when the axon is transected. The segment that has been isolated from the cell body degenerates together with its myelin sheath, and the fragments are eventually phagocytosed.
- The neuronal cell body initially reacts to axotomy with increased protein synthesis, accompanied by structural changes known as the axon reaction, or chromatolysis. In the absence of axonal regeneration, the cell body may later shrink or die. Axons severed in the peripheral nervous system can regrow and reinnervate their targets.
- In mammals, axons transected within the CNS fail to regenerate effectively. Synaptic rearrangements, however, can occur in partly denervated regions of gray matter, and some recovery of function occurs as a result of recruitment of alternative neuronal circuitry.
- The neuroglial cells of the normal CNS are astrocytes, oligodendrocytes, ependymal cells (derived from neural tube ectoderm), and microglia (derived from mesoderm). Astrocytes occur throughout the brain and spinal cord. Oligodendrocytes produce myelin and are also found next to the cell bodies of some neurons. Microglial cells become phagocytes when local injury or inflammation is present.
- The neuroglial cells of the peripheral nervous system are Schwann cells in nerves and satellite cells in ganglia.

Two classes of cells are present in the central nervous system (CNS) in addition to the usual cells found in blood vessel walls. **Neurons**, or **nerve cells**, are specialized for nerve impulse conduction and for exchanging signals with other neurons. They are, therefore, responsible for most of the functional characteristics of nervous tissue. **Neuroglial cells**, collectively known as the **neuroglia** or simply as **glia**, have important ancillary functions.

The CNS consists of gray matter and white matter. **Gray matter** contains the cell bodies of neurons, each with a nucleus, embedded in a **neuropil** made up predominantly of delicate neuronal and glial processes. **White matter**, on the other hand, consists mainly of long processes of neurons, the majority being surrounded by myelin sheaths; nerve cell bodies are lacking. Both the gray and the white matter contain large numbers of neuroglial cells and a network of blood capillaries.

Neurons

Neurons are cells specialized for sending and receiving chemically mediated electrical signals. The part of the cell that includes the nucleus is called the **cell body**, and its cytoplasm is known as the **perikaryon**. **Dendrites** are typically short branching processes that receive signals from other neurons. Most neurons of the CNS have several dendrites and are, therefore, multipolar in shape. By reaching out in various directions, dendrites increase the ability of a neuron to receive input from diverse sources. Each cell has a single **axon**. This process, which varies greatly in length from one type of neuron to another, typically conducts impulses away from the cell body. Some neurons have no axons, and their dendrites conduct signals in both directions. Axons of efferent neurons in the spinal cord and brain are included in spinal and cranial nerves. They end on striated muscle fibers or on nerve cells of autonomic ganglia. The term **neurite** refers to any neuronal process: axon or dendrite.

The fact that each neuron is a structural and functional unit is known as the **neuron doctrine**, proposed in the latter part of the 19th century in opposition to the then-prevailing view that nerve cells formed a continuous reticulum or syncytium. The unitary concept, conforming to the cell theory, was advanced by His on the basis of embryological studies, by Forel on the basis of the responses of nerve cells to injury, and by Ramón y Cajal from his histological observations. The neuron doctrine was given wide distribution in a review by Waldeyer of the individuality of nerve cells. The lack of cytoplasmic continuity between neurons at synapses was conclusively demonstrated in the 1950s when it became possible to obtain electron micrographs with sufficient resolution to show the structures of intimately apposed cell membranes.

DIFFERENT SHAPES AND SIZES OF NEURONS

Although all neurons conform to the general principles already outlined, a wide range of structural diversity exists. The size of the cell body varies from 5 μm across for the smallest cells in complex circuits to 135 μm for the largest motor neurons. Dendritic morphology, especially the pattern of branching, varies greatly and is distinctive for neurons that constitute a particular group of cells. The axon of a local circuit neuron may be as short as 100 μm, less than 1 μm in diameter, and devoid of a myelin covering. On the other hand, the axon of a motor neuron that supplies a muscle in the foot is nearly 1 m long, up to 10 μm in diameter, and encased in a myelin sheath up to 5 μm thick. (Much longer axons are present in large animals such as giraffes and whales.)

Neurons occur in **ganglia** in the peripheral nervous system and in either **laminae** (layers) or groups called **nuclei** in the CNS. The large neurons of a nucleus or comparable region are called Golgi type I or **principal cells**; their axons carry the encoded output of information from the region containing their cell bodies to other parts of the nervous system. The dendrites of a principal cell are contacted by axonal terminals of several other neurons. These neurons include principal cells of other areas and nearby small neurons. The latter are known variously as Golgi type II, internuncial, or local circuit neurons, or, more simply, as **interneurons**. In many parts of the brain, these neurons greatly outnumber the principal cells.

Examples of large and small neurons are shown in Figure 2-1, which shows the cells as they might appear in specimens stained by the Golgi method.

NEUROHISTOLOGICAL TECHNIQUES

Structural features of neurons and neuroglial cells are not well shown in sections prepared by general-purpose staining methods such as the alum-hematoxylin-eosin beloved of pathologists. Specialized staining methods are preferred

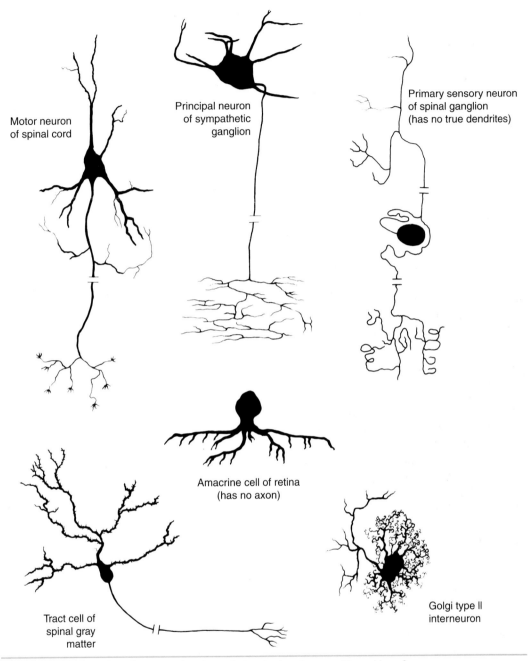

Motor neuron
of spinal cord

Principal neuron
of sympathetic
ganglion

Primary sensory neuron
of spinal ganglion
(has no true dendrites)

Amacrine cell of retina
(has no axon)

Tract cell of
spinal gray
matter

Golgi type II
interneuron

FIGURE 2-1   Examples of neurons, showing variations in size, shape, and branching of processes.

for light microscopy. Additional information is obtained with the electron microscope and from studies in which functionally significant chemical compounds are histochemically localized in the cells and parts of cells in which they are synthesized or stored.

Cationic dyes, called "Nissl stains" when applied to nervous tissue, bind to DNA and RNA.

Therefore, these stains demonstrate the nuclei of all cells and the cytoplasmic Nissl substance (RNA of rough endoplasmic reticulum) of neurons (Fig. 2-2).

Reduced silver methods produce dark deposits of colloidal silver in various structures, notably the proteinaceous filaments inside axons (Fig. 2-3). Other silver methods are avail-

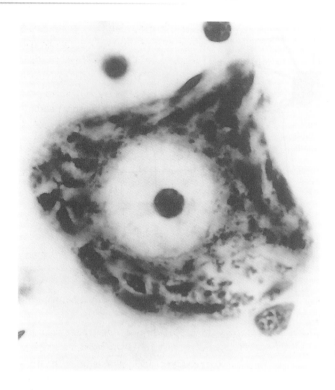

FIGURE 2-2 Motor neuron in the spinal cord, stained with cresyl violet to show the Nissl bodies and a prominent nucleolus (×800).

able for demonstration of different types of neuroglial cells.

Stains for myelin rely on the affinities of certain dyes for hydrophobic proteins and protein-bound phospholipids. They reveal the major tracts of fibers. Some of the photographs in this book (e.g., in Chapter 7) are of sections stained by Weigert's method for myelin.

The **Golgi method**, which has many variants, is valuable for the study of neuronal morphology, especially of dendrites. Insoluble salts of silver or mercury are precipitated within the cells in blocks of tissue that are then cut into thick sections. Some neurons, including the finest branches of their dendrites, stand out in black against a clear background (Fig. 2-4). Occasional neuroglial cells are similarly displayed,

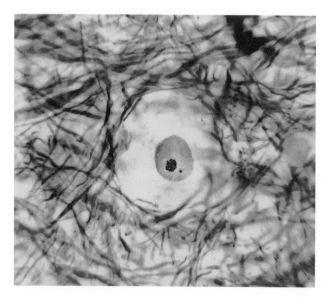

FIGURE 2-3 Cell body of a neuron in the brain, surrounded by axons. In addition, the nucleolus and a small accessory body of Cajal are seen in the nucleus. (Stained by one of Cajal's silver nitrate methods; ×1,000.)

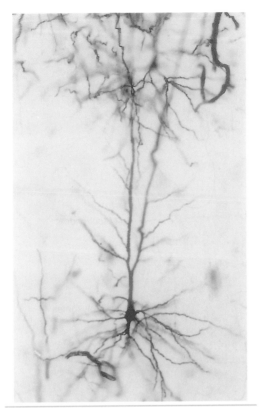

FIGURE 2-4 Pyramidal cell of the cerebral cortex, stained by the Golgi technique. The cell body is in the lower one third of the picture, and dendrites extend up toward the cortical surface. The axon is not visible. (×90; courtesy of Dr. E. G. Bertram.)

contained in specific populations of neurons. These substances include putative neurotransmitters and enzymes involved in their synthesis or degradation. Several previously unrecognized systems of neurons have been identified by the use of these methods. With immunohistochemistry, substances in tissues are detected by the binding of specific antibodies. Immunohistochemical methods for cell-specific proteins have largely replaced the traditional silver methods for staining axons and glial cells.

Electron microscopy reveals the detailed internal structure of neurons and the specializations that exist at synaptic junctions. The necessity of using very thin sections makes it difficult to reconstruct in three dimensions. Electron microscopy may be combined with staining by Golgi methods or with immunohistochemical procedures.

Confocal microscopy allows the examination of thin optical sections within thicker specimens prepared for light (usually fluorescence) microscopy. Resolution is enhanced, and images can be superimposed electronically to make pictures that are in focus for the whole depth of the specimen. In confocal images, immunohistochemical localizations can be combined with tracing based on filling or axonal transport.

but axons (especially if myelinated) are typically unstained. An important feature of these methods is the random staining of only a small proportion of the cells, enabling the resolution of structural details of the dendritic trees of individual neurons.

Filling techniques provide pictures similar to those obtained by the Golgi method but for individual neurons that have been studied physiologically. A histochemically demonstrable ion or enzyme or a fluorescent dye is injected into the neuron through a micropipette that has been used for intracellular electrical recording. Some other fluorescent dyes move laterally within cell membranes. These can be applied to fresh or even fixed tissue and used to trace neuronal connections over distances up to 5 mm.

Histochemical and immunohistochemical methods are available for localizing substances

NEURON CYTOLOGY

The parts of a generalized multipolar neuron are shown in Figure 2-5.

Cell Surface

The surface or limiting membrane of the neuron assumes special importance because of its role in the initiation and transmission of signals. The **plasma membrane**, or **plasmalemma**, is a double layer of phospholipid molecules whose hydrophobic hydrocarbon chains are all directed toward the middle of the membrane. Embedded in this structure are protein molecules, many of which pass through the whole thickness. Some transmembrane proteins provide hydrophilic **channels** through which inorganic ions may enter and leave the cell by diffusion. Each of the common ions (Na^+, K^+, Ca^{2+}, Cl^-) has its own specific type of molecular channel, and there are also mixed ion channels that allow passage of multiple

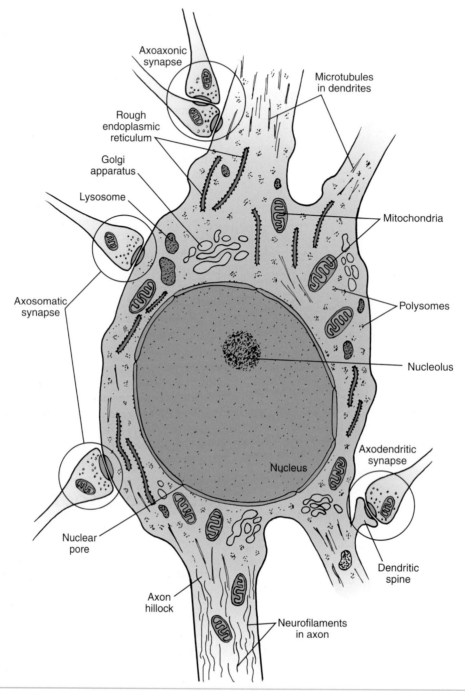

FIGURE 2-5   Components of a neuron, traced from an electron micrograph. Mitochondria are colored green and presynaptic terminals from other neurons yellow. (Modified from Heimer L. *The Human Brain and Spinal Cord,* 2nd ed. New York: Springer-Verlag, 1995.)

ions such as Na^+ and K^+ or Na^+, K^+, and Ca^{2+}. Some channels are voltage gated, which means that they open and close in response to changes in the electrical potential across the membrane. Other channels open in response to ligand, such as neurotransmitters, binding to specific receptors. Nerve impulses are propagated (conducted) along the cell membrane of the neuronal surface. **Pumps** are protein molecules of the cell membrane that consume energy (from adenosine triphosphate [ATP]) as they move ions against concentration gradients. A single pump, known as Na/K-ATPase, transports potassium ions into and sodium ions out of the cell, resulting in a net negative charge within the cell and contributing to the membrane potential. **Receptors** are protein molecules that respond to specific chemical stimuli, typically by causing the opening of associated channels.

The most abundant ions in extracellular fluid are sodium (Na^+) and chloride (Cl^-). Inside the cell, potassium (K^+) is the main positive ion; it is neutralized by organic anions of amino acids and proteins. Both the extracellular fluid and the cytoplasm are electrically neutral, and each has the same total osmotic pressure. A consequence of these conditions is that there is a potential difference across the membrane: The inside is negative (−70 mV) with respect to the outside when the neuron is not conducting a signal. This **resting membrane potential** opposes the outward diffusion of K^+ and the inward diffusion of Cl^- because unlike charges attract and like charges repel one another. The membrane is much less permeable to Na^+ because the voltage-gated channels for this cation are closed as a consequence of the resting membrane potential. The cytoplasmic anions are too large to pass through the membrane. The ionic concentrations are maintained by the activity of the **sodium pump**.

The signals carried by a neuron are changes in the potential difference across the plasmalemma. At rest, the cytoplasm is negative (about −70 mV) with respect to the extracellular fluid. This difference is reversed to about +40 mV inside when an axon is sufficiently stimulated. The reversal, known as an **impulse** or **action potential**, propagates along the axon. An action potential is an all-or-none phenomenon. In contrast, the dendrites and the cell body respond to stimuli with graded potential changes. Lowering of the membrane potential to a threshold level of −55 mV at the initial segment of the axon triggers an action potential.

Signaling in Neurons
Nucleus and Cytoplasm

The nucleus of a neuron is usually in the center of the cell body. In large neurons, it is vesicular (with finely dispersed chromatin), but in most small neurons, the chromatin is in coarse clumps. Typically, there is a prominent **nucleo-**

lus. The sex chromatin (see Fig. 2-5), present only in females, was first described in the large nuclei of motor neurons.

The cytoplasm of the cell body (Fig. 2-6) is dominated by the organelles of protein synthesis (rough endoplasmic reticulum and polyribosomes) and cellular respiration (mitochondria). Also present is a well-developed Golgi apparatus, where carbohydrate side chains are added to protein molecules packaged into membrane-bound vesicles destined to enter or pass through the surface membrane of the cell. In light microscopy, the rough endoplasmic reticulum is conspicuous as striated bodies of **Nissl substance** (see Fig. 2-2).

Filamentous organelles are most prominent in the neurites. **Neurofilaments** (diameter, 7.5 to 10 nm) are made of structural proteins similar to those of the intermediate filaments of other types of cells. When gathered into bundles, they form the **neurofibrils** of light microscopy. **Microtubules** (external diameter, 25 nm) are involved in the rapid transport of protein molecules and small particles in both directions along axons and dendrites. **Microfilaments** (4 nm) are molecules of the contractile protein actin. They are present on the inside of the plasmalemma and are particularly numerous in the tips of growing neurites.

Neuronal cytoplasm also contains small numbers of membrane-bound vesicles called **lysosomes**, which contain enzymes that catalyze the breakdown of unwanted large molecules. Neurons may also contain two types of pigment granules. **Lipofuscin** is a yellow-brown pigment formed from lysosomes that accumulates with aging. **Neuromelanin** is a black pigment seen only in neurons that use catecholamines (dopamine or noradrenaline) as neurotransmitters.

Neurites

Dendrites taper from the cell body and branch in its immediate environs. In some neurons, the smaller branches bear large numbers of minute projections, called **dendritic spines**, which participate in synapses. The surface of the cell body is also included in the receptive field of the neuron.

The single **axon** has a uniform diameter throughout its length. In **interneurons**, it is short and branches terminally to establish synaptic contact with adjacent neurons. Some interneurons have no axon, so they can conduct only graded changes of membrane potential. In **principal**

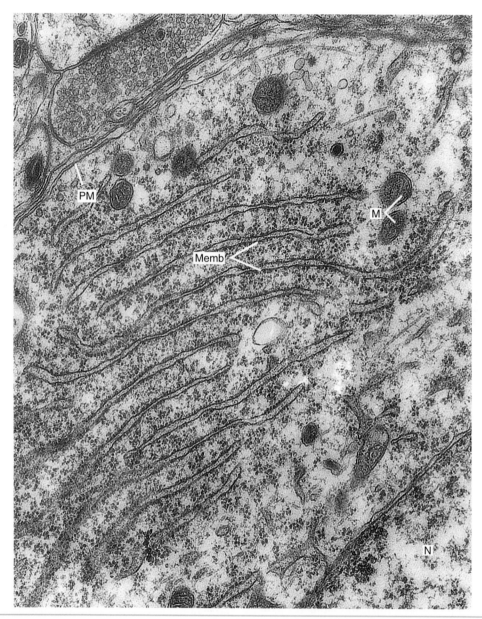

FIGURE 2-6   Electron micrograph of part of the cell body of a neuron in the preoptic area of a rabbit's brain. The series of membranes, together with the free polyribosomes between the membranes, constitute the Nissl material of light microscopy. M, mitochondria; Memb, membranes of endoplasmic reticulum; PM, plasma membrane at surface of cell. (×36,000; courtesy of Dr. R. Clattenburg.)

cells, the diameter of the axon increases in proportion to its length. **Collateral** branches may be given off at right angles to the axon. The terminal branches are known as **telodendria**; they typically end as **synaptic terminals** (also known as *boutons terminaux*) in contact with other cells. The cytoplasm of the axon is called **axoplasm**, and the surface membrane is known as the **axolemma**. The axoplasm includes neurofilaments, microtubules,

scattered mitochondria, and fragments of smooth endoplasmic reticulum.

Myelin

The axon of a principal cell is usually surrounded by a **myelin sheath**, which begins near the origin of the axon and ends short of its terminal branching. Myelin is laid down by neuroglial cells—Schwann cells in the peripheral nervous system and oligodendrocytes in the CNS. The sheath consists of closely apposed layers of glial plasma membranes. Interruptions called **nodes of Ranvier** indicate junctions between regions formed by different Schwann cells or oligodendrocytes. The ion movements of impulse conduction in a myelinated axon are confined to the nodes. This arrangement provides for **saltatory conduction** in which the action potential jumps electrically from one node to the next, so that signaling is much faster in a myelinated than in an unmyelinated axon. A **nerve fiber** consists of the axon and the surrounding myelin sheath or of the axon only in the case of an unmyelinated fiber. The greater the diameter of a nerve fiber, the faster is the conduction of the nerve impulse.

Myelin sheaths are laid down during the later part of fetal development and during the first postnatal year in the manner shown, for a peripheral fiber, in Figure 2-7. The ultrastructure of the sheath is seen in Figure 2-8. A Schwann cell myelinates only one axon, but in the CNS, each process of a single oligodendrocyte contributes to the myelination of a different axon (Fig. 2-9).

Experiments with peripheral nerves of animals show that all Schwann cells have the potential to

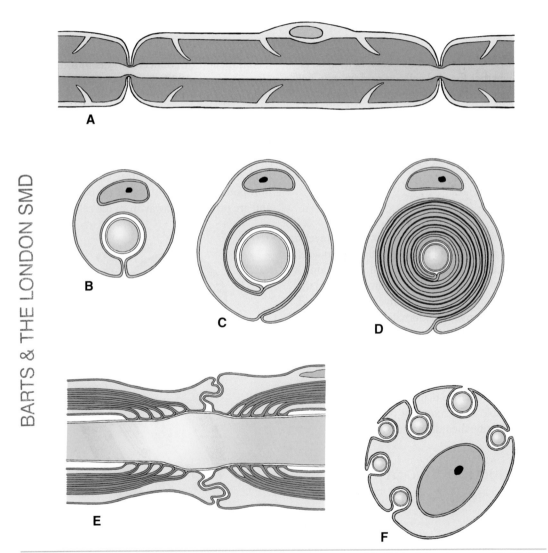

FIGURE 2-7 **(A)** The myelin sheath and Schwann cell as they are seen (ideally) by light microscopy. **(B–D)** Successive stages in the development of the myelin sheath from the plasma membrane of a Schwann cell. **(E)** Ultrastructure of a node of Ranvier, sectioned longitudinally. **(F)** Relation of a Schwann cell to several unmyelinated axons.

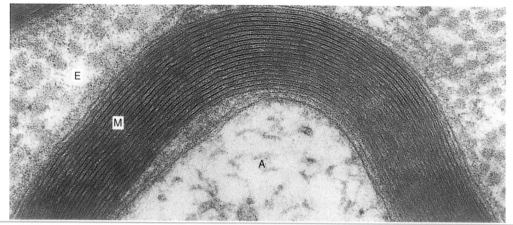

FIGURE 2-8   Ultrastructure of the myelin sheath (M) in a peripheral nerve. The dense and less dense layers alternate, and the latter includes a thin intraperiod line. A, axoplasm; E, endoneurium, with collagen fibers. (Electron micrograph, ×107,500; courtesy of Dr. R. C. Buck.)

make myelin sheaths and that each neuron determines whether the glial cells around its axon will or will not produce a myelin sheath.

Saltatory Conduction in Myelinated Axons

Nerve Fibers

A nerve fiber is an axon together with a myelin sheath, if present, and the ensheathing glial cells. The velocity of conduction of an impulse along a nerve fiber increases with the diameter. The largest axons have the thickest myelin sheaths and, therefore, the greatest external diameters. The axonal diameter is approximately two thirds of the total external diameter of the fiber. The thinnest, most slowly conducting axons are unmyelinated.

Peripheral nerve fibers are classified into groups according to external diameter and conduction velocity (Table 2-1). Axons in the CNS are not as easy to classify; their diameters vary greatly.

Conduction Velocity and the Compound Action Potential

Synapses

A neuron influences other neurons at junctional points, or synapses. The term *synapse*, meaning

a conjunction or connection, was introduced by Sherrington in 1897. An action potential can be propagated in either direction along the surface of an axon. The direction it follows under physiological conditions is determined by a consistent polarity at most synapses, where transmission is from the axon of one neuron to a dendrite or the perikaryon of another neuron. Consequently, action potentials are initiated at the axonal hillock and are propagated away from the cell body.

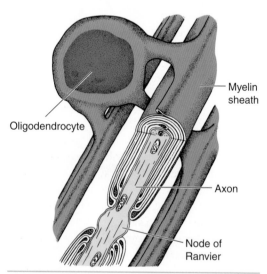

FIGURE 2-9   An oligodendrocyte with cytoplasmic extensions forming the myelin sheaths of axons in the central nervous system. (Modified from Bunge MB, Bunge RP, Ris H. Ultrastructural study of remyelinization in an experimental lesion in adult cat spinal cord. *J Biophys Biochem Cytol* 1961;10:67–94.)

TABLE 2-1 **Size and Conduction Velocity of Nerve Fibers**

Name and Function of Type of Fiber*	External Diameter (μm)	Conduction Velocity (m/sec)
Myelinated fibers		
Aα or IA Motor to skeletal muscle; sensory from muscle spindle proprioceptive endings (phasic, annulospiral type)	12–20	70–120
Aβ or IB Sensory from tendons (tension); also Ruffini endings in skin	10–15	60–80
Aβ or II Sensory from Meissner's and pacinian corpuscles and similar endings in skin and connective tissue; from large hair follicles and tonic proprioceptive endings (flower-spray type) of muscle spindles	5–15	30–80
Aγ Motor to intrafusal fibers of muscle spindles	3–8	15–40
Aδ or III Sensory from small hair follicles and from free nerve endings for temperature and pain sensations	3–8	10–30
B Preganglionic autonomic (white rami and cranial nerves 3, 7, 9, and 10)	1–3	5–15
Unmyelinated fibers		
C or IV Pain and temperature; olfaction; postganglionic autonomic	0.2–1.5	0.5–2.5

*Letters are used for any nerve; Roman numerals are used for sensory fibers in dorsal spinal roots.

CHEMICAL SYNAPSES

A point of functional contact between two neurons, or between a neuron and an effector cell, is a **synapse**. The structural details of synapses can be resolved only by electron microscopy. Most synapses in vertebrate animals are **chemical synapses**. The surface membranes of the two cells are thickened by deposition of proteins (receptors and ion channels) on their cytoplasmic surfaces. The intervening **synaptic cleft** contains an electron-dense glycoprotein that is absent from the general extracellular space.

The presynaptic neurite, which is most often a branch of an axon, is known as a **synaptic terminal** or **bouton terminal** ("terminal button"; the plural is *boutons terminax*. This French term recalls the appearance in light microscopy.). A synaptic terminal contains numerous mitochondria and a cluster of **synaptic vesicles**. The latter are membrane-bound organelles 40 to 150 nm in diameter (Fig. 2-10), which contain chemical neurotransmitters. The vesicles may be spherical (in Gray's type 1 synapses, which are generally excitatory) or ellipsoidal (in Gray's type 2 synapses, which use the inhibitory transmitter gamma-aminobutyrate [GABA]). Type 1 synapses are asymmetric, with deposits of fibrillary material that are conspicuously thicker on the postsynaptic than on the presynaptic membrane.

The postsynaptic structure is typically a dendrite. Often, it bears a pendunculated projection, a **dendritic spine**, that invaginates the presynaptic neurite. Commonly, synapses are grouped together on a dendrite or an axonal terminal to form a larger structure, known as a **synaptic complex** or **glomerulus**. In the CNS, the cytoplasmic processes of protoplasmic as-

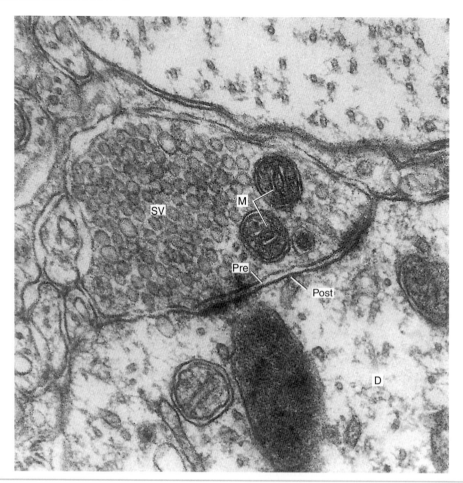

FIGURE 2-10   Electron micrograph of an axodendritic Gray's type I (asymmetrical) synapse in a rabbit's hypothalamus. D, dendrite; M, mitochondria; Pre, presynaptic membrane; Post, postsynaptic membrane; SV, synaptic vesicles. (×82,000; courtesy of Dr. R. Clattenburg.)

trocytes intimately invest synaptic complexes, restricting diffusion in the intercellular spaces of released transmitters and inorganic ions such as calcium and potassium. These small molecules and ions are absorbed into the cytoplasm of astrocytes and can then diffuse, by way of gap junctions, to adjacent astrocytes.

Some different types of chemical synapse are shown in Figure 2-11. The most common arrangements for transferring signals from one neuron to another are axodendritic and axosomatic synapses. Axoaxonal synapses are strategically placed to interfere either with the initiation of impulses at the initial segments of other axons or with the activities of other synaptic terminals. Dendrodendritic synapses can modify a neuron's responses to input at other synapses.

When the membrane potential of a presynaptic neurite is reversed by the arrival of an ac-

tion potential (or, in the case of a dendrodendritic synapse, adequately reduced by a graded fluctuation), calcium channels are opened and Ca^{2+} ions diffuse into the cell because they are present at a much higher concentration in the extracellular fluid than in the cytoplasm. Entry of calcium triggers the fusion of synaptic vesicles to the terminal plasmalemma, thereby releasing neurotransmitters and neuromodulators into the synaptic cleft. A classical **neurotransmitter** either stimulates or inhibits the postsynaptic cell. A **neuromodulator** has other actions, including modifying the responsiveness to transmitters.

Having crossed the synaptic cleft, the transmitter molecules combine with **receptors** on the postsynaptic cell. If the transmitter–receptor interaction is one that results in excitation, nonspecific cation channels are opened, allowing entry of Na^+ and Ca^{2+} and efflux of K^+ at postsynap-

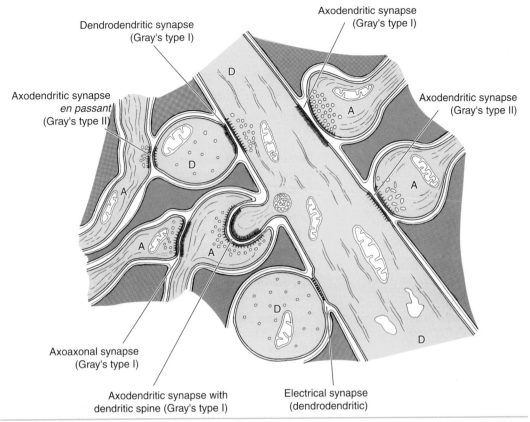

Dendrodendritic synapse
(Gray's type I)

Axodendritic synapse
(Gray's type I)

Axodendritic synapse
en passant
(Gray's type II)

Axodendritic synapse
(Gray's type II)

Axoaxonal synapse
(Gray's type I)

Axodendritic synapse with
dendritic spine (Gray's type I)

Electrical synapse
(dendrodendritic)

FIGURE 2-11 Ultrastructure of various types of synapses. The green areas represent the cytoplasmic processes of astrocytes. A, axons; D, dendrites.

tic sites. Inhibition, on the other hand, primarily involves the opening of chloride channels in the postsynaptic membrane, which is transiently hyperpolarized as a consequence of the diffusion of Cl^- ions into the cytoplasm. Some inhibition results from the opening of K^+ channels, which allows K^+ to leave the cell, thereby resulting in a net negative charge inside the neuron, similar to the effect of the entry of Cl^- ions. These changes in the membrane potential are additive over the whole receptive surface of the postsynaptic neuron. If the net electrical change reaches a threshold level of depolarization to about $-55\,mV$ at the axon hillock, an action potential will be initiated and will travel along the axon. Thus, the sum of the postsynaptic responses in the receptive field of a neuron determines whether, at any given moment, an impulse will be sent along the axon.

Some neurotransmitters act rapidly (within milliseconds) by combining with **ionotropic receptors**, which are also the ion channels in the membrane. Other substances, notably the peptides, have more protracted actions (within seconds, minutes, or hours). Slowly acting transmitters or modulators combine with **metabotropic receptors** associated with **G proteins**. The latter substances bind guanosine triphosphate and participate in intracellular second-messenger systems in the cytoplasm of the postsynaptic cell. The inhibitory transmitter GABA acts on ionotropic receptors associated with chloride channels and on G protein–associated receptors that induce opening of potassium channels. Glutamate, the most abundant excitatory transmitter, also acts on both ionotropic and metabotropic receptors.

The properties of some neurotransmitters and neuromodulators are summarized in Table 2-2. This table does not include the many peptides that serve as transmitters and modulators throughout the nervous system.

ELECTRICAL SYNAPSES

Electrical synapses are common in invertebrates and lower vertebrates and have been observed at a few sites in the mammalian nervous system.

TABLE 2-2   Neurotransmitters and Neuromodulators

Compound	Occurrence and Functions
Amino acids	
Glutamate	Excitatory neurotransmitter in all parts of the CNS
GABA	Inhibitory neurotransmitter in all parts of the CNS
Glycine	Inhibitory neurotransmitter in spinal cord and brain stem
Amines and related compounds	
Acetylcholine	Excitatory transmitter used by motor neurons and by all pre-ganglionic and some postganglionic autonomic neurons (see Chapter 24). In the CNS, acetylcholine is the transmitter or neuromodulator used by neurons in certain nuclei of the reticular formation (see Chapter 9) and in nuclei in the basal forebrain that project to the cerebral cortex.
Dopamine	Used by neurons in the hypothalamus, substantia nigra, and ventral tegmental area (see Chapters 11, 12, and 18). Modulatory actions in the corpus striatum, limbic system, and prefrontal cortex.
Noradrenaline (norepinephrine)	Transmitter used by most neurons of sympathetic ganglia (see Chapter24); actions vary with the receptors on the innervated cells.
	Noradrenaline-producing neurons in the locus coeruleus and other parts of the reticular formation (see Chapter 9) have neuromodulatory effects throughout the brain and spinal cord.
Histamine	Excitatory transmitter used by neurons in the tuberomamillary nucleus of the hypothalamus. These neurons have long, branched axons that go to most parts of the brain and are believed to be involved in maintaining consciousness.
Serotonin (5-hydroxytryptamine)	Neuromodulator used by neurons in the midline of the brain stem with long branching axons going to all parts of the CNS. Various actions include involvement in sleep (see Chapter 9), mood (see Chapter 18), and pain (see Chapter 19).

CNS, central nervous system; GABA, gamma-aminobutyrate.

Each consists of a close apposition (2 nm) of presynaptic and postsynaptic membranes, across which the cytoplasms of the two cells are joined by numerous tubules or **connexons**, formed from transmembrane protein molecules of both cells. Water and small ions and molecules move freely through the connexons. An electrical synapse offers a low-resistance pathway between neurons, and there is no delay because a chemical mediator is not involved. Unlike most chemical synapses, electrical synapses are not polarized, and the direction of transmission fluctuates with the membrane potentials of the connected cells. A cluster of connexons that joins cells is known by the general term **gap junction**.

Axonal Transport

Proteins, including enzymes, membrane lipoproteins, and cytoplasmic structural proteins, are transported distally within axons from their sites of synthesis in the perikaryon. Two major rates of transport have been identified by studying the distribution of proteins labeled by incorporation of radioactive amino acids. Most of the protein moves distally at a rate of about 1 mm/day. This component consists largely of structural proteins, including the subunits of neurofilaments and microtubules. A smaller proportion is transported much more rapidly at a mean velocity of 300 mm/day. Transport also occurs simultaneously in the reverse direction, from the synaptic terminals to the cell body. The retrogradely transported material includes proteins imbibed from the extracellular fluid by axonal terminals as well as proteins that reach the axon terminals by fast anterograde transport and are returned to the perikaryon. The rate of retrograde transport is variable, but most of the material moves at about two-thirds the speed of the fast component of the antero-grade transport.

The rapid components of axonal transport in both directions involve predominantly parti-cle-bound substances and require the integrity of the microtubules of the axoplasm. Particles move along the outsides of the tubules. It is an amazing feat of biological engineering that dif-ferent substances can move at different rates and in different directions at the same time within a tube as thin as an axon.

Responses of Neurons to Injury

Neurons may be injured physically or by dis-ease processes such as infarction caused by vas-cular occlusion. Whereas small interneurons are likely to suffer total destruction, injury to large neurons may result either in destruction of the cell body or transection of the axon with preservation of the cell body. When the cell body is destroyed, the axon is isolated from the synthetic machinery of the cell and soon breaks up into fragments, which are eventually phago-cytosed. Similar changes occur distally to the site of an axonal injury. The degeneration of an axon that has been detached from the remain-der of the cell is called **Wallerian degeneration**. This process affects not only the axon but also its myelin sheath, even though the latter is not part of the injured neuron.

REACTIONS IN THE CELL BODY

Changes in the cell body after axonal tran-section constitute the axon reaction. They vary according to the type of neuron. Cells in some locations degenerate and disappear. This happens to most

neurons when the injury occurs before or soon after birth. Conversely, the proximal portions of some adult neurons are not significantly altered by cutting the axon. In such cells, 24 to 48 hours after interruption of the axon, the normally coarse clumps of Nissl substance are changed to a finely granular dispersion, a change known as chromatolysis (Online Fig. 2-3). The nucleus assumes an eccentric position, and the whole cell body swells. These changes reach a maximum 10 to 20 days after axonal transection, and the closer the injury is to the cell body, the more severe the swelling. In a chromatolytic neuron, accelerated synthesis of RNA and proteins takes place that favors regrowth of the axon when conditions make such regeneration possible. Recovery commonly takes several months, and the cell body is eventually smaller than normal if the axon does not regenerate.

The changes described are most easily seen in motor neurons after transection of a pe-ripheral nerve. In cells confined to the CNS, the axon reaction is conspicuous only in some large neurons. Large cells may exhibit no axon reaction when collateral axonal branches that arise close to the cell body are spared.

Transneuronal degeneration is similar in appearance to the axon reaction, but it occurs in neuronal cell bodies that have been deprived of most of their afferents. For example, tran-section of the optic tract is followed after sev-eral weeks by atrophy of some of the neurons in the lateral geniculate body of the thalamus, which is where most of the optic fibers termi-nate. The postsynaptic neurons have not been directly injured, and their degeneration is at-tributed to withdrawal of a trophic substance normally supplied by the presynaptic neurons. Neurons in the CNS of immature animals are particularly susceptible to damage caused by deafferentation.

CONSEQUENCES OF CUTTING A PERIPHERAL NERVE

The axon does not last long when separated from the cell body. Phagocytes remove the re-sidual bits of axon and myelin, and they pre-pare the nerve to receive any axons that might regenerate into its distal stump. These events constitute Wallerian degeneration.

WALLERIAN DEGENERATION IN PERIPHERAL NERVES

Simultaneously, throughout its length, on the first day, the axon distal to the lesion becomes irregularly swollen. By the 3rd to 5th day, the axon has broken into fragments. Muscle contraction induced by electrical stimulation of a degenerating motor nerve ceases 2 to 3 days after the nerve is interrupted. The myelin sheath is converted into short ellipsoidal segments during the first few days and gradually undergoes complete disintegration. In the meantime, mononuclear leukocytes emigrate through the walls of blood vessels and accumulate in the cylindrical space within the basal lamina of the column of Schwann cells associated with each nerve fiber. The remains of the axon and its myelin sheath (or the axons only in the case of unmyelinated fibers) are phagocytosed. Thus, the distal stump of a degenerated nerve is filled with tubular formations, known as the bands of von Bungner, that contain phagocytes and Schwann cells.

AXONAL REGENERATION IN PERIPHERAL NERVES

If the axon of a large neuron is transected halfway along its length, the cell loses more than half of its cytoplasm. This lost part of the neuron can be regrown when the injury occurs within the territory of the peripheral nervous system. The reparative process is known as **axonal regeneration**. It is important to distinguish between this use of the word *regeneration* and the replacement of lost cells by mitosis and reorganization of tissue.

   In a severed nerve, the regeneration of axons requires surgical apposition of the cut ends. A crushing injury (or freezing a short length of nerve in a laboratory animal) transects the axons but leaves the connective tissue framework of the nerve intact to guide growing axons to their appropriate destinations.

AXONAL GROWTH AND MATURATION

The following description applies to nerves that have been cleanly cut through and repaired. During the first few days, phagocytes and fibroblasts fill the interval between the apposed ends. Regenerating axons and migrating

Schwann cells invade this region by about the 4th day, with each axon dividing into many filamentous branches, each with an enlarged tip known as a **growth cone**. The rate of axonal growth is slow at first; the growth cones may take up to 3 weeks to traverse the site of transection. Many axons grow into nearby connective tissue, but some find their way into the bands of von Bungner in the distal segment. If

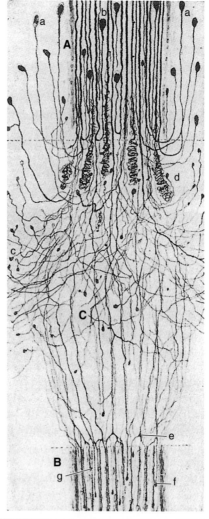

FIGURE 2-12 Longitudinal section of axons regenerating from the proximal stump (**A**) across the scar at a site of transection and repair (**C**) and into the distal stump (**B**) of a peripheral nerve. **a, b, c,** misdirected regenerating axons; **d,** coils formed by growing axons that fail to enter the scar; **e,** branching regenerated axon; **f, g,** axons growing into the peripheral stump. (Adapted from Cajal SR. *Degeneration and Regeneration of the Nervous System,* vol I. London: Oxford University Press, 1928:243.)

too many axons fail to enter the distal stump, a swelling or **neuroma** is formed and may become a source of spontaneous pain.

The invasion of a particular tube leading to a specific type of end organ appears to be determined only by chance. After crossing the region of the lesion (Fig. 2-12) and entering the bands of von Bungner, the axonal filaments grow along the clefts between columns of Schwann cells and the surrounding basal laminae. Usually, only one branch of each axon enters a single tube; other sprouts are drawn back into the shaft of the growing axon. The rate of growth within the nerve distal to the lesion is 2 to 4 mm/day.

Regenerating axons eventually reach motor and sensory endings; the proportion of correctly reinnervated endings depends on conditions at the site of the original injury. The time that will elapse between nerve suture and the beginning of functional return may be estimated on the basis of an average regeneration rate of 1.5 mm/day. This value takes into account the time required for the fibers to traverse the lesion and for the peripheral nerve endings to be reinnervated.

In a human limb, axonal regeneration can be monitored by testing for **Tinel's sign**—that is, when part of a nerve containing regenerating axons is tapped with a small hammer, the patient reports a tingling sensation in the area of skin that normally would be supplied by the nerve.

Each regenerating axon becomes surrounded by the cytoplasm of Schwann cells. For axons that are to be myelinated, the Schwann cells lay down myelin sheaths, starting near the lesion and proceeding distally.

Even years after injury and repair, the fiber diameters, internodal lengths, and conduction velocities are seldom more than 80% of the corresponding normal values. Regenerated motor axons supply more muscle fibers than they formerly did. There is less precise control of reinnervated muscles, and sensory function is also inferior to that mediated by uninjured nerves.

NERVE GRAFTS

When a substantial length of a nerve has been lost, the deficit can be repaired by inserting a graft taken from a thin cutaneous nerve that is functionally less important than the one to be repaired. Several strands of thin nerve are placed side by side, in the manner of a cable, for grafting into a large nerve. Axonal regeneration in a nerve graft is identical to that in a transected and sutured nerve, but the growing axons have to negotiate two sites of anastomosis. The functional recovery is, therefore, far from perfect. A nerve graft must be an autograft (i.e., taken from the same individual) or an isograft (i.e., taken from an identical twin), or it will be rejected by the immune system.

AXONAL DEGENERATION AND REGENERATION IN THE CENTRAL NERVOUS SYSTEM

The simplest lesion to visualize is an incised wound of the brain or spinal cord. The space made by the knife blade fills with blood and later with collagenous connective tissue, which is continuous with the pia mater. The astrocytes in the nervous tissue on each side of the collagenous scar generate longer and more numerous cytoplasmic processes, which form a tangled mass. The number of astrocytes does not increase appreciably, but there is a large increase in the total cell population caused mainly by emigration of monocytes from blood vessels to form phagocytic cells known as **reactive microglia**. The resting microglia that were present before the injury also transform into phagocytes.

The degeneration of severed central axons and their sheaths is different from the process of Wallerian degeneration in peripheral nerves. Degenerating fragments of myelinated axons are present as extracellular objects for several months after the original injury, and the reactive microglial cells that eventually phagocytose the debris persist in situ for many years, marking the positions of the degenerated fibers.

Axons that have been transected in a nerve regrow vigorously, as described earlier. In contrast, when axons are transected within the brain or spinal cord, their proximal stumps begin to regenerate, sending sprouts into the region of the lesion, but this growth ceases after about 2 weeks. This failure of axonal regeneration is attributed partly to inadequate provision of **growth factors**, which are proteins that promote survival of neurons and axonal growth. Growth factors are produced by various cell types, including neurons and glial cells. Some proteins inhibit axonal growth; the one best understood is present in oligodendrocytes and myelin.

In a few circumstances, axons regenerate successfully within the mammalian brain. For example, the unmyelinated neurosecretory axons of the pituitary stalk (see Chapter 11) can regenerate effectively in adult mammals. Axons of several kinds can regenerate across lesions made in the brain or spinal cord in newborn rodents or the pouch-young of marsupials. Both newly growing and regenerating axons cross the sites of transection and make appropriate synaptic connections with other neurons. These animals are at developmental stages equivalent to early and midfetal development in humans. Nevertheless, many neurons of immature animals die after axotomy. Central axons can regenerate and accurately reconnect with other neurons in adult fishes and amphibians.

PLASTICITY OF NEURAL CONNECTIONS

Considerable functional recovery commonly occurs after traumatic or pathological damage to the brain, especially when the lesion is not large. For example, destruction of a small area of cerebral cortex that had a well-defined motor or sensory function is followed by paralysis or loss of sensation, with recovery after several weeks. Similar recovery occurs after partial transection of tracts of fibers. Recovery from paralysis caused by occlusion of blood vessels in the cerebral hemispheres (i.e., stroke) is commonly seen in clinical practice, and functional recovery may even occur after incomplete transverse lesions of the spinal cord.

Functional recovery involves the taking over of the functions of damaged neurons by neurons that remain intact. The reorganization of connections within the brain is known as **plasticity**. This may be an extension of a normally present adaptability used in the learning of often-repeated tasks. Structural changes accompany the functional plasticity that occurs after injury to the nervous system. Thus, when a group of neurons is deprived of part of its afferent input, preterminal axons that come from quite different places grow new branches that then form synapses at the sites denervated by the original lesion. This event, known as **axonal sprouting**, may occur within a small group of neurons or over greater distances, as when the axons of intact dorsal root ganglion cells extend their axons for three or four segments up and down the spinal cord after transection of neighboring dorsal roots.

TRANSPLANTATION OF CENTRAL NEURONS

Neurons of the adult CNS die soon after removal from the body, presumably as the result of severance of their axons and dendrites. Axons can, however, grow into and out of fragments or isolated cells taken from the embryonic or fetal brain and transplanted into certain parts of the adult brain. In laboratory animals, transplanted fetal neurons can partly compensate for the effects of injuries and experimentally induced diseases. Many attempts have been made to try such grafts in people with Parkinson's disease (see Chapter 12), but no substantial or lasting benefits to the recipients have been found. Transplantation of fetal neurons into the human brain or spinal cord is unlikely to acquire therapeutic significance because (a) even with multiple fetal donors, the number of grafted neurons is unrealistically small in relation to the corresponding parts of the recipient brain; (b) neurons deposited in what would be the normal locations of their cell bodies are unlikely to generate axons that will grow several centimeters in the right direction through the host brain into appropriate populations of postsynaptic neurons; and (c) neurons deposited in regions their axons might normally innervate will not receive afferent synapses appropriate to the normal locations of their cell bodies.

Current research on transplantation into the brain is focused on stem cells, which may be induced to differentiate into neurons or neuroglial cells and on adult-derived glial cells such as Schwann cells and olfactory ensheathing cells, which can encourage axonal growth in the adult brain. There is also much interest in neural progenitor cells that occur in certain places in the brains of adult animals. These cells can be induced to migrate and differentiate into neurons; exploitation of this property may have therapeutic potential.

Neuroglial Cells

The term *neuroglia* originally referred only to cells in the CNS. It is now applied also to the nonneuronal cells that are intimately related to neurons and their processes in peripheral ganglia and nerves. The principal structural features of each type are shown in Figure 2-13. The developmental biology of neuroglial cells is reviewed in Chapter 1.

CENTRAL NEUROGLIA

Astrocytes

Astrocytes are variable cells with many cytoplasmic processes. Their cytoplasm contains intermediate filaments composed of **glial fibrillary acidic protein** (GFAP). Many astrocytic processes are closely applied to capillary blood vessels, where they are known as perivascular **end feet**. Other end feet are applied to the pia mater at the external surface of the CNS and beneath the single layer of ependymocytes that lines the ventricular system, forming, respectively, the **external** and the **internal glial limiting membranes**.

Two extreme types of astrocytes are easily recognized by light or electron microscopy. **Fibrous astrocytes** occur in white matter and have long processes with coarse bundles of GFAP filaments. **Protoplasmic** (or **velate**) **astrocytes** are found in gray matter, and their processes are greatly branching and flattened to form delicate lamellae around the terminal branches of axons, dendrites, and synapses.

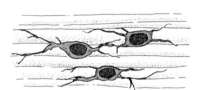

Interfascicular oligodendrocytes

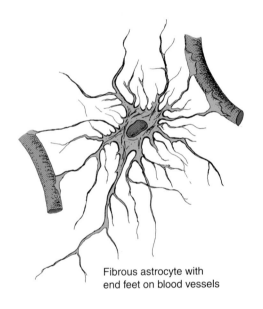

Fibrous astrocyte with end feet on blood vessels

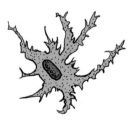

Resting microglial cell in gray matter

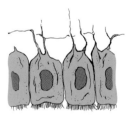

Ependymal cells

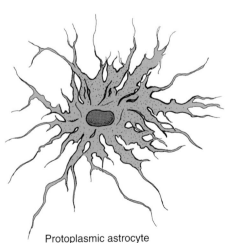

Protoplasmic astrocyte

FIGURE 2-13   Neuroglial cells of the central nervous system.

Müller cells (in the retina) and **pituicytes** (in the neurohypophysis; see Chapter 11) are varieties of protoplasmic astrocytes. **Olfactory ensheathing cells** occur in the olfactory nerves and in the olfactory bulb of the forebrain. They are derived from the olfactory placode and have properties in common with both astrocytes and Schwann cells.

Synapses and nodes of Ranvier are surrounded by the processes of protoplasmic astrocytes, which bear neurotransmitter-specific transporter molecules on their surfaces. Astrocytes can absorb some neurotransmitters, notably glutamate, thus terminating their actions on the postsynaptic membrane. The absorption of potassium ions by astrocytes around synapses, unmyelinated axons, and nodes of Ranvier restrains the spread of electrical disturbances within bundles of axons and regions of neuropil. The dissipation of potassium ions and other small molecules is further enhanced by the existence of gap junctions between adjacent astrocytes.

Corpora amylacea are spherical bodies 25 to 50 μm in diameter and are seen in the normal brains and spinal cords of most middle-aged and elderly people. The name is from a fancied similarity to starch grains. Most corpora amylacea are formed by accumulation of glycoproteins and lipoproteins within processes of astrocytes, although some contain proteins that are normally present in oligodendrocytes or neurons. Corpora amylacea are often extremely abundant, especially in the white matter of the spinal cord, and it is surprising that they do not interfere with function. At sites of degeneration of the cerebral cortex, a locally increased abundance of corpora amylacea sometimes occurs, but these bodies are not thought to be involved in the causation of disease.

Oligodendrocytes

The nuclei of oligodendrocytes are small. A rim of cytoplasm surrounds the nucleus, and the cell has a few long, thin processes. The cytoplasm is conspicuous because of its high electron density and because it contains much granular endoplasmic reticulum and many polyribosomes. Filaments and glycogen are absent, but numerous microtubules are present in the processes. **Interfascicular oligodendrocytes** occur in rows among myelinated axons, where their cytoplasmic processes form and remain continuous with the myelin sheaths (see Fig. 2-9). This function is equivalent to that of the Schwann cell in peripheral nerves. One oligodendrocyte is connected to several myelinated axons. **Satellite oligodendrocytes** are closely associated with the cell bodies of some large neurons. Astrocytes are also closely associated with neuronal cell bodies. A third type of oligodendrocyte, which does not form myelin, has cytoplasmic processes that contact the nodes of Ranvier in white matter, alongside processes of astrocytes.

Ependyma

The ependyma is the simple cuboidal-to-columnar epithelium that lines the ventricular system. Three cell types are recognized in the ependyma. **Ependymocytes** constitute the majority. Their cytoplasm contains all the usual organelles as well as filaments similar to those in astrocytes. Most ependymocytes bear cilia and microvilli on their free or apical surfaces. The bases of the cells have cytoplasmic processes that mingle with the astrocytic end feet of the internal glial limiting membrane. Ependymocytes line the ventricular system and are thus in contact with the cerebrospinal fluid (CSF). These cells are not connected by tight junctions, and molecules of all sizes are freely exchanged between the CSF and the adjacent nervous tissue.

Tanycytes differ from ependymocytes in having long basal processes. Most of these cells occur in the floor of the third ventricle. Their basal processes end on the pia mater and on blood vessels in the median eminence of the hypothalamus (see Chapter 11). It has been suggested that the tanycytes of the ventral hypothalamic region respond to changing levels of blood-derived hormones in the CSF by discharging secretory products into the capillary vessels of the median eminence. Such activity may be involved in the control of the endocrine system by the anterior lobe of the pituitary gland (see Chapter 11).

Choroidal epithelial cells cover the surfaces of the choroid plexuses. They have microvilli at their apical surfaces and invaginations at their basal surfaces, which rest on a basement membrane. Adjacent choroidal epithelial cells are joined by tight junctions, thus preventing the passive movement of plasma proteins into the CSF. These cells are metabolically active in controlling the chemical composition of the fluid, which is secreted by the choroid plexuses into the cerebral ventricles (see Chapter 26).

Microglia

About 5% of the total neuroglial population in the CNS is composed of **resting microglial cells**. These have small, elongated nuclei; scanty cytoplasm; and several short-branched processes with spiny appendages. Resting microglial cells are evenly spaced throughout the gray and white matter, with little overlapping or intertwining of their processes.

Resting microglial cells are equivalent to the resident macrophages of other tissues, and they can acquire phagocytic properties when the CNS is afflicted by injury or disease. They may also be involved in protecting the nervous tissue from viruses, microorganisms, and the formation of tumors.

Abnormal Central Neuroglia

When the brain or spinal cord is injured, the astrocytes near the lesion undergo hypertrophy. The cytoplasmic processes become more numerous and are densely packed with GFAP filaments. There may also be a small increase in the number of the cells caused by mitosis of mature astrocytes. These changes, known as **gliosis**, occur in many pathological conditions, and sometimes the reactive astrocytes acquire phagocytic properties.

Cells with structural and staining properties similar to those of resting microglial cells appear in large numbers at the sites of injury or inflammatory disease in the CNS. Experimental evidence indicates that some of these pathological cells, known as **reactive microglial cells**, are formed from resting microglial cells, which retract their processes, divide, exhibit amoeboid movement, and acquire phagocytic properties. The activation of resident microglia occurs immediately after almost any kind of insult. At a later stage, large numbers of monocytes enter the nervous system by passing through the walls of blood vessels, and these also assume the appearance of reactive microglial cells and phagocytose the remains of dead cells, bacteria, and other debris. This function is equivalent to that of macrophages in other parts of the body. Reactive microglial cells that are distended with lipid-rich phagocytosed material are known as **gitter cells**.

PERIPHERAL NEUROGLIA

Schwann Cells (Neurolemmocytes)

These tubular cells with elongated nuclei intimately ensheath all axons in all parts of the peripheral nervous system, including nerve roots and peripheral nerves. Each axon is suspended in the cytoplasm of its Schwann cell by a double layer of surface membrane, the **mesaxon**. The myelin sheaths in peripheral nerves are formed by Schwann cells. A myelinated axon is exposed to extracellular fluid at regular intervals along its length, where there are short gaps between adjacent neurolemmocytes. The gaps are called **nodes of Ranvier**. One Schwann cell ensheaths either one myelinated axon or several unmyelinated axons. The surface of an unmyelinated axon is in contact with extracellular fluid along its whole length, through the cleft between the layers of its mesaxon. (This cleft is closed off by the formation of a myelin sheath.) On the outside surface of each Schwann cell, a basal lamina is present.

Satellite Cells (Ganglionic Gliocytes)

In sensory and autonomic ganglia, these cells intimately surround the neuronal somata. Ganglia also contain Schwann cells around axons.

The enteric nervous system consists of small ganglia and interconnecting strands of mostly unmyelinated neurites in the wall of the gut (see Chapter 24). The neuroglial cells in this system have structural and chemical features in common with both astrocytes and peripheral gliocytes. No special name has been given to the enteric glial cells.

Suggested Reading

Altman J. Microglia emerge from the fog. *Trends Neurosci* 1994;17:47–49.

Bahr M, Bonhoeffer F. Perspectives on axonal regeneration in the mammalian CNS. *Trends Neurosci* 1994;17:473–479.

Borlongan CV, Sanberg PR. Neural transplantation for treatment of Parkinson's disease. *Drug Discov Today* 2002;7:674–682.

Brecknell JE, Fawcett JW. Axonal regeneration. *Biol Rev* 1996;71, 227–255.

Bruni JE. Ependymal development, proliferation, and functions: a review. *Microsc Res Tech* 1998;41:2–13.

Bunge RP. Glial cells and the central myelin sheath. *Physiol Rev* 1968;48:197–251.

Cajal SR. *Degeneration and Regeneration of the Nervous System*, vol I. London: Oxford University Press, 1928:243.

Del Bigio MR. The ependyma: a protective barrier between brain and cerebrospinal fluid. *Glia* 1995;14:1–13.

Jones K, ed. Olfactory ensheathing cells: therapeutic potential for spinal cord regeneration [special issue]. *Anat Rec Part B* 2003;271:39–85.

Kettenman N, Ransom BR, eds. *Neuroglia*, 2nd ed. New York: Oxford University Press, 2005.

Landau WM. Artificial intelligence: the brain transplant cure for parkinsonism. *Neurology* 1990;40:733–740.

Leitch B. Ultrastructure of electrical synapses: review. *Electron Microsc Rev* 1992;5:311–339.

Nicholls JG, Wallace BG, Fuchs PA, et al. *From Neuron to Brain*, 4th ed. Sunderland, MS: Sinauer, 2001.

Peters A, Palay SL, Webster HdeF. *The Fine Structure of the Nervous System: Neurons and Their Supporting Cells*, 3rd ed New York: Oxford University Press, 1991.

Ramsay HJ. Ultrastructure of corpora amylacea. *J Neuropathol Exp Neurol* 1965;24:25–39.

Schipper HM, Cisse S. Mitochondrial constituents of corpora amylacea and autofluorescent astrocytic inclusions in senescent human brain. *Glia* 1995;14:55–64.

Shepherd GM. *Neurobiology*, 3rd ed. New York: Oxford University Press, 1994.

Somjen GG. Nervenkitt: notes on the history of the concept of neuroglia. *Glia* 1988;1:2–9.

Thored P, Arvidsson A, Cacci E, et al. Persistent production of neurons from adult brain stem cells during recovery after a stroke. *Stem Cells* 2006;24:739–747.

Weiss S, Dunne C, Hewson J, et al. Multipotent CNS stem cells are present in the adult mammalian spinal cord and ventricular neuroaxis. *J Neurosci* 1996;16:7599–7609.

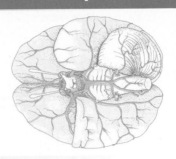

Chapter 3

PERIPHERAL NERVOUS SYSTEM

Important Facts

- Ganglia are the sites of all neuronal cell bodies in the peripheral nervous system. Motor and preganglionic autonomic neurons have their cell bodies in the spinal cord and brain stem.

- A nerve is a bundle of axons, together with the associated glia, myelin sheaths, and supporting connective tissue. A nerve fiber is one axon together with its myelin sheath and neuroglial (Schwann) cells. The most rapidly conducting fibers, those with the largest diameters, innervate extrafusal muscle fibers or serve the senses of discriminative touch, proprioception, and vibration. The smallest axons are for pain, olfaction, and visceral innervation.

- Sensory ganglia are present on the dorsal roots of spinal nerves and on some cranial nerves. These ganglia contain unipolar neurons with axons that enter the central nervous system (CNS).

- Skin contains a variety of types of sensory nerve endings for touch, temperature, pain, and other external sensations. Muscles, tendons, and joints contain proprioceptive endings. Muscle spindles inform the CNS of changes in the length of a muscle; tendon receptors respond to tension. Kinesthetic sensation (i.e., conscious proprioception) arises mainly from muscle spindles but partly from joints.

- Striated skeletal muscle is supplied by motor neurons, which have their cell bodies in the spinal cord and brain stem.

- The motor end plate is the structurally specialized effector ending in striated skeletal muscle. The synaptic transmitter is acetylcholine, which makes the muscle fibers contract.

- Preganglionic neurons have axons that synapse with the neurons in autonomic ganglia. Smooth muscle and glands are innervated by the neurons in autonomic ganglia.

- The endings of autonomic axons are swellings (varicosities) of unmyelinated axons, containing a variety of chemical transmitter substances that stimulate or inhibit smooth muscle, cardiac muscle, and secretory cells.

General Organization

Certain aspects of the peripheral nervous system are especially pertinent to a study of the brain and spinal cord. These include the sensory receptors, motor endings, histology of peripheral nerves, and structure of ganglia. The following introductory comments refer to all spinal nerves and to the cranial nerves that are not restricted to the special senses. The structures discussed in this chapter are shown in Figure 3-1, which represents a spinal nerve in the thoracic or upper lumbar region in which neurons for visceral innervation are included.

General sensory endings are scattered profusely throughout the body. They are biological transducers, in which physical or chemical stimuli create action potentials in nerve endings. The resulting nerve impulses, on reaching the central nervous system (CNS), produce reflex responses, awareness of the stimuli, or both. Sensory endings that are superficially located, such as those in the skin, are called **exteroceptors**; they respond to stimuli for pain, temperature, touch, and pressure. **Proprioceptors** in muscles, tendons, and joints provide data for reflex adjustments of muscle action and for awareness of position and movement.

Components of Nerves, Roots, and Ganglia

Signals from exteroceptors and proprioceptors are conducted centrally by primary sensory neurons, whose cell bodies are located in

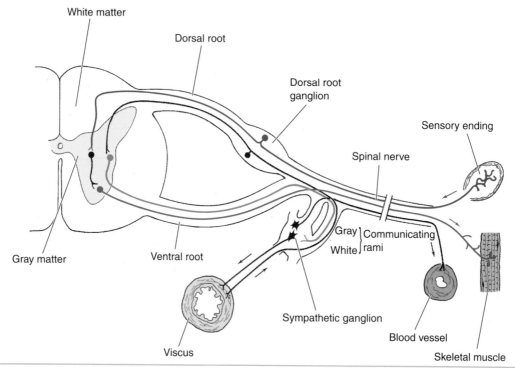

White matter

Dorsal root

Dorsal root
ganglion

Sensory ending

Spinal nerve

Gray matter

Ventral root

Gray ⎱ Communicating
White ⎰ rami

Sympathetic ganglion

Viscus

Blood vessel

Skeletal muscle

FIGURE 3-1   Functional components of a "typical" spinal nerve, in this case between levels T1 and L2. Color scheme: Red for somatic motor neurons; blue for primary sensory neurons; green for preganglionic autonomic (sympathetic) neurons; and black for interneurons in the spinal cord and for postganglionic sympathetic neurons.

dorsal root ganglia (or in an equivalent cranial nerve ganglion). On entering the spinal cord, the dorsal root fibers divide into ascending and descending branches; these are distributed as necessary for reflex responses (of which some are considered in Chapter 5) and for transmission of sensory data to the brain (pathways are reviewed in Chapter 19).

There is a third class of sensory endings, known as **interoceptors**, in the viscera. Central conduction occurs through primary sensory neurons like those already noted, except that the peripheral process follows a different route. For a receptor concerned with pain, the sensory axon reaches the sympathetic trunk through a white communicating ramus and continues to a viscus in a branch of the sympathetic trunk. For receptors concerned with the functional regulation of internal organs, some sensory axons may follow similar courses, but the best understood of these "physiological afferent" axons have their cell bodies in cranial nerve ganglia and are connected centrally with the brain stem. There are, therefore, two broad categories of sensory endings and afferent neurons: **somatic afferents**,

for the skin, bones, muscles, and connective tissue that makes up most of the mass of the body (soma), and **visceral afferents**, for the internal organs of the circulatory, respiratory, alimentary, excretory, and reproductive systems.

There are also two categories of efferent neurons. The cell bodies of **somatic efferent** neurons (also called **motor neurons**) are in the ventral gray horns of the spinal cord and motor nuclei of cranial nerves. The axons of ventral horn cells traverse the ventral roots and spinal nerves and terminate in motor end plates on skeletal muscle fibers. The **visceral efferent** or autonomic system has a special feature, in that at least two neurons participate in transmission from the CNS to smooth muscle, cardiac muscle, or secretory cells (Fig. 3-2).

Sensory Endings

The sensory endings are supplied by axons that differ in size and other characteristics. This is a matter of some interest because there is a correlation between fiber diameter and the rate of conduction

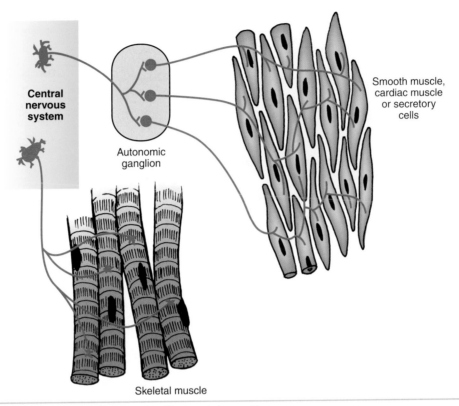

Central nervous system

Autonomic ganglion

Smooth muscle, cardiac muscle or secretory cells

Skeletal muscle

FIGURE 3-2 Comparison of autonomic with somatic innervation.

of the action potential and because functionally different sensory endings are supplied by fibers of specific sizes. A commonly used nomenclature for peripheral nerve fibers, using Roman and Greek letters, is given in Table 2-1. This table includes the functions associated with the categories.

CUTANEOUS SENSORY ENDINGS

On a structural basis, two classes of cutaneous and other sensory endings are recognized. **Nonencapsulated endings** are terminal branches of the axon that may either be closely applied to cells or lie freely in the extracellular spaces of connective tissue. **Encapsulated endings** have distinctive arrangements of nonneuronal cells that completely enclose the terminal parts of the axons. In the following account, the receptors are described according to location, with exteroceptors and some proprioceptors shown in Figures 3-3 and 3-4, respectively.

Most of the skin bears hairs that vary greatly in length, thickness, and abundance from one

part of the body to another. Glabrous skin, which lacks hairs, is present on the palmar surfaces of the hands and fingers, the soles, and parts of the face and external genitalia. Hairy and glabrous skin have different patterns of innervation.

HISTOLOGY OF CUTANEOUS INNERVATION

Cutaneous branches of spinal and cranial nerves pass through the subcutaneous connective tissue into the dermis, where the axons spread out horizontally to form three plexuses, which lie in the plane of the skin's surface. The **subcutaneous plexus** lies in the loose connective tissue deep to the skin, the **dermal plexus** is within the densely collagenous reticular layer that constitutes the deeper part of the dermis, and the **papillary plexus** lies in the papillary layer of the dermis, immediately beneath the epidermis. The axons of each plexus send branches into the adjacent tissues. The density of cutaneous innervation varies considerably from one region to another. For example, the

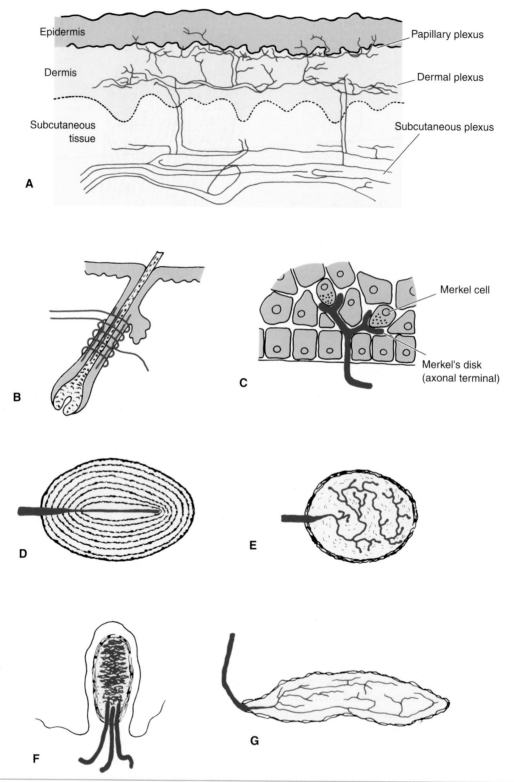

FIGURE 3-3   Sensory innervation of skin. **(A)** Plexuses. **(B)** Peritrichial ending. **(C)** Merkel ending in epidermis. **(D)** Pacinian corpuscle. **(E)** End bulb. **(F)** Meissner's corpuscle. **(G)** Ruffini ending.

face and hands are more richly innervated than is the dorsal aspect of the trunk.

Free nerve endings occur in the subcutaneous tissue and dermis, and some extend among the cells of the epidermis. They are the terminal branches of group C fibers and the unmyelinated terminal branches of group A fibers, and they are receptive to all modalities of cutaneous sensation. Although they are called "free endings," these axons are always invested with Schwann cells (the neuroglia of peripheral nerves) and do not contact the extracellular fluid directly. Indeed, it is impossible to identify the exact point of termination of an axon within the skin. The existence of free nerve endings is inferred from the functional sensitivity of regions of skin in which no other types of sensory ending can be recognized.

Merkel endings are found in the germinal layer (stratum basale) of the epidermis. Axonal branches end as flattened expansions, each being closely applied to a **Merkel cell**. This small cell differs from the other epidermal cells in having an indented nucleus and electron-dense cytoplasmic granules. Merkel cells are found in glabrous skin and in the outer root sheaths of hairs.

Peritrichial nerve endings are cagelike formations of axons that surround hair follicles. A single axon sends branches to many hair follicles, and each follicle is supplied by from 2 to 20 axons. The axons approach the follicle deep to its sebaceous gland and branch in the connective tissue outside the outer root sheath. Some branches encircle the follicle, others run parallel to its long axis, and some end on Merkel cells in the outer root sheath.

Skin contains several types of encapsulated ending. The **Ruffini ending**, typically about 1 mm long and 20 to 30 μm wide, is an array of terminal branches of a myelinated axon surrounded by capsular cells. The **pacinian corpuscle** (or Vater-Pacini corpuscle) consists of a single axon that loses its myelin sheath and is encapsulated by several layers of flattened cells with greatly attenuated cytoplasm. These ellipsoidal corpuscles are about 1 mm long and 0.7 mm wide. Ruffini endings and pacinian corpuscles are present in the subcutaneous tissue and dermis of both hairy and glabrous skin. **Meissner's tactile corpuscles** occur in large numbers in the dermal papillary ridges of the fingertips and are less abundant in other hairless regions. Each Meissner's corpuscle is supplied by three or four myelinated axons whose terminal branches form a complicated knot that is enclosed in a cellular and collagenous capsule. Meissner's corpuscles are about 80 μm by 30 μm in size and are oriented with their long axes perpendicular to the skin's surface. **End bulbs** vary in size and shape, and several types have been described (e.g., end bulbs of Krause, Golgi-Mazzoni endings, genital corpuscles, mucocutaneous endings), although all may be variants of the same structure. They are commonly spherical, about 50 μm in length, with each containing a coiled, branching axonal terminal in a thin cellular capsule. Most end bulbs occur in mucous membranes (mouth, conjunctiva, anal canal) and in the dermis of glabrous skin close to orifices (lips, external genitalia).

PHYSIOLOGIC CORRELATES

The types of sensation consciously perceived from the skin are called **modalities**. The different sensations are not always clear cut, but in medical practice, it is customary to recognize five modalities that are easily tested by clinical examination. These are fine (discriminative) touch, vibration, light touch, temperature (warmth or cold), and pain. Sensations of each modality also have **quality**. For example, pain may have an aching or a burning quality; temperature has quality that varies continuously, from painfully cold to painfully hot. The central pathways that process these sensations are fairly well known (see Chapter 19), but for other modalities (e.g., itch, tickle, rub, firm pressure), they are only poorly understood. Careful testing has revealed that the human skin is a mosaic of spots, each of which responds selectively to only one of the four elementary sensations of touch, warmth, cold, and pain. The response of any one of these spots is always the same, whatever the nature of the stimulus. For example, a feeling of coldness will be experienced from a "cold spot" even if it is heated or injured. The sensitivity is greatest (or in physiologists' parlance, the threshold is lowest) for the specific modality.

Attempts to correlate the modalities of sensation in humans with morphologically identified nerve endings have yielded inconclusive results.

Electrophysiological studies in animals, however, have shown that although no cutaneous receptors have absolute specificity, there is a high degree of selectivity for certain end organs.

An important physiological property of any receptor is **adaptation**, which is a reduced response to continued stimulation. A slowly adapting receptor reports continuously on the stimulus that activates it. A rapidly adapting receptor reports changes in the stimuli it receives. *Meissner's corpuscles* are sensitive to mechanical deformation, and they adapt rapidly (i.e., they do not continue to respond to a sustained deformation). These properties, associated with alignment in papillary ridges, allow an array of these receptors to identify with great accuracy the positions and movements of objects touching or moving across the surface of the skin. Thus, Meissner's corpuscles are the sense organs used when feeling the texture of a surface with the tips of the fingers. *Merkel endings* also respond preferentially to tactile stimuli but are much more slowly adapting than Meissner's corpuscles, so they respond to steady indentation of the surface of the skin. Their sensitivity to this stimulus is enhanced by their location in the epidermis. *Pacinian corpuscles* also initiate action potentials when they are deformed; they are the most rapidly adapting receptors, so they have a special sensitivity to vibration. The rapid adaptation is attributed to the fluid between the many layers of the corpuscle; a sustained deformation causes a change of shape without mechanically disturbing the axon in the center. The *Ruffini ending* responds to mechanical stimuli that pull on the collagen fibers attached to its capsule, when pressure on or stretching of the skin causes movement in the subcutaneous tissue. *Peritrichial endings* respond to mechanical displacement of the hair shaft, so that hair follicles serve as receptor organs for light touch. The various *end bulbs* are poorly understood but are presumed to respond to tactile stimuli.

For the modalities of warmth and cold (all skin) and touch (hairy skin that does not contain encapsulated endings), it is presumed that the receptors must be free nerve endings derived from the dermal and papillary plexuses. The physiological characteristics of some of these receptors have been ascertained from electrical recordings made from individual axons in peripheral nerves in animals and humans. The receptors for tactile sensation are **low threshold mechanoceptors**, a category that includes all encapsulated and some free nerve endings.

Painful sensations are received by free nerve endings, termed **nociceptors**. Three types are recognized. **High threshold mechanoreceptors** respond only to mechanical stimuli such as stretching or cutting. **Polymodal nociceptors** respond to both mechanical and thermal ($\geq 45°C$) stimuli and to chemical mediators released from injured cells. The third type of nociceptor responds only to chemical mediators and may contribute to the **hyperalgesia** (lowered pain threshold) associated with inflammation.

SENSORY ENDINGS IN MUSCLES, TENDONS, AND JOINTS

Proprioceptors in the capsules of joints, muscles, and tendons furnish the CNS with information required for the performance of properly coordinated movements through reflex action. In addition, proprioceptive information reaches consciousness so that there is awareness of the position of body parts and of their movements (**kinesthetic sense** or **conscious proprioception**). Pain that arises in muscles, tendons, ligaments, and bones is probably detected by free nerve endings in connective tissue. These nociceptive endings respond to physical injury and to local chemical changes such as those caused by inflammation or ischemia.

Muscles

The proprioceptive organs in skeletal muscles are the **neuromuscular spindles**, often simply called muscle spindles. They are innervated by both sensory and motor neurons.

Neuromuscular spindles are a fraction of a millimeter wide and up to 6 mm long. They lie in the long axis of the muscle, and their collagenous capsules are continuous with the fibrous septae that separate the muscle fibers. The fibrous septa are in mechanical continuity with the skeletal attachments of the muscle so that the spindles are lengthened whenever a muscle is passively stretched. Spindles are typically located near the tendinous insertions of muscles and are especially numerous in muscles that perform highly skilled movements, such as those of the hand.

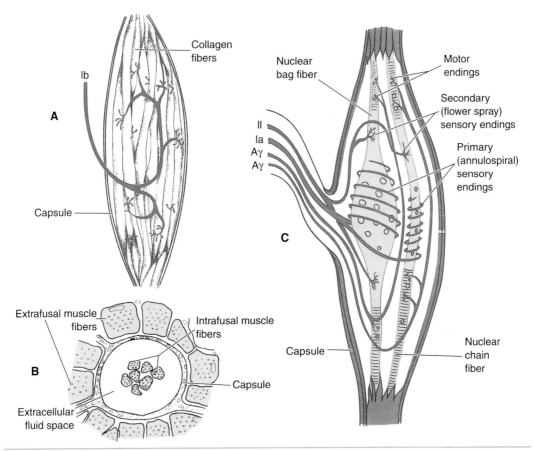

FIGURE 3-4   Specialized sensory endings in skeletal muscle and tendon. Sensory axons are shown in shades of blue, fusimotor axons in red, muscle fibers in yellow, and connective tissue in black and gray. **(A)** A Golgi tendon organ. **(B)** Neuromuscular spindle in transverse section. **(C)** Innervation of a muscle spindle.

Each spindle (see Fig. 3-4) consists of a capsule of connective tissue, with two to 14 **intrafusal** muscle fibers. The latter differ in several respects from the main or **extrafusal** fibers of the muscle. Intrafusal fibers are considerably smaller than the extrafusal; the equatorial region lacks cross striations and contains many nuclei that are not in the sub-sarcolemmal position characteristic of mature striated muscle.

A muscle spindle is supplied by two sensory axons. One of these is an Aα or Ia fiber (see Table 2-1); the axon loses its myelin sheath as it pierces the capsule, and then it winds spi-rally around the midportions of the intrafusal muscle fibers in the form of an **annulospiral ending**. The second, slightly smaller sensory fiber (Aβ or II) branches terminally and ends as varicosities on the intrafusal muscle fibers some distance from the midregion. The latter

terminals are called **flower spray endings**. The annulospiral and flower spray terminals are also known, respectively, as the primary and secondary sensory endings of the spindle.

The extrafusal fibers composing the main mass of a muscle are innervated by large motor cells (**alpha motor neurons**), whose axons are of Aα size. Smaller motor cells (**gamma motor neurons**), with Aγ axons, supply the intrafusal muscle fibers within the spindle.

The simplest role of the muscle spindle is that of a receptor for the **stretch reflex**. Slight stretching of a muscle lengthens the intrafusal fibers, and the sensory endings are stimulated. Action potentials are conducted to the spinal cord, where terminal branches of the sensory axons synapse with alpha motor neurons that supply the main mass of the muscle. The lat-ter thereupon contracts in response to stretch through a two-neuron reflex arc. Stimulation of the spindles ceases when the muscle contracts because the spindle fibers, in parallel with the other muscle fibers, return to their original lengths. The stretch reflex is in constant use in the adjustment of muscle tone. It also forms the basis of tests for **tendon reflexes**, such as the knee jerk (extension at the knee on tapping the patellar tendon), which are standard items in clinical examinations.

The spindles also have an important role in muscle action that results from the activity of the brain. The motor fibers that descend from the brain into the spinal cord influence both alpha and gamma motor neurons in the ventral gray horns by synapsing with them directly and through the mediation of interneurons. Contraction of the intrafusal muscle fibers in response to stimulation by gamma motor neurons lengthens the midportions and starts a volley of impulses in the sensory axons. This causes contraction of the regular muscle fibers through reflex stimulation of alpha motor neurons. The **gamma reflex loop** consists of the gamma motor neuron, muscle spindle, sensory neuron, and alpha motor neuron supplying extrafusal muscle fibers. It is an adjunct to the more direct control of muscles by descending fibers from the brain that control the alpha motor neuron. Activation of the gamma reflex loop can set the length of a muscle before the initiation of a movement.

Tendons

Golgi tendon organs, also known as **neurotendinous spindles**, are most numerous near the attachments of tendons to muscles. Each receptor has a thin capsule of connective tissue that encloses a few collagenous fibers of the tendon. The axon of an Aβ or Ib fiber (there may be more than one) breaks up into unmyelinated terminal branches after entering the spindle, and the branches end as varicosities on the intrafusal tendon fibers. This type of sensory ending is stimulated by *tension* in the tendon, in contrast to the muscle spindle, which responds to changes in the *length* of the region containing sensory nerve endings. Afferent signals from Golgi tendon organs reach interneurons in the spinal cord, which, in turn, have an inhibitory effect on alpha motor neurons, causing relaxation of the muscle to which the particular tendon is attached. The different functions of the

neuromuscular and neurotendinous spindles are in balance in the total integration of spinal reflex activity. As constant monitors of tension, the Golgi tendon organs also provide protection against damage that might result from an excessively strong muscular contraction.

Joints

Around the capsules of synovial joints, there are small pacinian corpuscles and formations similar to Ruffini cutaneous endings. They respond, respectively, to the cessation and initiation of movement. Receptors identical to Golgi tendon organs are present in the articular ligaments; they mediate reflex inhibition of muscles when excessive strain is placed on the joint. Free nerve endings are abundant in the synovial membrane, capsule, and periarticular connective tissues. They are believed to respond to potentially injurious mechanical stresses and to mediate the pain that arises in diseased or injured joints.

CONSCIOUS PROPRIOCEPTION

The various types of proprioceptors provides essential information for neuromuscular control at the subconscious level, including reflexes that involve the spinal cord, brain stem, cerebellum, and cerebral cortex. The roles of specific receptors in conscious proprioception (**kinesthesia**) are still debated. Observations made with human subjects indicate that the nerves from both joints and muscles carry signals that are consciously perceived as position and movement. Infiltration of a small joint with local anesthetic does not impair these sensations, but damage to major ligaments of a large joint, such as the knee, is followed by diminished position sense. The muscle spindles are considered to be the principal kinesthetic receptors.

SENSORY ENDINGS IN VISCERA

Except for pacinian corpuscles, most of which are in mesenteries, the sensory endings in viscera consist mainly of nonencapsulated terminal branches of axons, some of which are quite complicated. In general, visceral afferents function in physiological visceral reflexes; in the sensations of fullness of the stomach, rectum, and bladder; and in pain caused by visceral dysfunction or disease. Afferent fibers for pain generally travel in different nerves from those involved in functional control and have different connections in the CNS (see Chapter 24).

Effector Endings

The nervous system acts on muscle fibers and secretory cells. Control of these nonneural cells is effected by a mechanism similar to that of chemical synaptic transmission between neurons (see Chapter 2). At the neuroeffector endings, axons terminate in relation to skeletal, cardiac, and smooth muscle fibers and to the cells of exocrine and endocrine glands. Many endocrine organs are controlled, directly or indirectly, by hypothalamic neurosecretory neurons that discharge their products into blood vessels for subsequent delivery to the target cells.

MOTOR END PLATES

The **motor end plates**, or **myoneural junctions**, on extrafusal and intrafusal fibers of skeletal striated muscles are synaptic structures with two components: the ending of a motor axon and the subjacent part of the muscle fiber. The axon of an alpha motor neuron divides terminally to supply variable numbers of muscle fibers. A **motor unit** consists of one motor neuron and the muscle fibers that it innervates. The number of muscle fibers in a motor unit varies from fewer than 10 to several hundred, depending on the size and function of the muscle. Small muscles, such as the extraocular and intrinsic

hand muscles, must contract with greater precision, so their motor units include only a few muscle fibers. Large motor units occur in the muscles of the trunk and proximal parts of the limbs; they are necessary for sudden and powerful movements, with many muscle fibers contracting simultaneously.

Each branch of the motor nerve fiber gives up its myelin sheath on approaching a muscle fiber and ends as several branchlets that constitute the neural component of the end plate (Fig. 3-5). The end plate is typically 40 to 60 μm in diameter and is usually located midway along the length of the muscle fiber. The neurolemmal sheath (consisting of the nucleated cytoplasmic parts of Schwann cells) continues around the terminal branches of the motor axon but does not intervene between the nerve ending and the muscle fiber. The nerve fiber is surrounded outside the neurolemma by a thin sheath of endoneurial connective tissue, which blends at the motor end plates with the endomysium (the connective tissue that ensheaths each muscle fiber).

The axonal endings within the end plates contain mitochondria and synaptic vesicles. The latter contain **acetylcholine**, which is the neurotransmitter in motor end plates. Each axonal branchlet occupies a groove or "synaptic gutter" on the surface of the muscle fiber. The intervening synaptic cleft is 20 to 50 nm wide. The plasma membrane and associated basement membrane, which together constitute the sarcolemma of the muscle fiber, have a wavy outline where they appose the nerve terminal, with the irregularities known as junctional folds. This folded region of the sarcolemma, the **subneural**

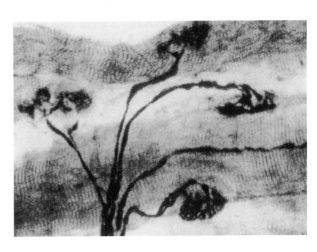

FIGURE 3-5 Motor end plates. (Gold chloride technique, ×800; courtesy of Drs. R. Mitchell and A. S. Wilson.)

apparatus, is demonstrable histochemically by its content of **acetylcholinesterase**, the enzyme that inactivates acetylcholine.

Acetylcholine, which is released from the synaptic vesicles when action potentials travel along the axon, binds to **acetylcholine receptor** molecules in the folded sarcolemma of the subneural apparatus. An adequate train of impulses releases enough acetylcholine to depolarize the postsynaptic membrane, and the resulting action potential is carried into the muscle fiber (by invaginations of the sarcolemma that constitute the transverse tubular system) to the contractile myofibrils.

POSTGANGLIONIC AUTONOMIC ENDINGS

The presynaptic effector nerve endings on smooth muscle, cardiac muscle, and secretory cells are swellings, usually called **varicosities**, along the courses and at the tips of unmyelinated axons. These swellings contain accumulations of mitochondria and clusters of synaptic vesicles. The terminals are applied to the effector cells, sometimes as closely as they are in skeletal muscle, but there are no obvious postsynaptic structural specializations. Whereas noradrenergic terminals of the sympathetic nervous system contain electron-dense synaptic vesicles, cholinergic terminals (typically parasympathetic) contain small electron-lucent vesicles. Other types of synaptic vesicles are also seen frequently, and immunohistochemical studies indicate that most autonomic nerve endings contain one or more peptides in addition to the two classical neurotransmitters.

Ganglia

Spinal ganglia are swellings on the dorsal roots of spinal nerves, located in the intervertebral foramina, just proximal to the union of dorsal and ventral roots. Spinal ganglia contain the cell bodies of primary sensory neurons, mainly in a large peripheral zone. The center of the ganglion is occupied by the proximal parts of the neurites. Dorsal root ganglia and ganglia of cranial nerves involved with general sensation have the same histological structure.

The neurons in sensory ganglia are at first bipolar, but the two neurites soon unite to form a single process. (The term *pseudounipolar* is often applied to the sensory ganglion cell, but this is a truly unipolar neuron after the two processes of the bipolar embryonic cell have fused.) The neurite divides into peripheral and central branches; the former terminates in a sensory ending, and the latter enters the spinal cord through a dorsal root. Action potentials pass directly from the peripheral to the central branch, bypassing the cell body. Both branches have the structural and electrophysiological characteristics of axons.

The spherical cell bodies in a sensory ganglion vary from 20 to 100 μm in diameter; their processes are similarly of graded size, ranging from small unmyelinated fibers in group C to the largest myelinated fibers in group A (see Table 2-1). The large neurons are for proprioception and discriminative touch; those of intermediate size are concerned with light touch, pressure, pain, and temperature; the smallest neurons transmit impulses for pain and tem-

---

CLINICAL NOTES

Myasthenia Gravis

An autoimmune disease is one in which there is production of antibodies that bind to cells or proteins that are normal components of the person's own body. In myasthenia gravis, such antibodies combine with the acetylcholine receptors at motor end plates, thereby blocking the normal action of acetylcholine. In many cases, the antibody-producing cells are derived from a benign tumor of the thymus. All skeletal muscles become weak and easily fatigued,

so the first signs of the disease appear in constantly used muscles, such as those that move the eyes and eyelids and those of respiration. Symptomatic relief is provided by drugs that inhibit acetylcholinesterase, allowing higher concentrations of the transmitter to accumulate in the synaptic cleft. Treatments that suppress the immune system (e.g., removal of the thymus, use of corticosteroids and other drugs) are also valuable in the management of patients with myasthenia gravis.

perature. Each cell body is closely invested by a layer of **satellite cells** that is continuous with the Schwann cell sheath that surrounds the axon External to this, the neurons are supported by connective tissue that contains collagen fibers and blood vessels.

Autonomic ganglia include those of the sympathetic trunks along the sides of the vertebral bodies, collateral or prevertebral ganglia in plexuses of the thorax and abdomen (e.g., the cardiac, celiac, and mesenteric plexuses), and certain ganglia near viscera. The **principal cells** of autonomic ganglia are multipolar neurons 20 to 45 μm in diameter. The cell body is surrounded by satellite cells similar to those of spinal ganglia. Several dendrites extend and branch outside the capsule of satellite cells and receive synaptic contacts from preganglionic axons. The thin, unmyelinated axons (group C fibers) of the principal cells leave the ganglia and eventually supply smooth muscle and gland cells in some viscera, cardiac muscle, the enteric plexuses, blood vessels throughout the body, and sweat glands and arrector pili muscles in the skin. Autonomic ganglia also contain small **interneurons** with short dendrites that are postsynaptic to the preganglionic axons and presynaptic to dendrites of principal cells.

Peripheral Nerves

ARRANGEMENT AND ENSHEATHMENT OF NERVE FIBERS

The constituent fibers of all but the smallest peripheral nerves are arranged in bundles or fascicles, and three connective tissue sheaths are recognized (Fig. 3-6). The entire nerve is surrounded by the **epineurium**. This is composed of ordinary connective tissue, and it also fills the spaces between the fascicles. Undulations in the epineurial collagen fibers around each fascicle allow for stretching of the nerve that accompanies flexion of joints and other movement. A nerve root within the vertebral canal does not have an epineurium; this ensheathing layer is acquired as the nerve pierces the dura mater on its way through an intervertebral foramen. (The dura mater is the outermost of the three meninges; these layers of connective tissue that envelop the brain and spinal cord are described in Chapter 26.)

The sheath that encloses each small bundle of fibers in a nerve consists of several layers of flattened cells, collectively known as the **perineurium**. Within the perineurium, individual nerve fibers have a delicate covering of connective tissue that constitutes the **endoneurium**, or sheath of Henle. The cells of all three connective tissue layers of peripheral nerves are derived from mesodermal cells rather than from the neuroectoderm. Within the endoneurium, the axons are intimately ensheathed by neuroglial cells (Schwann cells), which are derived from the neural crest and constitute the **neurolemma** (also spelled *neurilemma*) or sheath of Schwann.

MYELINATED NERVE FIBERS

A **nerve fiber** consists of the axon, the myelin sheath (of fibers in groups A and B), and the neurolemma (sheath of Schwann). The axon is no different from a long axon in the CNS. Its cytoplasm (axoplasm) contains neurofilaments, microtubules, patches of smooth-surfaced endoplasmic reticulum, and mitochondria. The plasma membrane of an axon is called

---

■CLINICAL NOTES■

Herpes Zoster

A common disorder involving spinal or cranial nerve ganglia is **herpes zoster** (or **shingles**), in which a viral infection of the ganglion causes pain and other sensory disturbances and a skin eruption in the area of distribution of the affected dorsal root or cranial nerve. The cutaneous inflammation is caused partly by spontaneous antidromic conduction of impulses in the group C fibers of the nerve. These release from their terminals peptides, including substance P (SP) and calcitonin gene-related peptide (CGRP). SP and CGRP dilate small arteries and make small veins permeable, causing exudation of plasma.

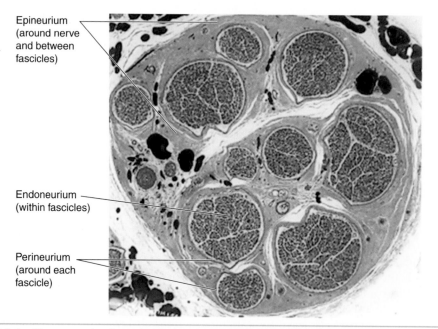

Epineurium
(around nerve
and between
fascicles)

Endoneurium
(within fascicles)

Perineurium
(around each
fascicle)

FIGURE 3-6 The connective tissue sheaths in a transversely sectioned nerve. This is a biopsy of human sural nerve. Fat cells are black (from treatment with osmium tetroxide), and other structures are blue, from staining of the thin resin-embedded section with alkaline toluidine blue. (Courtesy of Dr. William McDonald.)

the **axolemma**. The neurolemma and the **myelin sheath** are components of Schwann cells. The ultrastructure of myelin and its mode of formation from the Schwann cell membrane are described and illustrated in Chapter 2. The neurolemma consists of the cytoplasm of the Schwann cell, outside the myelin sheath. Most of the cytoplasm is in the region of the ellipsoidal nucleus, but traces of cytoplasm and the plasma membrane closely surround the myelin sheath.

The myelin sheath is interrupted at intervals by **nodes of Ranvier**. The distance between nodes varies from 100 μm to about 1 mm, depending on the length and thickness of the fiber, and there is one Schwann cell for each internode. Funnel-shaped clefts in myelin sheaths, the **incisures of Schmidt-Lanterman**, can be seen by light microscopy in longitudinal sections of nerves. In electron micrographs, these incisures are shown to be zones in which there are spaces between the layers, with occasional retention of Schwann cell cytoplasm between the membranes. This may aid the passage of materials through the myelin sheath to the axon.

The myelin sheath electrically insulates the internodal parts of the axon. At each node,

however, the cytoplasmic portions of the adjoining Schwann cells have irregular edges, and there is a narrow space between the two cells through which the axolemma at the node is in contact with extracellular fluid (see Fig. 2-7E). Voltage-gated sodium channels are present in the axolemma only at nodes. This arrangement allows action potentials to skip electrically (instantaneously) from node to node. This rapid transmission of action potentials along a myelinated fiber is called **saltatory conduction** (from the Latin *saltare*, to jump). The most rapidly conducting myelinated fibers in a nerve are those with the largest diameters and the longest internodes.

UNMYELINATED FIBERS

Nerves contain many axons that do not have myelin sheaths. A single Schwann cell envelops several (up to 15) such axons, as shown in Figure 2-7F. The cell and its included axons constitute a **Remak fiber**. Each axon is surrounded by a single layer of the glial cell's plasma membrane. It is, therefore, unmyelinated, and there are no nodes of Ranvier. The nerve impulse is a self-propagating action potential along the axolemma, without the accelerating factor of node-

Peripheral Nerve Diseases and Injuries

Peripheral neuropathy is a common cause of sensory loss and motor weakness. Loss of myelin is a typical feature of affected nerves. Distal parts of nerves are affected first, with symptoms in the hands and feet. There are many causes of peripheral neuropathy, including autoimmunity, nutritional deficiencies, toxic substances of various kinds (including ethanol), and metabolic disorders (notably, diabetes mellitus).

Nerve injuries may or may not cause transection of axons, with resulting loss of function. There may be failure of conduction in axons that have been injured but not transected. Patients with this condition, known as neurapraxia, usually recover quite quickly, but sometimes neurapraxia is permanent for unknown reasons. As explained in Chapter 2, severed axons regenerate vigorously in the peripheral nervous system, but many are misdirected to inappropriate places. Damage to a nerve by a penetrating wound may be followed by an incapacitating disorder known as causalgia. Severe pain is present in the affected limb, together with changes in skin texture. The symptoms of causalgia may be attributable, at least in part, to the formation in the injured nerve of abnormal excitatory contacts between sympathetic and sensory axons. The pain can often be relieved by surgical removal of the sympathetic ganglia that supply the affected skin.

If the proximal stump of a transected nerve is not connected to a distal stump, the axons go on regenerating and, with associated glial cells, form a neuroma in which there are many abnormal contacts between the surfaces of axons and other cells. The neuroma may account for painful sensations that are perceived as coming from an amputated limb, known as phantom limb pain. Phantom limb sensations also include feelings of size, position, and movement. They are experienced not only by amputees but also by about one third of people born without one of their limbs. Genetically determined circuitry in the CNS may, therefore, provide for conscious awareness of a map of the parts of the body that normally exist.

A nerve may be pressed on where it passes over a bony prominence or through a restricted aperture; for example, the ulnar nerve is subject to pressure at the elbow, and the median nerve can be squeezed in the carpal tunnel at the wrist. The resulting entrapment syndrome includes motor and sensory disturbances in the area of distribution of the nerve. The major plexuses, especially the brachial plexus, may be compressed (as in crutch palsy). Nerve roots are more fragile than nerves because they lack an epineurium. They may be irritated or compressed by inflamed meninges, by abnormally protruding parts of intervertebral disks (spondylosis), or by bony irregularities (spinal osteoarthritis). Clinical manifestations of nerve root lesions include weakness and wasting of muscles as well as pain in the affected cutaneous areas. The distribution of axons from segmental sensory nerve roots to the skin is discussed in association with the spinal cord in Chapter 5.

to-node or saltatory conduction. This accounts for the slow rate of conduction that is characteristic of unmyelinated (group C) axons.

The thinnest unmyelinated axons are those of the olfactory nerves. Here, each mesaxon envelops a bundle consisting of many unmyelinated axons. A somewhat similar arrangement exists in the enteric nervous system, which consists of ganglia and nerves in the wall of the alimentary canal and its associated organs. Olfactory ensheathing cells and enteric glial cells differ from the Schwann cells of ordinary nerves, and they contain some chemical components that are otherwise characteristic of astrocytes of the CNS (see Chapter 2).

Suggested Reading

Arroyo EJ, Scherer SS. On the molecular architecture of myelinated fibers. *Histochem Cell Biol* 2000;113:1–18.

Bunge MB, Wood PM, Tynan LB, et al. Perineurium originates from fibroblasts: demonstration in vitro with a retroviral marker. *Science* 1989;243:229–231.

Ferrell WR, Gandevia SC, McCloskey DI. The role of joint receptors in human kinesthesia when intramuscular receptors cannot contribute. *J Physiol (Lond)* 1987;386:63–71.

Fu SY, Gordon T. The cellular and molecular basis of peripheral nerve regeneration. *Mol Neurobiol* 1997;14:67–116.

Halata Z, Grim M, Christ B. Origin of spinal cord meninges, sheaths of peripheral nerves, and cutaneous receptors including Merkel cells: an experimental study with avian chimeras. *Anat Embryol* 1990;182:529–537.

Houk JC. Reflex control of muscle. In: Adelman A, ed. *Encyclopedia of Neuroscience*, vol 2. Boston: Birkhauser, 1987:1030–1031.

Iggo A, Andres KH. Morphology of cutaneous receptors. *Annu Rev Neurosci* 1982;5:1–31.

Janig W. Causalgia and reflex sympathetic dystrophy: in which way is the sympathetic nervous system involved? *Trends Neurosci* 1985;8:471–477.

Luff SE. Ultrastructure of sympathetic axons and their structural relationship with vascular smooth muscle. *Anat Embryol* 1996;193:515–531.

Matthews PBC. Where does Sherrington's muscular sense originate? *Annu Rev Neurosci* 1982;5:189–218.

Melzack R, Israel R, Lacroix R, et al. Phantom limbs in people with congenital limb deficiency or amputation in early childhood. *Brain* 1997;120:1603–1620.

Risling M, Dalsgaard C-J, Cukierman A, et al. Electron microscopic and immunohistochemical evidence that unmyelinated ventral root axons make U-turns or enter the spinal pia mater. *J Comp Neurol* 1984;225:53–63.

Schott GD. Mechanisms of causalgia and related clinical conditions: the role of the central and of the sympathetic nervous systems. *Brain* 1986;109:717–738.

Stolinski C. Structure and composition of the outer connective tissue sheaths of peripheral nerve. *J Anat* 1995;186:123–130.

Sunderland S. *Nerves and Nerve Injuries*, 2nd ed. Edinburgh: Churchill-Livingstone, 1978.

Swash M, Fox KP. Muscle spindle innervation in man. *J Anat* 1972;112:61–80.

Terenghi G. Peripheral nerve regeneration and neurotrophic factors. *J Anat* 1999;194:1–14.

Valeriani M, Restuccia D, Dilazzaro V, et al. Central nervous system modifications in patients with lesion of the anterior cruciate ligament of the knee. *Brain* 1996;119:1751–1762.

Winkelmann RK. Cutaneous sensory nerves. *Semin Dermatol* 1988;17:236–268.

Chapter 4

IMAGING TECHNIQUES AND NEUROANATOMICAL RESEARCH METHODS

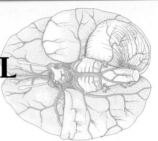

Important Facts

- Diagnostic images of the living brain can be made with radiographs. Computed tomography (CT) has largely supplanted pneumoencephalography and ventriculography. Angiography provides information about the condition and positions of blood vessels, especially arteries.

- Nuclear magnetic resonance imaging (MRI) provides images that are derived from the distribution and concentration of hydrogen atoms. Bone is invisible, and the anatomical resolution is superior to that attainable with x-ray tomography. Positron emission tomography (PET) and regional cerebral blood flow studies can localize metabolically active regions of the brain. PET images are anatomically less precise than those obtained by CT or MRI. Functional MRI is another technique for showing metabolically active areas.

- Exact information about connections between groups of neurons can be obtained only from experimental studies in animals.

- The distribution of fragments of degenerating axons can provide evidence for the former existence of neuronal connections in the injured or diseased brain or spinal cord.

- Investigations of neuronal activities, such as axonal transport and glucose or oxygen metabolism, are now widely used in the study of connectivity and function in the central nervous system. Tracer substances may be transported anterogradely or retrogradely along axons, and their distributions can be correlated with information obtained about neurotransmitters and their actions on postsynaptic cells. Certain viruses spread within neurons and across synapses, and these are used to identify chains of functionally connected neurons.

During the past 2 centuries, clinical investigators have been correlating disordered function with abnormalities found in different parts of the brain. Normal functions are deduced from the effects of destructive lesions. Experimentation with animals provides more precise information about the ways that populations of neurons are interconnected. If the same connections are seen in a variety of mammalian species, it is reasonable to suspect that the human nervous system is similarly organized.

Imaging the Nervous System

Since the 1970s, methods have been available to make images of the living human brain that are almost as accurate as the observations of a pathologist. Therefore, it is possible to record symptoms and physical signs and identify the affected parts at the same time. Images can also be made that show regions of the brain with increased metabolic activity associated with sensory, motor, or mental tasks.

The techniques used for obtaining structural and functional information about the living human brain are summarized in Table 4-1. Notes follow on the methods that provide the most anatomical and functional information.

RADIOGRAPHY

A plain radiograph of the head or spinal column provides hardly any information about the normal anatomy of the brain or spinal cord. In adults, displacement of the calcified pineal gland (see Chapter 11) can reveal displacement of midline structures. With contrast media, the images are more informative. In **angiography**, a radiopaque liquid injected into one of the carotid or vertebral arteries shows the branches of these vessels and, 1 or more seconds later,

49

TABLE 4-1 **Neuroimaging Methods**

Technique	Comments
Methods using radiographs	
Simple radiography of the skull and vertebral column	Nervous tissue is invisible. Injury or disease can be inferred from bony abnormalities. The calcified pineal gland of adults is visible, and its displacement from the midline can indicate a unilateral intracranial mass lesion.
Angiography	Detailed two-dimensional projections of blood vessels, including small branches of arteries. Abnormality of the brain can be deduced from displaced vessels.
Pneumoencephalography and ventriculography (air or radiopaque contrast medium makes the subarachnoid space and ventricles visible in radiographic images)	CT has replaced these procedures. Pneumoence-phaography is painful; ventriculography is unduly invasive.
Myelography (radiopaque contrast medium introduced into spinal subarachnoid space)	This investigation is still used to outline the spinal cord and nerve roots, especially where MRI is not available.
Computed tomography (CT)	Provides profiles of sectional images with 2-mm resolution, with enough contrast to recognize brain tissue, CSF, blood, and bone.
Methods using ultrasound	These techniques are used mainly to detect abnormal flow in arteries, especially the internal carotid artery.
Methods using nuclear magnetic resonance	
Magnetic resonance imaging (MRI)	Provides sectional images 3 to 5 mm thick with 0.5- to 1.0-mm resolution and considerable anatomical detail. Different imaging modes can emphasize gray and white matter, CSF, or major blood vessels (MRI angiography). Expensive; takes 30 min for images of the head, and images are spoiled by movement. MRI angiograms show less detail than radiographic angiograms.
MRI with contrast medium	An intravenously injected gadolinium compound provides enhancement of abnormal regions (such as tumors) that have permeable blood vessels.
Functional nuclear magnetic resonance imaging (fMRI)	Blood oxygenation level–dependent (BOLD) signals, based on local concentrations of oxygen, indicate parts of the brain that become more metabolically active during the completion of a physical or mental task.
Methods using radioactive isotopes	
Scans for vascular permeability	A compound that escapes from the abnormally permeable blood vessels of tumors is labeled with a gamma-emitting isotope. By scanning for gamma rays, the approximate position of the tumor can be determined.
Scans for regional blood flow	A compound that remains in the blood is labeled with a gamma-emitting isotope. Scanning the surface of the head reveals increased blood flow in active areas of the cerebral cortex, with a resolution of 5 to 10 mm.
Single photon emission computed tomography (SPECT)	Makes sectional images of the distribution of a gamma-emitting isotope, which is used to label a compound that concentrates in active regions or at sites of increased vascular permeability. Resolution is inferior to that obtained with PET, but less expensive equipment is needed.
Positron emission tomography (PET)	Sectional images indicate sites of concentration of short-lived positron-emitting isotopes, showing sites of concentration with a resolution of 5 to 10 mm. A cyclotron and a laboratory for rapid chemical syntheses must be adjacent to the imaging equipment. PET can be carried out only in major centers of research.

the veins. Some normal angiograms are shown in Chapter 25. The chief value of this technique is for detecting arterial disease (occlusion, stenosis, aneurysm) or displacements of blood vessels by lesions such as tumors. Computed tomography (CT) has replaced the older techniques of **pneumoencephalography** and **ventriculography** (see Table 4-1).

Computed Tomography

This application of radiographic imaging is based on scanning the head with a narrow, moving beam of radiographs and measuring the attenuation of the emerging beam. The density readings from thin "sections" (tomograms) of the head are processed by a computer to generate an image whose brightness depends on the absorption values of the tissues. The technique is valuable in clinical diagnosis because the density of many cerebral lesions is greater or less than the density of normal brain tissue.

To avoid irradiation of the eyes, the "axial" plane of the sections imaged by CT is oblique, being somewhat closer to horizontal than to coronal. Special neuroanatomical atlases are available in which CT scans are compared with photographs of slices of the brain cut in the same plane.

Nuclear Magnetic Resonance Imaging

This imaging technique was developed from nuclear magnetic resonance (NMR), a physical method used in chemical analysis. In a strong magnetic field, the nuclei of atoms absorb radiofrequency energy. The absorbed frequency is characteristic of the element and of the immediate molecular environment of its atoms. In diagnostic magnetic resonance imaging (MRI), a frequency is chosen that is absorbed mainly by the nuclei of the hydrogen atoms of water. The patient's head is put into a magnetic field and irradiated with the radiofrequency radiation for protons. The measured energy absorptions are integrated in a computer, which generates a series of images of sections through the head. The sections may be reconstructed in any plane. Horizontal sections (parallel to the plane passing through the anterior and posterior commissures), as well as sagittal and coronal sections, are commonly presented. The reconstructed slices are typically 4 or 5 mm thick.

Images are commonly prepared in three ways, taking advantage of different components of the NMR signal. A **T1-weighted image** emphasizes the difference between central nervous tissue (brighter) and other fluids and tissues (dark) and gives some discrimination between gray matter (brighter) and white matter (less bright). A **T2-weighted image** emphasizes the cerebrospinal fluid (CSF; bright) in the subarachnoid space and ventricles, providing crisp anatomical resolution but with poor contrast between gray and white matter. A **proton density image** emphasizes the difference between gray matter (bright) and white matter (darker). Examples of images of the brain are shown in Figures 4-1 to 4-3. Later chapters, especially Chapter 16, explain the anatomy displayed in these images. NMR data can also be processed to show the larger blood vessels (**MRI angiography**), but the images show less detail than conventional radiographic angiograms.

The advantages of MRI are that no potentially harmful radiation is used, and the anatomical resolution is greatly superior to that obtainable with radiographs. Bone and flowing blood are invisible in MRI images. Gray and white matter and CSF have different densities, and it is sometimes possible to identify regions of white matter that contain degenerating axons. A special contrast medium (a gadolinium compound) can be introduced into the circulation to reveal regions of the brain with abnormally permeable blood vessels, which often occur at sites of disease. The chief disadvantage is that MRI is a slow process, requiring about 1 hour in contrast to a few minutes for a CT scan.

Functional Nuclear Magnetic Resonance Imaging

Increased blood flow and oxygen usage accompany neuronal activity. In the course of NMR imaging, blood oxygen level–dependent (BOLD) signals can be collected that relate to oxygen concentration in the tissue being examined. Locally, high levels of metabolic activity can be translated into signals of high intensity in an image, thus rendering prominent any parts of the brain that are more active than the surrounding regions. Fine anatomical resolution and an indicator of function are obtained without the use of radiographs or radioactive isotopes. This technique is being

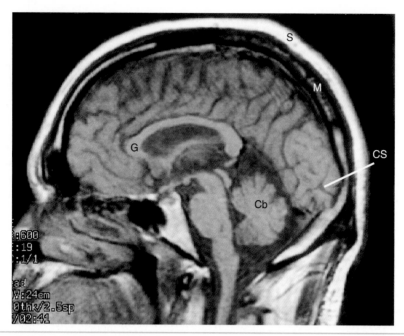

FIGURE 4-1   Sagittal T1-weighted nuclear magnetic resonance image of the normal brain. Note that compact bone and flowing blood are not visible. Many other neuroanatomical features can be seen, including the paracentral lobule, the fornix, a mamillary body, the cerebral aqueduct, the pons, and the medulla. Compare this image with Figure 1-3. CS, calcarine sulcus; Cb, cerebellum; G, genu of corpus callosum; M, marrow in parietal bone; S, scalp. (Courtesy of Dr. D. M. Pelz.)

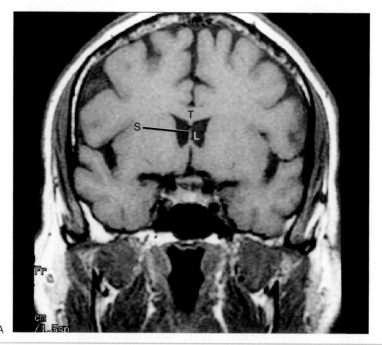

FIGURE 4-2   Three coronal magnetic resonance images of a plane that contains the insula, lentiform nucleus, internal capsule, and head of caudate nucleus. **(A)** T1-weighted image: T, trunk of corpus callosum; L, lateral ventricle; S, septum pellucidum. *(continued)*

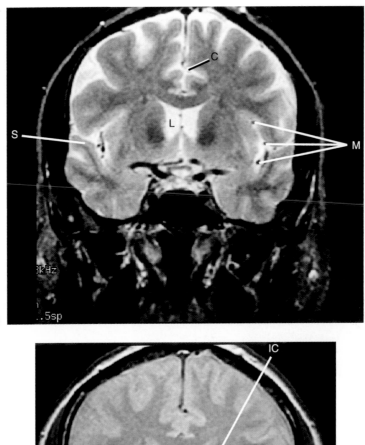

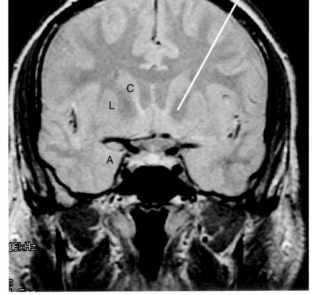

FIGURE 4-2   *(continued)* Three coronal magnetic resonance images of a plane that contains the insula, lentiform nucleus, internal capsule, and head of caudate nucleus. **(B)** T2-weighted image: C, cingulate sulcus with callosomarginal artery; L, lateral ventricle. M, middle cerebral vessels in subarachnoid space; S, superior temporal gyrus. **(C)** Proton density image: A, amygdaloid body; C, head of caudate nucleus; IC, internal capsule; L, lentiform nucleus. (Courtesy of Dr. D. M. Pelz.)

used extensively for studies of cerebral metabolism in normal mental and physical activities, and it may become important in the diagnosis of diseases.

Two types of BOLD signals can be exploited. In T_2* BOLD functional MRI (fMRI), the most frequently used type, the signal is due to deoxygenated hemoglobin, and "activation" is com-

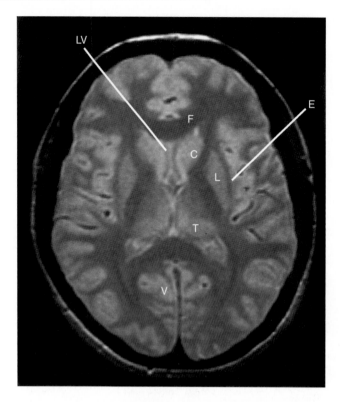

FIGURE 4-3 A proton density nuclear magnetic resonance image in a horizontal plane through the level of the insula. C, head of caudate nucleus; E, external capsule; F, forceps frontalis; L, lentiform nucleus; LV, lateral ventricle; T, thalamus; V, primary visual cortex. (Courtesy of Dr. D. M. Pelz.)

monly imaged in large veins as well as in nervous tissue. More accurate localization is achieved with Hahn spin-echo (HSE) BOLD fMRI, which detects movements of water into and out of red blood cells, with much stronger signals arising from capillaries than from larger vessels. The spatial resolution of HSE BOLD fMRI is about 0.1 mm, but this technique is available only in certain research institutes because it requires a stronger magnetic field (7 to 9 Tesla) than that ordinarily used (1.5 Tesla) for MRI.

FUNCTIONAL MAPPING WITH RADIOACTIVE TRACERS

Structure can be related to function by mapping the distribution of a metabolically significant substance that has been labeled with a radioactive isotope.

Regional Cerebral Blood Flow

Although the flow of blood through the whole brain does not change much, transient but conspicuous local increases in flow are associated with the activity of neurons. To monitor regional cerebral blood flow, a radioactive tracer such as ^{133}Xe is introduced into the blood, and

the intensities of the emitted gamma rays are measured by an array of detectors at the surface of the patient's head. The intensity of the radiation at any point varies with the vascular perfusion of the underlying tissues. The method is used for examining different parts of the cerebral cortex. A computer integrates the measurements of radioactivity and provides anatomical images of the functioning areas. Clinicians use this method to identify cortical regions in which the circulation is inadequate, and research with normal volunteers provides evidence of functional localization in the cerebral cortex.

Regional cerebral blood flow can also be studied by single-photon emission computed tomography (SPECT) using ^{133}Xe or ^{99}Tc as the tracer and by positron emission tomography (PET) using [^{15}O]carbon dioxide. SPECT and PET provide sets of reconstructed sections, thereby providing information about both the cerebral cortex and the interior of the brain.

Single-Photon Emission Computed Tomography

Each disintegrating atom of an ordinary gamma-emitting isotope emits one photon. The SPECT technique makes sectional maps based on the uptake into tissue and subsequent dispersal of radiolabeled compounds that have been introduced into the blood. Regional blood flow is represented as variations of intensity in the resulting images. The images have low resolution (2–3 cm), but they are obtained in only a fraction of the time needed for a PET scan and at much lower cost.

Positron Emission Tomography

Positrons are emitted by certain radioactive isotopes, of which ^{15}O, ^{13}N, ^{11}C, and ^{18}F are the most useful. A positron is immediately annihilated when it encounters an electron and two gamma-ray photons are emitted. Detection of these pairs of photons enables the computation of sites of concentration of the isotope, which is incorporated into a metabolically significant compound. For example, $[^{15}O]$water can indicate blood flow, and $[^{18}F]$fluorodeoxyglucose is taken up by cells as if it were real glucose. The images of slices of the brain built by PET scanning are based on such functions as blood flow, uptake of a glucose analog, metabolism of a neurotransmitter precursor, or the binding of a labeled drug to receptors on the surfaces of cells. The anatomical resolution of PET (5–10 mm) is superior to that of a cortical blood flow or a SPECT scan, but it is inferior to that attainable with CT (2 mm) or MRI (0.5–1.0 mm).

Positron-emitting isotopes have half-lives ranging from 2 minutes for ^{15}O to 2 hours for ^{18}F, during which time they must be made, incorporated into suitable compounds, and administered to the patient. This technique can, therefore, be used only in hospitals equipped with a cyclotron and a laboratory for rapid radiochemical syntheses. The images obtained by PET, some of which display the distributions of neurons that use or respond to particular synaptic transmitters, can be more informative to physicians than the purely anatomical images obtained with CT or MRI.

Methods for Investigating Neural Pathways and Functions

Clinicopathological correlations and functional imaging techniques show which parts of the brain and spinal cord are used for particular purposes, but they do not provide much information about the ways in which neurons, with their long axons, communicate between different parts of the nervous system.

In histological material from normal animals, it is seldom possible to follow an individual axon from its cell body of origin to the distant site in which it terminates. The small diameters and curved trajectories of axons, together with the fact that different pathways commonly occupy the same territory, make the direct tracing of most connections impossible. It is, therefore, necessary to use experimental methods to determine the connectivity of the many groups of neurons in the brain and spinal cord. Results obtained in laboratory animals, especially cats and monkeys, may be applicable to human brains. This transfer of data from animals to humans is usually justifiable when there are no major differences between the connections found in diverse groups of animals. Some injuries and diseases in the human nervous system can cause degeneration of particular tracts of axons. Postmortem examination of the degenerated fibers provides valuable information about human neural connections.

NEUROANATOMICAL METHODS BASED ON DEGENERATION

Until the introduction of methods based on axoplasmic transport, fiber tracts were traced by staining fibers undergoing Wallerian degeneration (see Chapter 2) after the placement of a destructive lesion at a selected site in the central nervous system (CNS) of an animal. The oldest staining method for anterograde degeneration is the **Marchi technique**, which selectively stains degenerating myelin with osmium tetroxide in the presence of an oxidizing agent. The course of a tract can be followed in sections taken at appropriate intervals (Fig. 4-4). The archi technique does not show the unmyelinated terminal branches of the degenerating axons, but it is the only method that can nevertheless give useful results when applied to human postmortem material. **Silver methods**, which can show degenerating unmyelinated axons and synaptic terminals, were much used for laboratory animals until about 1975. These methods are not suited to the human nervous system because the degenerating axons are de-

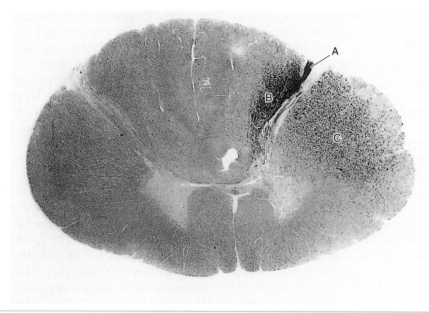

FIGURE 4-4   Section of the third cervical segment of a human spinal cord. The patient died 9 days after an injury that damaged the dorsal roots of the second, third, and fourth cervical nerves on the right side, together with the dorsal part of the right lateral funiculus in segment C2. The tissue was processed by the Marchi method, and degenerating myelin can be seen in entering fibers of the third right cervical dorsal root **(A)**, branches of fibers derived from dorsal roots C3 and C4 in the lateral part of the dorsal funiculus **(B)**, and descending corticospinal fibers in the lateral funiculus **(C)**.

monstrable only during a critical period of 4 to 8 days after placement of a lesion. Degenerating axonal terminals can also be recognized in **electron micrographs**.

NEUROANATOMICAL METHODS BASED ON AXOPLASMIC TRANSPORT

Research methods based on degenerating axons were replaced in the 1970s by much more sensitive techniques that reveal both the cells of origin and the sites of termination of axons. In these procedures, a tracer substance is injected into a region of gray matter. The tracer is taken up by axonal terminals or neuronal cell bodies (or both) and transported within the cytoplasm. **Retrograde tracers** accumulate in the cell bodies of neurons whose axons end in the injected region. **Anterograde tracers** enter cell bodies and are moved into the presynaptic terminals at the destinations of the axons. A tracer may be a radioactively labeled amino acid, a fluorescent dye, a histochemically demonstrable enzyme (notably horseradish peroxidase [HRP]), or a protein that has been chemically linked to a fluorescent dye or HRP.

MEMBRANE PROBES

Some hydrophobic fluorescent compounds, most notably a cyanine dye called **DiI**, enter the lipid domains of cell membranes, including the neuronal axolemma, and then diffuse in the plane of the membrane. This happens even in dead tissue, allowing the tracing of fiber tracts from a site of application of the dye. Diffusion within the axolemma is slow: several months are needed to trace axons over distances of less than a centimeter. This method has been applied to human postmortem material but has not yet yielded new neuroanatomical knowledge.

TRANSSYNAPTIC TRACING OF PATHWAYS

Certain viruses are used for experimental neuronal tracing because they replicate within neurons, are transported within the axon, and are passed from one cell to another at synapses. These viruses can be modified to make the cells that harbor them synthesize a histochemically detectable enzyme, or the viral protein may be stained immunohistochemically. Transsynaptic transfer of viruses occurs naturally in some diseases, notably rabies.

Metabolic Marking Methods

The sugar **2-deoxy-D-glucose**, an analog of ordinary D-glucose, enters cells but is not metabolized. Consequently, radioactively labeled 2-deoxyglucose accumulates in the cytoplasm of metabolically active cells and may be detected there by autoradiography. The deoxyglucose method can reveal structures in the brain that are active when a particular system of pathways is in use. Thus, it may be possible to determine which of a multitude of connections demonstrated by neuroanatomical tracing methods are the most important in relation to function.

The catalytic functions of certain enzymes used in the metabolic activities of all cells can be demonstrated histochemically. **Cytochrome oxidase** is a notable example, and in regions that contain active neurons, the activity of this enzyme is higher than in adjacent quiescent areas. Cytochrome oxidase histochemistry has been used with great success in the demonstration of columns of cells that respond to different visual stimuli in the cortex of the occipital lobe of the brain (see Chapter 14).

Physiological and Pharmacological Methods

Neuroanatomical studies are often supplemented by electrically stimulating neurons and recording the potentials evoked elsewhere. Timing of the response may help to determine the number of neurons, or synaptic delays, that are included in a pathway. Neuroanatomical tracing and electrophysiological experiments are frequently combined with immunohistochemistry to identify neurotransmitters and to ascertain their actions on postsynaptic neurons. Electrophysiological investigations of the human CNS are necessarily more limited in scope than experiments using animals. Nevertheless, a great deal has been learned from observation of the effects of stimulating the cerebral cortex. Such studies are reviewed in Chapter 15.

Several **toxic substances** are used in laboratory animals as adjuncts to the study of neuroanatomy. For example, **nicotine** was used a century ago by Langley to block synapses and thus establish their locations in autonomic ganglia. Local injection of **kainic acid** or **ibotenic acid** kills many types of neurons without causing transection of passing fibers. These substances are known as **excitotoxins** because they are analogs of the excitatory transmitter glutamic acid. When an excitotoxin binds to glutamate receptors, there is an unusually long activation of nonspecific ligand-gated cation channels of the postsynaptic cells. Calcium ions diffuse into the neurons and activate proteolytic enzymes that destroy the cytoplasm. The resulting lesion is more selective than one produced by physical methods. Cells that use monoamines as synaptic transmitters are selectively intoxicated by analogs of these substances or their metabolic precursors. Thus, neurons that make use of dopamine or noradrenaline are selectively poisoned by **6-hydroxydopamine**, and serotonin cells are similarly sensitive to **5,6-dihydroxytryptamine**.

Some toxic lectins (e.g., **ricin-60** from the castor bean) and other compounds (notably the antibiotic **doxorubicin**) are taken up by axonal endings and by injured axons of passage and transported retrogradely to the neuronal cell bodies, where they inhibit nucleic acid and protein synthesis. This strategy, known as **suicide transport**, produces selective lesions that can provide experimental models of diseases in which certain populations of neurons degenerate spontaneously.

Suggested Reading

DeYoe EA, Bandettini P, Neitz J, et al. Functional magnetic resonance imaging (FMRI) of the human brain. *J Neurosci Methods* 1994;54:171–187.

Frackowiak RSJ, ed. *Human Brain Function*, 2nd ed. Amsterdam: Elsevier, 2004.

Heimer L. Neuroanatomic Techniques. In Heimer L, ed. *The Human Brain and Spinal Cord*, 2nd ed. New York: Springer-Verlag, 1995:172–184.

Krassioukov AV, Bygrave MA, Puckett WR, et al. Human sympathetic preganglionic neurons and motoneurons retrogradely labelled with DiI. *J Autonom Nerv Syst* 1998; 70:123–128.

Lukas JR, Aigner M, Denk M, et al. Carbocyanine postmortem neuronal tracing: influence of different parameters on tracing distance and combination with immunocytochemistry. *J Histochem Cytochem* 1998;46: 901–910.

McLean JH, Shipley MT, Bernstein DI. Golgi-like trans-neuronal retrograde labelling with CNS injections of Herpes simplex virus type 1. *Brain Res Bull* 1989;22:867–881.

Purves D. Assessing some dynamic properties of the living nervous system. *Q J Exp Physiol* 1989;74:1089–1105.

Raichle ME. Functional brain imaging and human brain function. *J Neurosci* 2003;23:3959–3962.

Rajakumar N, Elisevich K, Flumerfelt BA. Biotinylated dextran: a versatile anterograde and retrograde neuronal tracer. *Brain Res* 1993;607:47–53.

Rao SM, Binder JR, Hammeke TA, et al. Somatotopic mapping of the human primary motor cortex with functional magnetic resonance imaging. *Neurology* 1995;45:919–924.

Ugurbil K, Toth L, Kim DS: How accurate is magnetic resonance imaging of brain function? *Trends Neurosci* 2003;26:108–114.

Vercelli A, Repici M, Garbossa D, et al. Recent techniques for tracing pathways in the central nervous system of developing and adult mammals. *Brain Res Bull* 2000;51:11–28.

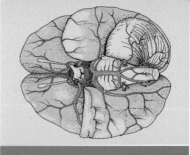

PART II

Regional Anatomy of the Central Nervous System

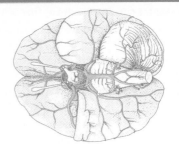

Chapter 5

SPINAL CORD

- The spinal cord is shorter than the spinal canal in which it is suspended. Except in the neck, spinal cord segments are rostral (superior) to the corresponding vertebrae; the caudal end of the cord is level with vertebra L2.

- Cerebrospinal fluid can be sampled by inserting a needle into the subarachnoid space below the level of the conus medullaris.

- The cross-sectional area of the central gray matter indicates the numbers of neurons, which are largest for segments supplying limbs.

- The cross-sectional area of the white matter decreases caudally, with fewer descending and ascending fibers.

- Motor neurons are in the ventral horn; sensory axons enter the dorsal horn and the dorsal funiculi. Preganglionic autonomic neurons are laterally placed, in segments T1–L2 and S2–S4.

- The ascending tracts include the uncrossed gracile and cuneate fasciculi (from sensory ganglia) and the crossed spinothalamic tract (from the dorsal horn). These are concerned with different types of sensation.

- The descending motor tracts include the uncrossed vestibulospinal and the crossed lateral corticospinal tract. Hypothalamospinal and some reticulospinal fibers influence autonomic functions.

- For most of the time, the stretch reflex and the flexor or withdrawal reflex are suppressed by activity in the descending pathways.

- Lesions in different parts of the spinal cord produce sensory and motor abnormalities appropriate to the functions of the tracts that have been transected. The segmental level of a lesion is indicated by the affected dermatomes and movements.

The spinal cord and dorsal root ganglia innervate most of the body. Afferent sensory fibers enter the spinal cord through the dorsal roots of spi-

nal nerves; motor and other efferent fibers leave by way of the ventral roots (the Bell-Magendie law). Signals originating in sensory endings initiate reflexes within the spinal cord and are relayed to the brain stem and cerebellum to contribute to circuits that influence motor performance and other functions. Sensory signals are also sent rostrally to the thalamus and cerebral cortex, where they enter conscious experience and may elicit immediate or delayed behavioral responses. Motor neurons in the spinal cord are excited or inhibited by impulses originating at various levels of the brain, from the medulla to the cerebral cortex. As the tracts of the spinal cord are identified, references are made to components of the brain that are discussed in later chapters. When the central nervous system (CNS) is described by regions, it is necessary to probe ahead of the region under immediate consideration. An appreciation of the major systems is acquired step by step. The general sensory and motor systems are reviewed in Chapters 19 and 23, respectively.

Gross Anatomy of the Spinal Cord and Nerve Roots

The spinal cord is a cylindrical structure, slightly flattened dorsoventrally, located in the spinal canal of the vertebral column. Protection for the cord is provided not only by the vertebrae and their ligaments but also by the meninges and a cushion of cerebrospinal fluid (CSF).

SPINAL CANAL AND MENINGES

The innermost meningeal layer is the thin **pia mater**, which adheres to the surface of the spinal cord. The outermost layer, the thick **dura** mater (or simply, **dura**) forms a tube extending from the level of the second sacral vertebra to the foramen magnum at the base of the skull, where it is continuous with the dura around the brain. The **arachnoid** lies against the inner surface of the dura, forming the outer boundary of the fluid-filled **subarachnoid space**. The spinal cord is suspended in the dural sheath by a **denticulate ligament** on each side. This ligament is made of pia–arachnoid tissue and is in the form of a ribbon attached to the cord midway between the dorsal and ventral roots (Fig. 5-1). The lateral edge of the denticulate ligament is serrated and is attached at 21 points to the dural sheath at intervals between the foramen magnum and the level at which the dura is pierced by the roots of the first lumbar spinal nerve. An **epidural space**, filled with fatty tissue that contains a venous plexus, intervenes between the dura and the wall of the spinal canal. The epidural space caudal to the second sacral vertebra also contains the roots of the most caudal spinal nerves.

SEGMENTS OF THE SPINAL CORD, ROOTS, AND VERTEBRAL COLUMN

The segmental nature of the spinal cord is demonstrated by the presence of 31 pairs of **spinal nerves**, but there is little indication of segmentation in its internal structure. Each dorsal root is broken up into a series of **rootlets** that are attached to the spinal cord along the corresponding segment (Fig. 5-2). The ventral root arises similarly as a series of rootlets.

Each spinal nerve divides into a dorsal and a ventral **primary ramus**. The dorsal primary ramus supplies the skin of the back and muscles that are attached at both ends to parts of the vertebral column. In the cervical, brachial, and lumbosacral **plexuses**, ventral primary rami join, exchange fibers, and branch into the mixed nerves that carry motor and sensory axons to the skin and muscles of the lateral and ventral trunk and the limbs. The numeric relations of spinal nerves and vertebrae are explained in Table 5-1.

EMBRYOLOGY AND GROWTH

The early development of the spinal cord from the neural tube and the caudal eminence is described in Chapter 1. Segments of the neural tube (neuromeres) correspond in position with segments of the vertebral column (scleromeres) until the third month of fetal development. The vertebral column elongates more rapidly than the spinal cord during the remainder of fetal life. By the time of birth, the caudal end of the spinal cord is opposite the disk between the second and third lumbar vertebrae. A slight difference in growth rate continues during childhood, such that the adult's cord ends opposite the disk between the first and second lumbar vertebrae (Fig. 5-3). This is an average level; the caudal end of the cord may be as high as the twelfth thoracic or as low as the third lumbar vertebral body. The subarachnoid space caudal to the end of the spinal cord is known as the **lumbar cistern**. It contains CSF and is traversed by the roots of lumbar and sacral nerves.

The rostral shift of the spinal cord during development determines the direction of spinal nerve roots in the subarachnoid space. As shown in Figure 5-3, spinal nerves from C1 through C7 leave the spinal canal through the intervertebral foramina above the corresponding

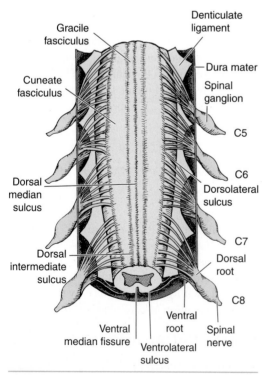

FIGURE 5-1 Dorsal view of the cervical enlargement of the spinal cord, showing the attachments of the denticulate ligament.

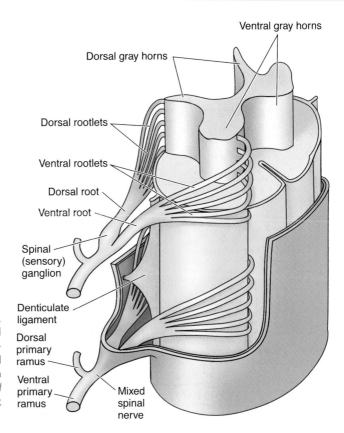

Ventral gray horns

Dorsal gray horns

Dorsal rootlets

Ventral rootlets

Dorsal root

Ventral root

Spinal
(sensory)
ganglion

Denticulate
ligament

Dorsal
primary
ramus

Ventral
primary
ramus

Mixed
spinal
nerve

FIGURE 5-2 A segment of the spinal cord, showing the dorsal and ventral rootlets and roots, sensory ganglia, and mixed spinal nerves. (Used with permission from Moore KL, Dalley AF. *Clinically Oriented Anatomy*, 5th ed. Philadelphia: Lippincott Williams & Wilkins, 2006.)

vertebrae. (The first and second cervical nerves lie on the vertebral arches of the atlas and axis, respectively.) The eighth cervical nerve passes through the foramen between the seventh cervical and first thoracic vertebrae because there are eight cervical cord segments and seven cervical vertebrae. From that point caudally, the spinal nerves leave the canal through foramina immediately below the pedicles of the corresponding vertebrae.

SPINAL AND VERTEBRAL LEVELS

The dorsal and ventral roots traverse the subarachnoid space and pierce the arachnoid and dura mater. At this point, the dura becomes

TABLE 5-1 Numbering of Spinal Nerves and Vertebrae*

Segmental Level	Number of Nerves	Level of Exit From Vertebral Column
Cervical	8	Nerve C1* (suboccipital nerve) passes *above* the arch of vertebra C1. Nerves C2–C7 go through foramina above the corresponding vertebrae.
		Nerve C8 passes through the foramen between the arches of vertebra C7 and vertebra T1.
Thoracic Lumbar	12 5	Nerves T1 to L5 also pass through foramina *below* the arches of the corresponding vertebrae.
Sacral	5	Nerves S1–S4 branch into primary rami within the sacrum, and the rami go through the dorsal and ventral sacral foramina.
Coccygeal	1	The fifth sacral and the coccygeal nerves pass through the sacral hiatus.

*The first cervical nerves lack dorsal roots in 50% of people, and the coccygeal nerves may be absent.

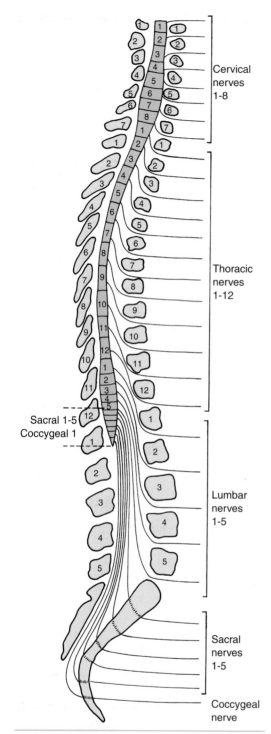

Cervical nerves 1-8

Thoracic nerves 1-12

Sacral 1-5
Coccygeal 1

Lumbar nerves 1-5

Sacral nerves 1-5

Coccygeal nerve

FIGURE 5-3   Relation of segments of the spinal cord and spinal nerves to the vertebral column. The vertebral bodies are on the right side, and the dorsal spines of the vertebrae on the left.

continuous with the epineurium. After passing through the epidural space, the roots reach the intervertebral foramina, where the dorsal root ganglia are located. The dorsal and ventral roots join immediately distal to the ganglion to form the spinal nerve. The length and obliqueness of the roots increase progressively in a rostrocaudal direction because of the increasing distance between cord segments and the corresponding vertebral segments (see Fig. 5-3). The lumbosacral roots are, therefore, the longest and constitute the **cauda equina** in the lower part of the subarachnoid space. The cord ends as the **conus medullaris**, which tapers rather abruptly into a slender filament called the filum terminale. The caudal 3 cm of the spinal cord contains most of the segments that communicate with the lower limb and perineum. Immediately below the conus medullaris are all the segmental nerve roots below L1.

The **filum terminale** lies in the middle of the cauda equina and has a distinctive bluish color that distinguishes it from the white nerve roots. It consists of pia mater surrounding neuroglial elements and is a vestige of the spinal cord of the embryonic tail. The filum terminale picks up a dural investment opposite the second segment of the sacrum, and the resulting **coccygeal ligament** attaches to the dorsum of the coccyx.

LIMB ENLARGEMENTS

The spinal cord is enlarged in two regions for innervation of the limbs. The **cervical enlargement** includes segments C4 to T1, with most of the corresponding spinal nerves forming the brachial plexuses for the nerve supply of the upper limbs. Segments L2 to S3 are included in the **lumbosacral enlargement**, and the corresponding nerves constitute most of the lumbosacral plexuses for the innervation of the lower limbs.

Internal Structure of the Spinal Cord

The surface of the spinal cord is marked by longitudinal furrows. The deep **ventral median fissure** contains connective tissue of the pia mater and the anterior spinal artery and its branches. The **dorsal median sulcus** is a shallow midline

Lumbar Disks and Spinal Nerves

All intervertebral foramina are slightly rostral to the levels of the intervertebral disks. If the nucleus of a lumbar disk herniates laterally through its fibrous outer ring, the protrusion presses on a spinal nerve that has not yet left the spinal canal. For example, herniation of the

disk between vertebrae L4 and L5 results in compression of spinal nerve L5 or S1.

It is helpful when examining a patient with a possible spinal cord or nerve root lesion to determine the location of the cord segments in relation to vertebral spines, vertebral bodies, and intervertebral disks. The corresponding levels are shown in Figure 5-3.

furrow. Many textbooks describe a dorsal septum, supposedly composed of pial tissue, that extends from the base of this sulcus almost to the gray matter. In fact, there is no collagenous connective tissue in the dorsal midline of the cord; the "dorsal septum" does not exist.

GRAY MATTER AND WHITE MATTER

In transverse sections, the gray matter has a roughly H-shaped outline (Figs. 5-4 to 5-6). The small **central canal** is lined by ependyma, and its lumen may be obliterated in places. The gray matter on each side consists of **dorsal** and **ventral horns** and an **intermediate zone**. A **lateral horn**, containing preganglionic sympathetic neurons, is added in the thoracic and upper lumbar segments.

There are three main categories of neurons in the spinal gray matter. **Motor cells** of the ventral horn supply the skeletal musculature and consist of alpha and gamma motor neurons, whose functions are described in Chapter 3. The cell bodies of **tract cells**, whose axons constitute the ascending fasciculi of the white matter, are located mainly in the dorsal horn. The cells, involved in local circuitry, are called **interneurons**, even though many of them have quite long axons (see under *Fasciculus Proprius*, later).

The white matter consists of three **funiculi** (see Figs. 5-4 to 5-6). (These are often called "columns," but this word is more appropriate for longitudinally aligned arrays of neuronal cell bodies in the gray matter.) The **dorsal funiculus** (posterior column) is bounded by the midline and the dorsal gray horn. It consists of a **gracile fasciculus**, present throughout the length of the cord, and above the midthoracic level is also a laterally placed **cuneate fasciculus**. The remainder of the white matter consists of **lateral** and **ventral funiculi**, between which there is no anatomical demarcation. Axons decussate in the **ventral white commissure**. The **dorsolateral tract** (tract of Lissauer) occupies the interval between the apex of the dorsal horn and the surface of the cord. The white matter consists of partially overlapping bundles (tracts or fasciculi) of fibers, as described later.

Although the general pattern of gray matter and white matter is the same throughout the spinal cord, regional differences are apparent in transverse sections (see Figs. 5-4 to 5-6). For example, the amount of white matter increases in a caudal-to-rostral direction because fibers are added to ascending tracts, and fibers leave descending tracts to terminate in the gray matter. The main variation in the gray matter is its increased volume in the cervical and lumbosa-

Lumbar Puncture

It may be necessary to insert a needle into the subarachnoid space to obtain a sample of CSF for analysis or for other reasons. A spinal lumbar puncture is the preferred method: the needle is inserted between the dorsal spines

of the third and fourth lumbar vertebrae to enter the lumbar cistern without risk of damaging the spinal cord. In the midline of the lumbar cistern, the needle does not touch the lumbosacral nerve roots.

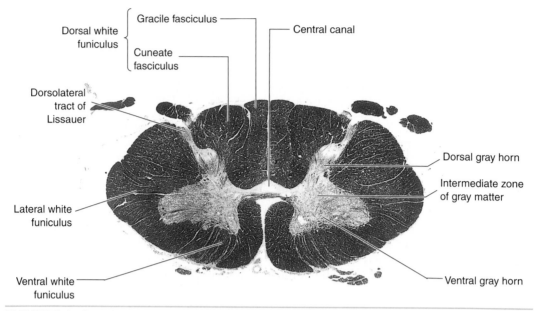

FIGURE 5-4   Seventh cervical segment. (Transverse section stained by Weigert's method for myelin, ×6.)

cral enlargements for innervation of the upper and lower limbs. The lateral horn of gray matter is characteristic of the thoracic and upper lumbar segments. Caudal to S2, the ventral median fissure is shallow, so the left and right ventral horns blend together in a wide band of gray matter ventral to the central canal.

NEURONAL ARCHITECTURE OF SPINAL GRAY MATTER

As with other parts of the CNS, the spinal gray matter is composed of several neuronal populations. The cell types are classified according to their appearances under the microscope, and

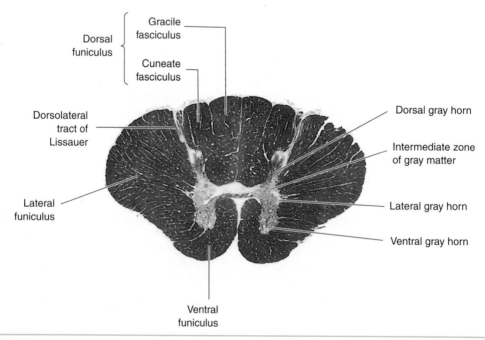

FIGURE 5-5   Second thoracic segment. (Weigert's stain, ×7.)

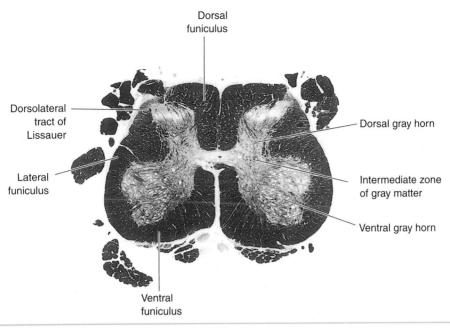

Dorsal
funiculus

Dorsolateral
tract of
Lissauer

Dorsal gray horn

Lateral
funiculus

Intermediate zone
of gray matter

Ventral gray horn

Ventral
funiculus

FIGURE 5-6   First sacral segment. (Weigert's stain, ×7.)

it has been found that cells of the same type are usually clustered together into groups. Because the architecture of the spinal gray matter is essentially the same along the length of the cord, the populations of similar neurons occur in long columns. When viewed in transverse sections of the spinal cord, many of the cell columns appear as layers, especially within the dorsal horn. Ten layers of neurons are recognized, known as the **laminae of Rexed**. Before the laminae were described in 1952, names were given to many of the cell columns, but they were used differently by different authors, and confusing synonyms existed. The laminar scheme is summarized in Figure 5-7. Descriptions of the laminae can be found in the extended chapter available online.

The spinal gray matter is organized in the following way. Sensory axons of dorsal roots end predominantly in the dorsal horn. Impulses concerned with pain, temperature, and touch reach the tract cells, most with cell bodies in the deeper laminae of the dorsal horn, from which the spinothalamic tract originates. The sensory information transmitted to the brain, especially for pain, is subject to modification (editing) by interaction with other modalities of sensation and by impulses that reach the dorsal horn by way of various descending pathways. Lamina II, the **substantia gelatinosa**, contains interneurons that have a prominent role in modifying the perception of pain (see Chapter 19). Motor neurons (lamina IX) supply the skeletal musculature. With the intervention of interneurons, the motor neurons usually come under the influence of dorsal root afferents for spinal reflexes and of several descending tracts for the control of motor activity by the brain. Of the columns of motor neurons that constitute lamina IX, those supplying axial musculature are present in the medial part of the ventral horn, and those supplying the limbs are located more laterally. Distinctive columns of motor neurons include the **phrenic** and **accessory nuclei** in the cervical segments (motor neurons for the phrenic and accessory nerves) and the **nucleus of Onuf** (innervation of pelvic floor muscles) in the sacral cord. Distinctive cell columns in the thoracic and upper lumbar segments (formally included with lamina VII) are the **nucleus dorsalis**, which gives rise to the dorsal spinocerebellar tract, and the **intermediolateral cell column**, which consists of preganglionic sympathetic neurons. The midsacral segments contain a less conspicuous intermediolateral column, the **sacral autonomic nucleus**. Scattered **spinal border cells**, at the

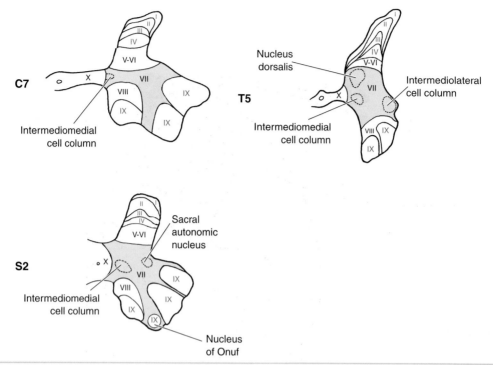

FIGURE 5-7 Positions of cytoarchitectonic laminae in the spinal gray matter at three levels of the human spinal cord. Roman numerals in blue are for laminae that receive input from dorsal roots; red is for the lamina that contains motor neurons. Lamina VII, which contains named cell columns, is colored yellow.

gray–white interface of the ventral horn in the lumbar segments, contribute to the ventral spinocerebellar tracts.

DORSAL HORN

Each dorsal root branches into six to eight rootlets as it approaches the spinal cord, and the axons become segregated into two divisions within each rootlet (Fig. 5-8). The lateral division contains most of the unmyelinated (group C) axons and some thin myelinated (group A) axons. These axons enter the **dorsolateral tract** (of Lissauer), where they divide into ascending and descending branches, each giving off collaterals that enter the dorsal horn. Most of these fibers terminate in their own or in immediately adjacent segments, synapsing with interneurons and with **tract cells** that give rise to spinothalamic fibers. Most of the tract cells are in the **nucleus proprius** in the deeper laminae of the dorsal horn.

The medial division of dorsal root fibers, for modalities of sensation other than pain and temperature, consists largely of myelinated axons, including all the large-caliber, rapidly conducting sensory fibers. These enter the spinal white matter medial to the dorsal horn where, similar to those of the lateral division, they divide into ascending and descending branches. The descending branches run caudally within the dorsal funiculi for varying distances and eventually terminate in the dorsal horn. (Some of the long descending fibers of the dorsal funiculi are in distinct bundles, the **septomarginal fasciculus** and the **interfascicular fasciculus**, whose positions are indicated in Fig. 5-9.) Many of the ascending sensory fibers in the dorsal funiculus terminate in the gracile and cuneate nuclei in the medulla. At the other extreme, axons from the medial division of the dorsal root enter the gray matter at their own segmental levels; such fibers are conspicuous in lamina IV of the dorsal horn (see Figs. 5-4 and 5-6). Primary sensory axons conveying signals from muscle spindles have some branches that terminate on motor neurons and are involved in the stretch reflex. Some of the synaptic arrange-

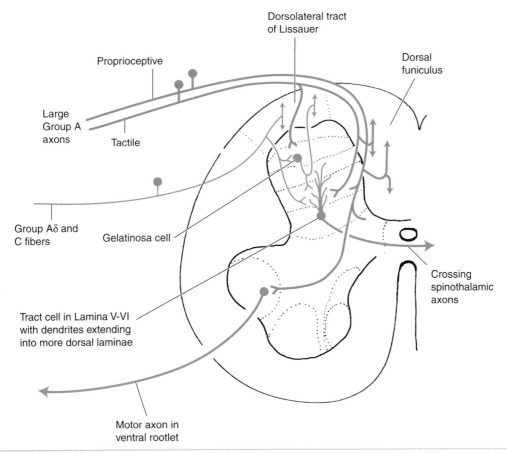

FIGURE 5-8 Neuronal circuitry of the dorsal horn of the spinal gray matter, showing afferent fibers in the medial (blue) and lateral (black) divisions of the dorsal root. Principal cells of the spinal cord are shown in red, and an interneuron of the substantia gelatinosa is green. Compare with Figure 5-11.

ments in the dorsal gray horn are summarized in Figure 5-8.

VENTRAL HORN

The columns of cells constituting lamina IX contain motor neurons of two types, named after the diameters (and therefore the conduction velocities) of their axons. The **alpha motor neurons** supply the ordinary (extrafusal) fibers of striated skeletal muscles. The smaller **gamma motor neurons** are less numerous and supply the intrafusal fibers of the neuromuscular spindles. The surfaces of both motor neuron types are densely covered with synaptic terminals, which release either excitatory or inhibitory transmitter substances. Each alpha motor neuron receives at least 20,000 synaptic contacts. The sources of the afferents are nu-

merous; some are from descending tracts of the spinal cord, and others are branches of axons of primary afferent neurons. The greatest numbers, however, are from intrinsic cells of the spinal gray matter, which behave physiologically as interneurons. The interneurons are located mainly in lamina VII. They receive their afferents from one another, from descending tracts, and from dorsal root ganglion neurons concerned with all modalities of sensation.

A special type of interneuron, from the physiological standpoint, is the **Renshaw cell**, which receives excitatory synaptic input from branches of the axons of nearby motor neurons. The branched axon of a Renshaw cell forms inhibitory synaptic junctions on motor neurons, including the same ones that are presynaptic to the Renshaw cell itself. By inhibiting nearby motor neurons, the Renshaw cell circuitry focuses

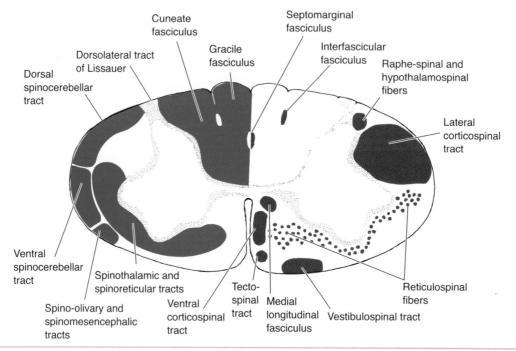

FIGURE 5-9   Major tracts of the spinal white matter at midcervical level. Ascending tracts *(blue)* are on the left; descending tracts *(red)* are on the right. The stippled areas adjacent to the gray matter indicate propriospinal fibers.

motor commands onto the muscles supplied by the most frequently firing motor neurons. The circuitry of the ventral horn is summarized in Figure 5-10.

TRACTS OF ASCENDING AND DESCENDING FIBERS

The spinal white matter is divided into longitudinally aligned **funiculi**, whose positions have already been described. Each funiculus contains tracts of ascending and descending fibers. The positions of the tracts have been approximately determined from clinical and pathological studies and from comparison of these clinical data with the more exact information obtained from animal studies. Most neuroanatomy and clinical neurology textbooks contain diagrams such as Figure 5-9, showing the positions of the major tracts. It is important to realize that the precise positions of some tracts are not known with certainty and that the territories of the different tracts overlap.

Dorsal Funiculus

The most important component of each dorsal funiculus is a large body of ascending axons derived from neurons located in the dorsal

root ganglia. Other ascending fibers are axons of neurons in the dorsal horn. The ascending fibers are all ipsilateral. They are especially concerned with the discriminative qualities of sensation, including the ability to recognize changes in the positions of tactile stimuli applied to the skin and conscious awareness of movement and of the positions of joints. It was formerly thought that conscious appreciation of vibration required the integrity of the dorsal funiculi, but clinical observations indicate that this is not so. Both the dorsal and the lateral funiculi conduct impulses initiated by vibratory stimuli.

As the spinal cord is ascended, axons are added to the lateral side of each dorsal funiculus. Consequently, in the upper cervical cord, the lowest levels of segmental innervation are represented in the most medial part of the gracile fasciculus, and the uppermost levels of segmental innervation are represented in the most lateral part of the cuneate fasciculus. These two fasciculi end, respectively, in the gracile and cuneate nuclei, which are located dorsally in the medulla. As a useful approximation, the gracile fasciculus and nucleus may be said to deal with sensations from the lower limb, and the cuneate fasciculus

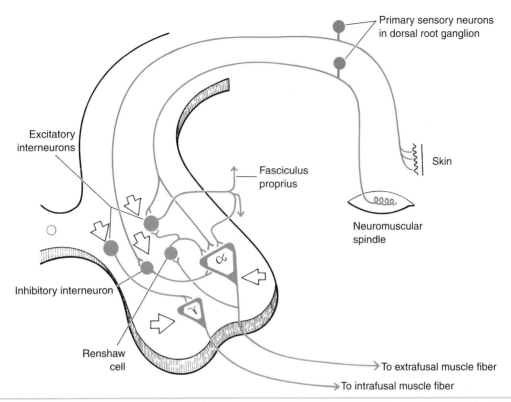

FIGURE 5-10 Neuronal circuitry of the ventral horn of the spinal gray matter, showing afferents (*blue*) to alpha (α) and gamma (γ) motor neurons (*red*). Large arrows point to the sites of termination of axons of descending tracts from the brain. Interneurons are green.

and nucleus may be said to deal with sensations from the upper limb. The orderly arrangement of different levels of the body in the dorsal funiculi is an example of **somatotopic lamination** in a tract. As will be seen, comparable lamination also exists in other tracts of the spinal cord and brain.

Lateral Funiculus

It is convenient to describe the dorsal and ventral halves of the lateral funiculus separately.

Dorsolateral Fasciculus

The most conspicuous tract in the dorsal half of the lateral funiculus is the **lateral corticospinal tract**, which consists of axons of neurons in the cortex of the frontal and parietal lobes of the contralateral cerebral hemisphere. These fibers pass through the internal capsule, the basis pedunculi of the midbrain, the pons, and the medullary pyramid before they decussate and enter the lateral funiculus of the cord. Corticospinal fibers from the frontal cortex terminate mainly in the intermediate gray matter and the ventral horn. Those from the parietal lobe end in the dorsal horn. The somatotopic lamination of the lateral corticospinal tract is such that fibers destined for the lowest levels of the spinal cord are the most laterally placed.

Experiments with animals indicate that a reticulospinal component of the dorsolateral funiculus arises in the nucleus raphes magnus in the reticular formation of the medulla and terminates in laminae I, II, and III. These unmyelinated fibers, constituting the **raphespinal tract** in the most dorsal part of the lateral funiculus, contain histochemically demonstrable quantities of serotonin, which they probably use as a neurotransmitter. The raphespinal tract modifies the transmission from the dorsal horn of impulses initiated by noxious stimuli, which produce painful sensations. Unmyelinated **hy-**

pothalamospinal fibers, similarly located, arise from the paraventricular nucleus of the hypothalamus and end among the preganglionic autonomic neurons in segments T1 to L3 and S2 to S4. Some hypothalamospinal axons contain the peptide oxytocin.

The largest body of ascending fibers in the dorsal part of the lateral funiculus is the superficially located **dorsal spinocerebellar tract**, which is present only above level L3. Its axons arise from the cells of the nucleus thoracicus (Clarke's column) in the same side of the spinal cord and terminate ipsilaterally in the cortex of the cerebellum, which they enter by way of the inferior cerebellar peduncle.

Ventrolateral Fasciculus

Several tracts are present in the ventral half of the lateral funiculus. The largest is the **spinothalamic tract**, which consists of the ascending axons of neurons located in the gray matter of the opposite half of the cord. The cells of origin are mostly in the nucleus proprius of the dorsal horn (laminae IV and V–VI). The axons cross the midline in the ventral white commissure close to the central canal and then traverse the ventral horn to enter the ventrolateral and ventral funiculi. The fibers of the spinothalamic tract end in thalamic nuclei. As they pass through the brain stem, some of these axons give off collateral branches to the reticular formation in the medulla and pons and to the periaqueductal gray matter in the midbrain. The spinothalamic tract conducts impulses concerned with tactile, thermal, and painful sensations. Its fibers are somatotopically arranged, with those for the lower limb lying most superficially and those for the upper limb lying closest to the gray matter. Distinct ventral and lateral spinothalamic tracts (for touch and for pain and thermal sensation, respectively) were formerly recognized, but there seems to be little justification for such a subdivision. The functions of the spinothalamic fibers are discussed in more detail in Chapter 19.

The **ventral spinocerebellar tract** is located superficially in the ventrolateral funiculus. It arises from the base of the dorsal horn and from the spinal border cells of the ventral horn of the lumbosacral segments and consists largely of crossed fibers. The tract ascends as far as the midbrain and then makes a sharp turn caudally

into the superior cerebellar peduncle. The fibers cross the midline for a second time within the cerebellum before ending in the cerebellar cortex. Thus, both spinocerebellar tracts convey sensory information (mainly proprioceptive) from one lower limb to the same side of the cerebellum. The other ascending components of the ventral half of the lateral funiculus are small. The axons composing the **spinotectal tract** (also known, more accurately, as the **spinomesencephalic tract**) originate in the same parts of the gray matter as the spinothalamic fibers, cross the midline, and then project rostrally to the periaqueductal gray matter, the superior colliculus, and various nuclei in the reticular formation of the midbrain. The **spinoreticular tract** is traditionally described as including crossed fibers that terminate in the pontine reticular formation and uncrossed fibers that end in the medullary reticular formation. In addition, many spinothalamic fibers have collateral branches that synapse with neurons of the reticular formation. These projections from the spinal cord to the brain stem form part of the ascending reticular activating system (see Chapter 9) and may also be involved in the perception of pain and of various sensations that originate in internal organs. It is customary to indicate a small **spino-olivary tract** in the human spinal cord, but its existence in primates is uncertain.

The ventrolateral funiculus also contains descending **reticulospinal fibers**. These are present also in the ventral funiculus, under which heading they are described below.

Ventral Funiculus

The long tracts in this part of the spinal white matter are all descending ones. The **ventral corticospinal tract** comprises a small proportion of the corticospinal fibers—those that did not cross the midline in the lower part of the medulla. Most ventral corticospinal fibers decussate at segmental levels and terminate next to those of the larger lateral corticospinal tract. In a few people, most of the corticospinal fibers fail to decussate in the medulla and, therefore, descend ipsilaterally in the ventral funiculus or, rarely, in the ventrolateral fasciculus.

The **vestibulospinal tract** is uncrossed. It arises from the lateral vestibular nucleus (of Deiters) in the medulla and descends in the ventrolateral and ventral white matter of the spinal cord, close to the surface (see Fig. 5-9). In the upper cervical cord, its fibers are located in the most medial part of the lateral funiculus. They then move medially so that in the lower cervical segments, they are close to the margin of the ventral median fissure. In the thoracic cord, the tract moves into a more lateral location in the ventral funiculus, among the axons that form the ventral rootlets, and it maintains this position at more caudal levels. Most vestibulospinal axons terminate in the medial part of the ventral horn. The tract's function is to mediate equilibratory reflexes, which are triggered by the activity of the vestibular apparatus of the internal ear and put into effect chiefly by the axial musculature and the extensors of the limbs.

Reticulospinal tracts originate in several nuclei of the reticular formation (see Chapter 9) of the midbrain, pons, and medulla. Most end by contacting interneurons in the ventral horn at all levels but most abundantly in the cervical segments. In the human spinal cord, reticulospinal fibers are present throughout the ventral funiculus and the ventral half of the lateral funiculus. The majority of the reticulospinal fibers are from the same side of the brain stem, and some of these axons cross the midline ventral to the central canal. Many reticulospinal fibers shift from the ventral into the lateral funiculus as they proceed down the spinal cord. The reticulospinal tracts constitute one of the descending pathways through which the brain directs and controls the activity of motor neurons. Whereas the corticospinal tract is concerned mainly with skilled volitional movements, the reticulospinal tracts control ordinary activities that do not require constant conscious effort. Other reticulospinal fibers influence the autonomic nervous system. The **descending bundle of the lateral horn** is a population of such axons that run alongside the lateral horn in the upper seven or eight thoracic segments. Clinical evidence indicates that these fibers, which probably originate ipsilaterally in the pons, are excitatory to the preganglionic sympathetic neurons that control blood vessels and sweat glands throughout the body. Degeneration studies (see Chapter 4) of human material support the preceding account of reticulospinal fibers and do not support the tradi-

tional notion of separate and distinct medullary and pontine reticulospinal tracts.

The remaining tracts of the ventral funiculus are small. The descending component of the **medial longitudinal fasciculus** (also called the **medial vestibulospinal tract**, in which case the vestibulospinal tract previously described is designated as lateral) arises in the medial vestibular nucleus in the medulla. It is involved in movements of the head required for maintaining equilibrium and probably does not descend below the upper cervical levels of the spinal cord. The few fibers that constitute the **tectospinal tract** from the contralateral superior colliculus do not descend below this level, either.

Fasciculus Proprius

The fasciculus proprius, a zone containing both myelinated and unmyelinated fibers, is present in all the funiculi immediately adjacent to the gray matter (see Fig. 5-9). It contains **propriospinal (spinospinalis) fibers**, which connect different segmental levels of the gray matter. The shorter axons are closer to the gray matter than the longer fibers. Propriospinal fibers run both rostrally and caudally and have collateral branches that end in the gray matter near their own cell bodies, providing the functional equivalent of interneurons for reflexes within segments. Some neurons with axons that ascend in the fasciculus proprius extend for almost the whole length of the spinal cord and serve as necessary components of intersegmental spinal reflexes. Descending propriospinal fibers seldom extend over more than two segments of the spinal cord.

Spinal Reflexes

Certain neuronal connections in the spinal cord form the bases of spinal reflexes. The stretch reflex and the flexor reflex are examples.

The **stretch reflex** has a two-neuron or monosynaptic reflex arc (Fig. 5-11). Slight stretching of a muscle stimulates the sensory endings in neuromuscular spindles, and the resultant excitation reaches the spinal cord by way of primary sensory neurons that have large (group A) axons. The proximal branches of these axons in the dorsal funiculus give off collateral branches that excite alpha motor

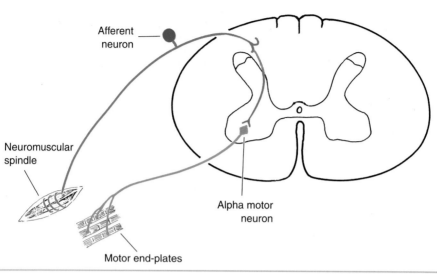

Afferent
neuron

Neuromuscular
spindle

Alpha motor
neuron

Motor end-plates

FIGURE 5-11   Afferent (*blue*) and efferent (*red*) limbs of the monosynaptic stretch reflex arc.

neurons, causing the stretched muscle to contract. This is an important postural reflex. The
neuromuscular spindles are delicate monitors
of change in the length of the muscle, and the
stretch reflex alters tension in such a way as to
maintain a constant length. The stretch reflex
forms the basis of the clinical **tendon jerk** tests
that are part of physical examinations. A sharp
tap on the tendon causes synchronous discharges from the spindles in the muscle, with
prompt reflex contraction. A diminished or absent tendon jerk indicates disease affecting either the afferent or the efferent neurons of the
stretch reflex. Exaggerated jerks indicate loss of
inhibition of motor neurons by activity in tracts
descending from the brain.

In addition to the simple monosynaptic
stretch reflex, a response with longer latency
occurs when a voluntarily contracting muscle
is stretched. Physiological studies indicate that
this slower reflex, which is most easily elicited
in the hand, passes through the somatosensory
and motor areas of the cerebral cortex.

The tension on a muscle is monitored
by Golgi tendon organs. When the tension
reaches a certain level, a distinct increase
takes place in the discharge from these receptors. The resulting action potentials reach in-

terneurons in the spinal gray matter, which in
turn inhibit alpha motor neurons. Relaxation
of the muscle follows. This reflex can prevent
excessive tension on the muscle and tendon.
When a muscle is abnormally contracting
(spasm or spasticity), passive stretching can
induce relaxation by stimulating the Golgi
tendon organs.

The **flexor reflex** is also protective. It consists of the withdrawal of a limb in response
to a painful stimulus. At least three neurons
are involved, so this is a polysynaptic reflex
(Fig. 5-12). The cutaneous receptors are free
nerve endings that respond to potentially injurious stimuli, and the proximal branches of
the afferent fibers synapse in the dorsal horn
with interneurons. These end on alpha motor cells in several segments because a withdrawal response requires the action of groups
of muscles. Some neurons in the dorsal horn
have axons that decussate and contact neurons in the contralateral ventral horn to
stimulate, in a fully developed response, extension of the contralateral limb: the **crossed
extensor reflex**.

Reflexes in Infancy

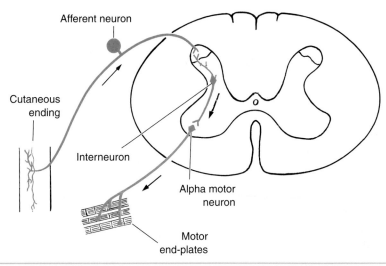

FIGURE 5-12   Afferent (*blue*) and efferent (*red*) neurons of the flexor reflex arc, which include an interneuron (*green*).

Anatomical and Clinical Correlations

Lesions of the spinal cord result from trauma, degenerative and demyelinating disorders, tumors, infections, and impairment of blood supply. The following notes on selected lesions show the necessity of understanding the intrinsic anatomy of the spinal cord to interpret signs and symptoms.

CLINICAL EXAMINATION

Testing for impairment or loss of cutaneous sensation is an important part of the neurological examination; it is particularly useful in detecting the site of a lesion that involves the spinal cord or nerve roots. The distribution of cutaneous areas (**dermatomes**) supplied by the spinal nerves is shown in Figure 5-13. Cutaneous areas supplied by adjacent spinal nerves overlap. For example, the upper half of the area supplied by T6 is also supplied by T5, and the lower half by T7. There is, therefore, little or no sensory loss after interruption of a single spinal nerve or dorsal root. The overlapping of dermatomes contrasts with the sharp delineation of the areas supplied by cutaneous nerves, which are formed in the limb plexuses by the mingling of fibers from various segmental nerve roots.

Reflex contraction of muscles is also used in testing for the integrity of segments of the cord and of the spinal nerves. The segments involved in four commonly tested **stretch or tendon reflexes** are as follows: biceps reflex, C5 and C6; triceps reflex, C6 to C8; quadriceps reflex (knee jerk), L2 to L4; and gastrocnemius reflex (ankle jerk), S1 to S2.

Before specific pathological conditions are mentioned, it should be noted that a distinction is made between the effects of a lesion involving motor neurons as opposed to those involving descending motor pathways. Destruction or atrophy of **lower motor neurons** (in the present context, those of the ventral horn) results in flaccid paralysis of the affected muscles, diminished or absent tendon reflexes, and progressive atrophy of the muscles deprived of motor fibers. The term **upper motor neuron lesion** is regularly used clinically but leaves much to be desired. The lesion may be in the cerebral cortex or in another part of the cerebral hemisphere, in the brain stem, or in the spinal cord. Thus, the term *upper motor neuron* is a collective term including all the descending pathways that control the activities of the neurons that supply the muscles. The following signs are associated with an upper motor neuron lesion after the acute effects have worn off: varying degrees of voluntary paralysis, which is most severe in the upper limb; a positive Babinski's sign (i.e., upturning of the great toe

(continued)

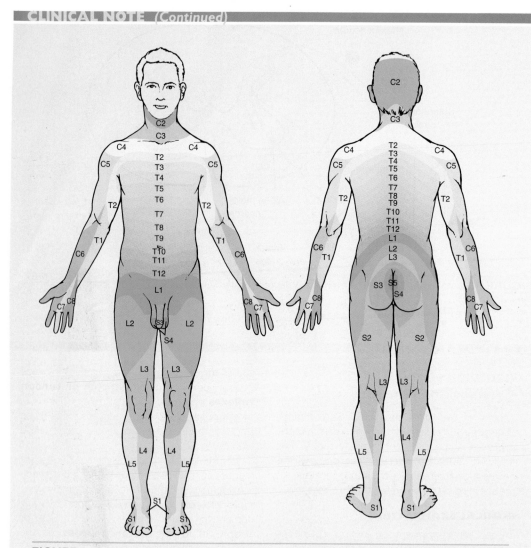

FIGURE 5-13   Cutaneous distribution of spinal nerves (dermatomes).

and spreading of the toes on stroking the sole); and spasticity with exaggerated tendon reflexes.

SPINAL CORD TRANSECTION

The spinal cord may be damaged by penetrating wounds (caused by stabbing or gunfire) or by spinal fracture or dislocation (especially from traffic accidents or diving into shallow water). Complete transection results in loss of all sensibility and voluntary movement below the lesion. The patient is **tetraplegic** (quadriplegic), with both arms and both legs paralyzed, if the upper cervical cord is transected, or **paraplegic** (both legs paralyzed) if the transection is between the cervical and lumbosacral enlargements. During

an initial period of **spinal shock**, lasting from a few days to several weeks, all somatic and visceral reflex activity is abolished. On return of reflex activity, spasticity of muscles and exaggerated tendon reflexes occur. The lower limbs assume positions of flexion because the vestibulospinal tract (which stimulates extensors) is one of the transected descending pathways. Bladder and bowel functions are no longer under voluntary control.

The events that occur after partial transection of the spinal cord depend on the size and location of the lesion. **Hemisection**, although unusual in the literal sense, is an instructive lesion anatomically. The neurological signs caudal to

(continued)

the hemisected region of the cord constitute the Brown-Séquard syndrome. Position sense, tactile discrimination, and the feeling of vibration are lost *on the side of the lesion* because of interruption of the dorsal and dorsolateral funiculi. Anesthesia for pain and temperature are provided *on the opposite side* because of interruption of the spinothalamic tract. Light touch is not much affected because of essentially bilateral conduction in the dorsal and lateral funiculi. Whereas the patient is **hemiplegic** (left or right upper and lower limbs paralyzed) if the lesion is in the upper cervical cord, hemisection of the thoracic cord results in paralysis of the leg (**monoplegia**). The paralysis is *ipsilateral* to the lesion and of the upper motor neuron type.

The immediate treatment of patients with incomplete spinal cord transection is largely directed to protection against further damage from fractured or dislocated vertebrae and suppression of an aggressive and destructive inflammatory reaction that occurs within the cord for several days after the injury. Long-term management includes prevention of bedsores in insensitive skin, avoidance of urinary tract infections, and maximization of any preserved motor functions.

Potentially curative treatments, such as ways to induce severed axons to grow across the scarred site of an injury, have been a goal of research for at least 100 years. Recent efforts include extracting olfactory ensheathing cells (see Chapters 2 and 17) from the olfactory mucosa of the patient's nose. These pluripotential glial cells can be propogated in culture and introduced into the injured spinal cord. In laboratory animals, the grafted cells appear to facilitate axonal growth, and with the recipient of the graft being also the donor, the cells are not rejected. Clinical trials of this procedure are in progress.

DEGENERATIVE DISEASES

The following degenerative diseases also illustrate the anatomical basis of neurological signs. In **subacute combined degeneration**, bilateral demyelination and loss of nerve fibers in the dorsal

and dorsolateral funiculi occur. The principal causative factor is vitamin B_{12} deficiency, and the disorder is typically encountered in association with pernicious anemia. The lesion results in loss of the senses of position, discriminative touch, and vibration. The gait is ataxic (i.e., without coordination) because the patient is unaware of the position of his or her legs.

Amyotrophic lateral sclerosis (also called motor neuron disease) is a bilateral degenerative disease. The degenerative process is largely restricted to the motor system, affecting the corticobulbar and corticospinal tracts (and perhaps other descending motor pathways) along with motor nuclei of cranial nerves and ventral horn motor cells. A combination of upper and lower motor neuron clinical signs are present, with the latter predominating in the terminal stages of the disease. **Poliomyelitis** is caused by a virus that infects motor neurons, killing many of them. Paralysis is of the lower motor neuron type and affects the muscles supplied by the infected neurons. Correlation of clinical data with postmortem findings in poliomyelitis has been the chief source of knowledge of the distribution in the human ventral horn of motor neurons that supply individual muscles.

Syringomyelia differs from the disorders already mentioned in that neuronal degeneration is not the primary pathological change. Central cavitation of the spinal cord is present, usually beginning in the cervical region, with a glial reaction (gliosis) adjacent to the cavity. Decussating fibers for pain and temperature in the ventral white commissure are interrupted early in the disease. The cavitation and gliosis spread into the gray and white matter as well as longitudinally, leading to variable signs and symptoms, depending on the regions involved. The classical clinical picture is that of "yokelike" anesthesia for pain and temperature over the shoulders and upper limbs accompanied by lower motor neuron weakness and consequent wasting of the muscles of the upper limbs. Spread of the cavitation and glial reaction into the lateral funiculi may result in voluntary paresis of the upper motor neuron type, particularly affecting the lower limbs.

Suggested Reading

Abdel-Maguid TE, Bowsher D. The gray matter of the dorsal horn of the adult human spinal cord, including comparisons with general somatic and visceral afferent cranial nerve nuclei. *J Anat* 1985;142:33–58.

Atkinson PP, Atkinson JLD. Spinal shock. *Mayo Clin Proc* 1996;71:384–389.

Coggeshall RE, Carlton SM. Receptor localization in the mammalian dorsal horn and primary afferent neurons. *Brain Res Rev* 1997;24:28–66.

Feron F, Perry C, Cochrane J, et al. Autologous olfactory ensheathing cell transplantation in human spinal cord injury. *Brain* 2005;128:2951–2960.

LaMotte C. Distribution of the tract of Lissauer and the dorsal root fibers in the primate spinal cord. *J Comp Neurol* 1977;172:529–561.

Martin JH. *Neuroanatomy: Text and Atlas*, 2nd ed. Stamford, CT: Appleton & Lange, 1996.

Matthews PBC. The human stretch reflex and the motor cortex. *Trends Neurosci* 1991;14:87–91.

Nathan PN, Smith MC, Deacon P. The corticospinal tracts in man: course and location of fibres at different segmental levels. *Brain* 1990;113:303–324.

Nathan PN, Smith MC, Deacon P. Vestibulospinal, reticulospinal and descending propriospinal nerve fibers in man. *Brain* 1996;119:1809–1833.

Norenberg MD, Smith J, Mercillo A. The pathology of human spinal cord injury: defining the problems. *J Neurotrauma* 2004;21:429–440.

Parkinson D, Del Bigio MR. Posterior 'septum' of human spinal cord: normal developmental variations, composition, and terminology. *Anat Rec* 1996;244:572–578.

Pullen AH, Tucker D, Martin JE. Morphological and morphometric characterization of Onuf's nucleus in the spinal cord in man. *J Anat* 1997;191:201–213.

Ralston DD, Ralston HJ. The terminations of corticospinal tract axons in the macaque monkey. *J Comp Neurol* 1985;242:325–337.

Renshaw B. Central effects of centripetal impulses in axons of spinal nerve roots. *J Neurophysiol* 1946;9:191–204.

Routal RV, Pal GP. A study of motoneuron groups and motor columns of the human spinal cord. *J Anat* 1999;195:211–224.

Routal RV, Pal GP. Location of the phrenic nucleus in the human spinal cord. *J Anat* 1999;195:617–621.

Smith MC, Deacon P. Topographical anatomy of the posterior columns of the spinal cord in man: the long ascending fibres. *Brain* 1984;107:671–698.

Wall PD, Noordenbos W. Sensory functions which remain in man after complete transection of dorsal columns. *Brain* 1977;100:641–653.

Willis WD, Coggeshall RE. *Sensory Mechanisms of the Spinal Cord*, 3rd ed. 2 vols. New York: Kluwer, 2004.

Wolf JK. *Segmental Neurology*. Baltimore: University Park Press, 1981.

Yezierski RP. Spinomesencephalic tract: projections from the lumbosacral spinal cord of the rat, cat and monkey. *J Comp Neurol* 1988;267:131–146.

BRAIN STEM: EXTERNAL ANATOMY

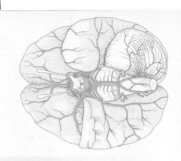

- Proceeding laterally from the ventral midline, the anatomical landmarks at different levels are as follows. Each represents a functionally important nucleus or tract within the brain stem. The student must also know the sites of emergence of cranial nerves III to XII in relation to these landmarks.

- **Medulla:** Pyramid, olive, inferior cerebellar peduncle; cuneate and gracile tubercles (below obex); floor of fourth ventricle (above obex).

- **Pons:** Basal part of pons, middle cerebellar peduncle, superior cerebellar peduncle, floor of fourth ventricle.

- **Midbrain:** Interpeduncular fossa, basis pedunculi, inferior or superior colliculus.

- In the floor of the fourth ventricle motor nuclei of cranial nerves are typically medial and sensory nuclei lateral to the sulcus limitans. There are named areas for hypoglossal, vagal, and vestibular nuclei. The facial colliculus contains fibers of the facial nerve that pass dorsal to the abducens nucleus.

- The superior and inferior medullary vela form the roof of the fourth ventricle, which narrows into the central canal caudally and the cerebral aqueduct rostrally.

- Cerebrospinal fluid enters the fourth ventricle from the aqueduct and leaves by way of the median and lateral apertures.

The **brain stem** consists of the medulla oblongata, pons, and midbrain. Each region has special features, including nuclei of cranial nerves, but long tracts of fibers are present at all levels. The **fourth ventricle** is partly in the medulla and partly in the pons. This chapter is concerned with the surface landmarks of the brain stem. For more details of the internal features of the brain stem (e.g., certain nuclei and tracts), see Chapter 7 or refer to the Index. The central connections and functions of the cranial nerves are explained in Chapter 8.

Medulla Oblongata

The medulla oblongata (or medulla) is about 3 cm long and widens gradually in a rostral direction. It rests on the midline part of the occipital bone and is covered dorsally by the cerebellum. The junction of the spinal cord and medulla is level with the foramen magnum. The rostral limit of the medulla is marked ventrally by a prominent sulcus (Figs. 6-1 and 6-2). On the dorsal surface, the junction is an imaginary transverse line that joins the caudal margins of the middle cerebellar peduncles (Fig. 6-3). The dorsal surface, therefore, contains the caudal half of the fourth ventricle; this rostral end of the medulla is known as the **open part** because the thin roof of the fourth ventricle is usually removed in the course of dissection. The caudal part of the medulla is called the **closed part**; it contains a continuation of the central canal of the spinal cord.

The surface of the medulla is marked by several bulges or eminences, outlined by sulci. Ventrally, the **pyramid** (see Fig. 6-1) consists of corticospinal fibers. This is the origin of the term *pyramidal tract* as a synonym for corticospinal tract. In the most caudal part of the medulla, most of the pyramidal fibers cross the midline; the decussating fibers obscure the ventral median sulcus at this level. Lateral to the pyramid, the **olive** (see Fig. 6-2) is an oval swelling that marks the position of the inferior olivary nucleus. Lateral to the olive, the **inferior cerebellar peduncle** is a body of white matter that connects the medulla with the cerebellum and forms the

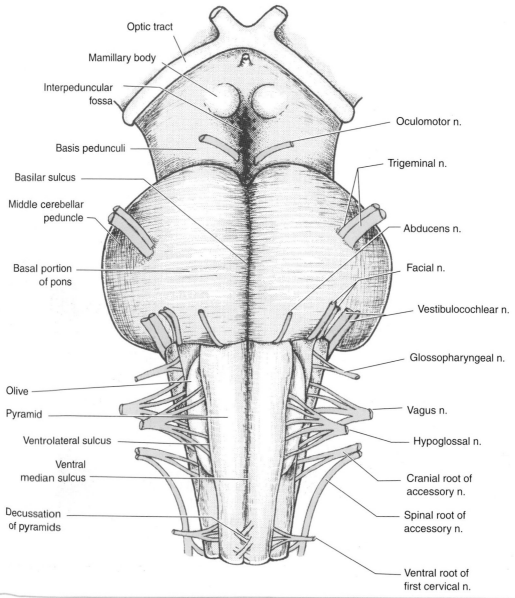

Optic tract

Mamillary body

Interpeduncular fossa

Basis pedunculi

Basilar sulcus

Middle cerebellar peduncle

Basal portion of pons

Olive

Pyramid

Ventrolateral sulcus

Ventral median sulcus

Decussation of pyramids

Oculomotor n.

Trigeminal n.

Abducens n.

Facial n.

Vestibulocochlear n.

Glossopharyngeal n.

Vagus n.

Hypoglossal n.

Cranial root of accessory n.

Spinal root of accessory n.

Ventral root of first cervical n.

FIGURE 6-1   Ventral aspect of the brain stem.

side wall of the caudal half of the fourth ventricle. On the dorsal surface of the closed part of the medulla, the **gracile** and **cuneate fasciculi** continue from the spinal cord (see Figs. 6-2 and 6-3). The axons in the fasciculi terminate in the gracile and cuneate nuclei, which cause slight elevations, the **gracile** and **cuneate tubercles**. The apex of the V-shaped boundary of the inferior part of the fourth ventricle, which is folded caudally over the most rostral 1 to 2 mm of the central canal, is known as the **obex**.

Seven cranial nerves are attached to the medulla or to the junction of the medulla and pons (see Figs. 6-1 to 6-3). The **abducens nerve** emerges near the midline between the pons and the pyramid. The **facial** and **vestibulocochlear nerves** are attached to the lateral aspect of the brain stem at the caudal border of the pons. The facial nerve, which is the more medial, has two roots. The smaller sensory and parasympathetic root lies between the larger motor root and the vestibulocochlear nerve; therefore, it is known

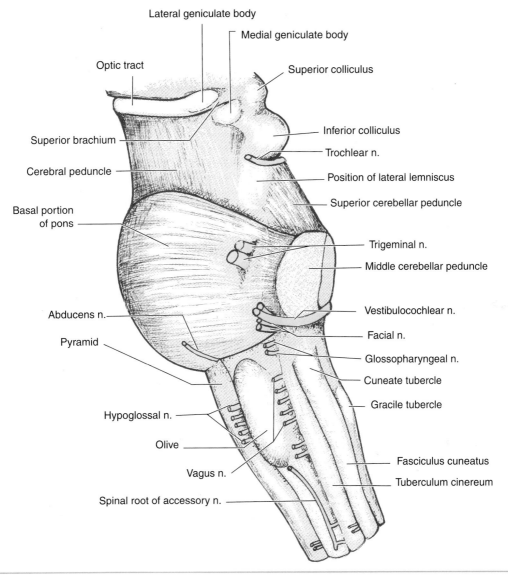

FIGURE 6-2   Lateral aspect of the brain stem.

as the **nervus intermedius**. The cochlear division of the vestibulocochlear nerve ends in the dorsal and ventral cochlear nuclei, which are situated on the base of the inferior cerebellar peduncle. The vestibular division penetrates the brain stem deep to the root of the inferior cerebellar peduncle.

Roots of the **glossopharyngeal** and **vagus nerves** as well as those of the cranial division of the **accessory nerve** are attached to the medulla rostral and dorsal to the olive. The cranial root of the accessory nerve is joined by the spinal root, and the glossopharyngeal, vagus, and

accessory nerves all leave the posterior cranial fossa through the jugular foramen. Rootlets of the **hypoglossal nerve** emerge along the sulcus between the pyramid and the olive.

Pons

This part of the brain stem is about 2.5 cm long. It owes its name to the appearance of its ventral surface (see Fig. 6-1), which is that of a bridge connecting the right and left cerebellar hemispheres. (This appearance is deceptive, as noted later.) The

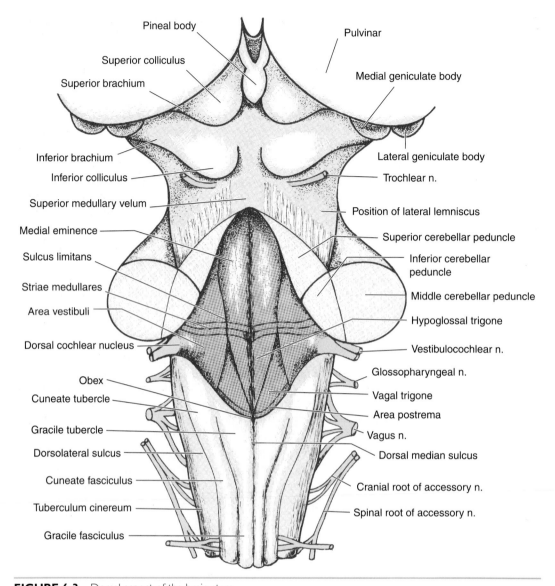

FIGURE 6-3   Dorsal aspect of the brain stem.

pons consists of quite different basal (ventral) and dorsal parts (see Figs. 7-9 and 7-10).

The **basal part** is indented along its ventral surface in the midline by a shallow groove, the **basilar sulcus**, which accommodates the basilar artery. The basal pons blends laterally into the **middle cerebellar peduncles**, with the attachment of the **trigeminal nerve** marking the transition between the pons and the peduncle (see Figs. 6-1 and 6-2). The motor root of the trigeminal nerve is rostromedial to the larger sensory root. Fibers from the cerebral cortex terminate ipsilaterally on neurons that com-

pose the pontine nuclei, and axons of the latter cells cross the midline and then constitute the contralateral middle cerebellar peduncle. The basal pons thus serves as a large synaptic relay station, providing a connection from the cortex of each cerebral hemisphere to the opposite cerebellar hemisphere. The corticospinal tracts traverse the basal part of the pons before they enter the pyramids (see Fig. 7-9).

The **dorsal part** or **tegmentum** of the pons is similar to much of the medulla and midbrain in that it contains ascending and descending tracts and nuclei of cranial nerves. The dorsal surface of the pons is formed by the floor of the fourth ventricle. The most rostral part of the pons is known as the **isthmus of the brain stem**; it is situated immediately below the cerebral peduncles and inferior colliculi of the midbrain (see Fig. 6-2).

Fourth Ventricle

When the cerebellum is removed by cutting through its six peduncles, the thin roof of the fourth ventricle comes off with it, exposing the **floor of the ventricle** on the dorsal aspect of the brain stem (see Fig. 6-3).

The diamond-shaped floor of the fourth ventricle, also called the **rhomboid fossa**, narrows toward the obex caudally and the aqueduct of the midbrain rostrally (see Fig. 6-3). The floor is divided into symmetrical halves by a median sulcus. The **sulcus limitans** further divides each half into medial and lateral areas. The lateral area is known as the **vestibular area** because there the vestibular nuclear complex lies beneath most of the floor of the ventricle.

Motor and parasympathetic nuclei are located beneath the floor of the medial area. The caudal part of the rhomboid fossa is marked by two triangles or trigones. The **vagal trigone** (or ala cinerea) marks the site of the rostral ends of the dorsal nucleus of the vagus nerve and the rostral end of the solitary nucleus. The **hypoglossal trigone** is a landmark for the rostral end of the **hypoglossal nucleus**. The **facial col-** liculus, a swelling at the lower end of the **medial eminence** (see Fig. 6-3), is formed by fibers from the motor nucleus of the facial nerve looping over the abducens nucleus.

A pigmented area, the **locus coeruleus**, is situated at the rostral end of the sulcus limitans, indicating the site of a cluster of noradrenergic neurons that contain melanin pigment. In the middle of the floor of the fourth ventricle, delicate strands of nerve fibers emerge from the median sulcus, run laterally as the **striae medullares**, and enter the inferior cerebellar peduncle. The connections of these fibers, which are more conspicuous in some brains than in others, are explained in Chapter 7.

The tent-shaped roof of the fourth ventricle protrudes dorsally toward the cerebellum. The rostral part of the roof is formed on each side by the **superior cerebellar peduncles**, which consist mainly of fibers proceeding from cerebellar nuclei into the midbrain. The V-shaped interval between the converging peduncles is bridged by the **superior medullary velum**, a thin sheet of white matter. The remainder of the roof consists of a thinner pial–ependymal membrane, the **inferior medullary velum**, which adheres to the undersurface of the cerebellum. A deficiency of variable size in the inferior medullary velum constitutes the **median aperture** of the fourth ventricle, also called the **foramen of Magendie**. This hole provides the principal communication between the ventricular system and the subarachnoid space (Fig. 6-4).

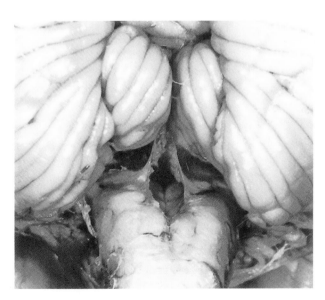

FIGURE 6-4 Median aperture of the fourth ventricle (foramen of Magendie) opening from the fourth ventricle into the cerebellomedullary cistern of the subarachnoid space (×2.5).

The lateral walls of the fourth ventricle include the **inferior cerebellar peduncles**, which curve from the medulla into the cerebellum on the medial aspects of the middle peduncles (see Fig. 6-3). Lateral recesses of the ventricle extend around the sides of the medulla and open ventrally as the **lateral apertures** of the fourth ventricle (the **foramina of Luschka**), which are two other channels through which cerebrospinal fluid enters the subarachnoid space (Fig. 6-5). These foramina are situated at the junction of the medulla, pons, and cerebellum (the cerebellopontine angles) near the attachment to the brain stem of the vestibulocochlear and glossopharyngeal nerves.

The **choroid plexus** of the fourth ventricle is suspended from the inferior medullary velum; the plexus extends into the lateral recesses, and a small tuft usually protrudes through each lateral aperture. Choroid plexus is the tissue that secretes cerebrospinal fluid (see Chapter 26). Most of the fluid is produced in the lateral and third ventricles and flows into the fourth ventricle by way of the cerebral aqueduct. The choroid plexus of the fourth ventricle makes a small addition to the volume of the cerebrospinal fluid in the cavity of the ventricle and di-

rectly into the subarachnoid space of the pontocerebellar angle (see Fig. 6-5).

Midbrain

The midbrain is about 1.5 cm long. Its ventral surface extends from the pons to the mamillary bodies of the diencephalon (see Fig. 6-1). The robust column of white matter on each side is the **basis pedunculi** (crus cerebri), composed of corticospinal, corticobulbar, and corticopontine fibers. The deep depression between these two columns is the **interpeduncular fossa**. Many small blood vessels penetrate the midbrain in the floor of the interpeduncular fossa; therefore, this region is known as the **posterior perforated substance**. The **oculomotor nerve** emerges from the side of the interpeduncular fossa.

The lateral surface of the midbrain (see Fig. 6-2) is formed mainly by the **cerebral peduncle**, which constitutes the major part of this region of the brain stem on each side. The cerebral peduncle comprises the basis pedunculi and some internal structures, the substantia nigra, and the tegmentum, which are described in Chapter 7.

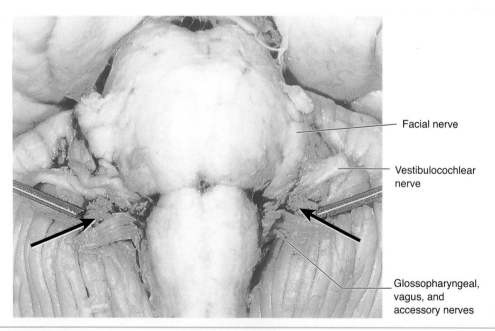

Facial nerve

Vestibulocochlear nerve

Glossopharyngeal, vagus, and accessory nerves

FIGURE 6-5   Lateral apertures of the fourth ventricle (formina of Luschka). Tufts of choroid plexus (*arrows*) occupy the foramina, into which metal marker sticks have been inserted.

The dorsal surface of the midbrain bears four rounded elevations, the paired **inferior** and **superior colliculi** (also called the **corpora quadrigemina**). These colliculi (see Figs. 6-2 and 6-3) make up the **tectum** and indicate the extent of the midbrain on the dorsal surface. Fibers that connect the inferior colliculus with the medial geniculate body (part of the thalamus) form a ridge known as the **inferior brachium** (see Figs. 6-2 and 6-3). The superior colliculus is involved in the control of movements of the eyes and head in response to visual and other stimuli. The **superior brachium** contains fibers proceeding from the cerebral cortex and the retina to the superior colliculus. Other fibers in the superior brachium terminate in the **pretectal area** ventral and just rostral to the superior colliculi; these fibers are part of a pathway from the retina for the pupillary light reflex. The **trochlear nerve** emerges from the brain stem immediately caudal to the inferior colliculus and curves around the midbrain on its way toward the orbit.

The posterior part of the thalamus projects caudally beyond the plane of transition between the diencephalon and the midbrain (see Fig. 6-3). Consequently, transverse sections at the level of the superior colliculi include thalamic nuclei, in particular those of the medial and lateral geniculate bodies, and a prominent part of the thalamus known as the pulvinar (see Figs. 6-3, 7-14, and 7-15).

Suggested Reading

Barr ML. Observations on the foramen of Magendie in a series of human brains. *Brain* 1948;71:281–289.

England MA, Wakely J. *Color Atlas of the Brain and Spinal Cord. An Introduction to Normal Neuroanatomy*, 2nd ed. Orlando, FL: Mosby, 2005.

Haines DE. *Neuroanatomy: An Atlas of Structures, Sections and Systems*, 5th ed. Philadelphia: Lippincott, Williams & Wilkins, 2000.

Montemurro DG, Bruni JE. *The Human Brain in Dissection*, 2nd ed. New York: Oxford University Press, 1988.

Noback CR, Strominger NL, Demarest RJ, et al. *The Human Nervous System: Structure and Function*, 6th ed. Totowa, NJ: Humana Press, 2005.

Smith CG. *Serial Dissections of the Human Brain*. Baltimore: Urban & Schwarzenberg, 1981.

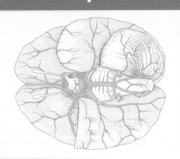

Chapter 7

BRAIN STEM: NUCLEI AND TRACTS

Important Facts

- The brain stem contains ascending and descending tracts, cranial nerves and other nuclei, and fibers connecting with the cerebellum.

- The spinothalamic tract, which crosses into the spinal cord, is laterally located throughout the length of the brain stem.

- The medial lemniscus is formed from axons that arise in the contralateral gracile and cuneate nuclei. The lemniscus is near the midline in the medulla, shifts laterally in the pons, and is laterally situated in the tegmentum of the midbrain.

- Corticopontine and corticospinal fibers occupy the basis penduculi. Corticopontine fibers end in the pontine nuclei. Corticospinal fibers continue caudally, forming the pyramid. Most pyramidal fibers decussate at the caudal end of the medulla.

- The inferior olivary complex of nuclei and the pontine nuclei project across the midline to the cerebellum into the inferior and middle cerebellar peduncles, respectively.

- The superior cerebellar peduncles consist largely of fibers leaving the cerebellum. These decussate at the level of the inferior colliculi, and some end in the red nucleus at the level of the superior colliculus.

- The substantia nigra and the periaqueductal gray matter are present at all levels of the midbrain.

- The seven motor nuclei of cranial nerves are the oculomotor and trochlear nuclei in the midbrain, trigeminal motor nucleus in the pons, facial motor and abducens nuclei at the pontomedullary junction, and nucleus ambiguus and hypoglossal nucleus in the medulla.

- Preganglionic parasympathetic nuclei include the Edinger-Westphal nucleus, the dorsal nucleus of the vagus, and some of the neurons in the nucleus ambiguus.

- The only general somatic sensory nuclei are the three components (spinal, pontine, and mesencephalic) of the trigeminal nuclear complex. The only visceral sensory nucleus is the solitary nucleus, the most rostral part of which is the gustatory nucleus (for taste).

- The two cochlear and four vestibular nuclei receive special somatic sensory fibers. The lateral lemniscus extends for the length of the pons. The medial longitudinal fasciculus maintains its dorsomedial position throughout the brain stem.

- The level of a lesion in the brain stem is indicated by involvement of cranial nerves and their nuclei. The position of the lesion at a particular level is indicated by disordered function of ascending or descending tracts.

The principal nuclei and fiber tracts of the brain stem are described and illustrated in this chapter. Long tracts that traverse the brain stem are noted successively in the medulla, pons, and midbrain. Some pathways are also reviewed as functional systems in Chapters 19 and 23. The nuclei of cranial nerves are included among the cell groups identified, but systematic descriptions of the functional components of the cranial nerves are reserved for Chapter 8.

Sections stained by Weigert's method are used as illustrations; the levels of the sections are shown in Figure 7-1. Some tracts do not stand out as distinct entities in such sections; their locations and functions have been established from clinicopathological correlations in humans and from experimental work with laboratory animals.

The **reticular formation** is mentioned briefly here because the term is used in several contexts in this chapter. The reticular formation is a region in the dorsal parts of the medulla and pons, and it extends rostrally into the tegmentum of the midbrain. It is traversed by small bundles of myelinated axons that course in all directions, and it contains overlapping populations of neu-

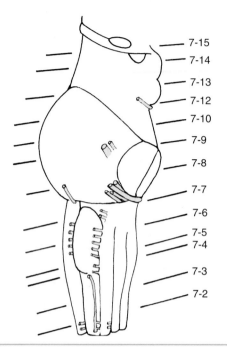

7-15
7-14
7-13
7-12
7-10
7-9
7-8
7-7
7-6
7-5
7-4
7-3
7-2

FIGURE 7-1   Key to the levels of the series of Weigert-stained sections of the brain stem that illustrate this
chapter.

rons that are not easily classified into groups,
although numerous nuclei are recognized. The
reticular formation has several functions of primary importance, including an influence on
levels of consciousness and degrees of alertness
(ascending reticular activating system); a role
in the control of movement through efferents
to the spinal cord and to motor nuclei of cranial
nerves; and contributions to visceral and other
involuntary activities through groups of neurons that function as cardiovascular and respiratory "centers." In view of its special histological characteristics and functional importance,
the reticular formation is discussed separately
in Chapter 9, along with several smaller nuclei
of the brain stem.

Medulla

At the level of the pyramidal decussation, there
is an extensive rearrangement of gray matter
and white matter in the transitional zone between the spinal cord and the medulla. The
ventral gray horns continue into the region of
the decussation, where they include motor cells
for the first cervical nerve and the spinal root

of the accessory nerve. There, the gray matter
is traversed obliquely by bundles of fibers that
pass from the pyramids to the lateral corticospinal tracts (Figs. 7-2 and 7-3). The dorsal gray
horns of the spinal cord are replaced by the
spinal trigeminal nuclei. At the rostral ends of
the dorsal funiculi, at the level of the pyramidal
decussation, are the caudal ends of the **gracile**
and **cuneate nuclei.** Above the decussation, the
medulla has a complex structure that is entirely
different from that of the spinal cord (Figs. 7-4
to 7-7). The **inferior olivary nucleus,** which is
dorsal and lateral to the pyramid, is the most
prominent feature of the rostral half of the medulla, and the base of the **inferior cerebellar
peduncle** appears as a prominent area of white
matter in the dorsolateral part of the medulla
(see Fig. 7-7).

ASCENDING PATHWAYS

Medial Lemniscus System

The dorsal funiculus of the spinal cord transmits impulses for ipsilateral discriminative
touch and proprioception. The **gracile fasciculus** is concerned with sensations from the leg
and lower trunk, and the **cuneate fasciculus**
carries signals from the upper trunk, arm, and
neck. The **gracile nucleus,** in which fibers of
the corresponding fasciculus terminate, is present throughout the closed portion of the medulla. The fibers of the cuneate fasciculus end
in the **cuneate nucleus,** which is located laterally and slightly rostrally to the gracile nucleus
(see Fig. 7-3).

The myelinated axons of the cells in the gracile and cuneate nuclei pursue a curved course to
the midline as **internal arcuate fibers,** which are
clearly shown in Figure 7-4. After crossing the
midline in the **decussation of the medial lemnisci,** these fibers turn rostrally in the **medial
lemniscus.** This is one of the most conspicuous
tracts of the brain stem, occupying the interval
between the midline and the inferior olivary
nucleus in the medulla (see Figs. 7-6 and 7-7).
Fibers that conduct sensory signals from the
contralateral foot are most ventral (i.e., adjacent to the pyramid). The opposite side of the
body is then represented sequentially, so that
fibers for the neck are in the most dorsal part of
the medial lemniscus. After traversing the pons
and midbrain, the tract ends in the lateral divi-

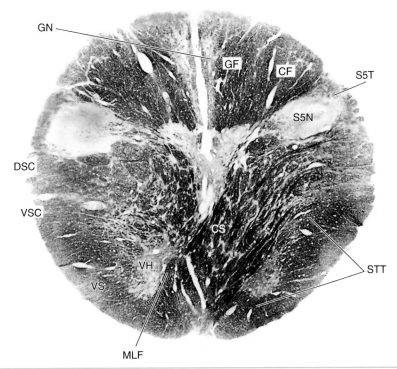

FIGURE 7-2   Junction of the medulla and spinal cord. Corticospinal fibers are passing from the pyramidal decussation into the lateral corticospinal tract (Weigert stain). **(See inside back cover of book for abbreviations used in figures in this chapter.)**

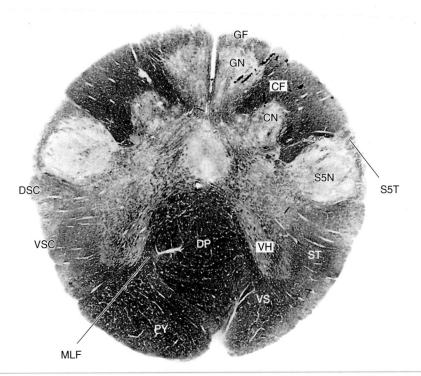

FIGURE 7-3   Medulla at the rostral end of the pyramidal decussation (Weigert stain). **For abbreviations see inside back cover of book.**

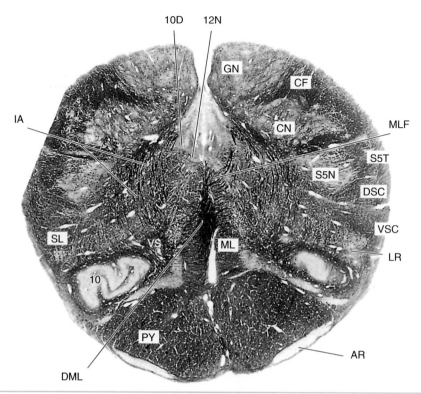

FIGURE 7-4   Medulla at the caudal end of the inferior olivary nucleus (Weigert stain). **For abbreviations see inside back cover of book.**

sion of the ventral posterior (VPl) nucleus of the thalamus. This is the thalamic nucleus for general somatic sensation.

Spinothalamic and Spinotectal Tracts

The spinothalamic tract for pain, temperature, and touch on the opposite side of the body continues into the medulla without appreciable change in position. This is also true of the spinotectal (or spinomesencephalic) tract, which conveys somesthetic data to the superior colliculus and the reticular formation of the midbrain. The two tracts soon merge to form the **spinal lemniscus**, which traverses the lateral area of the medulla dorsal to the inferior olivary nucleus (see Figs. 7-4 to 7-7). The spinothalamic fibers continue to the ventral posterior nucleus of the thalamus and send branches also to the intralaminar and posterior groups of nuclei of the thalamus. (The thalamic nuclei are described in Chapter 11.)

Spinoreticular Fibers

The spinoreticular tracts in the ventral and lateral white matter of the spinal cord continue into the brain stem, where their constituent axons synapse with cells of the reticular formation. They transmit sensory data, especially from the skin and internal organs. Some spinoreticular fibers are collateral branches of fibers of the spinothalamic tract. Axons of cells in the reticular formation project caudally to the spinal cord and rostrally to the thalamus.

There are at least three routes from the spinal cord to the thalamus and cerebral cortex. The **medial lemniscus system** proceeds without interruption, mainly to the ventral posterior thalamic nucleus, which, in turn, projects to the primary somatosensory area of the cerebral cortex. The **neospinothalamic system**, a mammalian pathway, consists of the axons of the tract cells that do not have collateral branches to the reticular formation. Sensory signals also reach the intralaminar group of thalamic nuclei through the **paleospinothalamic system**, which exists in all vertebrate animals. This less direct pathway consists of spinoreticular fibers (i.e., ones that are not collaterals of the spinothalamic tract) and reticulothalamic fibers, which are the rostrally projecting axons of neurons of the reticular formation. These as-

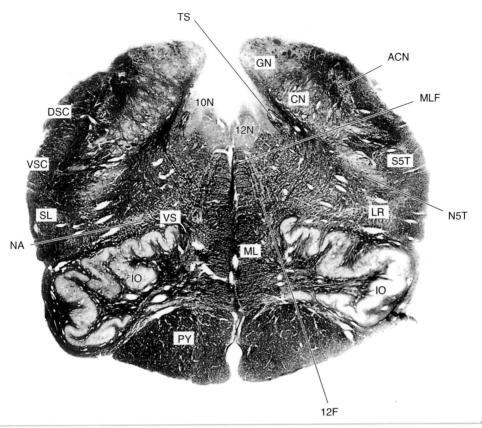

FIGURE 7-5   Medulla at the level of transition between its closed and open parts (Weigert stain). **For abbreviations see inside back cover of book.**

cending fibers form the reticular formation end in the intralaminar nuclei, which project to the cerebral cortex generally. This diffuse pathway influences levels of consciousness and degrees of alertness, and it is also involved in the awareness (but not the localization) of pain.

Spinocerebellar Tracts

The **dorsal** and **ventral spinocerebellar tracts**, which carry proprioceptive signals mainly from the lower limb, are located near the lateral surface of the medulla (see Figs. 7-2 to 7-6). The dorsal tract, which is uncrossed, originates in the nucleus thoracicus (nucleus dorsalis or Clarke's column) of the thoracic and upper lumbar segments of the spinal cord. The ventral tract, on the other hand, is largely crossed, and most of its cells of origin are in the lumbosacral enlargement of the spinal cord. The dorsal spinocerebellar fibers enter the inferior cerebellar peduncle (see Figs. 7-7 and 7-8), and the ventral spinocerebellar tract continues through the pons and enters the cerebellum

by way of the superior cerebellar peduncle. The spinocerebellar tracts serve the lower limb. For the upper limb, equivalent pathways involve the external cuneate nucleus.

MEDULLARY NUCLEI CONNECTED WITH THE CEREBELLUM

External Cuneate Nucleus

The external or accessory cuneate nucleus is lateral to the cuneate nucleus (see Fig. 7-5). The afferents to the external cuneate nucleus are fibers that enter the spinal cord in cervical dorsal roots, and many of them are collateral branches of axons that end in the cuneate nucleus. Efferents from the external cuneate nucleus enter the cerebellum by way of the inferior peduncle. These **cuneocerebellar fibers** provide a pathway to the cerebellum from proprioceptive and other sensory endings in the neck and upper limb. The functions of the

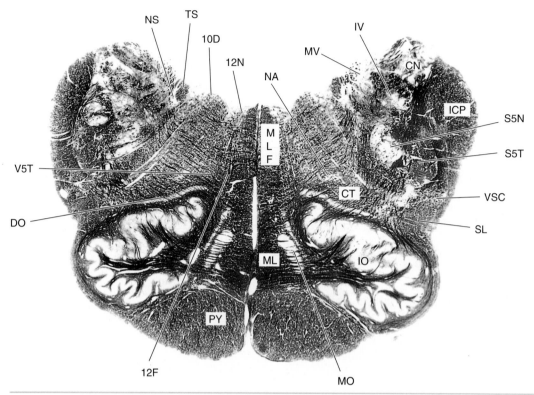

FIGURE 7-6   Medulla at the mid-olivary level (Weigert stain). **For abbreviations see inside back cover of book.**

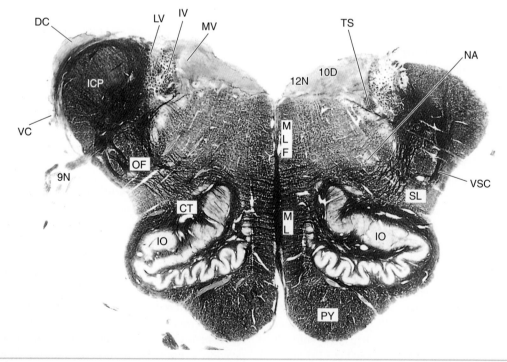

FIGURE 7-7   Rostral end of the medulla (Weigert stain). **For abbreviations see inside back cover of book.**

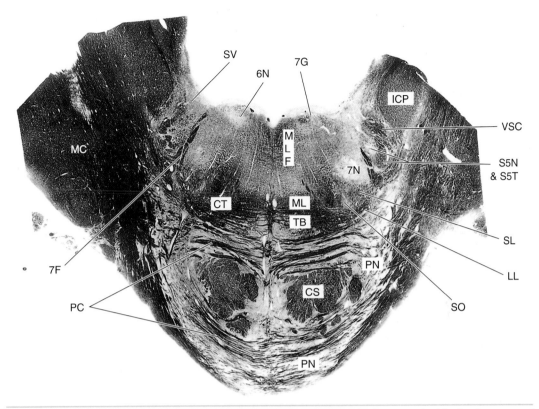

FIGURE 7-8 Caudal region of the pons (Weigert stain). **For abbreviations see inside back cover of book.**

external cuneate nucleus and cuneocerebellar tract are equivalent to those of the nucleus thoracicus and the dorsal spinocerebellar tract: both transmit proprioceptive signals along rapidly conducting axons to areas of cortex in and near the midline of the cerebellum (see Chapter 10).

Inferior Olivary Complex of Nuclei

Several groups of neurons in the medulla and pons are known as **precerebellar nuclei**. They receive afferents from various sources and project to the cerebellum. These nuclei include the components of the inferior olivary complex. The largest component is the **inferior olivary nucleus**, which is shaped like a crumpled bag or purse with the hilus facing medially (see Figs. 7-5 to 7-7). The inferior olivary complex receives afferents from the contralateral dorsal horn of all levels of the spinal cord and from the ipsilateral red nucleus (in the midbrain) and cerebral cortex.

The **central tegmental tract** is in part a pathway from the red nucleus and the periaqueductal gray matter of the midbrain to the inferior olivary complex. The terminal part of the central tegmental tract forms a dense layer on the dorsal surface of the inferior olivary nucleus, best seen in Figure 7-7. The tract also contains fibers that ascend to the diencephalon from the reticular formation of the brain stem and from the solitary nucleus (of the medulla).

Olivocerebellar fibers constitute the projection from the inferior olivary complex. Fibers from the principal nucleus occupy its interior and leave through the hilus. After decussating in the midline, the strands of myelinated olivocerebellar fibers curve in a dorsolateral direction through the reticular formation and enter the inferior cerebellar peduncle, of which they are the largest single component (see Fig. 7-7). The inferior olivary complex is the source of **climbing fibers**, which terminate on and excite the Purkinje cells in all parts of the cerebellar cortex. Physiological studies indicate that the inferior olivary complex of nuclei channels into the cerebellum programs of instructions for subsequent use in the coordination of learned patterns of movement.

Arcuate Nucleus

The arcuate nucleus on the surface of the pyramid (see Fig. 7-4) receives collateral branches of corticospinal fibers. The axons of cells in the arcuate nucleus enter the cerebellum by way of the inferior cerebellar peduncle, which they reach by two routes. Some travel over the lateral surface of the medulla as the **external arcuate fibers**; the remainder run dorsally in the midline of the medulla and then laterally in the **striae medullares** in the floor of the fourth ventricle. The connections of the arcuate nucleus are similar to those of the pontine nuclei (in the ventral part of the pons; see Chapter 10). Both receive afferents from the ipsilateral cerebral cortex and project across the midline to the cerebellum.

Lateral Reticular Nucleus

This exceptionally distinct group of cells of the reticular formation is dorsal to the inferior olivary nucleus and medial to the spinal lemniscus, near the surface of the medulla (see Figs. 7-4 to 7-6). It receives afferents from the spinal cord and projects to the cerebellum. Other precerebellar reticular nuclei are described in Chapter 9.

DESCENDING TRACTS

Corticospinal (Pyramidal) Tract

The parent cell bodies of the corticospinal (pyramidal) tract are located in an area of cerebral cortex that occupies adjoining regions of the frontal and parietal lobes. Their axons traverse the subcortical white matter, the internal capsule, and the brain stem. In the medulla, each corticospinal tract is a compact body of white matter in the pyramid (see Figs. 7-4 to 7-7).

In most people, about 85% of corticospinal fibers cross over in the **decussation of the pyramids**. The rostral end of this decussation appears in Figure 7-3, and a bundle of axons passing through the gray matter from a pyramid to the opposite **lateral corticospinal tract** is shown in Figure 7-2. The 15% of nondecussating fibers continue into the ventral funiculus of the cord as the **ventral corticospinal tract**.

Corticospinal fibers terminate in the base of the dorsal horn, the intermediate gray matter, and the ventral horn; a few synapse directly with motor neurons. Each pyramid contains approximately 1 million axons of varying size. The widest and most rapidly conducting ones come from the giant pyramidal cells of Betz in the primary motor area; these are the fibers believed to end in synaptic contact with the cell bodies of spinal motor neurons.

The corticospinal tracts are often thought of as having an exclusively motor function, and this is, indeed, their major function. Many axons of cortical origin arise in the primary somatosensory area (see Chapter 15); however, these modulate the transmission of sensory signals to the brain, by synapsing with neurons in the gracile and cuneate nuclei and in the dorsal horn of the spinal cord.

Tracts That Originate in the Midbrain

The **central tegmental tract** has already been mentioned as arising from the ipsilateral red nucleus and other gray areas of the midbrain. It terminates in the inferior olivary complex. A tiny bundle of axons from the contralateral red nucleus continues caudally as the **rubrospinal tract**, which comes to occupy a position ventral to the lateral corticospinal tract. In humans, this tract ends in the upper two cervical segments of the spinal cord.

The **tectospinal tract** originates in the superior colliculus of the midbrain, and the fibers cross at that level to the opposite side of the brain stem. The tract (see Fig. 5-10) is probably insignificantly small in humans. **Tectobulbar fibers** go from the superior colliculus to the reticular formation of the pons and upper medulla. They are involved in the control of eye movements (see Chapter 8).

NUCLEI OF CRANIAL NERVES AND ASSOCIATED TRACTS

Hypoglossal, Accessory, Vagus, and Glossopharyngeal Nerves

The **hypoglossal nucleus**, which contains motor neurons for the tongue muscles, is near the midline throughout most of the medulla in the central gray matter of the closed part (see Fig. 7-4) and beneath the hypoglossal trigone of the rhomboid fossa (see Figs. 7-5 to 7-7). The axons leaving the nucleus pass ventrally between the medial lemniscus and the inferior olivary nucleus (see Figs. 7-5 and 7-6) and then continue lateral to the pyramid, emerging as the rootlets of the hypoglossal nerve along the sulcus between the pyramid and the olive. The **nucleus ambiguus** lies within the reticular formation, dorsal to the inferior olivary nucleus (Figs. 7-5 to 7-7). This important cell column supplies the muscles of the soft palate, pharynx, larynx, and upper esophagus through the cranial root of the accessory nerve and the vagus and glossopharyngeal nerves. It also contains parasympathetic neurons whose axons end in the cardiac ganglia and control the heart rate. The **dorsal nucleus of the vagus nerve** is the largest parasympathetic nucleus in the brain stem; it contains the cell bodies of preganglionic neurons that regulate the activities of smooth muscle and glandular elements of the thoracic and abdominal viscera. The nucleus lies lateral to the hypoglossal nucleus in the gray matter that surrounds the central canal (see Fig. 7-4) and extends rostrally beneath the vagal trigone of the rhomboid fossa (see Figs. 7-5 to 7-7).

A bundle of visceral afferent fibers known as the **solitary tract** lies along the lateral side of the dorsal nucleus of the vagus nerve (see Figs. 7-5 to 7-7). This tract consists of caudally directed axons from the inferior ganglia of the vagus and glossopharyngeal nerves and the geniculate ganglion of the facial nerve. The fibers terminate in the **solitary nucleus** (nucleus of the solitary tract), a column of cells that lies adjacent to and partly surrounds the tract. The vagal and glossopharyngeal afferents to the caudal part of the solitary nucleus have important roles in visceral reflexes. Fibers mediating the sense of taste (mostly from ganglia of the facial and glossopharyngeal nerves) go to the rostral end of the nucleus.

Vestibulocochlear Nerve

Nuclei in the rostral part of the medulla receive afferent axons from the cochlear and vestibular divisions of the eighth cranial nerve. The **dorsal cochlear nucleus**, lying on the base of the inferior cerebellar peduncle, is shown in Figure 7-7, and part of the **ventral cochlear nucleus** appears lateral to the peduncle in the same

figure. Fibers leaving the cochlear nuclei are noted later in the description of the pons.

The **vestibular nuclei**, beneath the vestibular area of the rhomboid fossa, comprise the **superior, lateral, medial,** and **inferior vestibular nuclei,** which differ in their cytoarchitecture and connections. Whereas the superior nucleus is located in the pons (see Fig. 7-8), the remaining nuclei are located in the medulla (see Figs. 7-6 and 7-7). The vestibular nerve penetrates the brain stem ventral to the inferior cerebellar peduncle and medial and slightly rostral to the attachment of the cochlear nerve. Most vestibular nerve fibers end in the vestibular nuclei, but a few enter the cerebellum through the inferior peduncle. In addition to the primary vestibulocerebellar fibers, numerous secondary fibers proceed from the vestibular nuclei into the cerebellum through the inferior peduncle.

Vestibular nuclei project to the spinal cord by way of two tracts. The larger is the **vestibulospinal tract** (sometimes called the lateral vestibulospinal tract), for which the cells of origin are in the lateral vestibular nucleus. Vestibulospinal fibers run caudally, dorsal to the inferior olivary nucleus, in the position indicated in Figures 7-4 and 7-5. The tract is deflected ventrally at the level of the pyramidal decussation (see Figs. 7-2 and 7-3) and continues into the ipsilateral ventral funiculus of the spinal cord.

Fibers from the left and right medial vestibular nuclei account for most of those in each **medial longitudinal fasciculus**, a bundle that extends rostrally and caudally adjacent to the midline (see Figs. 7-2 to 7-7). The ascending fibers will be identified later in the discussion of the pons and midbrain. The small bundle of descending fibers, which are mainly from ipsilateral cell bodies, is sometimes called the medial vestibulospinal tract. Below the pyramidal decussation, it is joined by the nearby ventral corticospinal and tectospinal tracts.

Trigeminal Nerve

The trigeminal nerve contributes a tract and associated nucleus to the internal structure of the medulla. Many fibers of the trigeminal sensory root turn caudally on entering the pons. They constitute the **spinal trigeminal tract**, so named because many of these axons extend as far as the third cervical segment of the spinal cord. The spinal tract transmits data for pain, temperature, and touch from the extensive area of distribution of the trigeminal nerve (most of the head; see Chapter 8). The tract also receives primary afferent fibers from the other three cranial nerves (facial, glossopharyngeal, and vagus) that have general somatic sensory functions. Axons leave the tract at all levels from the caudal pons to the second or third cervical segment of the spinal cord. They terminate in the **spinal trigeminal nucleus** (nucleus of the spinal trigeminal tract), which is located alongside and medial to the tract. The spinal trigeminal tract and its nucleus share several structural and functional characteristics with the dorsolateral tract of Lissauer and the outermost four laminae of the dorsal horn of the spinal gray matter, with which the nucleus is continuous.

The longest descending fibers in the spinal trigeminal tract are unmyelinated or thinly myelinated, and they carry signals relating to pain and temperature. The first synapses in the pathway for these types of sensation are, therefore, located in the most caudal part of the spinal trigeminal nucleus in the closed medulla and the uppermost cervical levels of the spinal cord.

The **ventral trigeminothalamic tract** (see Fig. 7-6) is a crossed fasciculus that arises from neurons in the spinal (and pontine) trigeminal nuclei and in the adjacent part of the reticular formation. It ends in the medial division of the ventral posterior nucleus of the thalamus (VPm). Conducting sensory signals from the opposite side of the head, the ventral trigeminothalamic tract is functionally comparable to the spinothalamic tract for the parts of the body below the neck.

Dorsal Pons (Tegmentum)

The main features seen in sections through the pons are its division into basal (ventral) and tegmental (dorsal) regions and the prominent cerebellar peduncles (see Figs. 7-8 and 7-9). The pontine tegmentum is structurally simi-

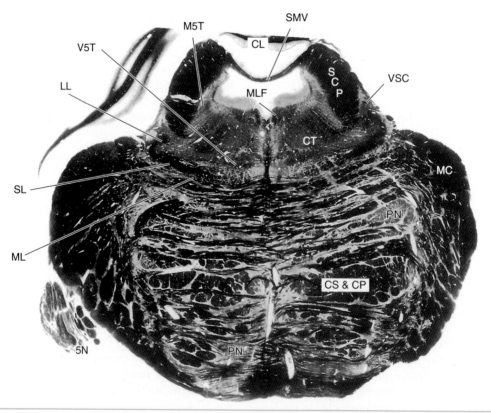

FIGURE 7-9 Section through the middle of the pons (Weigert stain). **For abbreviations see inside back cover of book.**

lar to the medulla and midbrain. There are, therefore, tracts that were encountered in the medulla, together with components of several cranial nerves.

TRACTS AND CEREBELLAR PEDUNCLES

The **medial lemniscus** twists as it leaves the medulla, rotating in such a way that in the ventral pontine tegmentum, the fibers from the cuneate nucleus are medial to those from the gracile nucleus. Therefore, the somatotopic representation is neck, arm, trunk, and leg, in a medial-to-lateral sequence. The **spinal lemniscus** is near the lateral edge of the medial lemniscus throughout the pons (see Figs. 7-8 to 7-10). The **ventral spinocerebellar tract** traverses the most lateral part of the tegmentum (see Fig. 7-8) and then curves dorsally and enters the cerebellum through the superior peduncle (see Figs. 7-9 and 7-11).

With respect to descending tracts, the **central tegmental tract** is medial to the fibers of the superior cerebellar peduncle at the level of the pon-

tine isthmus (see Fig. 7-10), in the central area of the tegmentum at midpontine levels (see Fig. 7-9), and dorsal to the medial lemniscus in the caudal region of the pons (see Fig. 7-8). As in the medulla and spinal cord, the **medial longitudinal fasciculus** is located near the midline in the pontine tegmentum (see Figs. 7-8 to 7-10).

The **inferior cerebellar peduncles** enter the cerebellum from the caudal part of the pons. At this level, they lie medial to the middle cerebellar peduncles and form the lateral walls of the fourth ventricle (see Fig. 7-8). Olivocerebellar fibers are the most numerous in the inferior peduncle, followed by fibers of the dorsal spinocerebellar tract. The region of the inferior cerebellar peduncle immediately adjoining the fourth ventricle consists of fibers that enter the cerebellum from the vestibular nerve and vestibular nuclei, together with fibers that arise in the parts of the cerebellum concerned with maintaining equilibrium. Most of the latter fibers terminate in the vestibular nuclei.

The **superior cerebellar peduncles** (see Fig. 7-9) consist mainly of fibers that originate in

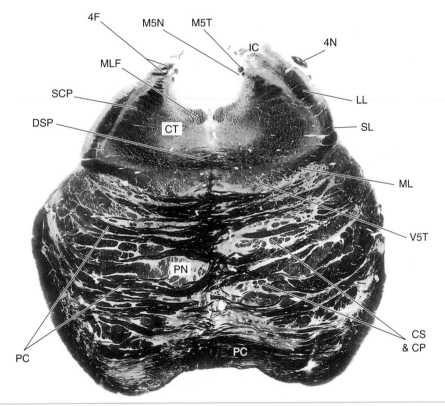

FIGURE 7-10 Rostral part of the pons, including the isthmus region of the pontine tegmentum (Weigert stain). **For abbreviations see inside back cover of book.**

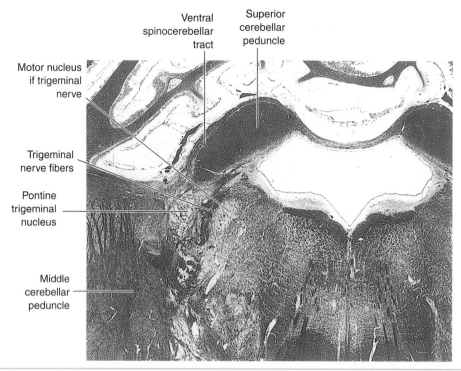

FIGURE 7-11   Part of a section through the middle of the pons at the level of the pontine and motor trigeminal nuclei (Weigert stain).

cerebellar nuclei and enter the brain stem immediately caudal to the inferior colliculi of the midbrain. The fibers cross the midline at the level of the inferior colliculi in the **decussation of the superior cerebellar peduncles** (see Figs. 7-10, 7-12, and 7-13). Most of these fibers continue rostrally to the thalamus, and the remainder end in the red nucleus and in the reticular formation. The superior cerebellar peduncle also contains fibers that enter the cerebellum: the ventral spinocerebellar tract and some axons from the mesencephalic trigeminal nucleus and the red nucleus.

NUCLEI OF CRANIAL NERVES AND ASSOCIATED TRACTS

Vestibulocochlear Nerve

Fibers from the dorsal and ventral cochlear nuclei cross the pons to ascend in the lateral lemniscus of the opposite side. Most of the decussating fibers constitute the **trapezoid body** (see Fig. 7-8), which intersects the medial lemnisci. It is difficult to distinguish these slender bundles of acoustic fibers from nearby bundles

of pontocerebellar fibers. The axons from the ventral cochlear nuclei end in the **superior olivary nucleus** (see Fig. 7-8), from which more ascending fibers are added to the auditory pathway. Fibers from the dorsal cochlear and superior olivary nuclei turn rostrally in the lateral part of the tegmentum to form the **lateral lemniscus** (see Fig. 7-8). This tract is lateral to the medial lemniscus in the first part of its course (see Fig. 7-9) and then moves dorsally to end in the inferior colliculus of the midbrain (see Figs. 7-10 and 7-12). The auditory pathway, which continues to the thalamus and cerebral cortex, is more fully described in Chapter 21.

One of the four vestibular nuclei, the **superior vestibular nucleus**, extends into the pons (see Fig. 7-8). Fibers from the vestibular nuclei, some crossed and some uncrossed, ascend in the **medial longitudinal fasciculus**, which is next to the midline and close to the floor of the fourth ventricle throughout the pons (see Figs. 7-8 to 7-12). The fibers terminate mainly in the abducens, trochlear, and oculomotor nuclei, establishing connections that coordinate movements of the eyes with movements of the head.

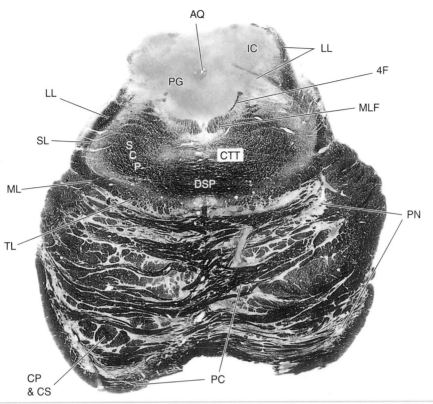

FIGURE 7-12   Section that passes through the rostral end of the basal pons and the caudal ends of the inferior colliculi of the midbrain (Weigert stain). **For abbreviations see inside back cover of book.**

The medial longitudinal fasciculus also contains other groups of fibers concerned with eye movements; these are discussed in Chapter 8.

Facial and Abducens Nerves

The **facial motor nucleus**, which supplies the muscles of expression, is a prominent group of typical motor neurons in the ventrolateral part of the tegmentum (see Fig. 7-8). Axons arising from the nucleus course dorsomedially and then form a compact bundle, the **internal genu**, which loops over the caudal end of the abducens nucleus beneath the facial colliculus of the rhomboid fossa. The bundle of fibers that forms the genu then runs forward along the medial side of the abducens nucleus and curves again over its rostral end (see right side of Fig. 7-8). After leaving the genu, the fibers pass between the nucleus of origin and the spinal trigeminal nucleus, emerging as the motor root of the facial nerve at the junction of the pons and medulla.

The **abducens nucleus** innervates the lateral rectus muscle of the eye and also contains

internuclear neurons. It is located beneath the facial colliculus, as noted previously (see Fig. 7-8). The efferent motor fibers of the nucleus proceed ventrally with a caudal inclination and leave the brain stem as the abducens nerve between the pons and the pyramid of the medulla (see Fig. 6-1). The **internuclear neurons** have axons that travel in the contralateral medial longitudinal fasciculus to the division of the oculomotor nucleus that supplies the medial rectus muscle. This arrangement provides for simultaneous contraction of the lateral rectus and contralateral medial rectus when the eyes move in the horizontal plane.

Trigeminal Nerve

The **spinal trigeminal tract** and **nucleus** are located in the lateral part of the tegmentum of the caudal half of the pons (see Fig. 7-8), lateral to the fibers of the facial nerve. The pontine tegmentum also contains two other trigeminal nuclei (see Fig. 7-11). The **pontine trigeminal nucleus** (also known as the chief or principal

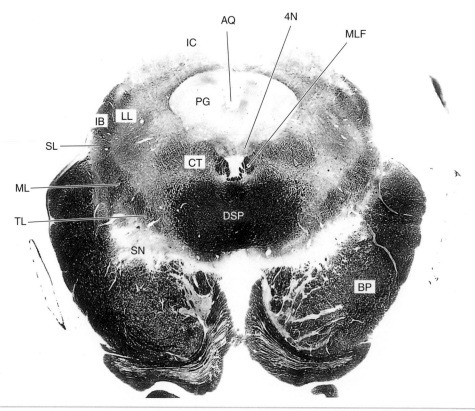

FIGURE 7-13   Midbrain at the level of the rostral ends of the inferior colliculi (Weigert stain). **For abbreviations see inside back cover of book.**

nucleus) is located at the rostral end of the spinal trigeminal nucleus. It receives fibers for touch, especially discriminative touch. Fibers from the pontine trigeminal nucleus project to the thalamus, along with fibers from the spinal nucleus, in the **ventral trigeminothalamic tract** (see Figs. 7-9 and 7-10). A **dorsal trigeminothalamic tract**, consisting of crossed and uncrossed fibers, originates exclusively in the pontine trigeminal nuclei. (Alternatively, all the trigeminothalamic fibers are said to compose the **trigeminal lemniscus**.) The **motor nucleus**, which is medial to the pontine trigeminal nucleus (see Fig. 7-11), contains the motor neurons that supply the muscles of mastication and a few other muscles.

The **mesencephalic trigeminal nucleus** is a slender column of cells beneath the lateral edge of the rostral part of the fourth ventricle (see Figs. 7-9 and 7-10), extending into the midbrain. These unipolar cells are unusual because they are cell bodies of primary sensory neurons and the only such cells in the central nervous

system. The axons of the unipolar neurons form the **mesencephalic tract of the trigeminal nerve** (see Figs. 7-9 and 7-10); most are distributed through the mandibular division of the nerve to proprioceptive endings in the muscles of mastication.

Ventral or Basal Pons

The basal or ventral part of the pons (see Figs. 7-8 to 7-10) is especially large in humans because of its connections with the cortices of the cerebral and cerebellar hemispheres. The basal part of the pons consists of longitudinal and transverse fiber bundles and the pontine nuclei, which are collections of neurons that lie among the bundles. The longitudinal bundles are numerous and small at rostral levels (see Figs. 7-9 and 7-10), but many coalesce as they approach the medulla (see Fig. 7-8).

The longitudinal fasciculi are descending fibers that enter the pons from the basis pedunculi of the midbrain. Many are **corticospinal fibers** that pass through the pons to reassemble as the pyramids of the medulla. Numerous **corticopontine fibers**, which originate in widespread areas of cerebral cortex and establish synaptic contact with cells of the **pontine nuclei** of the same side, are also present. Except in the caudal one third of the pons, where large regions of pontine gray matter are present (see Fig. 7-8), the pontine nuclei are small groups of cells scattered among the longitudinal and transverse fasciculi (see Figs. 7-9 and 7-10). The axons of the neurons of the pontine nuclei cross the midline, forming the conspicuous transverse bundles of **pontocerebellar fibers**, and enter the cerebellum through the **middle cerebellar peduncle**. The activities of the cerebral cortex are thus made available to the cerebellar cortex through the relay in the pontine nuclei. The cerebellar cortex influences motor areas in the frontal lobe of the cerebral hemisphere through a pathway that includes the dentate nucleus of the cerebellum and the ventral lateral nucleus of the thalamus. The well-developed circuit linking the cerebral and cer-

ebellar cortices contributes to the precision and efficiency of voluntary movements.

Midbrain

The internal structure of the midbrain is shown in Figures 7-12 to 7-15. The sections shown in Figures 7-12 and 7-13 are through the inferior colliculi. The planes of the sections are such that Figure 7-12 includes the basal pons, and Figure 7-13 shows the extreme rostral lip of the basal pons (see Fig. 7-1). Figures 7-14 and 7-15 show more rostral levels that include the superior colliculi and certain thalamic nuclei that are in the same transverse plane.

For descriptive purposes, the midbrain is divided into the following regions (see Fig. 7-14): the **tectum**, which consists of the paired inferior and superior **colliculi** (corpora quadrigemina); the **basis pedunculi**, which is a dense mass of descending fibers; and the **substantia nigra**, which is a prominent zone of gray matter immediately dorsal to the basis pedunculi. The remainder of the midbrain comprises the **teg-**

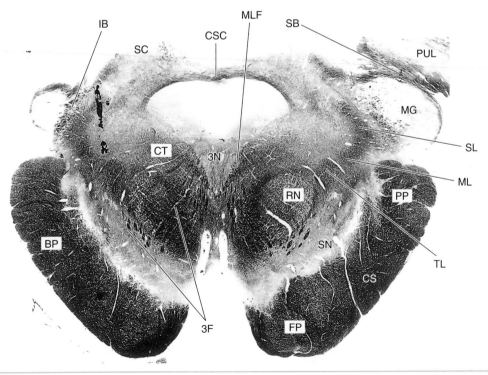

FIGURE 7-14   Midbrain at the level of the superior colliculi (Weigert stain). **For abbreviations see inside back cover of book.**

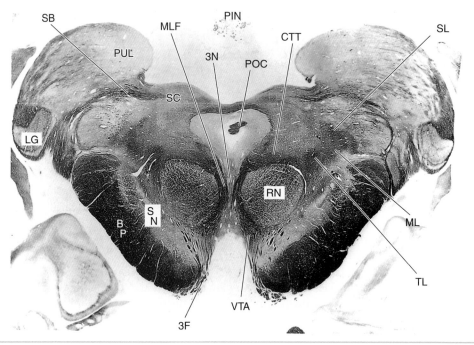

FIGURE 7-15   Midbrain at the level of the rostral ends of the superior colliculi. The section also includes parts of the thalamus and some cortex of the temporal lobes (Weigert stain). **For abbreviations see inside back cover of book.**

mentum, which contains fiber tracts, the prominent red nuclei, and the periaqueductal gray matter surrounding the cerebral aqueduct. The term **cerebral peduncle** refers to all of the midbrain on each side, exclusive of the tectum.

TECTUM AND ASSOCIATED TRACTS

Inferior Colliculus

The inferior colliculus is a large nucleus of the auditory pathway. Fibers of the lateral lemniscus envelop and enter the nucleus (see Fig. 7-12). Fibers leaving the inferior colliculus traverse the inferior brachium to reach the medial geniculate body of the thalamus (see Figs. 7-13 to 7-15), which, in turn, projects to the auditory cortex in the temporal lobe. Commissural fibers are present between the inferior colliculi, accounting partly for the bilateral cortical projection from each ear.

Some axons from the inferior colliculus pass forward into the superior colliculus. From the latter site, through a polysynaptic pathway described in Chapter 8, auditory signals reach cranial nerve nuclei that supply the extraocular muscles, and a few tectospinal fibers influence spinal motor neurons in the cervical region. A pathway is thereby established for reflex turning of the eyes and head toward the source of an unexpected sound.

Superior Colliculus

The superior colliculus (see Figs. 7-14 and 7-15) has a complex structure consisting of seven alternating layers of white and gray matter; its connections are with the visual system. Corticotectal fibers come from the visual cortex in the occipital lobe, from adjacent parietal cortex, and from an area of the frontal lobe called the frontal eye field. The corticotectal fibers (which are ipsilateral) make up most of the **superior brachium**, which reaches the superior colliculus by passing between the pulvinar and the medial geniculate body of the thalamus (see Figs. 7-14 and 7-15). Through collicular efferents (to be described), this connection between the cortex and the superior colliculus is responsible for both voluntary and involuntary movements of the eyes and head, as when rapidly shifting the direction of gaze (saccadic movements) or when following objects passing across the visual field (smooth pursuit movements). Corticotectal fibers that originate in the occipital cortex also participate in the ocular response of accommodation (i.e., thickening of the lens and constriction of the pupil), which accompanies convergence of the eyes when viewing a near object.

Some fibers of the optic tract reach the superior colliculus by way of the superior brachium and constitute the afferent limb of a reflex pathway that assists in turning the eyes and head to follow an object moving across the field of vision. In addition, spinotectal fibers terminate in the superior colliculus and transmit data from general sensory endings, especially those in the skin. These connections presumably serve to direct the eyes and head toward sources of cutaneous stimuli. Another source of afferents to the superior colliculus is the pars reticulata of the substantia nigra, which thereby connects the corpus striatum (see Chapter 12) with the parts of the midbrain that control movements of the eyes and head.

Efferents from the superior colliculus are distributed to the spinal cord and nuclei of the brain stem. The few fibers destined for the spinal cord curve around the periaqueductal gray matter, cross to the opposite side in the **dorsal tegmental decussation**, and continue caudally near the midline as the tectospinal tract. Efferents to the brain stem, known as **tectobulbar fibers**, are, for the most part, directed bilaterally. They go to the pretectal area, the accessory oculomotor nuclei, and the paramedian pontine reticular formation. These regions project to the nuclei of the nerves that supply the eye muscles. (Neural control of these muscles is discussed in Chapter 8.) Other efferent fibers from the superior colliculus terminate in the reticular formation near the motor nucleus of the facial nerve, providing a reflex pathway for protective closure of the eyelids when there is a sudden visual stimulus.

The superior colliculi are interconnected by the **commissure of the superior colliculi** (see Fig. 7-14). The **posterior commissure** is a robust bundle that runs transversely, just dorsal to the transition between the cerebral aqueduct and the third ventricle. A small piece of this commissure is included in the section shown in Figure 7-15. Fibers in the posterior commissure come from the superior colliculus and from the following nearby smaller nuclei: pretectal area,

habenular nuclei (in the epithalamus of the diencephalon), and the accessory oculomotor nuclei of the midbrain (which are reviewed in Chapter 9).

Pretectal Area

The pretectal area consists of four pairs of small nuclei rostral to the lateral edge of the superior colliculus. One of the pretectal nuclei, the **olivary pretectal nucleus**, receives fibers from both retinas by way of the ipsilateral optic tract and the superior brachium. Axons arising in the olivary pretectal nucleus go to the Edinger-Westphal nucleus of each side. The latter nucleus is the source of the preganglionic parasympathetic fibers in the oculomotor nerve. The pretectal area is thereby included in a reflex pathway for constriction of the pupils in response to increased intensity of light. The pretectal area also has connections that implicate it in pathways for the control of eye movements, including convergence (see Chapter 8).

TEGMENTUM

Fasciculi Proceeding to the Thalamus

The **medial lemniscus** traverses the midbrain in the lateral area of the tegmentum to its termination in the ventral posterior nucleus of the thalamus (see Figs. 7-13 to 7-15). The **spinal lemniscus** is dorsolateral to the medial lemniscus; this spatial relation is continued from the pontine tegmentum. Spinotectal fibers leave the spinal lemniscus to enter the superior colliculus and the periaqueductal gray matter. The spinothalamic fibers continue into the diencephalon, where they end in the ventral posterior and other thalamic nuclei. Some spinothalamic fibers send branches into the periaqueductal gray matter of the midbrain.

Red Nucleus and Associated Tracts

The red nucleus is egg shaped (round in transverse section) and extends from the caudal limit of the superior colliculus into the subthalamic region of the diencephalon. The nucleus is more vascular than the surrounding tissue and is named for its pinkish hue in a fresh specimen. Myelinated axons that pass through the red nucleus give it a punctate appearance in Weigert-stained sections (see Figs. 7-14 and 7-15).

Afferent fibers from the contralateral cerebellum reach the red nucleus by way of the superior cerebellar peduncle and its decussation (see Fig. 7-13). Corticorubral fibers come from the motor areas of the ipsilateral cerebral hemisphere. Many other afferents to the red nucleus have been detected in animals, but their significance in the human brain is not known.

The red nucleus gives rise to a small number of axons that cross the midline in the **ventral tegmental decussation** and continue through the brain stem into the lateral funiculus of the spinal cord as the rubrospinal tract. This is a minor pathway in the human brain, and its few fibers terminate in the first two segments of the cervical spinal gray matter. In laboratory animals, some descending fibers from the red nucleus end in the facial motor nucleus and in those nuclei of the reticular formation that project to the cerebellum. In addition to these crossed projections, large numbers of **rubroolivary fibers** travel in the ipsilateral **central tegmental tract** to terminate in the inferior olivary complex of nuclei, which projects across the midline to the cerebellum.

NUCLEI OF CRANIAL NERVES AND ASSOCIATED TRACTS

The midbrain contains nuclei of three cranial nerves as well as certain tracts that originate in the sensory nuclei of cranial nerves in the medulla and pons.

Vestibulocochlear Nerve

The **lateral lemniscus** was identified in the discussion of the inferior colliculus. The **medial longitudinal fasciculus** is adjacent to the midline (see Figs. 7-12 to 7-15) in the same general position as at lower levels. Most of its fibers originate in vestibular nuclei, and those that reach the midbrain end in the trochlear, oculomotor, and accessory oculomotor nuclei. The fasciculus also contains the axons of **internuclear neurons**, which connect the abducens, trochlear, and oculomotor nuclei.

Trigeminal Nerve

The **trigeminal lemniscus**, comprising fibers from the spinal and pontine trigeminal nuclei, is medial to the medial lemniscus (see Figs. 7-12 to 7-15). The **mesencephalic nucleus** of the trigeminal nerve continues from the pons into the lateral region of the periaqueductal gray matter up to the level of the superior colliculus.

Trochlear and Oculomotor Nerves

The **trochlear nucleus** is located in the periaqueductal gray matter at the level of the inferior colliculus, where it lies just dorsal to the medial longitudinal fasciculus (see Fig. 7-13). Fibers from the nucleus curve dorsally around the periaqueductal gray matter, with a caudal slope (see Figs. 7-10 and 7-12). On reaching the dorsal surface of the brain stem, the fibers decussate in the superior medullary velum and emerge as the trochlear nerve just below the inferior colliculi. The trochlear nerve supplies the superior oblique muscle of the eye.

The **oculomotor nucleus** is actually a group of subnuclei in and adjacent to the midline in the ventral part of the periaqueductal gray matter at the level of the superior colliculus. The paired nuclei have a V-shaped outline in sections (see Figs. 7-14 and 7-15). Bundles of axons from the nucleus curve ventrally through the tegmentum, with many of them passing through the red nucleus (see Fig. 7-14), and then emerge along the side of the interpeduncular fossa to form the oculomotor nerve (see Figs. 6-1 and 7-15). The oculomotor nerve supplies four of the six extraocular muscles (all except the lateral rectus and superior oblique) and the striated fibers of the levator palpebrae superioris muscle, which raises the upper eyelid. Distinct subnuclei supply the individual muscles. The oculomotor nuclear complex includes a functionally different parasympathetic component, the **Edinger-Westphal nucleus**, concerned with the ciliary and sphincter pupillae muscles of the eye (see Chapter 8).

SUBSTANTIA NIGRA

The substantia nigra is a large nucleus situated between the tegmentum and the basis pedunculi throughout the midbrain (see Figs. 7-13 to 7-15) and extending into the subthalamic region of the diencephalon. The black color is caused by the dopaminergic neurons of the **pars compacta**, adjacent to the tegmentum. These cells contain cytoplasmic inclusion granules of melanin pigment. The melanin granules are few at birth; their numbers increase rapidly during childhood and then more slowly throughout life. The pigment, which is present in albinos, is also known as neuromelanin to distinguish it from the pigment of skin. It is probably a by-product of the metabolism of **dopamine**, which is the neurotransmitter used by these cells. The substantia nigra is connected with the corpus striatum, a large body of gray matter in the forebrain, and it is included in the functional system known as the **basal ganglia**.

The major source of fibers afferent to the pars compacta is the striatum (a part of the cor-

---

CLINICAL NOTE

Parkinson's Disease

The importance of the substantia nigra is apparent when the disturbances of motor function in **Parkinson's disease** (paralysis agitans) are considered. The clinical features of this crippling disorder are muscular rigidity, a slow tremor, and bradykinesia (or poverty of movement). The last is manifest as a masklike face, difficulty in initiating movements, and loss of associated involuntary movements such as swinging the arms when walking. All three features combine to cause a shuffling gait, with a tendency to fall forward and difficulty in stopping. The most consistent pathological finding in Parkinson's disease is degeneration of the melanin-containing cells in the pars compacta of the substantia nigra. Most cases of Parkinson's disease have no known cause, but a few are caused by poisons, including manganese compounds (industrial exposure in some mines) and MPTP (1-methyl-4-phenyl-1,2,4,6-tetrahydropyridine), a compound present in illegally manufactured heroin. Some drugs (see below) can cause transient parkinsonian symptoms by blocking the normal actions of dopamine at synapses.

Biochemical and histochemical research in the 1960s provided the basis for modern medical therapy. The normally high concentrations of dopamine in the substantia nigra and striatum are greatly reduced in patients with Parkinson's disease. Administration of dopamine might replace the regulatory action of the substantia nigra on the striatum, but this amine does not cross the blood–brain barrier. Therefore, a metabolic precursor that does gain access to brain tissue is used instead. This precursor is L-dopa (L-dihydroxyphenylalanine; also called levodopa), and its conversion to dopamine occurs in the surviving neurons of the pars compacta. The administration of L-dopa does not stop the loss of neurons, but it does relieve the motor abnormalities in Parkinson's disease until there are not enough nigral neurons left to deliver dopamine to the striatum.

Other drugs used to treat parkinsonism include anticholinergic agents and inhibitors of an enzyme that degrades dopamine. The former work indirectly by suppressing the actions of the cholinergic interneurons of the striatum.

The traditional surgical treatment of Parkinson's disease consists of destroying parts of the brain that are overactive when there is not enough dopaminergic modulation of the striatum. Clinical experimentation in the 1940s and 1950s led to the adoption of either the globus pallidus or the ventral lateral nucleus of the thalamus as the site of choice for such lesions, but transient relief of parkinsonian symptoms followed either surgical or spontaneous pathological damage almost anywhere in the base of the cerebral hemisphere. Magnetic resonance imaging (MRI; see Chapter 4) allows for electrical recording and stimulation at anatomically known sites in the diencephalon and corpus striatum, so it is now possible to locate lesions more accurately than in earlier years of the disease process. Surgical ablations in the thalamus **(thalamotomy)** relieve tremor and rigidity but not bradykinesia. With lesions in the ventral medial part of the globus pallidus **(pallidotomy)**, relief of rigidity and bradykinesia takes place. In recent years, symptomatic relief has been achieved with stimulating electrodes chronically implanted in the pallidum, thalamus, or subthalamic nucleus.

In the 1980s and 1990s, many attempts were made to treat patients with Parkinson's disease by transplanting cells potentially capable of secreting dopamine (taken from aborted human fetuses) into the corpus striatum. Clinical follow-up and postmortem studies, which became available in the early 1990s, showed that symptomatic relief was usually transient. Experimentation with human fetal transplants has continued, and it is now generally agreed that any resulting clinical improvement is minor and seldom lasts for more than a few months except in some younger patients. Trials involving sham-operated patients indicate that transient improvement is a placebo effect. Other current research in the field of therapeutic grafting is directed toward the potential use of genetically modified cells that might produce dopamine and form appropriate synaptic connections in the corpus striatum.

pus striatum comprising the caudate nucleus and the putamen of the lentiform nucleus). The efferent fibers from the pars compacta go to the striatum. These connections form part of a larger piece of neuronal circuitry, discussed in Chapters 12 and 23.

The region of the substantia nigra bordering the basis pedunculi consists of cells that lack pigment and is called the **pars reticulata**. It is a detached part of the internal segment of the globus pallidus, which is part of the corpus striatum (see Chapter 12). The pars reticulata contains neurons that project to the same thalamic nuclei that receive input from the pallidum, and it also sends fibers to the superior colliculus, providing a pathway whereby the basal ganglia participate in the control of eye movements.

Ventral Tegmental Area

The ventral tegmental area is another population of dopaminergic neurons, on the medial aspect of the cerebral peduncle, between the substantia nigra and the red nucleus (see Fig. 7-15). The axons of these cells end in the hypothalamus, amygdala, hippocampal formation, nucleus accumbens, and elsewhere. These projections, sometimes called the **mesolimbic dopaminergic system**, have been intensively studied in animals because their actions are blocked by drugs that are used in the clinical management of patients with schizophrenia and other mental disorders. The drugs antagonize dopamine at its postsynaptic receptors, and their most serious adverse effect is a syndrome that resembles Parkinson's disease.

BASIS PEDUNCULI

The basis pedunculi (crus cerebri) consists of fibers of the pyramidal and corticopontine systems (see Figs. 7-13 to 7-15 and Chapter 23).

Corticospinal fibers constitute the middle three fifths of the basis pedunculi; the somatotopic arrangement is that of fibers for the neck, arm, trunk, and leg in a medial-to-lateral direction.

Corticobulbar (corticonuclear) fibers are located between the corticospinal and frontopontine tracts, but many leave the basis pedunculi and continue to their destinations through the tegmentum of the midbrain and pons. The majority of the corticobulbar fibers end in the reticular formation near the motor nuclei of cranial nerves (the trigeminal and facial motor nuclei, nucleus ambiguus, and hypoglossal nucleus). A few of the fibers make direct synaptic contacts with the motor neurons in these nuclei. In addition to these pathways, which have obvious motor functions, corticobulbar fibers to the pontine and spinal trigeminal nuclei and to the solitary nucleus are present. Axons of cortical origin that end in the gracile and cuneate nuclei are also classified as corticobulbar. Thus, corticobulbar connections are involved in modulating the transmission of sensory information rostrally from the brain stem as well as in the control of movement.

Corticopontine fibers are divided into two large bundles. The **frontopontine tract** occupies the medial one-fifth of the basis pedunculi. The lateral one fifth consists of the **parietotemporopontine tract**, which contains fibers from the parietal, occipital, and temporal lobes. Corticopontine fibers end in the basal pons, synapsing with the neurons of the pontine nuclei.

Visceral Pathways in the Brain Stem

The **ascending visceral pathways** in the spinal cord are situated in the ventral and ventrolateral funiculi. They may be considered to be parts of the spinothalamic and spinoreticular tracts. Signals of visceral origin reach the reticular formation, thalamus, and hypothalamus.

Physiologically important visceral sensory fibers reach the **solitary nucleus** in the medulla by way of the vagus and glossopharyngeal nerves (see Chapter 8). The solitary nucleus also receives afferents for taste, mainly through the glossopharyngeal and facial nerves. Ascending fibers from the solitary nucleus travel ipsilaterally in the **central tegmental tract** and terminate in the hypothalamus and in the most medial part of the ventral posterior medial nucleus of the thalamus. From the latter site, information with respect to taste is relayed to a cortical taste area in the parietal and insular lobes. A small **solitariospinal tract**, which originates in the solitary nucleus and nearby parts of the reticular formation, terminates on

Anatomical and Clinical Correlations

Vascular lesions are among the more important causes of damage to the brain. **Hemorrhage** into the brain stem usually has serious consequences (such as sudden death or coma) because the escaping blood destroys regions of the reticular formation that control the vital functions of respiration, circulation, and consciousness. Some effects of large lesions in the brain stem are discussed in Chapter 9. **Vascular occlusion** can cause smaller destructive lesions, resulting in neu-

rological signs that depend on the location and size of the affected region. Symptoms and clinical signs can indicate the level of a lesion in the brain stem as well as the medial, lateral, dorsal, or ventral location of the lesion. The level is deduced largely from the anatomy of the nuclei of the affected cranial nerves. Interruption of motor or sensory pathways or connections with the cerebellum can establish the lateral, medial, dorsal, or ventral position of a lesion. Clinical imaging of the brain stem, especially MRI, is valuable but is less precise and, consequently, less accurate than deductions based on knowledge of neuroanatomy.

preganglionic autonomic neurons in the spinal cord and possibly also on neurons that supply respiratory muscles. Some axons ascend from nuclei of the reticular formation to the hypothalamus in the **dorsal longitudinal fasciculus**, which also contains descending fibers (see next paragraph and Chapter 11).

There are two descending pathways whose cells of origin are located in the hypothalamus. **Mamillotegmental fibers** originate in the mamillary body of the hypothalamus; they terminate in the reticular formation of the midbrain, which projects to autonomic nuclei in the brain stem and spinal cord. Fibers from other hypothalamic nuclei, notably the paraventricular nucleus, run caudally in the **dorsal longitudinal fasciculus**, a bundle of mostly unmyelinated fibers in the periaqueductal gray matter of the midbrain. Some terminate in the reticular formation of the brain stem and the dorsal nucleus of the vagus nerve, and the hypothalamospinal fibers proceed to autonomic nuclei in the spinal cord. Thus, impulses of hypothalamic origin reach the preganglionic sympathetic and sacral parasympathetic neurons both directly and through relays in the reticular formation. Clinical evidence indicates that fibers influencing the sympathetic nervous system descend ipsilaterally through the lateral part of the medulla.

The following examples are presented to show the correlation between clinical syndromes and the locations of some lesions in the brain stem. Table 7-1 provides a summary. Information contained in Chapters 8, 9, and 10 is needed in order to appreciate all the data in the table.

The **medial medullary syndrome** results from occlusion of a medullary branch of the vertebral artery; the size of the infarction depends on the distribution of the particular artery involved. In the example shown in Figure 7-16, the affected area includes the pyramid and most of the medial lemniscus on one side. The lesion extends far enough laterally to include fibers of the hypoglossal nerve as they pass between the medial lemniscus and the inferior olivary nucleus. A patient with this lesion has contralateral hemiparesis as well as impairment of the sensations of position and movement and of discriminative touch on the opposite side of the body. Paralysis of the tongue muscles is ipsilateral. This is an example of "crossed" or "alternating" paralysis, in which whereas the body below the neck is affected on the side opposite the lesion, muscles supplied by a cranial nerve are affected on the same side as the lesion.

Occlusion of a vessel supplying the lateral area of the medulla results in the **lateral medullary (Wallenberg's) syndrome**. Typically, the occluded vessel is a medullary branch of the posterior inferior cerebellar artery. The infarcted area (Fig. 7-17) includes (a) the base of the inferior cerebellar peduncle and vestibular nuclei, causing dizziness, cerebellar ataxia, and nystagmus; (b) the spinal trigeminal tract and its nucleus, causing ipsilateral loss of pain and temperature sensibility in the area of distribution of the trigeminal nerve; (c) the spinothalamic tract, causing contralateral loss of pain and temperature sensation below the neck; or (d) the nucleus ambiguus, causing paralysis of the muscles of the soft palate, pharynx, and

TABLE 7-1 **Some Clinical Syndromes Caused by Localized Lesions in the Brain Stem**

Clinical Features	Site of Lesion	Name of Syndrome and Other Comments
Ipsilateral hypoglossal palsy with contralateral hemiplegia	Ventromedial medulla, including pyramid and axons of hypoglossal nerve	Medial medullary syndrome (see Fig. 7-16)
Vertigo, ataxia, paralysis of the ipsilateral palate and vocal cord, loss of pain and thermal sensation on the same side of face and opposite side of body, ipsilateral Horner's syndrome, and loss of facial sweating	Lateral medulla (territory of posterior inferior cerebellar artery), including the vestibular nuclei inferior cerebellar peduncle, nucleus ambiguus, spinal trigeminal tract and nucleus, spinothalamic tract, and fibers descending to preganglionic sympathetic neurons	Wallenberg's syndrome (see Fig. 7-17 and Chapters 8 and 24); smaller lesions cause partial syndromes (see next row of this table for an example)
Paralysis of the ipsilateral palate and vocal cord and loss of pain and thermal sensation on same side of face and opposite side of body	Lateral medulla, including nucleus ambiguus, spinal trigeminal tract and nucleus, and spinothalamic tract	Avellis' syndrome; caused by a lesion in the ventral part of the shaded area in Fig. 7-17
Ipsilateral lower motor neuron facial paralysis with contralateral hemiplegia	Pons, including facial motor nucleus and descending motor fibers	Millard-Gübler syndrome (see Fig. 7-19)
Ipsilateral lower motor neuron facial paralysis, ipsilateral conjugate gaze paralysis, and transient contralateral hemiparesis	Dorsomedial pons, including abducens nucleus, facial motor nucleus and axons, dorsal to the descending motor fibers	Foville's syndrome (see Figs. 7-20 and 8-5)
Ipsilateral abducens nerve palsy with contralateral hemiparesis	Ventral pons, including axons (not the nucleus) of the abducens nerve and descending motor fibers	Raymond's syndrome (see Fig. 7-18)
Ipsilateral oculomotor nerve palsy with contralateral hemiplegia or hemiparesis	Ventral part of cerebral peduncle, including axons of oculomotor nerve and descending motor fibers in the basis pedunculi	Weber's syndrome (see Fig. 7-21)
Ipsilateral oculomotor nerve palsy with contralateral hemiparesis and tremor	Cerebral peduncle, with oculomotor axons and descending motor fibers and extending dorsally to include the red nucleus and fibers from the contralateral side of the cerebellum	Benedikt's syndrome (see Fig. 7-21 and Chapter 10); the tremor resembles a cerebellar tremor
Paralysis of conjugate upward gaze without paralysis of convergence	Dorsal midbrain; typically a pineal tumor pressing on the posterior commissure, pretectal area, and superior colliculi	Parinaud's syndrome (see Chapter 8 and Fig. 8-6)

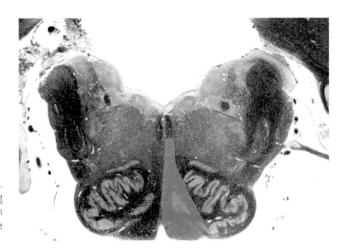

FIGURE 7-16   Site of a lesion producing the medial medullary syndrome. This lesion transects axons of the medial lemniscus, the pyramid, and the hypoglossal nerve.

larynx on the side of the lesion, with difficulty in swallowing and phonation. The descending pathway to the intermediolateral cell column of the spinal cord is usually included in the area of degeneration, thereby causing **Horner's syndrome** (i.e., constricted pupil and drooping of the upper eyelid [ptosis]) and warm, dry skin of the face, all on the side of the lesion. Cerebellar signs are more pronounced if infarction of part of the cerebellum is added to that of the medulla (posterior inferior cerebellar artery thrombosis). Partial syndromes such as that of Avellis (see Table 7-1) are caused by smaller lesions in the lateral part of the medulla.

Lesions in the basal region of the pons or the midbrain may produce alternating paralysis, similar to that described for the medial medullary syndrome. Figure 7-18 shows an area of infarction in one side of the caudal region of the pons, resulting from occlusion of a pontine

branch of the basilar artery, causing **Raymond's syndrome**. Interruption of corticospinal and other descending motor fibers causes contralateral hemiparesis. Inclusion of abducens nerve fibers in the lesion causes paralysis of the lateral rectus muscle on the ipsilateral side, resulting in a medial strabismus or squint. More laterally and dorsally located lesions (Fig. 7-19) involve descending motor fibers and the motor nucleus and axons of the facial nerve. In the resulting **Millard-Gübler syndrome**, contralateral hemiparesis and ipsilateral facial paralysis are present.

A more dorsally and medially located pontine lesion can involve the abducens nucleus together with the nearby motor fibers of the facial nerve or the facial motor nucleus (see Fig. 7-8). In the resulting **Foville's syndrome**, patients have ipsilateral paralysis of the facial muscles and of the lateral rectus muscle, which is sup-

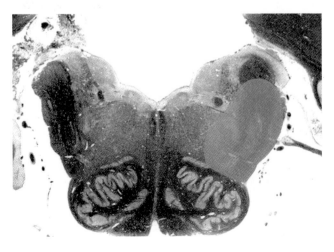

FIGURE 7-17   Site of a lesion producing a lateral medullary syndrome. This lesion (the one described by Wallenberg) involves the vestibular nuclei and inferior cerebellar peduncle, spinal trigeminal tract and nucleus, spinothalamic tract, and nucleus ambiguus and descending fibers that control the sympathetic innervation of the eye and face. Smaller lesions spare certain functions such as those of the vestibular system and cerebellum, the laryngeal and pharyngeal muscles, or the sympathetic control of the iris.

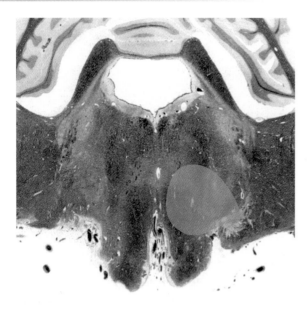

FIGURE 7-18 Site of a lesion in the basal pons involving corticospinal and other descending motor fibers and fibers of the abducens nerve. This lesion results in Raymond's syndrome. This lesion spares the abducens nucleus and the nucleus and axons of the facial nerve.

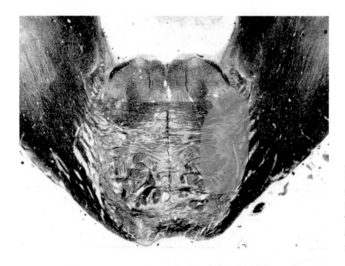

FIGURE 7-19 Site of a lesion in the caudal part of the pons involving descending motor fibers and the axons and nucleus of the facial nerve but sparing the nucleus and axons of the abducens nerve. This lesion results in the Millard-Gübler syndrome.

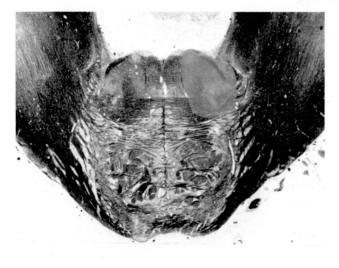

FIGURE 7-20 Site of a lesion causing Foville's syndrome. Involvement of the abducens nucleus causes paralysis of the contralateral medial rectus in addition to the ipsilateral lateral rectus muscle. The motor nucleus and axons of the facial nerve are also destroyed, and the lesion extends ventrally to cause partial damage to corticospinal and other descending motor tracts.

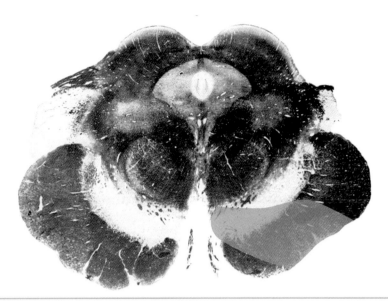

FIGURE 7-21   Site of a lesion in the rostral midbrain involving corticospinal and other descending motor fibers and the axons of the oculomotor nerve. This lesion results in Weber's syndrome.

plied by the abducens nerve. In addition, the medial rectus muscle of the contralateral eye fails to contract when a conjugate lateral eye movement is attempted but does contract when the eyes converge to look at a near object. The effect of the lesion on the contralateral medial rectus is caused by destruction of internuclear neurons. These, which occur alongside the motor neurons in the abducens nucleus, have axons that cross the midline, ascend in the medial longitudinal fasciculus, and stimulate the motor neurons in the oculomotor subnucleus for the medial rectus muscle. (The complex neural connections for conjugate eye movements are explained in Chapter 8 and summarized in Fig. 8-5.) Sensory and motor tracts are ventral to a lesion causing Foville's syndrome and, typically, there is a contralateral hemiparesis of brief duration caused by transient ischemia or pressure (Fig. 7-20).

The position of a vascular lesion in the basal region of a cerebral peduncle, which can follow occlusion of a branch of the posterior cerebral artery, is shown in Figure 7-21. This causes **Weber's syndrome**, consisting of contralateral hemiparesis caused by interruption of corticospinal and other descending motor fibers and ipsilateral paralysis of ocular muscles because of inclusion of oculomotor nerve fibers in the infarcted area. Affected patients have paralysis

of all the extraocular muscles except the lateral rectus and superior oblique. The most obvious signs are loss of ability to raise the upper eyelid and lateral strabismus, together with dilatation of the pupil because of interruption of parasympathetic fibers that control the sphincter pupillae muscle. A lesion that extends farther dorsally than the one in Figure 7-21 involves cerebellar efferent fibers, causing a tremor, similar to that associated with cerebellar disorders, in the paretic contralateral limbs. The condition is then known as **Benedikt's syndrome**.

Suggested Reading

Bassetti C, Bogousslavsky J, Mattle H, Bernasconi A. Medial medullary stroke: report of seven patients and review of the literature. *Neurology* 1997;48:882–890.

Damier P, Hirsch EC, Agid Y, et al. The substantia nigra of the human brain. *Brain* 1999;122:1421–1448.

Defer GL, Geny C, Ricolfi F, et al. Long-term outcome of unilaterally transplanted Parkinsonian patients, 1: clinical approach. *Brain* 1996;119:41–50.

Finnis KW, Starreveld YP, Parrent AG, et al. Three-dimensional database of subcortical electrophysiology for image-guided stereotactic functional neurosurgery. *IEEE Trans Med Imaging* 2003;22:93–104.

Freed CR, Greene PE, Breeze RE, et al. Transplantation of embryonic dopamine neurons for severe Parkinson's disease. *N Engl J Med* 2001;344:710–719.

Hirsch WL, Kemp SS, Martinez AJ, et al. Anatomy of the brainstem: correlation of in vitro MR images with histologic sections. *Am J Neuroradiol* 1989;10:923–928.

Landau WM. Artificial intelligence: the brain transplant cure for parkinsonism. *Neurology* 1990;40:733–740.

Nathan PW, Smith MC. The rubrospinal and central tegmental tracts in man. *Brain* 1982;105:223–269.

Nathan PW, Smith MC. The location of descending fibres to sympathetic neurons supplying the head and neck. *J Neurol Neurosurg Psychiatr* 1986;49:187–194.

Nieuwenhuys R, Voogd J, van Huijzen C. *The Human Central Nervous System. A Synopsis and Atlas*, 3rd ed. Berlin: Springer-Verlag, 1988.

Olszewski J, Baxter D. *Cytoarchitecture of the Human Brain Stem*, 2nd ed. Basel: S Karger, 1954; reprint, 1982.

Riley HA. *An Atlas of the Basal Ganglia, Brain Stem and Spinal Cord*. New York: Hafner, 1960.

Vuilleumier P, Bogousslavsky J, Regli E. Infarction of the lower brainstem: clinical, aetiological and MRI-topographical correlations. *Brain* 1995;118:1013–1025.

Wolf JK. *The Classical Brain Stem Syndromes*. Springfield, IL: Thomas, 1971.

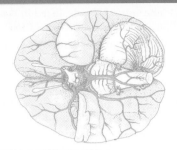

Chapter 8

CRANIAL NERVES

- The cranial nerves (I–XII) have motor, parasympathetic, and sensory functions.

Eye Movements

- Cranial nerves III, IV, and VI supply the extraocular muscles, which can be paralyzed by transection of motor axons in the nerves or in the brain stem.

- Voluntary saccadic eye movements are controlled by the frontal eye field, and smooth pursuit movements are controlled by the posterior parietal and occipital cortex.

- The pathways for conjugate horizontal gaze descend from the cortex and superior colliculus to the contralateral paramedian pontine reticular formation (PPRF) and abducens nucleus and then ascend in the ipsilateral medial longitudinal fasciculus (MLF) to the medial rectus subnucleus of the oculomotor nucleus. Lateral gaze palsies follow damage to the PPRF or nucleus of VI; internuclear ophthalmoplegia follows interruption of the MLF.

- Nuclei in the rostral midbrain are involved in vertical eye movements.

Other Motor Functions

- The trigeminal motor nucleus supplies masticatory and a few other muscles through the mandibular division of cranial nerve V.

- The facial motor nucleus supplies the facial muscles and the stapedius. The lower half of the face is controlled by the contralateral cerebral hemisphere. The upper half is bilaterally controlled and therefore not paralyzed by an "upper motor neuron" lesion.

- The muscles of the larynx, pharynx, and upper esophagus are supplied by neurons in the nucleus ambiguus, mostly by way of cranial nerve X.

- Cranial nerve XI consists largely of motor fibers from spinal cord segments C1 to C5 for the trapezius and sternocleidomastoid muscles.

- The protruded tongue deviates toward the abnormal side if the patient has weakness of the muscles supplied by XII.

Preganglionic Parasympathetic Fibers

- Cranial nerve III contains preganglionic fibers from the Edinger-Westphal nucleus. They end in the ciliary ganglion, which supplies the sphincter pupillae and ciliary smooth muscles. Loss of the light reflex is the first sign of compression of cranial nerve III.

- The salivary and lacrimal glands are supplied by parasympathetic ganglia, which receive preganglionic innervation from cranial nerves VII and IX. Preganglionic axons in cranial nerve X are from two nuclei in the medulla.

General Sensory Functions

- All general somatic sensory fibers from cranial nerve ganglia (V and IX; some from VII and X) end in trigeminal nuclei.

- Touch sensation is relayed through the pontine trigeminal nucleus and the rostral part of the spinal trigeminal nucleus.

- Pain and temperature fibers descend ipsilaterally in the spinal trigeminal tract and end in the caudal part of its nucleus.

- Trigeminothalamic fibers cross the midline in the brain stem and ascend to the contralateral thalamus (ventral posterior medial [VPm] nucleus).

- The caudal part of the solitary nucleus receives visceral afferent fibers (IX and X) for cardiovascular and respiratory reflexes.

Special Senses

- Cranial nerves I, II, and VIII are discussed in Chapters 17 and 20 to 22.

- Taste fibers (cranial nerves VII, IX, and a few from X) go in the solitary tract to the rostral end of the solitary nucleus. Solitariothalamic fibers go to the most medial part of the VPm thalamic nucleus.

The cranial nerves, listed in the order in which numbers are assigned to them, are as follows. These numbers were introduced by von Sömmering in 1798.

1. (or I) Olfactory
2. (or II) Optic
3. (or III) Oculomotor
4. (or IV) Trochlear
5. (or V) Trigeminal
6. (or VI) Abducens
7. (or VII) Facial
8. (or VIII) Vestibulocochlear
9. (or IX) Glossopharyngeal
10. (or X) Vagus
11. (or XI) Accessory
12. (or XII) Hypoglossal

An extremely thin **nervus terminalis**, which lies along the medial side of the olfactory bulb and tract, is sometimes numbered as cranial nerve 0. The nervus terminalis serves as the conduit along which a population of neurons migrates from the olfactory placode (a region of ectoderm of the embryonic nose) into the preoptic area and hypothalamus. These neurons are essential for reproductive function in both sexes (see Chapter 11).

Cranial nerves I, II, and VIII serve the olfactory, visual, auditory, and vestibular systems and are therefore discussed in Chapters 17, 20, 21, and 22, respectively. The special sense of taste (i.e., from the gustatory system) is dealt with in this chapter because the primary sensory neurons for taste are located in the same ganglia as sensory neurons that have other functions in cranial nerves VII, IX, and X.

This chapter has two major parts. The first is devoted to eye movements, and it includes information about the control of muscles supplied by cranial nerves III, IV, and VI. The second part of the chapter is concerned with the other cranial nerves, with the exceptions of I, II, and VIII, noted in the preceding paragraph. The central gustatory pathway is described in association with the facial nerve.

The Ocular Motor System

The control of eye movements, a complicated subject, is treated partly in this chapter and partly in Chapter 22. For the benefit of those who are unfamiliar with the anatomy of the muscles that move the eyeball, the actions of

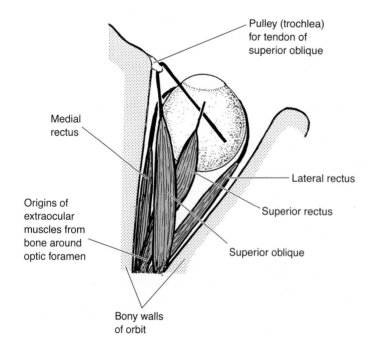

FIGURE 8-1 Muscles acting on the right eye, viewed from above. (The inferior rectus and inferior oblique are not visible.) Note that with the eye looking forward, as shown, contraction of the superior oblique muscle will cause the pupil to move downward and laterally. If the eye were looking medially, the superior oblique muscle would move the pupil downward. If the eye were looking laterally, the superior oblique muscle would rotate the eyeball but would not change the direction of gaze.

these muscles are reviewed in Figure 8-1. The lateral rectus muscle is supplied by the abducens nerve, and the superior oblique muscle is supplied by the trochlear nerve. All the other muscles are supplied by branches of the oculomotor nerve, which also supplies the levator palpebrae superioris.

Cranial nerves III, IV, and VI provide motor innervation of the extraocular muscles. Their nuclei of origin, collectively called the **ocular motor nuclei**, contain motor neurons and **internuclear neurons**, with axons that contact the motor neurons for muscles that move the opposite eye in the same direction. Internuclear neurons constitute part of the circuitry that coordinates the conjugate (yoked) movements of the two eyes. The oculomotor nucleus also includes a parasympathetic component. Functional impairment of any of the extraocular muscles causes misalignment of the eyes with consequent double vision (diplopia).

OCULOMOTOR NERVE

The **oculomotor nucleus** is in the periaqueductal gray matter of the midbrain, ventral to the aqueduct at the level of the superior colliculus (see Figs. 7-14, 7-15, and 8-2). Myelinated axons from each oculomotor nucleus curve ventrally through the tegmentum and emerge from the medial side of the cerebral peduncle, in the interpeduncular fossa. The nerve traverses the subarachnoid space, the cavernous sinus, and the superior orbital fissure. In the orbit, branches supply the superior, medial, and inferior rectus muscles; the inferior oblique muscle; and the levator palpebrae superioris muscle (which lifts the upper eyelid).

In the oculomotor nucleus, the motor neurons for individual muscles are localized in distinct groups or subnuclei. The small sizes of the motor units, in which about six muscle fibers are supplied by one neuron, attest to the high degree of precision required for coordinated movement of the eyes in binocular vision.

The **Edinger-Westphal nucleus** is situated dorsally to the main oculomotor nucleus, and its smaller cells are preganglionic parasympathetic neurons. Axons from the Edinger-Westphal nucleus accompany the other oculomotor fibers into the orbit, where they terminate in the **ciliary ganglion**, behind the eye. Postganglionic fibers (the axons of the neurons in the ganglion) pass through the **short ciliary nerves** to the eyeball, where they supply the sphincter pupillae muscle of the iris and the ciliary muscle.

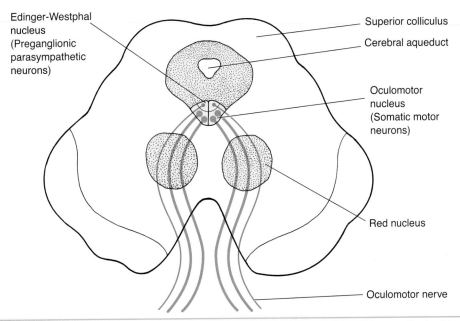

Edinger-Westphal nucleus (Preganglionic parasympathetic neurons)

Superior colliculus

Cerebral aqueduct

Oculomotor nucleus (Somatic motor neurons)

Red nucleus

Oculomotor nerve

FIGURE 8-2   Origins of the oculomotor nerves in the midbrain at the level of the superior colliculus. Motor neurons are red; preganglionic parasympathetic neurons are green.

TROCHLEAR NERVE

The **trochlear nucleus** for the superior oblique muscle is immediately caudal to the oculomotor nucleus, at the level of the inferior colliculus (see Figs. 7-13 and 8-3). Trochlear nerve fibers have an unusual course, and this is the only nerve to emerge from the dorsum of the brain stem. Small bundles of fibers curve around the periaqueductal gray matter with a caudal slope and decussate in the superior medullary velum. The slender nerve emerges immediately caudal to the inferior colliculus. The function of the superior oblique muscle is to depress and inwardly rotate the eyeball (see Fig. 8-1). If the eye is initially looking forward, the superior oblique also causes abduction.

ABDUCENS NERVE

The **abducens nucleus** for the lateral rectus muscle is situated beneath the facial colliculus in the floor of the fourth ventricle (see Figs. 7-8 and 8-4). A bundle of facial nerve fibers (known as the internal genu) curves over the nucleus, contributing to the facial colliculus. The motor neurons in the abducens nucleus give rise to axons that pass through the pons in a ventrocaudal direction, emerging from the brain stem at the junction of the pons and the pyramid. The abducens nucleus also contains internuclear neurons whose axons cross into the contralateral medial longitudinal fasciculus and travel rostrally to the oculomotor subnucleus that supplies the medial rectus muscle (Fig. 8-5).

COORDINATED MOVEMENTS OF BOTH EYES

Voluntarily initiated conjugate movements of the eyes include those that occur when scanning a landscape or reading a printed page. These movements, known as **saccadic eye movements**, are rapid, with each being completed in 20 to 50 msec. A saccade serves to aim the eye at a seen or remembered object in the visual field. Frequent saccades, made when the image on the retina is continuously changing, are called **optokinetic movements**. Slower

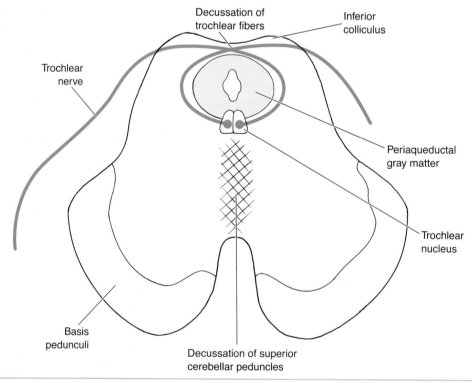

FIGURE 8-3   Origins of the trochlear nerves in the midbrain. The axons from the left and right trochlear nuclei are directed dorsally and caudally; they decussate in the superior medullary velum, which is below the inferior colliculi.

Extraocular Muscle Weakness

All the extraocular muscles are sensitive to diseases that afflict the skeletal muscle in a general way. Myasthenia gravis is a disease in which neuromuscular transmission is inhibited (see Chapter 3). Weakness of the levator palpebrae superioris is often the first symptom, causing ptosis. Weaknesses of the other extraocular muscles follow.

Sometimes cranial nerves III, IV, and VI are all involved in a single destructive lesion. This can be caused by inflammation of unknown cause in the region of the superior orbital fissure or by compression of the nerves in the cavernous sinus (see Chapter 26).

Defective alignment of the eyes is called squint or strabismus. Most often, squint is not caused by paralysis or weakness of muscles. In such cases, both eyes can move through a full range of positions. If one eye fails to converge, it will do so if the other eye is covered. This common condition is called a concomitant squint.

A malfunction of one or more of the extraocular muscles causes a paralytic squint. If paralysis is complete, it is not usually difficult to decide which muscle or group of muscles is not working. When only weakness (paresis) is present, however, the squint may be apparent only when the eye is attempting to move in the direction of action of the affected muscle. The first symptom is diplopia (double vision), which occurs because the central foveae of the two eyes cease to receive images of the same object. With time, the brain suppresses the false image, so the symptom of diplopia disappears. The two golden rules in the diagnosis of diplopia are:

1. The separation of the images increases with the amount of movement in the direction of pull of the weak muscle (or muscles).
2. The false image (the one in the abnormally moving eye) is displaced in the direction of action of the weak or paralyzed muscle (or muscles).

If the patient cannot be sure which eye produces which image, the uncertainty can be resolved by placing colored glass in front of one eye.

THIRD NERVE PALSY

"Palsy" is an old word for paralysis, often used for disorders of single nerves or muscles. A lesion that interrupts fibers of the oculomotor nerve causes paralysis of all extraocular muscles except the superior oblique and lateral rectus muscles. The sphincter pupillae muscle in the iris and the ciliary muscle in the ciliary body are functionally paralyzed, although they are not denervated. The consequences of such a lesion are:

1. drooping of the upper eyelid (ptosis);
2. lateral strabismus caused by unopposed action of the lateral rectus muscle;
3. inability to direct the eye medially or vertically; and
4. dilatation of the pupil, enhanced by unopposed action of the dilator pupillae muscle in the iris, which has a sympathetic innervation.

The pupil no longer constricts, either in response to an increase of light intensity or in accommodation for near objects. The ciliary muscle does not contract to allow the lens to increase in thickness for focusing on near objects.

The preganglionic parasympathetic fibers run superficially in the nerve and are therefore the first axons to suffer when a nerve is affected by external pressure. Consequently, the first sign of compression of the oculomotor nerve is ipsilateral slowness of the pupillary response to light.

FOURTH NERVE PALSY

Paralysis of the superior oblique muscle, as in the rare occurrence of an isolated lesion of the trochlear nerve, causes vertical diplopia, which is maximal when the eye is directed downward and inward. A person so affected experiences difficulty in walking down stairs. The condition can occur as a manifestation of a peripheral neuropathy (e.g., in diabetes mellitus). It is an occasional persistent complication of head injury. Tiny vascular lesions in the midbrain may be the most common cause of isolated, nontraumatic oculomotor and trochlear palsies in the elderly.

SIXTH NERVE PALSY

The **abducens nerve** may be affected by a peripheral neuropathy, or the lateral rectus muscle itself may degenerate for an unknown reason. The consequence is a medial squint with an inability to direct the affected eye laterally because the lateral rectus is the principal muscle that abducts the eyeball. Destruction of the **abducens nucleus** also causes paralysis of the contralateral medial rectus muscle, so that the patient cannot direct his or her gaze to the side of the lesion. A nuclear lesion may also involve the nearby nucleus or axons of the facial nerve, causing paralysis of all the ipsilateral facial muscles.

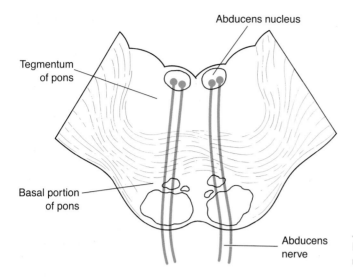

FIGURE 8-4   Origins of the abducens nerves in the caudal part of the pons.

conjugate movements of the eyes are possible only when tracking a moving object in the visual field. These largely involuntary **smooth pursuit movements** are mentioned later in connection with visual fixation. **Vergence movements**, in which both eyes move medially to look at a near object or laterally to look into the distance, can also occur slowly. **Vestibular eye**

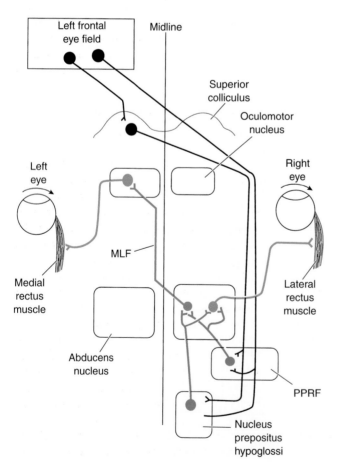

FIGURE 8-5   Some pathways involved in conjugate lateral movements of the eyes. Motor neurons are red, internuclear neurons are green, other preoculomotor neurons are blue, and other neurons are black.

movements, which are driven by sensory input from the vestibular apparatus of the inner ear, are described in Chapter 22.

The precise timing of contractions of extraocular muscles is determined by activity of neurons whose axons end in the nuclei of cranial nerves III, IV, and VI. An understanding of the neuroanatomical basis of ocular movements, discussed later in this chapter and in Chapter 22, is essential for the clinical analysis of impairments more complex than damage to a single muscle or cranial nerve.

Voluntary Eye Movements

The area of the cerebral cortex that controls voluntary eye movements is the **frontal eye field**, located anterior to the general motor cortex and known as Brodmann's area 8 (see Chapter 15). Stimulation of the frontal eye field results in conjugate deviation of the eyes to the opposite side. The voluntary control of eye movements is mediated by a polysynaptic pathway that involves the prefrontal cortex; frontal eye field; superior colliculus; various other groups of neurons in the brain stem; and the oculomotor, trochlear, and abducens nuclei (see Fig. 8-5). The "various other groups of neurons in the brain stem" include the pretectal area, superior colliculus, paramedian pontine reticular formation (PPRF), nucleus prepositus hypoglossi, rostral interstitial nucleus of the medial longitudinal fasciculus, and interstitial nucleus of Cajal. These nuclei, whose locations are illustrated in Chapter 9, are variously involved in maintaining the position of the eyes (tonic activity), generating saccades (phasic activity), and determining whether the eyes will move in the horizontal or vertical plane.

The **PPRF** has been called a "center for lateral gaze." It receives afferents from the contralateral cerebral cortex (including the frontal eye field), contralateral superior colliculus, and ipsilateral vestibular nuclei. Some of its neurons send their axons into the ipsilateral abducens nucleus, and the axons terminate on both motor neurons and internuclear neurons (see Fig. 8-5). The internuclear neurons have axons that cross the midline and ascend through the contralateral medial longitudinal fasciculus to the cells of the contralateral oculomotor nucleus that supply the medial rectus muscle. The actions of the medial and lateral recti are thereby coordinated in horizontal movements of the eyes.

Neurons in the PPRF send *bursts* of impulses (as many as 1,000/sec) to the motor and internuclear neurons, causing rapid contraction of the lateral rectus and contralateral medial rectus muscles. Slower *tonic* stimulation of the ocular motor neurons, with impulses at a rate just sufficient to maintain the direction of gaze, comes from the **nucleus prepositus hypoglossi**, which is rostral to the hypoglossal nucleus in the medulla. The neurons in this nucleus receive afferents from the contralateral cerebral cortex and superior colliculus and have axons that project rostrally in the medial longitudinal fasciculus to all the ocular motor nuclei.

Conjugate movement of the eyes in the vertical plane is controlled by cell groups in the upper midbrain. Bursts of impulses that stimulate vertical saccades arise in the **rostral interstitial nucleus of the medial longitudinal fasciculus** (see Fig. 9-7), which contains neurons with axons that end in the trochlear nucleus and the oculomotor subnuclei for the superior and inferior rectus and inferior oblique muscles. The axons that go to contralateral ocular motor nuclei decussate in the posterior commissure. Tonic neurons that maintain the vertical component of the direction of gaze are located in the **interstitial nucleus of Cajal** (see Fig. 9-7). Some of the neural connections mediating voluntary vertical eye movements are shown in Figure 8-6.

Smooth Pursuit Movements

The eyes are normally directed toward some object in the center of the field of vision. If the object moves, both eyes will execute smooth pursuit movements to maintain **visual fixation**, which contributes importantly to awareness of the position of the head and, integrated with other sensory information, helps in the maintenance of the body's equilibrium. These slow eye movements are largely involuntary. They are controlled principally by the **posterior parietal eye field**, which is adjacent to the visual association cortex of the lateral aspect of the occipital lobe. The descending connections of this parietal eye field are essentially the same as those of the frontal eye field (see Fig. 8-5). The direct visual input from the retina to the superior colliculus is also involved in reflex eye movements for visual fixation. The neural circuitry for pursuit movements involves the **cerebellum** and **vestibular nuclei**. The connections are summarized in Figure 8-7. This diagram includes some connections of the **pretectal area** that me-

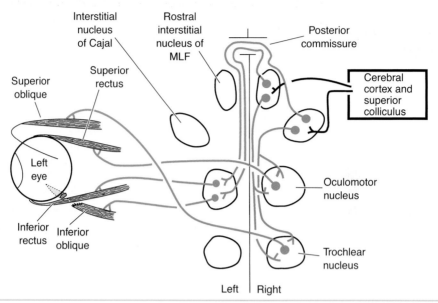

FIGURE 8-6   Some pathways involved in vertical eye movements. The connections are shown for only the left eye. Motor neurons are red, preoculomotor neurons are blue, and other neurons are black.

diate the short saccades (optokinetic movements) that occur when the point of visual fixation is continuously shifting, as when looking out of the side window of a moving vehicle. Eye movements driven primarily by sensory input from the vestibular nerve are explained in Chapter 22.

Vergence Movements

Convergence occurs when both eyes are focused on a near object. This nonconjugate movement is accompanied by constriction of the pupil and accommodation (focusing) of the lens. The neuronal pathways of convergence are similar to those described for visual fixation. Convergence requires the integrity of the occipital cortex but not that of the frontal eye field or the PPRF. Visual guidance is also provided through the superior colliculus. This projects to the **pretectal area**, which contains at least one group of cells (the **nucleus of the optic tract**) with axons that contact medial rectus motor neurons in the oculomotor nuclei of both sides (see Fig. 8-7).

LIGHT AND ACCOMMODATION REFLEXES

The **Edinger-Westphal nucleus** contains preganglionic parasympathetic neurons concerned with reflex responses of the smooth muscles of

the eye to light and accommodation. The **light reflex** occurs when an increased intensity of light falling on the retina causes constriction of the pupil. The afferent limb of the reflex arc involves fibers in the optic nerve and optic tract that reach one of the nuclei of the pretectal area (the **olivary pretectal nucleus**) by way of the superior brachium (Fig. 8-8). This part of the pretectal area projects to the Edinger-Westphal nucleus, from which fibers traverse the oculomotor nerve to the ciliary ganglion in the orbital cavity. Postganglionic fibers travel through the short ciliary nerves to the sphincter pupillae muscle of the iris. Some pretectal neurons send their axons across the midline in the posterior commissure to the contralateral Edinger-Westphal nucleus.

Both pupils constrict when a light is shone into only one eye. The response of the contralateral iris is known as the **consensual light reflex**. There are two reasons for the response of the other eye: (a) each optic tract contains fibers from both retinas (see Chapter 20) and (b) the pretectal area projects to the contralateral as well as to the ipsilateral Edinger-Westphal nucleus.

Accommodation of the lens accompanies ocular convergence produced by visual fixation on a near object. Both actions are trig-

Cortical Lesions Affecting Conjugate Gaze

Destruction of the frontal eye field causes deviation of both eyes toward the side of the lesion. Voluntary (saccadic) movements of the eyes away from the side of the cortical lesion cannot be made. Commonly, this condition is caused by ischemic damage to a larger area of cerebral cortex, which also includes the motor and premotor areas, with consequent paralysis of the limbs and lower half of the face on the contralateral side. The deviated eyes look away from the paralyzed side of the body.

A destructive lesion in the posterior parietal lobe can impair the ability to make smooth pursuit movements away from the side of the lesion. Voluntary saccades are unaffected, and the attempt to pursue a target in the visual field becomes a series of small, rapid movements of the eyes.

LESIONS IN THE BRAIN STEM THAT AFFECT GAZE

Lesions that destroy the **abducens nucleus** have already been described and contrasted with the consequence of severing the motor axons of the abducens nerve, either in the ventral part of the pons or in the nerve itself. **Foville's syndrome**, which is caused by a dorsally located infarction in the caudal part of the pons, comprises ipsilateral nuclear sixth nerve palsy and lower motor neuron facial palsy, with contralateral hemiplegia. The limb paralysis recovers because most of the descending motor fibers are ventral to the infarct.

Internuclear ophthalmoplegia is caused by a tiny lesion in one medial longitudinal fasciculus at a level between the nuclei of cranial nerves III and VI. The usual cause is multiple sclerosis. Interruption of the fibers going from the abducens nucleus of the opposite side to the oculomotor nucleus of the same side causes an inability to adduct the eye on the side of the lesion. The patient will also have nystagmus of the abducting eye, which is a useful diagnostic sign even though the mechanism producing the nystagmus is not fully understood. These abnormalities are evident only when the patient is asked to gaze to the side opposite that of the lesion; contraction of the medial rectus occurs normally with convergence of the eyes for looking at a near object. A somewhat larger lesion can involve both medial longitudinal fasciculi, causing bilateral internuclear ophthalmoplegia.

A lesion that destroys the PPRF prevents saccadic contractions of the lateral rectus and the contralateral medial rectus muscles, but pursuit and vergence movements are preserved. An incomplete lesion causes abnormally small, slow saccades.

Paralysis of vertical gaze is caused by a lesion in the rostral midbrain. Causes include pressure from a nearby tumor and isolated lesions of various diseases that produce widespread changes in the brain. A tumor arising from the pineal gland compresses the posterior commissure and nearby structures and causes paralysis of upward gaze (**Parinaud's syndrome**). In monkeys, a tiny lesion confined to the rostral interstitial nucleus of the medial longitudinal fasciculus causes selective paralysis of downward gaze; this condition has been described in humans but is extremely rare.

---

gered by signals that originate in the retina and in the occipital cortex and are relayed through the superior colliculus to the Edinger-Westphal nucleus. The efferent part of the pathway consists of preganglionic and postganglionic fibers from the Edinger-Westphal nucleus and the ciliary ganglion, respectively. The postganglionic fibers supply the ciliary muscle, which, on contraction, allows the lens to increase in thickness and thereby increases refractive power for focusing on a near object. The sphincter pupillae muscle contracts at the same time, sharpening the image by decreasing the diameter of the pupil and reducing spherical aberration in the refractive media of the eye.

Other Cranial Nerves

TRIGEMINAL NERVE

The trigeminal nerve is so named because it branches intracranially into three divisions. These provide general sensory innervation for most of the head (Fig. 8-9) and motor fibers to the muscles of mastication and several smaller muscles.

Sensory Components

The cell bodies of most of the primary sensory neurons are located in the **trigeminal** (semilunar or gasserian) **ganglion**, with the remainder located in the mesencephalic trigeminal

CLINICAL NOTE

Abnormal Pupillary Reflexes

No pupillary reflexes can be elicited by light shone into an eye that is blind for any reason. Both pupils constrict briskly when light is shone in the normal eye, however. If the light is then quickly moved to the blind eye (the "swinging flashlight test"), both pupils dilate. This apparently paradoxical light reflex is known as the **Marcus Gunn pupil**. It is seen especially in patients with **optic neuritis**, a condition in which a demyelinating lesion in an optic nerve causes visual failure in one eye, developing in the course of a few days. Optic neuritis is often a manifestation of **multiple sclerosis**, a disease in which foci of demyelination occur in scattered locations in the brain and spinal cord.

The most common abnormal visual reflex is impairment of the pupillary reaction to light in patients with deteriorating conscious level after a **head injury**. The usual cause is compression of the oculomotor nerve by the uncus, which is forced over the free edge of the tentorium cerebelli as a result of pressure from a subdural or extradural hemorrhage (see Chapter 26).

An **aneurysm of the posterior communicating artery** can injure the nearby oculomotor nerve.

The **Holmes-Adie pupil**, seen most frequently in young women, responds more slowly than the other pupil to both light and accommodation. It is attributed to the death of some neurons in the ciliary ganglion, perhaps as a result of viral infection, and it may be associated (for no known reason) with sluggish stretch reflexes throughout the body. The small pupil of **Horner's syndrome** is explained in Chapter 24.

The different pathways for pupillary responses to light and accommodation may be differently affected by disease. For example, in the **Argyll Robertson pupil**, constriction occurs when attention is directed to a near object, but no pupillary constriction occurs in response to light. The Argyll Robertson pupil is characteristically seen in patients with syphilitic disease of the central nervous system (CNS). Loss of the pupillary light reflex alone is probably the result of a small lesion in the pretectal or periaqueductal region, but pathological changes cannot always be found in these sites. An Argyll Robertson pupil is irregular and smaller than normal, probably because of disease in the iris itself.

nucleus. The peripheral processes of trigeminal ganglion cells constitute the ophthalmic and maxillary nerves and the sensory component of the mandibular nerve. The trigeminal nerve is responsible for sensation from the skin of the face and forehead, the scalp as far back as the vertex of the head, the mucosa of the oral and nasal cavities and the paranasal sinuses, and the teeth (see Fig. 8-9). The trigeminal nerve also contributes sensory fibers to most of the dura mater (see Chapter 26) and to the cerebral arteries.

Trigeminal Sensory Nuclei

The central processes of trigeminal ganglion cells make up the large sensory root of the nerve; these fibers enter the pons and terminate in the pontine and spinal trigeminal nuclei. The **pontine trigeminal nucleus** (also called the chief, principal, or superior sensory nucleus) is located in the dorsolateral area of the tegmentum at the level of entry of the sensory axons (see

Figs. 7-11 and 8-10). Large-diameter fibers for discriminative touch terminate in the pontine trigeminal nucleus. Other entering axons divide, with one branch ending in the pontine trigeminal nucleus and the other turning caudally in the spinal tract and ending in the rostral end of the spinal trigeminal spinal nucleus. These afferents are mainly for light touch, and both nuclei, therefore, participate in this sensory modality. The pontine trigeminal nucleus also receives some branches of the axons of neurons of the mesencephalic trigeminal nucleus.

Large numbers of sensory root fibers of intermediate size and many fine, unmyelinated fibers turn caudally on entering the pons. These fibers for pain, temperature, and light touch form the **spinal trigeminal tract** (see Fig. 8-10). The tract also acquires incoming fibers from the facial, glossopharyngeal, and vagus nerves. These are for general somatic sensation from part of the external ear, the mucosa of the posterior part of the tongue, the pharynx, and

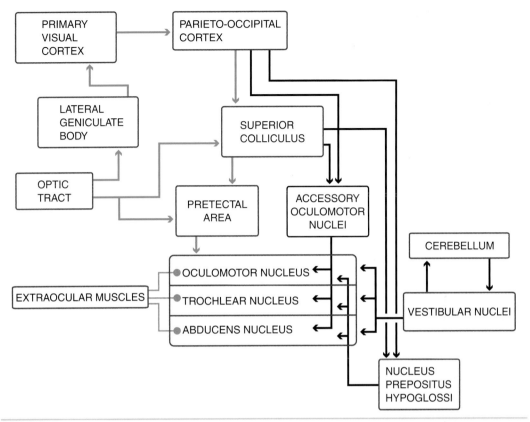

FIGURE 8-7   Some pathways involved in ocular pursuit and vergence movements. The pathways marked with green are used when the eyes converge to look at a near object.

the larynx. Some fibers of the spinal tract descend as far as the upper two or three segments of the cord, where they intermingle with axons in the dorsolateral tract of Lissauer.

The axons in the spinal tract terminate in the subjacent **spinal trigeminal nucleus** (see Fig. 8-10). The spinal nucleus extends from the pontine trigeminal nucleus to the caudal limit of the medulla, where it blends with the dorsal horn of the spinal gray matter. Based on cytoarchitecture, the spinal nucleus is divided into three parts (see Fig. 8-10). The **pars caudalis**, which extends from the level of the pyramidal decussation to spinal segment C3, receives fibers for pain and temperature. The integrity of the pars caudalis and of the caudal end of the spinal trigeminal tract is essential for the perception of pain that originates in the same side of the head. The **pars interpolaris** extends from the level of the rostral third of the inferior olivary nucleus to that of the pyramidal decussation. The **pars oralis** extends from the pars

interpolaris rostrally to the pontine trigeminal nucleus, which it resembles in its cellular architecture and its involvement in tactile sensation.

Some efferent fibers from the sensory trigeminal nuclei terminate in motor nuclei of the trigeminal and facial nerves, the nucleus ambiguus, and the hypoglossal nucleus. These mediate reflex responses to stimuli applied to the area of distribution of the trigeminal nerve. An example is the **corneal reflex**: touching the cornea causes both of the eyelids to close; the afferent fibers are located in the ophthalmic nerve, and the efferent fibers of the reflex arc are located in the facial nerve. Bilateral closure (blinking) follows a noxious stimulus anywhere near the eyes. Studies of patients with small lesions in the brain stem indicate that the reflex pathway begins in the caudal part of the spinal trigeminal nucleus and passes in the lateral parts of the tegmentum to both facial motor nuclei. The projection to the contralateral facial

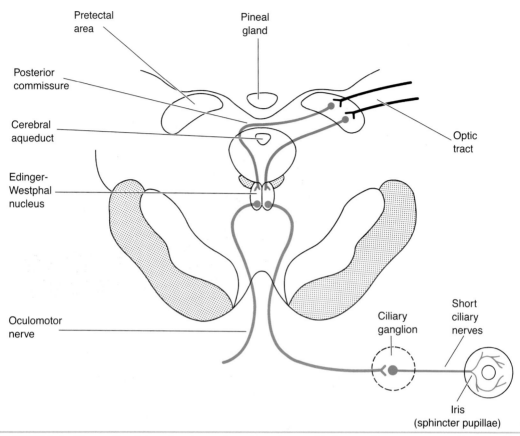

FIGURE 8-8 The pupillary light reflex. Axons from the retinas are black, central interneurons are blue, preganglionic parasympathetic neurons are red, and postganglionic neurons are green.

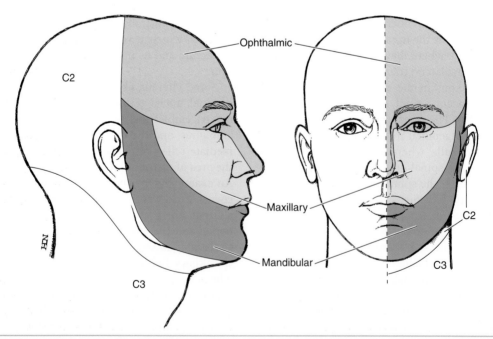

FIGURE 8-9 Cutaneous innervation of the head and neck. The boundaries between the territories of the three divisions of the trigeminal nerve do not overlap appreciably, as do the boundaries between spinal dermatomes.

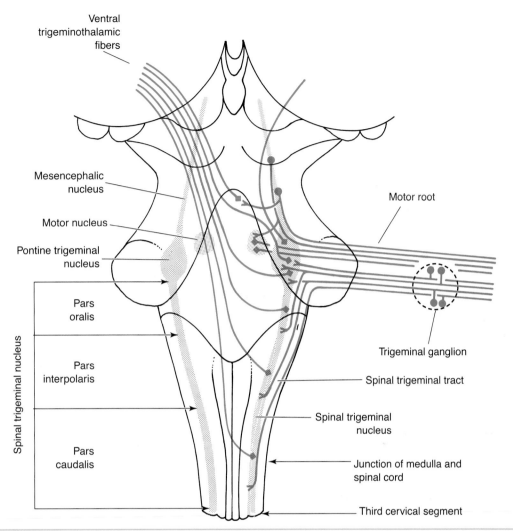

Ventral
trigeminothalamic
fibers

Mesencephalic
nucleus

Motor root

Motor nucleus

Pontine trigeminal
nucleus

Pars
oralis

Trigeminal ganglion

Spinal trigeminal nucleus

Pars
interpolaris

Spinal trigeminal tract

Spinal trigeminal
nucleus

Pars
caudalis

Junction of medulla and
spinal cord

Third cervical segment

FIGURE 8-10   Nuclei of the trigeminal nerve and their connections. Primary sensory neurons are blue, trigemino-thalamic neurons are green, and motor neurons are red.

motor nucleus crosses the midline in the lower medulla. As a further example, irritation of the nasal mucosa causes **sneezing**. For this reflex, afferent impulses in the maxillary nerve are relayed to motor nuclei of the trigeminal and facial nerves, the nucleus ambiguus, the hypoglossal nucleus, and (through a reticulospinal relay) the phrenic nucleus and motor cells in the spinal cord that supply the intercostal and other respiratory muscles.

The principal pathway from the pontine and spinal trigeminal nuclei to the thalamus is the crossed **ventral trigeminothalamic tract** (see Fig. 8-10 and Chapter 7), which ascends close to the medial lemniscus. Smaller numbers of

fibers, crossed and uncrossed, proceed from the pontine trigeminal nucleus to the thalamus in the **dorsal trigeminothalamic tract**. In the rostral pons and midbrain, the combined tracts are commonly called the **trigeminal lemniscus**. These axons end in the medial division of the VPm of the thalamus, which projects to the inferior end of the primary somatosensory area of the cerebral cortex.

The slender **mesencephalic trigeminal nucleus** is a strand of large unipolar neurons extending from the pontine trigeminal nucleus into the midbrain (see Fig. 8-10). These cells are primary sensory neurons in an unusual location; they are the only such cells that are incorporated into the CNS rather than being in ganglia. Their myelinated axons constitute the **mesencephalic tract** of the trigeminal nerve, which runs alongside the nucleus. Each axon divides into a peripheral and a central branch. Most of the peripheral branches enter the motor root of the trigeminal nerve and are distributed within the mandibular division. These fibers end in deep proprioceptive-type receptors adjacent to the teeth of the lower jaw and in neuromuscular spindles in the muscles of mastication. Some axons from the mesencephalic nucleus enter the maxillary division and go to endings around the roots of the upper teeth. Central branches of the axons of mesencephalic trigeminal neurons end in the motor nuclei of the trigeminal nerve. This connection establishes the stretch reflex that originates

in neuromuscular spindles in the masticatory muscles, together with a reflex for control of the force of the bite. Other central branches synapse with neurons in the reticular formation and the pontine trigeminal nucleus, and a few enter the cerebellum through its superior peduncle.

Motor Component

The **trigeminal motor nucleus** is medial to the pontine trigeminal nucleus (see Figs. 7-11 and 8-10). The axons of its neurons enter the motor root, which joins sensory fibers of the mandibular nerve just distal to the trigeminal ganglion. This nerve supplies the muscles of mastication (i.e., masseter, temporalis, and lateral and medial pterygoid muscles) and several smaller muscles (i.e., tensor tympani, tensor

---

CLINICAL NOTE

Disorders Affecting the Trigeminal Nerve and Its Nuclei

Of the diseases that affect the trigeminal nerve, **trigeminal neuralgia**, or **tic douloureux**, is of special importance. In this disorder, demyelination of axons in the sensory root takes place, caused in most cases by pressure of a small aberrant artery. There are paroxysms of excruciating pain in the area of distribution of one of the trigeminal divisions, usually with periods of remission and exacerbation. The maxillary nerve is most frequently involved, then the mandibular nerve, and, least frequently, the ophthalmic nerve. The paroxysm is often set off by touching an especially sensitive area of skin. The abnormal signaling of pain is thought to be amplified by ephaptic (electrical) communication among the demyelinated axons, which are tightly packed, without intervening glial cytoplasm. In most patients, the symptoms are relieved by carbamazepine, a drug otherwise used to treat epilepsy. If medical treatment fails, intracranial surgery is warranted because of the severity of the pain. Moving the aberrant artery away from the sensory root of the nerve is usually curative. Other procedures interrupt the pain pathway from the affected cutaneous area to the spinal trigeminal nucleus. Lesions may be placed in the trigeminal ganglion or in the sensory root of the nerve, but these can impair corneal sensitivity,

which affords protection from damage that might lead to corneal ulceration. Transection of the spinal trigeminal tract in the lower medulla abolishes the ability to feel pain in the face. The somatotopic lamination of the tract permits placement of a small lesion that restricts the analgesic area to the territory of a single division of the trigeminal nerve.

Another painful disorder that commonly affects the trigeminal nerve is **herpes zoster** (see Chapters 3 and 19).

The sensory and motor nuclei and the intracranial fibers of the trigeminal nerve may be included in areas damaged by vascular occlusion, trauma, tumor growth, or the presence of lesions in or near the brain stem. Interruption of the motor fibers causes paralysis and eventual atrophy of the muscles of mastication. The mandible deviates to the affected side because of the unopposed action of the contralateral lateral pterygoid muscle, which protrudes the jaw. Interruption of corticobulbar fibers does not cause paralysis of the masticatory muscles on the side opposite the lesion because the motor nucleus also receives some uncrossed fibers from the motor cortex. Laterally located lesions in the medulla interrupt the spinal trigeminal tract and impair facial and oral sensation of pain and temperature; this is part of Wallenberg's syndrome (explained in Chapter 7).

The Facial Nerve and the Middle Ear

The facial nerve is vulnerable in the middle ear, which is a region commonly invaded by bacteria and surgery. The exact site of a lesion can be determined by applying knowledge of the branches containing different functional components (Fig. 8-11).

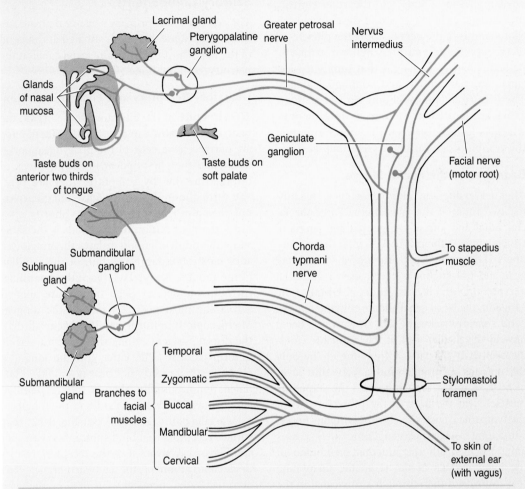

FIGURE 8-11 Components of the peripheral parts of the facial nerve. Primary sensory neurons are blue, motor neurons are red, and preganglionic and postganglionic parasympathetic neurons are green.

veli palatini, anterior belly of digastric, and mylohyoid). The motor nucleus receives descending afferents from the cortex of both cerebral hemispheres by way of the corticobulbar tract.

Afferents for reflexes come mainly from the sensory trigeminal nuclei, including the mesencephalic nucleus. The bilateral stretch reflexes of the jaw-closing muscles are tested clinically as the **jaw jerk**, elicited by tapping downward on the chin; the reflex arc passes through the mandibular nerve and the mesencephalic and motor trigeminal nuclei. In the **jaw-opening reflex**, the contractions of the masseter, temporalis, and medial pterygoid muscles are inhibited as a result of painful pressure applied to the teeth. This reflex passes through the pars caudalis of the spinal trigeminal nucleus and the motor nucleus, with intervening neurons in the reticular formation. Cells that supply the tensor tympani muscle receive acoustic fibers from the superior olivary nucleus. The tensor tympani, by reflex contraction, checks excessive movement of the tympanic membrane caused by loud sounds.

FACIAL NERVE

The facial nerve has two sensory components: one supplies taste buds, and the other contributes cutaneous fibers to part of the external ear. Motor axons in the nerve supply the muscles of facial expression, and preganglionic parasympathetic fibers go to ganglia that supply the lacrimal, submandibular, and sublingual glands. The sensory and preganglionic parasympathetic axons are located in the **nervus intermedius**, which is located between the motor root and the vestibulocochlear nerve (see Chapter 6).

Branches of the Facial Nerve

After traversing the internal acoustic meatus, the two roots of the facial nerve enter the **facial canal** and join at the **geniculate ganglion**, which contains the cell bodies of all the sensory fibers. The **greater petrosal nerve**, containing taste and preganglionic fibers, leaves the facial nerve at the level of this ganglion. Distal to the ganglion, the facial canal and its contained nerve bend sharply backward and downward, being now in the medial wall of the tympanic (middle ear) cavity, separated from the air by only the mucous membrane and a very thin layer of bone. A motor branch goes to the **stapedius** muscle. Near the floor of the posterior part of the tympanic cavity, the **chorda tympani nerve**, containing taste and preganglionic fibers, passes anteriorly beneath the mucous membrane of the inner surface of the tympanic membrane (ear drum) and then through a tiny canal in the tympanic part of the temporal bone to the infratemporal fossa. The main trunk of the facial nerve descends from the middle ear into the stylomastoid foramen, within which the single somatic sensory branch passes into the surrounding bone and joins small branches of the glossopharyngeal and vagus nerves. These three intermingled small populations of axons supply some of the skin of the tympanic membrane and external acoustic meatus as well as a small area of nearby skin behind the ear. After the departure of these sensory fibers, all the axons in the facial nerve are those of motor neurons. On emerging from the base of the skull between the styloid and mastoid processes, the facial nerve sends branches to the stylohyoid and the posterior belly of the digastric muscle and then splits into five branches (temporal, zygomatic, buccal, marginal mandibular, and cervical), which are distributed to the muscles of the scalp and face.

Sensory Components

The cell bodies of primary sensory neurons are in the **geniculate ganglion**, situated at the bend of the nerve as it traverses the facial canal in the petrous temporal bone.

Gustatory Receptors and Their Innervation

The structure of the gustatory sense organ, the **taste bud**, is shown in Figure 8-12. Taste buds are derived from cells of the pharyngeal endoderm, and they first appear in the 8th week of intrauterine life. By 5 months, they are present throughout the oral cavity and pharynx, but the numbers then decrease. Shortly after birth, the distribution of taste buds is the same as in the adult: the soft palate; the epiglottis; and, most abundantly, certain of the papillae of the tongue. About 10 large **vallate papillae**, each surrounded by deep trench, are aligned across the most posterior part of the tongue. Microscopic **fungiform papillae** occur all over the dorsal surface, among the more numerous filiform papillae. The latter give the tongue a rough texture and do not bear taste buds. Flattened, longitudinally aligned **foliate papillae** support taste buds on the sides of the tongue.

The cilia of the taste cells (see Fig. 8-12) bear surface receptors that bind substances with specific flavors. Activation of the receptors results in depolarization of the cell membrane. This event activates chemical transmission: the taste cells are presynaptic to the sensory axons that innervate them. Individual taste buds respond to different kinds of chemical stimuli. Physiological, pharmacological, and biochemical studies indicate that individual taste cells respond to one of five elementary flavors: salty (e.g., sodium ions), sour (acidity), sweet (e.g., sugar), bitter (alkalinity, also many organic compounds), and umami (amino acids, especially glutamate). Taste buds that respond to sweetness are most abundant on the tip of the tongue. Sour tastes are detected especially at the lateral edges, and bitter substances at the back of the tongue. Receptors for other flavors are generally

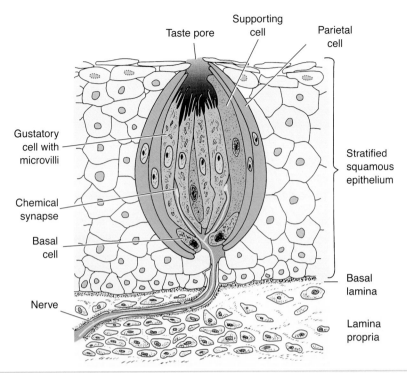

FIGURE 8-12   Structure of a taste bud. The chemical sensors are the apical microvilli of the taste cells. Chemical synapses communicate with the sensory axons. Taste cells and supporting cells are renewed every few days from the population of dividing basal cells.

distributed. Ordinary tastes are thought to result from mixed neural signals from at least four types of taste buds, integrated in the brain with the input from the olfactory system.

The sense of taste is served by cranial nerves VII, IX, and X. Primary sensory neurons for taste account for most of the cell bodies in the geniculate ganglion. The peripheral branches of their axons enter either of two branches of the facial nerve (Fig. 8-11):

1. The **greater petrosal** branch proceeds into the pterygopalatine fossa above the palate, where the taste axons join palatine branches of the maxillary division of the trigeminal nerve and are distributed to palatal taste buds, most of which are in the mucosa of the soft palate (see Fig. 8-11).

2. The **chorda tympani** branch of the facial nerve joins the lingual branch of the mandibular nerve. These fibers are distributed to taste buds in the anterior two thirds of the tongue, most of which are on its tip and along its lateral border. (Other gustatory nerves are reviewed in conjunction with the glossopharyngeal and vagus nerves, later in this chapter.)

The axons of geniculate ganglion cells that subserve taste enter the brain stem in the **nervus intermedius** and turn caudally in the **solitary tract** (see Figs. 7-6 and 8-13). The facial nerve fibers in this fasciculus are joined more caudally by gustatory axons from the glossopharyngeal and vagus nerves. Fibers from all three sources terminate in the **solitary nucleus**, a column of cells adjacent to and partly surrounding the tract. Only the large-celled rostral part of the solitary nucleus receives taste fibers; this part is sometimes called the **gustatory nucleus**. (The caudal part, whose cells are smaller, receives general visceral afferents.)

Ascending Pathway for Taste

Fibers from the gustatory nucleus run rostrally in the ipsilateral **central tegmental tract**, through the midbrain and subthalamic region, to their site of termination in the most medial part of the **ventral posterior nucleus of the thalamus**. This thalamic nucleus projects to

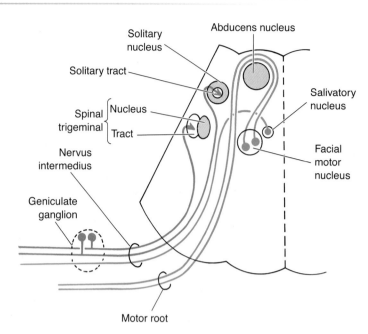

FIGURE 8-13 Components of the facial nerve in the brain stem. Primary sensory neurons are blue, motor neurons are red, and preganglionic and postganglionic parasympathetic neurons are green.

the **cortical area for taste**, which is adjacent to the general sensory area for the tongue and extends onto the insula and forward to the frontal operculum. Physiological evidence has shown that in animals, gustatory stimuli influence the hypothalamus, amygdala, and cortex of the limbic system but probably not through specific ascending projections from the brain stem. Similar to the functionally related olfactory system (see Chapter 17), the pathway for taste does not cross the midline (Fig. 8-14).

Cutaneous Fibers

Cutaneous sensory axons leave the facial nerve at the junction of the facial canal with the stylomastoid foramen (see Fig. 8-11). These fibers are distributed to the skin of the concha of the auricle, a small area behind the ear, the wall of the external acoustic meatus, and the external surface of the tympanic membrane. The central processes of the geniculate ganglion cells for cutaneous sensation enter the brain stem in the nervus intermedius. They continue into the spinal trigeminal tract (see Fig. 8-13) and terminate in the subjacent spinal trigeminal nucleus.

Efferent Components

For Supply of Striated Muscles

The motor component is the most important part of the nerve from the clinical viewpoint. The **facial motor nucleus** is located in the caudal

one third of the ventrolateral part of the pontine tegmentum (see Figs. 7-8 and 8-13). Axons leaving the nucleus pursue an unexpected course. Directed initially toward the floor of the fourth ventricle, these fibers loop over the caudal end of the abducens nucleus, run forward along its medial side, and loop again over the rostral end of the nucleus. The axons then proceed to the point of emergence of the motor root of the facial nerve by passing between their nucleus of origin and the spinal trigeminal nucleus. The configuration of the fiber bundle around the abducens nucleus is called the **internal genu**. (The external genu of the facial nerve is located in the facial canal at the level of the geniculate ganglion.)

The motor root of the facial nerve consists entirely of fibers from the motor nucleus. These fibers supply the muscles of expression (mimetic muscles), the platysma and stylohyoid muscles, and the posterior belly of the digastric muscle. The facial nerve also supplies the stapedius muscle of the middle ear; by reflex contraction in response to loud sounds, this small muscle prevents excessive movement of the stapes.

The facial motor nucleus receives afferents from several sources, including important connections for reflexes:

1. Tectobulbar fibers from the superior colliculus complete a reflex pathway that provides for closure of the eyelids in re-

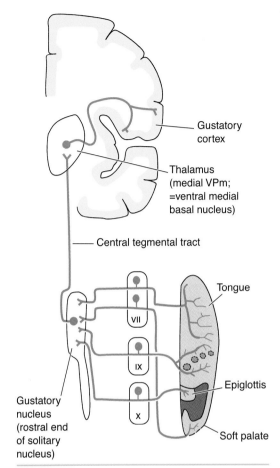

FIGURE 8-14   Central pathway for taste sensation, from taste buds to the ipsilateral cerebral cortex.

Labels in figure:
- Gustatory cortex
- Thalamus (medial VPm; =ventral medial basal nucleus)
- Central tegmental tract
- Tongue
- VII
- IX
- X
- Epiglottis
- Soft palate
- Gustatory nucleus (rostral end of solitary nucleus)

3. Fibers from the superior olivary nucleus (which is part of the auditory pathway) permit reflex contraction of the stapedius muscle.

Parasympathetic Nucleus

The salivary and lacrimal glands are supplied by parasympathetic ganglia. Neurons in the brain stem that supply these ganglia have been identified in laboratory animals, and structurally similar cells with the same histochemical properties (they contain the enzymes acetylcholinesterase and NADPH diaphorase) occur in corresponding locations in the human brain. Most are located dorsomedial and ventrolateral to the facial motor nucleus (Fig. 8-13). These groups of cells constitute the **salivary nucleus**, which is the probable source of preganglionic parasympathetic fibers in the facial and glossopharyngeal nerves. (Traditionally a lacrimal nucleus and superior and inferior salivatory nuclei, in vaguely specified positions, were named as the sources of preganglionic fibers to the pterygopalatine, submandibular, and otic ganglia. The traditional notion is not supported by observations or experimental data.)

The salivatory nucleus contains the cell bodies of preganglionic parasympathetic fibers that control the submandibular and sublingual salivary glands and the lacrimal gland. Axons from the salivatory nucleus leave the brain stem in the nervus intermedius and continue in the facial nerve until branches are given off in the facial canal in the petrous temporal bone (see Fig. 8-11). The preganglionic fibers follow devious routes to their destinations, running part of the way in branches of the trigeminal nerve.

sponse to intense light or a rapidly approaching object.

2. Fibers from trigeminal sensory nuclei function in the corneal reflex and in chewing or sucking responses on placing food in the mouth.

Descending Control of Facial Movements

Corticobulbar afferents are crossed, except for those that terminate on cells supplying the frontalis and orbicularis oculi muscles, which receive both crossed and uncrossed fibers. **Contralateral voluntary paralysis of only the lower facial muscles is, therefore, a feature of upper motor neuron lesions.** Under such circumstances, however, the facial muscles continue to respond involuntarily—and often excessively—to changing moods and emotions. In contrast, emotional changes of facial expression are typically lost in patients with Parkinson's disease (masklike face), although voluntary use of the facial muscles is retained. The neuroanatomical basis of controlling voluntary and emotionally driven facial movement is not known; it must involve different descending pathways from the cerebral hemispheres.

Fibers that control lacrimal secretion pass into the **greater petrosal nerve** and terminate in the pterygopalatine ganglion (also called the sphenopalatine ganglion) in the pterygopalatine fossa. Postganglionic fibers, which stimulate secretion and cause vasodilation, reach the lacrimal gland through the zygomatic branch of the maxillary nerve. Other secretomotor postganglionic fibers are distributed to mucous glands in the mucosa that lines the nasal cavity and the paranasal sinuses.

Other axons from the salivatory nucleus leave the facial nerve in the **chorda tympani** branch and are then carried in the lingual branch of the mandibular nerve to the floor of the oral cavity. There they terminate in the **submandibular ganglion** and on scattered neurons within the submandibular gland. Short postganglionic fibers are distributed to the parenchyma of the submandibular and sublingual glands, where they stimulate secretion and cause vasodilation.

The salivatory nucleus is influenced by the hypothalamus, perhaps through the dorsal lon-gitudinal fasciculus, and by the olfactory system through relays in the reticular formation. Taste and general sensation from the mucosa of the oral cavity promote salivation through connections of the solitary nucleus and sensory trigeminal nuclei, respectively.

GLOSSOPHARYNGEAL, VAGUS, AND ACCESSORY NERVES

Cranial nerves IX, X, and XI have much in common functionally and share certain nuclei in the medulla. To avoid repetition, it is convenient to consider them together.

Sensory Components

The glossopharyngeal and vagus nerves include sensory fibers for the special visceral sense of taste; general visceral afferents from baro- and chemoreceptors and from viscera of the thorax and abdomen; and general sensory fibers for pain, temperature, and touch from the back of the tongue, pharynx and nearby regions, the skin of part of the ear, and parts of the dura mater. The cell bodies of primary sensory neurons

---

CLINICAL NOTE

Facial Paralysis

Facial paralysis commonly accompanies hemiplegia caused by occlusion of an artery supplying the contralateral internal capsule or the motor areas of the cerebral cortex. For reasons already stated, only the lower half of the face is affected. When a unilateral facial paralysis involves the musculature around the eyes and in the forehead in addition to that around the mouth, the lesion must involve either the cell bodies in the facial nucleus or their axons. In a common condition known as **Bell's palsy**, the facial nerve is affected as it traverses the facial canal in the petrous temporal bone, with rapid onset of weakness (paresis) or paralysis of all the facial muscles on the affected side. The cause is edema (perhaps caused by a viral infection) of the facial nerve and adjacent tissue in the facial canal. The signs of Bell's palsy depend not only on the severity of the axonal compression but also on where the nerve is affected in its passage through the facial canal (see Fig. 8-11). All functions of the nerve are lost if the damage is at or proximal to the geniculate ganglion. In addition to the paralysis of facial muscles, there is a loss of taste (**ageusia**) in the anterior two thirds of the tongue and in the palate of the affected side, together with impairment of secretion by the submandibular, sublingual, and lacrimal glands. Also, sounds seem abnormally loud (**hyperacusis**) because of paralysis of the stapedius muscle. In contrast, compression near the stylomastoid foramen affects only the motor fibers of the nerve.

In mild cases of Bell's palsy, the axons are not damaged severely enough to result in Wallerian degeneration, and the prognosis is favorable. Recovery is slow and frequently incomplete when it must rely on axonal regeneration. There is no regeneration into the brain stem of sensory fibers that have been interrupted on the central side of the geniculate ganglion. In the case of such a lesion in the proximal part of the nerve, some regenerating salivatory fibers may find their way into the greater petrosal nerve and reach the pterygopalatine ganglion. This results in lacrimation (**crocodile tears**) instead of salivation when aromas and taste sensations cause stimulation of cells in the superior salivatory nucleus.

are located in the superior and inferior ganglia of cranial nerves IX and X.

Visceral Afferents

The unipolar cell bodies for the **gustatory fibers** are situated in the two **glossopharyngeal ganglia** (a tiny superior ganglion and a larger inferior ganglion) and in the **inferior ganglion of the vagus nerve**. The last of these is frequently called the **nodose ganglion**. The distal axonal branches are distributed through the glossopharyngeal nerve to taste buds on the posterior two thirds of the tongue as well as to the few that occur in the pharyngeal mucosa. Vagal fibers supply taste buds present on the epiglottis. Central processes of the ganglion cells join the solitary tract and terminate in the rostral portion of the solitary nucleus, the **gustatory nucleus** (see Fig. 7-6 and 8-15). The ascending pathway for taste is described and illustrated in Figure 8-14 in conjunction with the visceral afferent component of the facial nerve.

General visceral afferent neurons receive signals used for reflex regulation of cardiovascular, respiratory, and alimentary function. Their cell bodies are located in the glossopharyngeal and inferior vagal ganglia, together with the neurons for taste. These fibers in the glossopharyngeal nerve supply the carotid sinus at the bifurcation of the common carotid artery and the adjacent carotid body. Sensory endings in the wall of the **carotid sinus** function as **baroreceptors**, which monitor arterial blood pressure. The **carotid body** contains **chemoreceptors**, which monitor the concentration of oxygen in the circulating blood. Vagal fibers similarly supply baroreceptors in the **aortic arch** and chemoreceptors in the small **aortic bodies** adjacent to the aortic arch. The vagus nerve also contains many afferent fibers that are distributed to the **viscera of the thorax and abdomen**; impulses conveyed centrally are important in reflex control of cardiovascular, respiratory, and alimentary functions. The central branches of the axons of the general visceral afferent neurons descend in the solitary tract and end in the more caudal part of the **solitary nucleus** (see Figs. 8-15 and 8-16). Connections from the latter site are established bilaterally with several regions of the reticular formation. Reticulobulbar and reticulospinal projections, together with a small solitariospinal tract, provide pathways for reflex responses mediated by the parasympathetic and sympathetic nervous systems and by somatic motor neurons that supply the muscles of respiration.

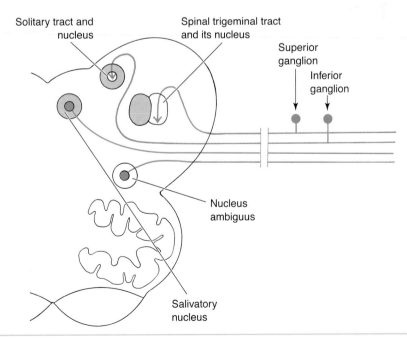

FIGURE 8-15   Components of the glossopharyngeal nerve in the medulla. Primary sensory neurons are blue, motor neurons are red, and preganglionic parasympathetic neurons are green.

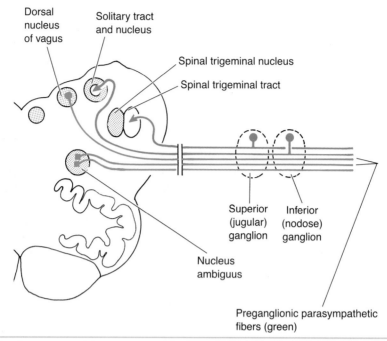

FIGURE 8-16   Components of the vagus nerve in the medulla. Primary sensory neurons are blue, motor neurons are red, and preganglionic parasympathetic neurons are green.

Some axons from the solitary nucleus proceed rostrally to the hypothalamus. Others probably go to the ventral posteromedial nucleus of the thalamus, providing for conscious sensations other than pain, such as fullness or emptiness of the stomach.

Somatic Afferent Fibers

The **glossopharyngeal nerve** includes fibers for the general sensations of pain, temperature, and touch in the mucosa of the posterior one third of the tongue, upper part of the pharynx (including the tonsillar area), auditory or eustachian tube, and middle ear. The **vagus nerve** carries fibers with the same functions to the lower part of the pharynx, the larynx, and the esophagus. The cell bodies of these sensory neurons are located in the **glossopharyngeal ganglia** and in the **superior ganglion of the vagus nerve**, which is also called the **jugular ganglion**. The central branches of their axons enter the **spinal trigeminal tract** and terminate in the **spinal trigeminal nucleus** (see Figs. 8-15 and 8-16). The afferents for touch from the pharynx are important in the **gag reflex**: touching the pharynx causes elevation of the soft palate and movement of the tongue through a path-

way that includes the nucleus ambiguus and the hypoglossal nucleus.

The **vagus nerve** sends general sensory (pain) fibers to the dura that lines the posterior fossa of the cranial cavity. Through its auricular branch, it contributes sensory fibers to the concha of the external ear, a small area behind the ear, the wall of the external acoustic meatus, and the tympanic membrane. The cell bodies are located in the superior ganglion of the nerve, and the central processes join the spinal trigeminal tract. The area of skin and tympanic membrane supplied by the auricular branch of the vagus nerve is coextensive with that supplied by the facial nerve. The vagus nerve also sends general sensory fibers to the larynx, trachea, bronchi, and esophagus.

Efferent Components

Cranial nerves IX, X, and XI include motor fibers for striated muscles, and cranial nerves IX and X contain parasympathetic efferents.

For Supply of Striated Muscles

The **nucleus ambiguus** is a slender column of motor neurons situated dorsal to the inferior olivary nucleus (see Figs. 7-5 to 7-7 and 8-15 to 8-17). Axons from this nucleus are directed dorsally at first. They then turn sharply to mingle with other fibers in the glossopharyngeal and vagus nerves, and some of them constitute the entire cranial root of the accessory nerve. The nucleus ambiguus supplies muscles of the soft palate, pharynx, and larynx, together with striated muscle fibers in the upper part of the esophagus. (The only muscle in these regions not supplied by this nucleus is the tensor veli palatini, which is innervated by the trigeminal nerve.)

A small group of cells in the rostral end of the nucleus ambiguus supplies the stylopharyngeus muscle through the **glossopharyngeal nerve** (see Fig. 8-15). A large region of the nucleus supplies the remaining pharyngeal muscles, the cricothyroid (an external muscle of the larynx), and the striated muscle of the esophagus, through the **vagus nerve** (see Fig. 8-16). Fibers from the caudal part of the nucleus ambiguus leave the brain stem in the **cranial root of the accessory nerve** (see Fig. 8-17). These fibers temporarily join the spinal root of the accessory nerve and then constitute the internal ramus of the nerve, which passes over to the vagus nerve in the region of the jugular foramen. These fibers supply muscles of the soft palate and the intrinsic muscles of the larynx.

The nucleus ambiguus receives afferents from sensory nuclei of the brain stem, most importantly from the spinal trigeminal and solitary nuclei. These connections establish reflexes for coughing, gagging, and vomiting, with the stimuli arising in the mucosa of the respiratory and alimentary passages. *Corticobulbar afferents are both crossed and uncrossed; muscles supplied by the nucleus ambiguus are, therefore, not paralyzed in the event of a unilateral lesion of the upper motor neuron type.* The nucleus ambiguus is

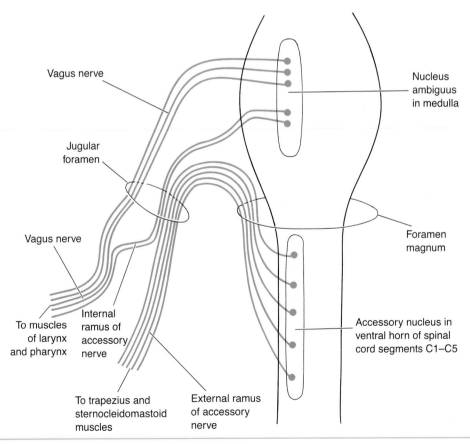

FIGURE 8-17   Spinal and cranial roots of the accessory nerve.

not composed solely of motor neurons. As described later, some of its cells are preganglionic parasympathetic neurons for control of the heart rate.

Motor neurons for the sternocleidomastoid and trapezius muscles are located in the spinal cord (segments C1 to C5) and constitute the **accessory nucleus** in the ventral gray horn. Arising as a series of rootlets along the side of the spinal cord, just dorsal to the denticulate ligament, the **spinal root of the accessory nerve** ascends next to the spinal cord (see Fig. 8-17). On reaching the side of the medulla by passing through the foramen magnum, the spinal and cranial roots unite and continue as the accessory nerve, but only as far as the jugular foramen. Fibers from the nucleus ambiguus then join the vagus nerve, as already noted. Those of spinal origin proceed through the posterior triangle of the neck and supply the sternocleidomastoid and trapezius muscles.

Parasympathetic Nuclei

Preganglionic parasympathetic fibers are present in the glossopharyngeal and vagus nerves. The **salivatory nucleus** consists of groups of neurons located lateral and medial to the facial motor nucleus and is the source of preganglionic fibers in the facial and glossopharyngeal nerves. (There is no evidence for the existence of distinct superior and inferior salivatory nuclei.) Axons from the salivatory nucleus pass into the tympanic branch of the glossopharyngeal nerve, the tympanic plexus, and the lesser petrosal nerve to the **otic ganglion**, which lies beneath the foramen ovale, close to the mandibular division of the trigeminal nerve. The neurons in the otic ganglion have axons (i.e., postganglionic fibers) that join the auriculotemporal branch of the mandibular nerve and thus reach the **parotid gland**. The parasympathetic supply to the parotid gland stimulates secretion and vasodilation. The salivatory nucleus is influenced by stimuli from the hypothalamus, olfactory system, solitary nucleus, and sensory trigeminal nuclei.

The largest parasympathetic nucleus is the **dorsal nucleus of the vagus nerve** (also called *dorsal motor nucleus*, but it does not directly innervate muscles). This column of cells is situated in the gray matter lateral to the central canal and extending beneath the vagal triangle in the floor of the fourth ventricle (see Figs. 7-4 to 7-7). The axons of the cells in the dorsal nucleus constitute the majority of the preganglionic parasympathetic fibers of the vagus nerve. They end in tiny ganglia in the **pulmonary plexus** and in **abdominal viscera**, notably the stomach. For details, see Chapter 24.

Other vagal parasympathetic neurons have their cell bodies near and among the motor neurons of the **nucleus ambiguus**. The axons of these neurons terminate in small ganglia associated with the **heart**. In some laboratory animals, about 10% of the cardioinhibitory neurons are located in the dorsal nucleus of the vagus. In others, the cardiac ganglia receive all their afferent fibers from the nucleus ambiguus and none from the dorsal nucleus. It seems likely that the nucleus ambiguus contains most or all of the vagal neurons that control the human heart.

The dorsal nucleus of the vagus nerve and the visceral efferent neurons of the nucleus am-

---

CLINICAL NOTE

Accessory Nerve Palsy

If the accessory nerve is injured (typically by an object falling onto the back of the shoulder or neck), the sternocleidomastoid and trapezius muscles will be paralyzed or weakened ipsilaterally.

Corticospinal fibers that control the spinal accessory neurons are both crossed and uncrossed. Those for the trapezius are from the contralateral cerebrum. Those for the sternocleidomastoid are from the ipsilateral cerebrum, an arrangement consistent with the action of this muscle, which turns the head toward the opposite side. *An upper motor neuron lesion, therefore, causes weakness (paresis) of the contralateral trapezius and of the ipsilateral sternocleidomastoid muscle.*

Hypoglossal Nerve Palsy

Destruction of the hypoglossal nucleus or interruption of the motor axons in the medulla or in the nerve is followed by paralysis and eventual atrophy of the affected muscles. The tongue *deviates to the weak side* on protrusion because of the unopposed action of the contralateral genioglossus muscle.

Corticobulbar afferents to the hypoglossal nucleus are predominantly but not exclusively crossed. A unilateral upper motor neuron lesion causes paresis of the opposite side of the tongue, which usually recovers quite quickly as the ipsilateral cerebral hemisphere assumes the functions of the damaged descending pathway.

biguus are influenced, directly or indirectly, by the solitary nucleus, hypothalamus, olfactory system, and autonomic "centers" in the reticular formation (see Chapter 9). Despite the functional importance of the visceral afferent and preganglionic parasympathetic fibers, transection of the vagus nerve does not cause cardiovascular symptoms. Vagal denervation of the stomach suppresses acid secretion there and causes gastric distention caused by inadequate emptying through the pylorus.

HYPOGLOSSAL NERVE

The **hypoglossal nucleus** lies between the dorsal nucleus of the vagus nerve and the midline of the medulla (see Figs. 7-4 to 7-7 and 8-18). The hypoglossal triangle in the floor of the fourth ventricle marks the position of the rostral part of the nucleus. The axons of hypoglossal neurons course ventrally on the lateral side of the medial lemniscus and emerge along

the sulcus between the pyramid and the olive. The hypoglossal nerve supplies the intrinsic muscles of the tongue and the three extrinsic muscles (genioglossus, styloglossus, and hyoglossus). The nucleus receives afferents from the solitary nucleus and the sensory trigeminal nuclei for reflex movements of the tongue in swallowing, chewing, and sucking in response to gustatory and other stimuli from the oral and pharyngeal mucosae.

Summary of Cranial Nerve Nuclei and Components

Distinct functions are associated with the nuclei of origin or termination of the component fibers of cranial nerves. Table 8-1 summarizes the functions of the nuclei and emphasizes the sharing of nuclei by different cranial nerves.

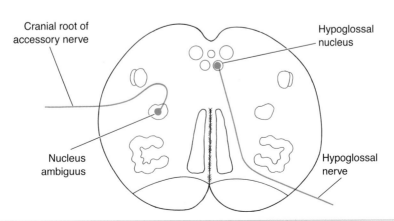

FIGURE 8-18   Right hypoglossal nerve and origin of the cranial root of the left accessory nerve in the medulla.

TABLE 8-1 **Cranial Nerve Nuclei, Associated Ganglia, and Their Functions**

Nucleus	Nerve	Ganglion	Muscles, Glands, or Sensory Functions
Oculomotor	III		Levator palpebrae superioris and all extra-ocular muscles except superior oblique and lateral rectus
Edinger-Westphal	III	Ciliary	Sphincter pupillae and ciliary muscle
Trochlear	IV		Superior oblique muscle
Motor trigeminal	V (mandibular)		Chewing muscles; tensor tympani
Mesencephalic trigeminal	V (maxillary and mandibular)	None	Proprioception from muscles of mastication and temporomandibular joint; pressure around roots of teeth
Pontine trigeminal	V (all divisions)	Trigeminal	Touch (face, mouth, and so on)
Spinal trigeminal	V (all divisions)	Trigeminal	Touch, pain, temperature (face, mouth, and so on)
	VII	Geniculate	Cutaneous sensation from parts of external ear (together with cranial nerve X)
	IX	Glossopharyngeal ganglia	General sensation from pharynx, posterior third of tongue, middle ear
	X	Superior vagal (jugular) ganglion for ear; inferior (nodose) ganglion for others	General sensation from parts of external ear, larynx, and so on
Abducens	VI		Lateral rectus muscle
Facial motor	VII		Facial muscles and stapedius
Salivatory	VII (greater petrosal and nervus inter-medius)	Pterygopalatine	Lacrimal and nasal glands
	VII (chorda tympani and nervus inter-medius)	Submandibular	Submandibular and sublingual glands
	IX	Otic	Parotid gland
Cochlear nuclei	VIII (cochlear)	Spiral	Hearing (see Chapter 21)
Vestibular nuclei	VIII (vestibular)	Vestibular	Equilibration (see Chapter 22)
Nucleus ambiguus	IX X and cranial root of XI		Stylopharyngeus Muscles of larynx, pharynx, esophagus
Solitary: rostral end (gustatory nucleus)	VII (greater petrosal and chorda tympani branches and nervus inter-medius)	Geniculate	Taste, soft palate and anterior two thirds of tongue
	IX	Glossopharyngeal	Taste, posterior third of tongue

(continued)

TABLE 8-1 **Cranial Nerve Nuclei, Associated Ganglia, and Their Functions (continued)**

Nucleus	Nerve	Ganglion	Muscles, Glands, or Sensory Functions
Solitary: caudal end	IX X	Glossopharyngeal Inferior vagal (nodose)	Carotid sinus and body Regulatory sensation (not pain) from thoracic and abdominal organs
Dorsal nucleus of vagus	X	Numerous, near thoracic and abdominal organs	See Chapter 24
Nucleus ambiguus	X	Cardiac ganglia	Heart (reduced rate and output)
Accessory nucleus	XI (spinal root)		Sternocleidomastoid and trapezius
Hypoglossal	XII		Tongue muscles

Suggested Reading

Bear MF, Connors BW, Paradiso MA. *Neuroscience: Exploring the Brain.* Philadelphia: Lippincott, Williams & Wilkins, 2007:252–263.

Beckstead RM, Morse JR, Norgren R. The nucleus of the solitary tract in the monkey: projections to the thalamus and brain stem nuclei. *J Comp Neurol* 1980;190:259–282.

Bender MB. Brain control of conjugate horizontal and vertical eye movements: a survey of the structural and functional correlates. *Brain* 1980;103:23–69.

Bianchi R, Rodella L, Rezzani R, et al. Cytoarchitecture of the abducens nucleus of man: a Nissl and Golgi study. *Acta Anat* 1996;157:210–216.

Blessing WW. Lower brain stem regulation of visceral, cardiovascular and respiratory function. In: Paxinos G, Mai JK, eds. *The Human Nervous System*, 2nd ed. Amsterdam: Elsevier Academic Press, 2004: 464–478.

Cagan RH, ed. *Neural Mechanisms in Taste.* Boca Raton, FL: CRC Press, 1989.

Cruccu G, Berardelli A, Inghilleri M, et al. Corticobulbar projections to upper and lower facial motorneurons: a study by magnetic transcranial stimulation in man. *Neurosci Lett* 1990;117:68–73.

Davies AM, Lumsden A. Ontogeny of the somatosensory system: origins and early development of primary sensory neurons. *Annu Rev Neurosci* 1990;13:61–73.

Gai WP, Blessing WW. Human brainstem preganglionic parasympathetic neurons localized by markers for nitric oxide synthesis. *Brain* 1996;119:1145–1152.

Horn AKE, Büttner-Ennever JA. Premotor neurons for vertical eye movements in the rostral mesencephalon of monkey and human: histologic identification by parvalbumin immunostaining. *J Comp Neurol* 1998;392:413–427.

Horn AKE, Büttner-Ennever JA, Suzuki Y, et al. Histological identification of premotor neurons for horizontal saccades in monkey and man by parvalbumin immunostaining. *J Comp Neurol* 1995;359:350–363.

Ito S, Ogawa H. Cytochrome oxidase staining facilitates unequivocal visualization of the primary gustatory area in the fronto-operculo-insular cortex of macaque monkeys. *Neurosci Lett* 1991;130:61–64.

Jenny A, Smith A, Decker J. Motor organization of the spinal accessory nerve in the monkey. *Brain Res* 1988;441:352–356.

Keller EL, Heinen SJ. Generation of smooth pursuit eye movements: neuronal mechanisms and pathways. *Neurosci Res* 1991;11:79–107.

Kourouyan HD, Horton JC. Transneuronal retinal input to the primate Edinger-Westphal nucleus. *J Comp Neurol* 1997;381:68–80.

Lekwuwa GU, Barnes GR. Cerebral control of eye movements, 1: the relationship between cerebral lesion sites and smooth pursuit deficits. *Brain* 1996;119:473–490.

Love S, Coakham HB. Trigeminal neuralgia: pathology and pathogenesis. *Brain* 2001;124:2347–2360.

Lui F, Gregory KM, Blanks RHI, et al. Projections from visual areas of the cerebral cortex to pretectal nuclear complex, terminal accessory optic nuclei, and superior colliculus in macaque monkey. *J Comp Neurol* 1995;363:439–460.

May M, ed. *The Facial Nerve.* New York: Thieme, 1986.

O'Rahilly R. On counting cranial nerves. *Acta Anat* 1988;133:3–4.

Plecha DM, Randall WC, Geis GS, et al. Localization of vagal preganglionic somata controlling sinoatrial and atrioventricular nodes. *Am J Physiol* 1988;255:R703–R708.

Pritchard TC, Norgren R. Gustatory System. In: Paxinos G, Mai JK, eds. *The Human Nervous System*, 2nd ed. Amsterdam: Elsevier Academic Press, 2004:1171–1196.

Robinson FR, Phillips JO, Fuchs AF. Coordination of gaze shifts in primates: brainstem inputs to neck and extraocular motoneuron pools. *J Comp Neurol* 1994;346:43–62.

Routal RV, Pal GP. Location of the spinal nucleus of the accessory nerve in the human spinal cord. *J Anat* 2000;196:263–268.

Ruskell GL, Simons T. Trigeminal nerve pathways to the cerebral arteries in monkeys. *J Anat* 1987;155:23–37.

Tarozzo G, Peretto P, Fasolo A. Cell migration from the olfactory placode and the ontogeny of the neuroendocrine compartments. *Zool Sci* 1995;12:367–383.

Tehovnik E, Sommer MA, Chou IH, et al. Eye fields in the frontal lobes of primates. *Brain Res Rev* 2000;32:413–448.

Thömke F. Brainstem diseases causing isolated ocular motor palsies. *Neuro-Ophthamology* 2004;28:53–67.

Urban PP, Hopf HC, Connemann B, et al. The course of cortico-hypoglossal projections in the human brainstem: functional testing using transcranial magnetic stimulation. *Brain* 1996;119:1031–1038.

Wilson-Pauwels L, Akesson EJ, Stewart PA, et al. *Cranial Nerves in Health and Disease*, 2nd ed. Toronto, British Columbia, Canada: Dekker, 2002.

Witt M, Reutter K. Innervation of developing human taste buds: an immunohistochemical study. *Histochem Cell Biol* 1998;109:281–291.

Zakrzewska JM. *Trigeminal Neuralgia*. London: Saunders, 1995.

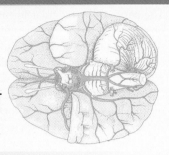

Chapter 9

RETICULAR FORMATION

Important Facts

- The reticular formation of the brain stem contains several populations of neurons with long dendrites surrounded by interlacing bundles of myelinated axons.
- The **precerebellar reticular nuclei** are probably concerned with coordination of muscle contractions.
- The **raphe nuclei** include many serotonergic neurons, with extensively distributed axons. Rostrally projecting serotonergic neurons are active in sleep. Caudally projecting neurons, which receive afferents from the periaqueductal gray matter, modulate pain sensation.
- The **central group** of nuclei includes the cells of origin of motor reticulospinal fibers. Rostral projections are concerned with eye movements and with the conscious state.
- **Cholinergic reticular nuclei** influence stereotyped movements through connections with the central group and the basal ganglia of the forebrain. They are also active in rapid eye movement sleep. Neuronal circuitry for consciousness and sleep also involves the hypothalamus, thalamus, and cerebral cortex.
- **Catecholaminergic neurons** in the locus coeruleus and elsewhere have axons that go to most parts of the brain and spinal cord, probably to increase the speed of reflex responses and the general level of alertness.
- Through connections with appropriate sensory, motor, and autonomic neurons, the laterally located parvocellular, parabrachial, and superficial medullary reticular areas are concerned with the regulation of feeding and of the respiratory and circulatory systems.
- The area postrema, which contains permeable blood vessels, is a chemoreceptor that mediates some physiological responses to bloodborne stimuli, including drug-induced vomiting.
- The paramedian pontine reticular formation, the perihypoglossal nuclei, and the accessory oculomotor nuclei are involved in the control of eye movements.

This chapter describes the anatomy and connections of the groups of neurons that constitute the reticular formation of the brain stem and reviews the involvement of the reticular formation in sleep and consciousness as well as in sensory and motor functions. The chapter also provides descriptions of a few other nuclei in the brain stem that are not discussed in Chapters 7 and 8.

Broadly defined, the **reticular formation** consists of a substantial part of the dorsal part of the brain stem in which the groups of neurons and intersecting bundles of fibers present a netlike (reticular) appearance in transverse sections. It excludes nuclei of cranial nerves, long tracts that pass through the brain stem, and the more conspicuous masses of gray matter. Some "excluded" structures, however, such as the medial lemniscus and the nucleus ambiguus, are located within the territory of the reticular formation. The neurons of the reticular nuclei all have unusually long dendrites that extend into parts of the brain stem remote from the cell bodies. Their architecture enables them to receive and integrate synaptic inputs from most or all of the axons that project to or through the brain stem.

Through its direct and indirect connections with all levels of the central nervous system (CNS), the reticular formation contributes to several functions, including the sleep–arousal cycle, perception of pain, control of movement, and regulation of visceral activity. Although such adjectives as "primitive" and "diffuse" have been applied to the reticular formation, it is not a mass of randomly interconnected neurons.

The parts of the reticular formation differ from one another in their cytoarchitecture, connections, and physiological functions. Aggregations of neurons are thereby recognized and are called nuclei, even though not all are as clearly circumscribed as nuclei elsewhere. As in every part of the nervous system, information obtained through research continues to reveal higher and higher degrees of orderly structural organization than were previously thought to exist.

Nuclei of the Reticular Formation

The nuclei of the reticular formation (Fig. 9-1) can be classified as follows: the precerebellar nuclei, the raphe nuclei, the central group of nuclei, the cholinergic and catecholamine cell groups, the lateral parvocellular reticular area, the parabrachial area, and the superficial medullary neurons. Ad-

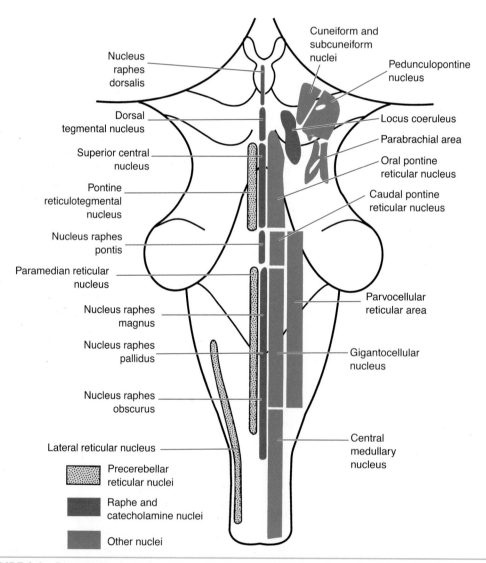

FIGURE 9-1   Diagram showing the positions of the larger nuclei of the reticular formation of the brain stem.

ditionally functionally designated "centers," recognized mainly from experiments in animals, are present that do not always correspond to anatomically defined populations of neuronal cell bodies.

PRECEREBELLAR RETICULAR NUCLEI

The **lateral reticular nucleus** (see Figs. 9-1 and 9-2A), the **paramedian reticular nucleus** (see Fig. 9-2A), and the **pontine reticulotegmental nucleus** (see Figs. 9-1 and 9-2D) project to the cerebellum. These precerebellar reticular nuclei are functionally quite separate from the rest of the reticular formation; they are briefly considered in Chapter 10, which deals with the cerebellum.

RAPHE NUCLEI

The raphe nuclei are groups of neurons either in or adjacent to the midline (raphe) of the brain stem, interspersed among bundles of decussating axons. Raphe nuclei with different cytoarchitecture and efferent projections are recognized at different levels (see Figs. 9-1 and 9-2). Many raphe neurons synthesize and secrete **serotonin** (5-hydroxytryptamine), and this amine is believed to be their principal synaptic transmitter. The axons of the serotonergic raphe neurons are thin, unmyelinated, and greatly branched. They are distributed to gray matter throughout the CNS. Their most prominent projections are summarized in Figure 9-3.

The connections of the medullary raphe nuclei with the periaqueductal gray matter and the spinal dorsal horn (and trigeminal sensory nuclei) are important from a clinical standpoint because activity of this pathway can suppress the conscious awareness of pain (see Chapter 19). The pontine and mesencephalic raphe nuclei project to the cerebellum and with all parts of the cerebrum, including the cerebral cortex, basal ganglia, and limbic system.

The best understood functions of the more rostrally located raphe nuclei are those related to sleep. They are discussed later in this chapter.

CENTRAL GROUP OF RETICULAR NUCLEI

The central group includes medially located nuclei in the medulla and pons and the **cuneiform** and **subcuneiform nuclei** in the midbrain

(see Figs. 9-1 and 9-2). The latter two are laterally located but are included in the central group because of their similar connections and functions. The **paramedian pontine reticular formation (PPRF)**, which is importantly involved in conjugate lateral movements of the eyes (see Chapter 8), includes neurons in the medial parts of the two pontine reticular nuclei. The gigantocellular reticular nucleus (Fig. 9-2B) includes some serotonin neurons, which have projections similar to those of neurons in the nearby nucleus raphes magnus.

The central nuclei receive afferents from all the general and special sensory systems and from the reticular formation of the midbrain, the cholinergic reticular nuclei (see below), the hypothalamus, and the premotor area of the cerebral cortex (Fig. 9-4).

Neurons of the central reticular nuclei typically have axons with long ascending and descending branches. In the brain stem, these axons also have numerous horizontally directed collateral branches, which synapse with the long dendrites of other reticular neurons (Fig. 9-5), including those of the raphe and catecholamine nuclei. The long descending axons constitute the **reticulospinal tracts**, located in the ventral and lateral funiculi of the spinal white matter (see Fig. 5-10). The reticulospinal tracts are important motor pathways (discussed later in this chapter and in Chapters 5 and 23). Ascending axons from the central group of reticular nuclei travel in the **central tegmental tract**. The involvement of the ascending projections in maintaining consciousness is reviewed later in this chapter. The reticulothalamic projection also provides an interaction with the corpus striatum, which has motor and other functions (see Chapters 12 and 23).

CHOLINERGIC NEURONS

The rostral part of the reticular formation contains two groups of neurons that use acetylcholine as their synaptic transmitter. The larger of these is in the **pedunculopontine nucleus** (see Figs. 9-1, 9-2, and 9-6) in the rostral pons and caudal midbrain. The smaller **lateral dorsal tegmental nucleus** is nearby, extending from the pontine periventricular gray matter into the periaqueductal gray matter. These nuclei receive afferents from nearby

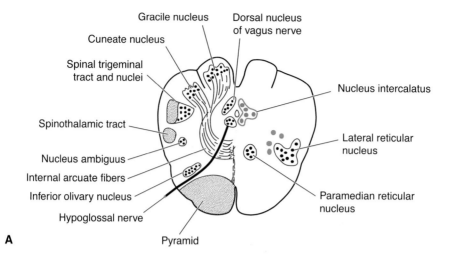

A

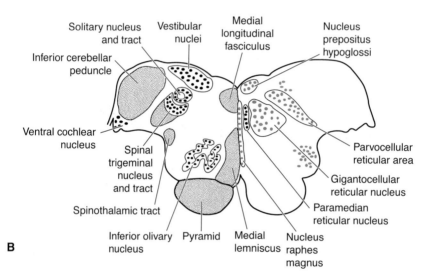

B

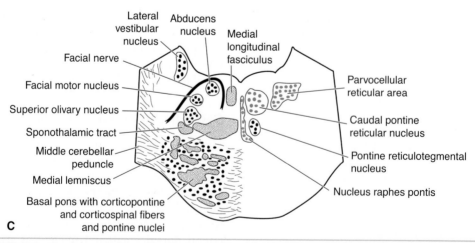

C

FIGURE 9-2   Transverse sections of the brain stem. The left side of each figure shows nuclei and tracts that are major anatomical landmarks. The right side shows the positions of reticular and other nuclei discussed in this chapter. Black dots indicate precerebellar nuclei, red dots indicate groups of serotonin- and catecholamine-containing neurons, and blue dots indicate other nuclei.

(continued)

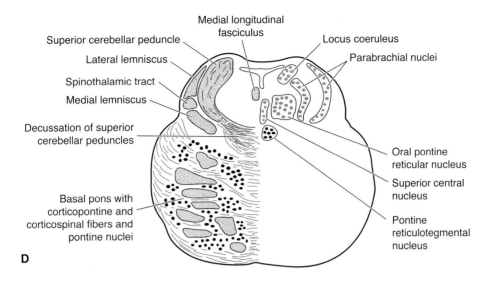

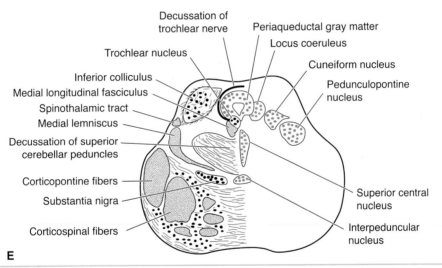

FIGURE 9-2 *(continued)* Transverse sections of the brain stem. The left side of each figure shows nuclei and tracts that are major anatomical landmarks. The right side shows the positions of reticular and other nuclei discussed in this chapter. Black dots indicate precerebellar nuclei, red dots indicate groups of serotonin- and catecholamine-containing neurons, and blue dots indicate other nuclei. **(A)** Nuclei at the level of the caudal pole of the inferior olivary nucleus, in the closed part of the medulla. (The unlabeled red dots indicate scattered adrenergic neurons.) **(B)** Nuclei at the level of the rostral pole of the inferior olivary nucleus, in the open part of the medulla. (The unlabeled red dots indicate groups of noradrenergic and adrenergic neurons. The blue dots dorsolateral to the inferior olivary nucleus indicate the probable position of the ventral superficial reticular area of the medulla.) **(C)** Nuclei in the caudal pontine tegmentum, at the level of the internal genu of the facial nerve. **(D)** Pontine tegmentum at a level rostral to the trigeminal motor nucleus. **(E)** Nuclei at the level of the caudal end of the inferior colliculus.

noradrenergic (locus coeruleus) and serotonergic (raphe) nuclei, from histaminergic neurons in the hypothalamus and inhibitory (gamma-aminobutyrate [GABA]) descending fibers from the pallidum (see Chapter 12), and from the preoptic area. The cholinergic neurons of the reticular formation have long, branching axons, which synapse with neurons in the central group of pontine reticular nuclei and the locus coeruleus. Axons of pontine cholinergic neurons have also been traced rostrally to the substantia nigra, subthalamic nucleus, intralaminar thalamic nuclei, and basal cholinergic nuclei of the forebrain (see

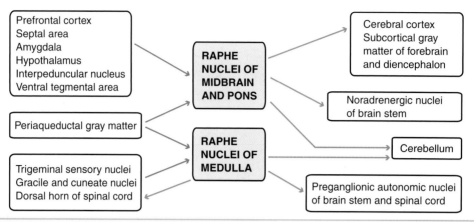

FIGURE 9-3   Major connections of the serotonergic raphe nuclei.

Chapter 12). Electrophysiological studies implicate cholinergic reticular nuclei in stereotyped motor functions, such as locomotion, and in consciousness and arousal.

CATECHOLAMINE NUCLEI

The catecholamines are noradrenaline (norepinephrine), adrenaline (epinephrine), and dopamine. The largest group of central noradrenergic neurons, and the only one easily seen in ordinary anatomical preparations, is the **locus coeruleus** or nucleus pigmentosus (see Figs. 9-2C and 9-2D), at the pontomesencephalic junction. Six smaller groups of noradrenergic neurons are present in the lateral part of the reticular formation in the medulla, pons, and midbrain. Two groups of adrenergic neurons are present in the medulla, one in the ventro-

lateral reticular formation and the other within the solitary nucleus (see Figs. 9-2A and 9-2B).

The afferent connections of the locus coeruleus and other noradrenergic nuclei of the human brain stem are unknown. Experimental work (mostly with nonprimate animals) suggests that the noradrenergic neurons fire spontaneously but are modulated by neurons in other parts of the reticular formation and in the hypothalamus. Noradrenergic projections are better known, even in primates, because the axons and their terminal branches are histochemically demonstrable.

Each noradrenergic neuron has an unmyelinated axon with numerous long branches. These branches go to many regions of the CNS. Most of the efferent axons of the locus coeruleus travel rostrally in the central tegmental tract and the medial forebrain bundle. Descending noradrenergic axons arise predominantly from

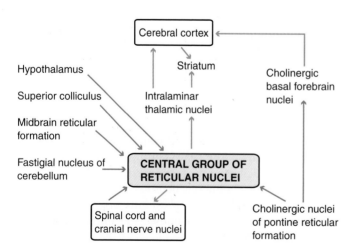

FIGURE 9-4   Major connections of the central group of reticular nuclei.

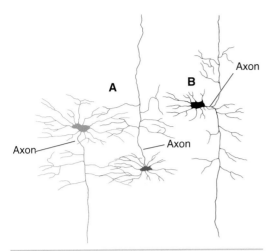

FIGURE 9-5 Neurons of the reticular formation. **(A)** Interaction between dendrites and collateral axonal branches of neurons with ascending *(blue)* and descending *(red)* projections. **(B)** A neuron whose axon divides into long ascending and descending branches.

the lateral medullary catecholamine nuclei. The distribution of the central noradrenergic system is summarized in Figure 9-7.

The noradrenaline released by axons from the locus coeruleus and related cell groups probably acts mainly as a modulator of synapses between other neurons. The effects on spinal reflexes and on alertness are generally excitatory. Destructive lesions of the locus coeruleus do not cause unconsciousness.

PARVOCELLULAR RETICULAR AREA

The parvocellular reticular area is located in the medulla and pons, lateral to the central group and medial to the trigeminal nuclei (see Figs. 9-1 and 9-2). Afferent fibers come from these sensory nuclei and from the cerebral cortex. The neurons in the parvocellular reticular area send their axons to the motor nuclei of the hypoglossal, facial, and trigeminal nerves. These connections indicate involvement in reflexes concerned with feeding. An "**expiratory center**" identified by electrical stimulation in animals is located within the medullary parvocellular reticular area. Stimulation in this region can also cause acceleration of the heart and increased arterial blood pressure.

PARABRACHIAL AREA

Rostral to the parvocellular reticular area, the medial and lateral **parabrachial nuclei** are situated in the lateral part of the reticular formation of the caudal midbrain, close to the superior cerebellar peduncle. This area has many connections. Afferent fibers are from the solitary nucleus and from the cortex of the insula and adjoining parts of the parietal lobe. The axons of parabrachial neurons project rostrally to the hypothalamus, preoptic area, intralaminar tha-

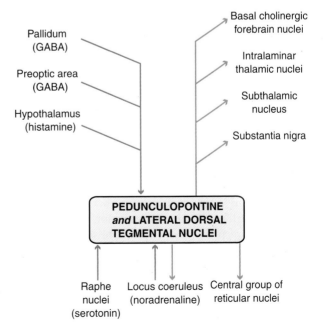

FIGURE 9-6 Major connections of the cholinergic nuclei of the brain stem.

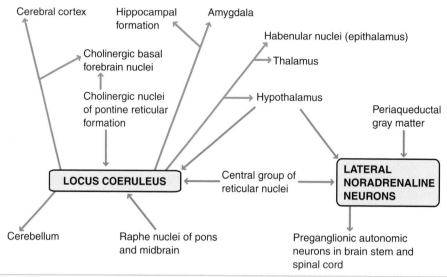

FIGURE 9-7   Major connections of the noradrenergic nuclei of the brain stem.

lamic nuclei, and amygdala. In many mammals, but not in primates, the parabrachial nuclei also form part of the sensory pathway for taste. Thus, the parabrachial area serves as a relay station in ascending pathways for visceral sensations. This region may also include the "**pneumotaxic center**," which is recognized by physiologists as a region concerned with the regulation of respiratory rhythm. Dorsal pontine lesions can cause **apneustic respiration**, in which a pause of a few seconds takes place between full inspiration and the beginning of expiration.

SUPERFICIAL MEDULLARY RETICULAR NEURONS

The ventral superficial reticular area in the medulla is another region concerned with cardiovascular and respiratory regulation. **Afferents** are from the spinal cord and solitary nucleus. They include fibers activated by the baroreceptors of the carotid and aortic sinuses and by the oxygen-sensitive chemoreceptors of the carotid and aortic bodies. Some of these medullary neurons respond directly to changes in the pH or carbon dioxide concentration in the nearby cerebrospinal fluid. The ventral superficial reticular area has **efferent projections** to the hypothalamus and to preganglionic autonomic neurons in the medulla and spinal cord. Functional connections also exist with the motor neurons that supply the muscles of respiration.

Functions of the Reticular Formation

SLEEP AND AROUSAL

Physiological Aspects of Consciousness

Consciousness, which is awareness of oneself and one's surroundings, is accompanied by neuronal activity in the whole cerebral cortex. Loss of consciousness occurs normally in sleep and abnormally with injuries or diseases that affect the brain. Profound loss of consciousness may be caused by extensive damage to the cerebral cortex or by localized destructive lesions in certain parts of the brain stem that have extensive divergent projections to the cortex. Impairment of consciousness is evaluated clinically by testing responses to sensory stimuli (see clinical note on the **Glasgow coma scale**).

The sleeping and awake states normally follow a rhythm with the same periodicity as the alternation of night and day. Within the nocturnal phase, sleep may be light (easily awakened) or deep (requiring a strong sensory stimulus for arousal). In addition, there are episodes of sleep in which there are rapid eye movements (**REM sleep**). At such times, the muscles of the trunk and limbs are relaxed, and a substantial sensory stimulus is needed for arousal, but the cerebral cortex is very active. A person suddenly awakened from REM sleep usually reports dreaming. The resistance to arousal in REM sleep is attributed to inhibition of transmission from the thalamus to the cerebral cortex in all the specific sensory pathways (e.g., somatic, auditory). The muscular relaxation is mediated by neurons in the reticular formation that inhibit motor neurons in the spinal cord.

Varying levels of consciousness are paralleled by changes in the **electroencephalogram (EEG)**, which is a crude indicator of the activity of the cerebral cortex. The fluctuations in voltage recorded from a point on the scalp are the sum of the variations in the membrane potentials of the dendrites of neurons in the underlying cerebral cortex (see also Chapter 14). Dendritic potentials are responses to activity of afferent axons, most of which come from neurons in the thalamus. Whereas large potentials are recorded when groups of thalamic neurons fire synchronously, low-voltage activity indicates that each cortical neuron is responding differently to its thalamic afferents. The EEG waves of a fully alert person are of low voltage and high frequency, indicating **desynchronization** of thalamocortical circuits. With progressive deepening of sleep, the waves become taller (synchronization) and longer ("slow-wave sleep"). In REM sleep, the EEG is desynchronized despite the fact that such sleep is deep in the sense of being resistant to sensory stimulation. Various abnormalities—notably, reduced voltage and frequency—are seen in the EEGs of comatose patients. The absence of recordable electrical activity (flat EEG) indicates death of the cerebral cortex.

Neuroanatomical Correlates of Consciousness and Sleep

The generalized activity of the cerebral cortex that constitutes an alert or wakeful condition occurs only when there is adequate cortical

---

CLINICAL NOTE

The Glasgow Coma Scale

This simple quantitative assessment of impaired consciousness is made by scoring for opening of the eyes and for vocal and motor responses to stimuli of graded intensity (Table 9-1).

The maximum (fully conscious) score of 15 is recorded as E4 V5 M6. With a state of **coma**, a term reserved for unconsciousness with little or no response to stimuli, the total Glasgow score is 8 or below. The three components are recorded separately because it is not always possible to evaluate all of them. For example, facial injuries

and swelling may prevent opening of the eyes, intubation of the trachea prevents the testing of vocal responses, and a concurrent spinal injury or multiple fractures may prevent motor responses. Meaningful scores cannot usually be obtained in children younger than age 2 years.

The Glasgow coma scale is useful because of its simplicity and because the scores correlate well with clinical outcome in cases of brain injury. Not surprisingly, deep coma is commonly associated with a poor prognosis.

TABLE 9-1 The Glasgow Coma Scale

Eye Opening (E)	Vocal Response (V)	Motor Response (M)
Spontaneous = 4	Conversation normal = 5	Normal = 6
To voice = 3	Converses but disoriented = 4	Localized response to pain = 5
To pain = 2	Says words but incoherent = 3	Withdrawal from pain (flexion) = 4
Absent = 1	Makes incomprehensible sounds = 2	Rigidity with limb flexion ("decorticate posture") = 3
	Absent = 1	Rigidity with limb extension ("decerebrate posture") = 2
		Absent = 1
		Total = E + V + M

excitation by neurons whose cell bodies are in the brain stem and thalamus. The ascending pathways that stimulate the whole cortex are anatomically separate from the specific sensory systems (see Chapters 17 and 19 to 22) and from the corticopetal projections of the cerebellum (see Chapter 10) and basal ganglia (see Chapters 12 and 23). Irreversible coma follows bilateral destruction of the medial parts of the brain stem at or above the upper pontine levels. Transmission in the more laterally located sensory pathways is not interrupted by medially located lesions that cause coma. The integrity of the rostral pontine reticular formation and of the central tegmental tract is essential for maintaining the conscious state. At the level of the midbrain and rostral pons, the central tegmental tract contains three populations of axons from the reticular formation that directly or indirectly stimulate the whole cerebral cortex:

1. **Noradrenergic neurons** (see Fig. 9-7) provide an ascending projection that excites neurons throughout the cerebral cortex. The cells of the locus coeruleus are most active in awake, attentive animals; they are less active in non-REM sleep and inactive in REM sleep.

2. **Cholinergic neurons** of the pedunculopontine nucleus (see Fig. 9-6) project to the hypothalamus, basal cholinergic nuclei of the forebrain (see later), and intralaminar thalamic nuclei, which, in their turn, have extensive although sparse projections to all parts of the cerebral cortex. These neurons are active in the awake state and in REM sleep but are quiescent in non-REM sleep.

3. The **central group of reticular nuclei** (especially the oral pontine reticular nucleus) sends axons to the intralaminar nuclei of the thalamus and to the basal cholinergic nuclei of the forebrain (see later). The central reticular neurons are a mixed population, differently active in all states of consciousness.

Groups of neurons in the diencephalon and telencephalon stimulate the cerebral cortex in a general way. The **intralaminar thalamic nuclei** (see Chapter 11) provide an essential link in most of the ascending pathways concerned with both arousal and REM sleep (Fig. 9-8). In addition to the connections already mentioned, the intralaminar nuclei receive collateral branches from all the sensory tracts that go to other nuclei of the thalamus. Sensory stimuli that cause arousal from sleep may do so by way of these branches. Lesions that bilaterally damage the intralaminar nuclei cause coma. The posterior part of the **hypothalamus** (see Chapter 11) contains the **tuberomamillary nucleus**, which is composed of **histamine-secreting neurons** with axons that branch profusely in the thalamus and also extend to many parts of the CNS, including the cerebral cortex. Pharmacological studies indicate that histamine of neuronal origin participates in arousal. The sedative side effects of traditional antihistaminic drugs (H1-receptor blockers) are probably caused by competitive inhibition of the action of histamine on cortical neurons. The **basal cholinergic nuclei of the forebrain** (see Chapter 12) also stimulate neurons throughout the cerebral cortex.

Deep (non-REM) sleep is associated with diminished activity of the systems just described. In addition, some neurons in the brain stem and hypothalamus actively promote sleep:

1. The **serotonergic raphe neurons** have axons that go to all parts of the CNS. The raphe neurons are active in deep sleep, which may be caused partly by a widespread inhibitory action of serotonin in the thalamus and cerebral cortex. Serotonergic neurons are less active in REM sleep, which may be caused partly by occasional release of the telencephalic neurons from serotonergic inhibition. A simultaneous reduction of inhibition of the caudal pontine reticular nucleus (the PPRF) may account for the accompanying movements of the eyes.

2. In the **lateral hypothalamus**, some neurons produce a pair of peptides, orexin-A and orexin-B, which are active in the awake state. The **orexins** are also called **hypocretins-1 and -2**. The long axons of orexin neurons extend to most parts of the brain. One of their actions is stimulation of the cholinergic neurons of the pedunculopontine nucleus. Deficiency of orexin in dogs, mice, and humans is associated with **narcolepsy**, a condition in which the waking state is frequently

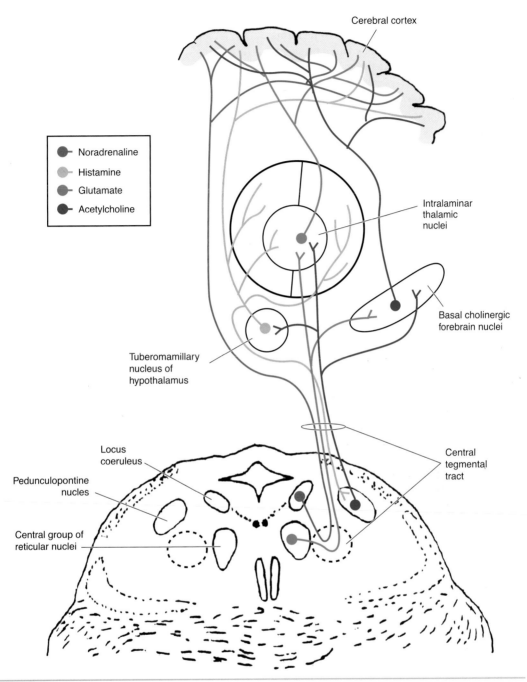

FIGURE 9-8   The ascending reticular-activating system. This diagram shows the groups of neurons that are more active in the alert state and less active during slow-wave (non-REM) sleep. With the notable exception of the locus coeruleus, these neurons are active also in REM sleep.

interrupted by brief episodes of REM sleep.

3. The **suprachiasmatic nucleus** of the hypothalamus (see Chapter 11) contains neurons whose patterns of firing follow a 24-hour cycle, serving as an internal clock for the brain. Axons from the suprachiasmatic nucleus contact the orexin neurons of the lateral hypothalamus and the dorsomedial hypothalamic nucleus

(see Fig. 11-14), which projects caudally to the locus coeruleus. These connections provide circuitry that may facilitate sleeping during the night rather than during the day.

4. The **cholinergic neurons** of the pedunculopontine and lateral dorsal tegmental nuclei are as active in REM sleep as they are in the awake state.

5. In the **preoptic area**, immediately anterior to the hypothalamus, a population of GABA-ergic neurons contains a peptide, galanin. These inhibitory neurons are active in deep (non-REM) sleep. Their axons go to the tuberomamillary nucleus, the locus coeruleus, and the cholinergic reticular nuclei. Destructive lesions in the preoptic area cause insomnia, indicating that this region is essential for the occurrence of sleep.

In REM sleep, suppression of transmission in specific sensory pathways takes place, accounting for the high threshold for arousal by sensory stimuli. This is believed to be mediated by rostrally projecting cholinergic neurons (Fig. 9-9) that stimulate the reticular nucleus of the thalamus (see also Chapter 11). This nucleus contains GABA-ergic neurons that inhibit transmission from the other thalamic nuclei to the cerebral cortex. The relaxation of limb muscles in REM sleep is mediated by reticulospinal fibers, some of which use glycine as an inhibitory transmitter.

PAIN

Through spinal afferents and projections to the thalamus, the central group of reticular nuclei forms part of an **ascending pathway** for the poorly localized perception of pain. Such sensation persists after transection of the spinothalamic tracts (see Chapter 19).

A **descending inhibitory pathway** consists of the axons of serotonergic raphe neurons that project to the dorsal horn and spinal trigeminal nucleus. This system inhibits the rostral transmission of action potentials that report pain. Electrical stimulation of the periaqueductal gray matter (which projects to the raphe nuclei in the medulla) results in loss of the ability to experience pain from sites of injury or disease.

This descending pathway is discussed in Chapter 19.

SOMATIC MOTOR FUNCTIONS

The reticulospinal tracts constitute one of the major descending pathways involved in the control of movement; the others are the corticospinal and vestibulospinal tracts. Equivalent reticulobulbar connections supply the motor nuclei of the cranial nerves. Animal experiments indicate that many reticulospinal fibers are the axons of cells in the caudal and oral pontine reticular nuclei and the gigantocellular nucleus of the medulla. Most of these fibers descend to the spinal cord without crossing the midline. Some end ipsilaterally in the ventral horn, and others decussate before terminating. The reticulospinal tracts, consequently, project both ipsilaterally and bilaterally to the spinal gray matter. They end on interneurons and influence the motor neurons indirectly through synaptic relays within the spinal cord.

With respect to motor functions, important afferents to the central group of reticular nuclei come from the motor cortex of the cerebral hemispheres, the cholinergic pedunculopontine nucleus (see Figs. 9-2D and 9-6), the cerebellar nuclei, and the spinal cord.

The **raphespinal tract** is a reticulospinal pathway best known for the involvement of its serotonergic neurons in the modulation of pain sensation. Raphespinal projections may also modulate the activities of motor neurons, which are made more excitable by serotonin. Drugs that block the action of serotonin have been used clinically to alleviate the spasticity that follows damage to the major descending motor pathways.

VISCERAL ACTIVITIES

Certain regions in the reticular formation regulate **visceral functions** and **breathing** through connections rostrally with the amygdala and hypothalamus and caudally with nuclei of the autonomic outflow and with respiratory motor neurons in the phrenic nucleus and thoracic cord. The functions of the superficial medullary reticular neurons in mediating reflex responses to the systemic blood pressure and the degree of oxygenation of the

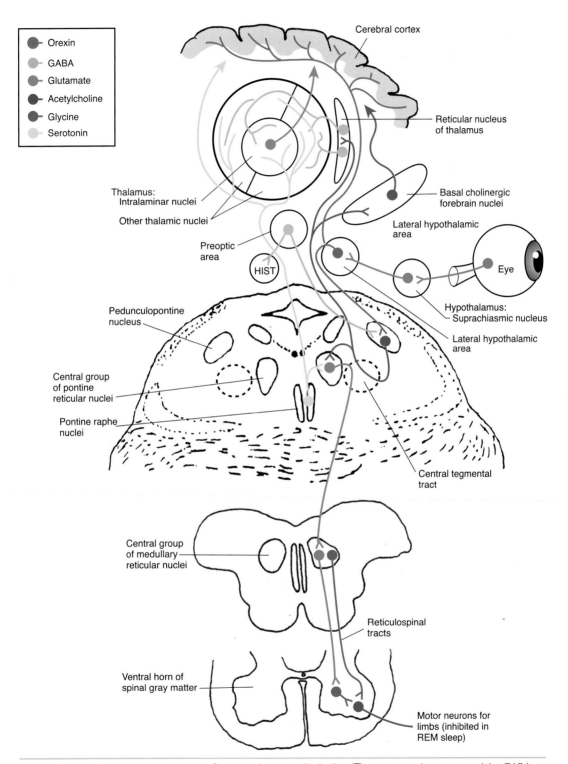

FIGURE 9-9   Diagram showing groups of neurons that are active in sleep. The serotonergic neurons and the GABA-ergic hypothalamic neurons are more active in slow-wave (non-REM) sleep. The other pathways are active in REM sleep though the physiological role of the orexin neurons is still uncertain. The arrows pointing up indicate extensive distribution of axonal branches to the cortex. The descending pathways mediate the inhibition of motor activity during periods of REM sleep.

blood were mentioned earlier in this chapter. Other cardiovascular and respiratory regions, commonly referred to as "centers," have been identified by electrical stimulation within the brain stem in laboratory animals. Some of these centers are fields within the network of dendrites in the reticular formation rather than compact collections of cell bodies. Maximal **inspiratory and expiratory responses** are obtained from the gigantocellular nucleus and the parvocellular reticular area, respectively, in the medulla, and respiratory rhythm is controlled by the pneumotaxic center in the parabrachial area.

Stimulation in the medial part of the reticular formation of the medulla has a depressor effect on the **circulatory system**, with slowing of the heart rate and lowering of blood pressure. The opposite effects are produced by stimulation in laterally located sites. Damage to the brain stem is life threatening because of the presence of these regions involved in the control of vital functions.

Miscellaneous Nuclei of the Brain Stem

The **area postrema** is a narrow strip of neural tissue in the caudal part of the floor of the fourth ventricle near the obex (see Fig. 6-3). The blood–brain barrier, which elsewhere prevents certain substances from entering nervous tissue from the blood, is lacking here. Among other connections, the area postrema has reciprocal connections with the solitary nucleus. The area has been shown experimentally to be a chemoreceptor region for emetic drugs such as apomorphine and digoxin. It may, therefore, function in the physiology of vomiting.

The **perihypoglossal nuclei** are three quite conspicuous groups of neurons in the caudal medulla: the nucleus intercalatus (see Fig. 9-2A), the nucleus of Roller (ventrolateral to the hypoglossal nucleus), and the nucleus prepositus hypoglossi (see Fig. 9-2B). The nucleus prepositus hypoglossi is the largest of the three, and it is continuous at its rostral end with the PPRF (see Fig. 8-5).

These nuclei receive afferents from several sources, including the cerebral cortex, vestibular nuclei, accessory oculomotor nuclei, and PPRF. Efferent fibers proceed mainly to the nuclei of cranial nerves III, IV, and VI, which they reach by passing into the medial longitudinal fasciculus. The perihypoglossal nuclei form part of the complex circuitry for movements of the eyes. Lesions in the nucleus prepositus hypoglossi impair the ability to keep the eyes fixed on a visual target, although conjugate movements are still performed accurately.

The **accessory oculomotor nuclei** are the interstitial nucleus of Cajal, nucleus of Darkschewitsch, nucleus of the posterior commissure, and rostral interstitial nucleus of the medial longitudinal fasciculus. They are situated at the junction of the midbrain and the diencephalon (Fig. 9-10) and are concerned with movements of the eyes in the vertical plane (see Chapter 8).

The **periaqueductal gray matter** surrounds the cerebral aqueduct of the midbrain. In laboratory animals, afferent and efferent connections have been traced with regions ranging from the spinal cord to parts of the telencephalon, but the periaqueductal gray matter's physiological role is largely obscure. As mentioned earlier, electrical stimulation of the periaqueductal gray matter causes analgesia, and this effect is mediated by way of the descending projection of the nucleus raphes magnus in the medulla. The nucleus of Darkschewitsch is located within the territory of the periaqueductal gray matter, but it is generally considered to be one of the accessory oculomotor nuclei.

The **interpeduncular nucleus** is located in the midline, ventral to the periaqueductal gray matter and near the roof of the most rostral part of the interpeduncular fossa. This nucleus lies on a pathway through which the limbic system projects to autonomic nuclei in the brain stem and spinal cord. Lateral to the interpeduncular nucleus, in the medial part of the cerebral peduncle, is a population of dopamine-secreting neurons known as the **ventral tegmental area**. This, too, has connections with the limbic system and is discussed in Chapter 18.

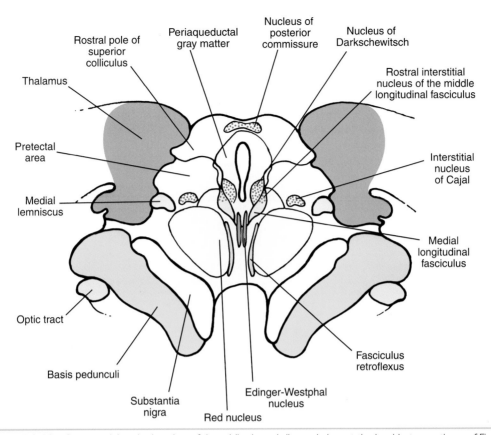

FIGURE 9-10   Some nuclei at the junction of the midbrain and diencephalon, at the level between those of Figures 7-15 and 11-7. The accessory oculometer nuclei are shown in red and the parasympathetic Edinger-Westphal nucleus in green. Parts of the thalamus (light blue) are included in the section, and some major tracts of fibers are colored yellow.

Suggested Reading

Aston-Jones G, Chen S, Zhu Y, et al. A neural circuit for circadian regulation of arousal. *Nature Neurosci* 2001;4:732–738.

Bogen JE. On the neurophysiology of consciousness, 1: an overview. *Conscious Cogn* 1995;4:52–62.

Crabtree JW. Intrathalamic sensory connections mediated by the thalamic reticular nucleus. *Cell Mol Life Sci* 1999;56: 683–700.

Ferguson AV. The area postrema: a cardiovascular control centre at the blood-brain interface? *Can J Physiol Pharmacol* 1991;69:1026–1034.

Huang XF, Paxinos G. Human intermediate reticular zone: a cyto- and chemoarchitectonic study. *J Comp Neurol* 1995;360:571–588.

Inglis WL, Winn P. The pedunculopontine tegmental nucleus: where the striatum meets the reticular formation. *Prog Neurobiol* 1995;47:1–29.

Manning KA, Wilson JR, Uhlrich D. Histamine-immunoreactive neurons and their inervation of visual regions in the cortex, tectum and thalamus in the primate Macaca mulatta. *J Comp Neurol* 1996;373:271–282.

Maquet P, Peters JM, Aerts J, et al. Functional neuroanatomy of human rapid eye-movement sleep and dreaming. *Nature* 1996;383:163–166.

Nieuwenhuys R, Voogd J, van Huijzen C. *The Human Central Nervous System. A Synopsis and Atlas*, 3rd ed. Berlin: Springer-Verlag, 1988.

Olszewski J, Baxter D. *Cytoarchitecture of the Human Brain Stem*, 2nd ed. Basel: Karger, 1982.

Paxinos G, Tork I, Halliday G, et al. Human homologs to brainstem nuclei identified in other animals as revealed by acetylcholinesterase activity. In: Paxinos G, ed. *The Human Nervous System*. San Diego: Academic Press, 1990:149–202.

Saper CB, Chou TC, Scammell TE. The sleep switch: hypothalamic control of sleep and wakefulness. *Trends Neurosci* 2001;24:726–731.

Siegel JM, Lai YY. Brainstem systems mediating the control of muscle tone. In: Mallick BN, Singh R, eds. *Environment and Physiology*. New Delhi: Narosa, 1994:62–78.

Taheri S, Zeiter JM, Mignot E. The role of hypocretins (orexins) in sleep regulation and narcolepsy. *Annu Rev Neurosci* 2002;25:283–313.

Wada H, Inagaki N, Yamatodani A, et al. Is the histaminergic neuron system a regulatory center for whole-brain activity? *Trends Neurosci* 1991;14:415–418.

Wainberg M, Barbeau H, Gauthier S. The effects of cyproheptadine on locomotion and on spasticity in patients with spinal cord injuries. *J Neurol Neurosurg Psychiatry* 1990;53:754–763.

Willie JT, Chemelli RM, Sinton CM, et al. To eat or to sleep? Orexin in the regulation of feeding and wakefulness. *Annu Rev Neurosci* 2001;24:429–458.

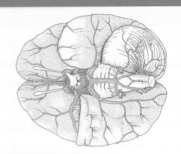

Chapter 10

CEREBELLUM

- The hemispheres, vermis, flocculus, nodule, and tonsil are major landmarks of the cerebellar cortex.

- Afferent fibers end in the three-layered cerebellar cortex. The Purkinje cells have axons that end in the cerebellar nuclei.

- The fastigial, interposed, and dentate nuclei receive branches of all cerebellar afferent fibers and the output of the cortex. These nuclei contain the cerebellar efferent neurons.

- The superior cerebellar peduncle contains cerebellar efferent fibers, the ventral spinocerebellar tract, and tectocerebellar fibers. The middle cerebellar peduncle consists of fibers from the contralateral pontine nuclei, and the inferior cerebellar peduncle contains olivocerebellar and dorsal spinocerebellar fibers and the vestibulocerebellar and fastigiobulbar connections.

- The vestibular system is connected ipsilaterally with the vestibulocerebellum, which comprises the flocculonodular lobe and the fastigial nucleus. This nucleus projects to the ipsilateral vestibular nuclei and to the reticular formation.

- Proprioceptive signals are carried ipsilaterally to the spinocerebellum, which consists of vermis, paravermal zones, and interposed nuclei. These nuclei project to the contralateral red nucleus and to the posterior division of the contralateral ventrolateral (VLp) thalamic nucleus. The VLp projects to the primary motor cortex.

- All parts of the cerebral cortex and the tectum influence the contralateral cerebellar hemisphere and dentate nucleus (pontocerebellum) by way of relays in the pontine nuclei. The dentate nucleus projects to the contralateral VLp thalamic nucleus.

- These connections determine that each side of the body is represented ipsilaterally in the cerebellum and that postural functions are localized in and near the midline.

- The cerebellum learns and executes instructions for movements, ensuring coordination of the force, extent, and duration of the contractions of muscles.

- Whereas a lesion in or near the midline causes disorders of posture and gait, a lesion in a hemisphere causes defective control of movements of the ipsilateral limbs (neocerebellar syndrome). The word **ataxia** refers to inaccurately controlled movements, including those caused by cerebellar disorders.

- The pontocerebellum participates also in nonmotor functions, and a neocerebellar syndrome can be associated with abnormalities of cognition and affect.

The cerebellum is best known as a motor part of the brain, serving to maintain equilibrium and coordinate muscle contractions. The cerebellum makes a special contribution to synergy of muscle action (i.e., to the synchronized contractions and relaxations of different muscles that make up a useful movement). The cerebellum ensures that contraction of the proper muscles occurs at the appropriate time, each with the correct force. There is reason to believe that the cerebellum participates in learning patterns of neuronal activity needed for carrying out movements and in the execution of the encoded instructions.

Despite their complexity, the activities of the cerebellum have long been thought to occur without conscious awareness because cerebellar diseases cause disturbed motor function without voluntary paralysis. This traditional viewpoint may not be entirely correct: imagined movements are accompanied by an increase in cerebellar blood flow that is larger than the increase detected in the motor areas of the cerebral cortex. Evidence also suggests that the cerebellum has sensory and cognitive functions.

The cerebellum consists of a cortex, or surface layer, of gray matter contained in transverse folds or folia plus a central body of white matter. Four pairs of central nuclei are embedded in the cerebellar white matter. Three pairs of cerebellar peduncles, composed of myelinated axons, connect the cerebellum with the brain stem.

Gross Anatomy

The superior cerebellar surface conforms to the dural reflection or tentorium, which forms a roof for the posterior cranial fossa. The inferior surface is deeply grooved in the midline; the re-

mainder of this surface is convex on each side and rests on the floor of the posterior cranial fossa (Fig. 10-1).

Certain terms are useful to identify regions of the cerebellar surface. The region in and near the midline is known as the **vermis**, and the remainder is known as the **hemispheres**. The superior vermis blends into the hemispheres, but the inferior vermis lies in a deep depression (the vallecula) and is well delineated. The **paravermal zone** is the medial parts of the hemispheres for 1 to 2 cm on either side of the vermis.

Three major regions or lobes are recognized in the horizontal plane (see Fig. 10-1). The flocculonodular lobe (or lobule) is a small component that lies at the rostral edge of the inferior surface. If the cerebellum were unrolled, this would be its most caudal part. The

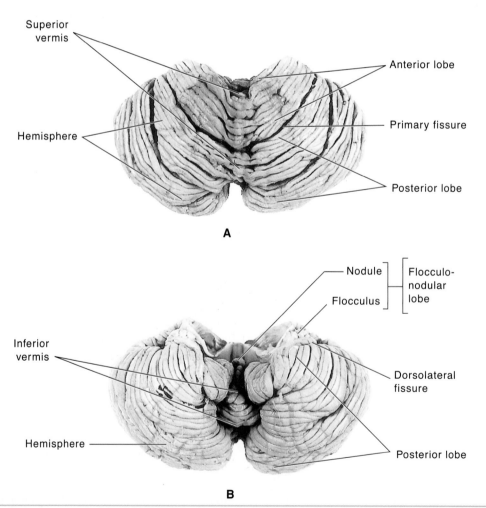

FIGURE 10-1   The cerebellum. **(A)** Superior surface. **(B)** Inferior surface.

nodule is the end portion of the inferior vermis, and the flocculi are irregularly shaped masses on each side. Several transverse fissures indent the cerebellum. The dorsolateral (or posterolateral) fissure is the first of these to appear during embryonic development; it demarcates the flocculonodular lobe. The main mass of the cerebellum (all but the flocculonodular lobe) consists of anterior and posterior lobes. The anterior lobe is the part of the superior surface rostral to the primary fissure. The remainder of the cerebellum on both surfaces constitutes the large posterior lobe.

The roof of the rostral part of the fourth ventricle is formed by the superior cerebellar peduncles and by the superior medullary velum that bridges the interval between them (Fig. 10-2; see also Fig. 7-10). The remainder of the roof consists of the thin inferior medullary velum, formed by pia mater and ependyma. This membrane (see Fig. 6-4) commonly adheres to the inferior vermis. The three pairs of peduncles are attached to the cerebellum in the interval between the flocculonodular and anterior lobes.

Other fissures outline further subdivisions or lobules, especially in the posterior lobe. Figure 10-3 is provided for reference if smaller subdivisions of the cerebellum need to be identified. The position of the **tonsils** is clinically significant because these parts of the cerebellar hemispheres are close to the medulla and can compress this vital part of the brain stem if the contents of the posterior fossa of the skull are displaced downward into the foramen magnum. The tonsil is also an angiographic landmark, associated with a characteristic curve in the course of the posterior inferior cerebellar artery.

Cerebellar Cortex

The cerebellar surface is folded into many narrow folia, with 85% of the cortical surface concealed in the intervening sulci. The cortical area is about three-quarters the size of the cerebral cortex.

Neuronal Organization

Three layers are seen in sections (Fig. 10-4). The Purkinje cell layer consists of a single row of bodies of Purkinje cells, the large principal cells of the cerebellar cortex. Superficial to these is the molecular layer, which is a synaptic zone, containing the dendrites of the Purkinje cells, which branch profusely in a plane perpendicular to the long axis of the folium. The granule cell

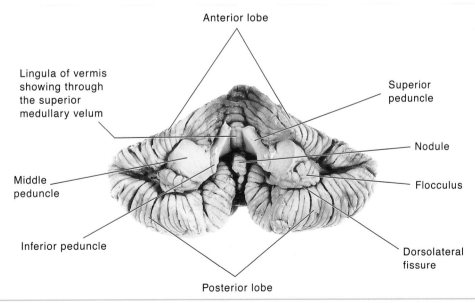

FIGURE 10-2 The cerebellum viewed from in front and below, showing the cut surfaces of the cerebellar peduncles.

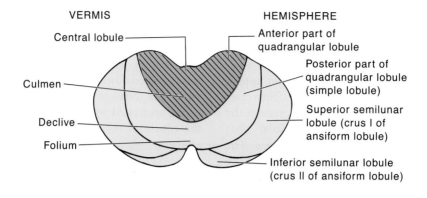

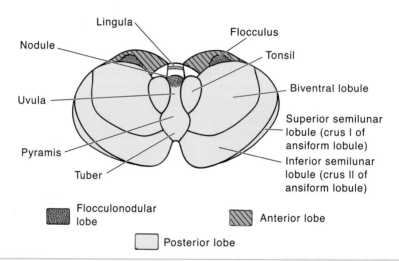

FIGURE 10-3   Anatomical names of parts of the cerebellum. (The lingula, not seen in these figures, is a small, flattened portion of the superior vermis beneath the central lobule and adherent to the superior medullary velum; see Fig. 10-2.)

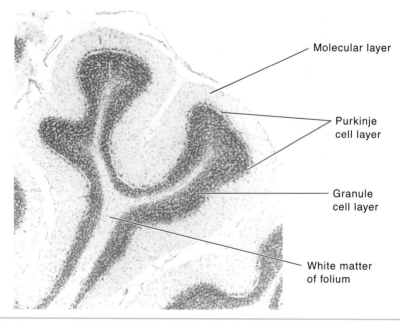

FIGURE 10-4   Transverse section of cerebellar folia showing the three layers of the cortex and the underlying white matter (stained with cresyl violet).

layer, deep to the layer of Purkinje cells, contains closely packed interneurons with axons that extend into the molecular layer. Other cerebellar interneurons (Fig. 10-5) have their cell bodies in the molecular and granular layers.

Of the afferent fibers to the cortex, climbing fibers originate in the inferior olivary complex of nuclei and synapse with the proximal parts of the dendritic trees of Purkinje cells. Cerebellar afferents from other sources end as mossy fibers, each synapsing with the neurons in the granular layer in a formation known as a glomerulus (Fig. 10-6). The axons of the granule cells have branches known as parallel fibers that run in the long axis of the folium in the molecular layer. Whereas each Purkinje cell is contacted by a single climbing fiber, parallel fibers are much more numerous, with each one contacting many Purkinje cells. (Noradrenergic and serotonergic projections to the cerebellum from the brain stem are also present; these are mentioned in Chapter 9 but are not discussed here.) The only axons that leave the cortex are those of the Purkinje cells. These terminate in central nuclei of the cerebellum, with the exception of some fibers from the cortex of the flocculonodular lobe that proceed to the brain stem.

The cerebellar cortex was one of the first regions of the brain to be thoroughly studied with microelectrodes to determine whether synapses between specific types of neurons produced excitatory (EPSP) or inhibitory (IPSP) postsynaptic potentials. The observations have since been supplemented by immunohistochemical and pharmacological studies of neurotransmitters and their receptors.

The axons afferent to the cerebellum all make excitatory connections. Before reaching the cortex, all afferent axons give off collateral branches that contact the neurons in the cerebellar nuclei. The granule cells also make excitatory synapses with the Purkinje cells. The excitatory transmitter is glutamate. All the other cerebellar neurons make inhibitory synapses, with gamma-aminobutyric acid (GABA) as the transmitter. The excitatory input to the cortex is thereby modified by intracortical circuits that inhibit Purkinje cells and suppress transmission from the cortex to central nuclei. The granule cells are the most numerous cerebellar interneurons; others are the Golgi cells and basket cells shown in Figure 10-5. For example, activation of parallel fibers elicits EPSPs in basket cells, but synapses between basket cells and Purkinje cells cause IPSPs. Parallel fibers also excite Golgi cells, which inhibit granule cells. Whereas each parallel fiber contacts the dendrites of many Purkinje cells along the

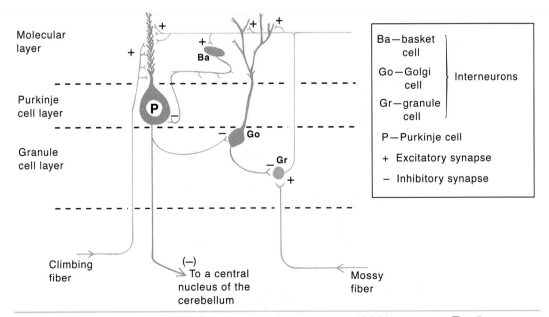

FIGURE 10-5 Neurons in the cerebellar cortex, showing excitatory and inhibitory synapses. The diagram represents a longitudinally sectioned folium, with an edge-on view of the dendritic tree of the Purkinje cell. Glutamatergic (excitatory) neurons are red; GABA-ergic (inhibitory) neurons are blue.

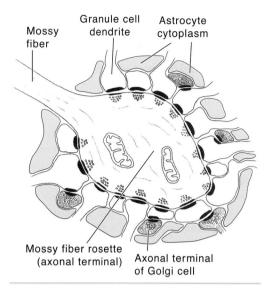

FIGURE 10-6   Ultrastructure of a synaptic glomerulus in the granule cell layer. The astrocyte processes *(yellow)* prevent diffusion of neurotransmitters to adjacent synapses.

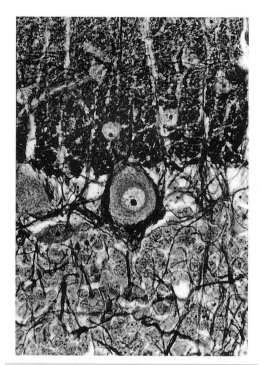

FIGURE 10-7   Cell body of a Purkinje cell situated between the molecular layer *(above)* and the granule cell layer of the cerebellar cortex. Most of the fibers surrounding the Purkinje cell are preterminal branches of basket cell axons. (Stained by one of Cajal's silver nitrate methods.)

length of a folium, the axon of each basket cell contacts several Purkinje cells across the width of a folium (see Figs. 10-5 and 10-7). Inhibitory circuits, which include more synapses than do the excitatory relays, serve to limit the area of cortex excited and the degree of excitation resulting from a volley of impulses delivered by a mossy fiber.

Central Nuclei

Four pairs of nuclei are embedded deep in the cerebellar white matter; in a medial to lateral direction, they are the fastigial, globose, emboliform, and dentate nuclei (Fig. 10-8).

The **fastigial nucleus** is close to the midline, almost in contact with the roof of the fourth ventricle. The **interposed nucleus** (comprising two cell clusters, the globose and the emboliform nuclei) is situated between the fastigial and dentate nuclei. The prominent **dentate nucleus** has the irregular shape of a crumpled purse, similar to that of the inferior olivary nucleus, with the hilus facing medially. Its efferent fibers occupy the interior of the nucleus and leave through the hilus.

The input to the cerebellar nuclei is from (a) sources outside the cerebellum and (b) the

Purkinje cells of the cortex. The extrinsic input consists of pontocerebellar, spinocerebellar, and olivocerebellar fibers, together with fibers from the precerebellar reticular nuclei. Most of these afferents are collateral branches of fibers proceeding to the cerebellar cortex. A few rubrocerebellar fibers end in the interposed nucleus, and the fastigial nucleus receives afferents from the vestibular nerve and nuclei. Whereas the fastigial nucleus projects to the brain stem through the inferior cerebellar peduncle, efferents from the other nuclei leave the cerebellum through the superior peduncle and end in the brain stem and thalamus.

Whereas the input to the central nuclei from outside the cerebellum is excitatory, the input from Purkinje cells, which use GABA as their transmitter, is inhibitory. Crudely processed information in the central nuclei is refined by the inhibitory signals received from the cortex. The combination of the two inputs maintains a tonic discharge from the central nuclei to

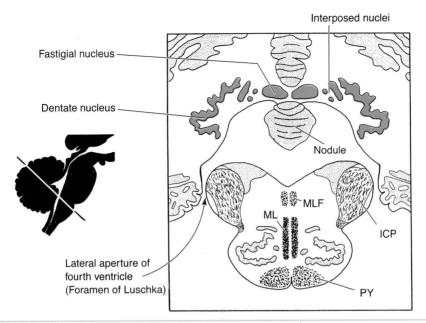

FIGURE 10-8   Central nuclei of the cerebellum, as seen in a transverse section that also passes through the open part of the medulla. ICP, inferior cerebellar peduncle; ML, medial lemniscus; MLF, medial longitudinal fasciculus; PY, pyramid.

the brain stem and thalamus. This discharge changes constantly according to the afferent input to the cerebellum at any given time.

Cerebellar Peduncles

The white matter in the region of the vermis produces a branching treelike pattern (the *arbor vitae cerebelli*) in a sagittal section (Fig. 10-9). Each hemisphere contains a large body of white matter in which the dentate nucleus is embedded (Fig. 10-10). The white matter consists of afferent and efferent fibers of the cortex and nuclei. The afferent and efferent systems are discussed in connection with the functional divisions of the cerebellum. They are identified at this point only as components of the cerebellar peduncles.

The inferior cerebellar peduncle consists mainly of fibers entering the cerebellum, with the largest contingent being from the contralateral inferior olivary complex of nuclei. The other components are the dorsal spinocerebellar tract and fibers from the vestibular nerve and nuclei and from various other nuclei of the medulla (Table 10-1). Efferent fibers in the inferior cerebellar peduncle proceed from the

flocculonodular lobe and fastigial nucleus to the vestibular nuclei and to reticular formation of the medulla and pons.

The middle cerebellar peduncle consists of pontocerebellar fibers that originate in the contralateral pontine nuclei.

The superior cerebellar peduncle consists mainly of efferent fibers from the interposed and dentate nuclei. These axons end in the thalamus. Smaller contingents of fibers in the superior peduncle are summarized in Table 10-1.

Functional Anatomy

Three divisions of the cerebellum are recognized on the basis of comparative anatomy. These are the archicerebellum, which is the only component of the cerebellum in fishes and in lower amphibians; the paleocerebellum, which is present in higher amphibians and is larger in reptiles and birds; and the neocerebellum, which is found only in mammals and is largest in humans. These phylogenetic divisions of the cerebellum (Fig. 10-11) correspond in large part with functional divisions (Fig. 10-12), based on the major

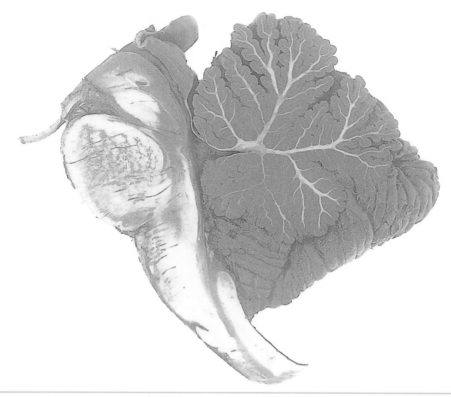

FIGURE 10-9   Midline structures of the brain stem and cerebellum, showing the arbor vitae cerebelli in the vermis. The cut surface of the specimen has been stained by a method that differentiates gray matter *(dark)* from white matter *(light)*.

sources of afferent mossy fibers. (Olivocerebellar climbing fibers are distributed to all parts of the cortex.)

The functional divisions are as follows. The vestibulocerebellum is the flocculonodular lobe and receives input from the vestibular nerve

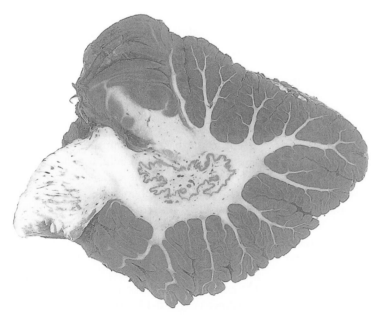

FIGURE 10-10   Section cut in a sagittal plane through a cerebellar hemisphere, stained to differentiate gray matter *(dark)* from white matter *(light)*. The dentate nucleus is shown, embedded in the white matter of the hemisphere.

TABLE 10-1 **Composition of the Cerebellar Peduncles**

Name of Peduncle	Cerebellar Afferents	Cerebellar Efferents
Inferior cerebellar peduncle	Olivocerebellar fibers Dorsal spinocerebellar tract Cuneocerebellar fibers Vestibulocerebellar fibers (from vestibular nerve and nuclei) Arcuate nucleus (see Chapter 7) Trigeminal sensory nuclei (pontine and spinal) Precerebellar reticular nuclei	Cerebellovestibular fibers (to vestibular nuclei) Cerebelloreticular fibers (to central group of reticular nuclei in medulla and pons)
Middle cerebellar peduncle	Pontocerebellar fibers	(None)
Superior cerebellar peduncle	Ventral spinocerebellar tract Trigeminothalamic fibers (from mesencephalic trigeminal nucleus) Tectocerebellar fibers (from superior and inferior colliculi) Noradrenergic fibers from the locus coeruleus	Cerebellothalamic fibers (to ventral lateral nucleus of contralateral thalamus) Cerebellorubral fibers (mostly from interposed nucleus, going to ipsilateral red nucleus)

and nuclei. The spinocerebellum consists of the vermis of the anterior lobe together with the adjacent medial or paravermal zones of the hemispheres; the spinocerebellar tracts and cuneocerebellar fibers, which convey proprioceptive and other sensory information, terminate here. The pontocerebellum comprises the large lateral parts of the hemispheres and the superior vermis

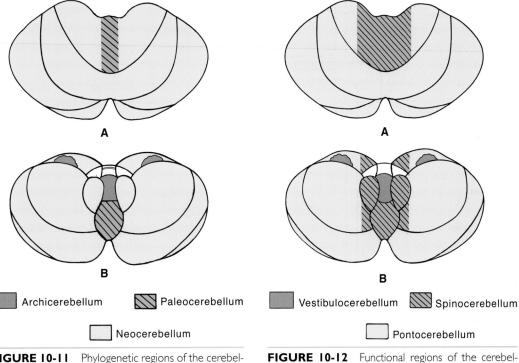

Archicerebellum   Paleocerebellum   Neocerebellum

Vestibulocerebellum   Spinocerebellum   Pontocerebellum

FIGURE 10-11   Phylogenetic regions of the cerebellum. **(A)** Superior surface. **(B)** Inferior surface.

FIGURE 10-12   Functional regions of the cerebellum. **(A)** Superior surface. **(B)** Inferior surface

in the posterior lobe; afferents are from the contralateral pontine nuclei. There is some overlapping of the divisions; for example, both spinocerebellar and pontocerebellar fibers terminate in the cortex of the paravermal zones.

VESTIBULOCEREBELLUM

The vestibulocerebellum receives afferent fibers from the vestibular ganglion and from the vestibular nuclei of the same side (Fig. 10-13). Some of the afferent fibers from these sources terminate in the fastigial nucleus, which also receives collateral branches of the axons destined for the cortex of the vestibulocerebellum. The vestibulocerebellum also receives afferents from the contralateral accessory olivary nuclei. These fibers have collateral branches to the fastigial nucleus and end as climbing fibers in the cortex of the flocculonodular lobe.

Some Purkinje cell axons from the vestibulocerebellar cortex proceed to the brain stem (an exception to the general rule that such fibers end in central nuclei), but most terminate in the fastigial nucleus. Fibers from the cortex and the fastigial nucleus traverse the inferior cerebellar peduncle to their termination in the vestibular nuclear complex and in the central group of reticular nuclei (see Fig. 10-13).

In summary, the vestibulocerebellum influences motor neurons through the vestibulospinal tract, the medial longitudinal fasciculus, and reticulospinal fibers. It is concerned with adjustment of muscle tone in response to vestibular stimuli. It coordinates the actions of muscles that maintain equilibrium and participates in other motor responses, including those of the eyes, to vestibular stimulation (see Chapter 22). The posterior vermis also contributes to the cerebellar control of eye movements.

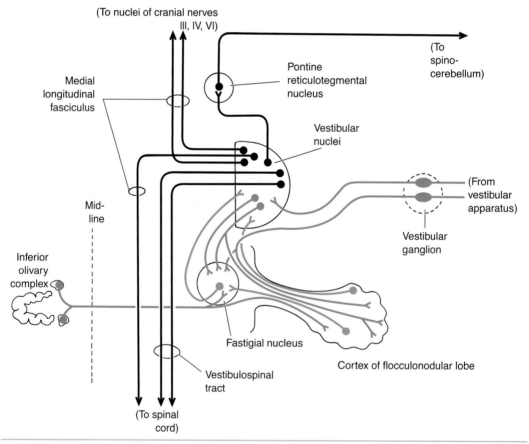

FIGURE 10-13   Connections of the vestibulocerebellum and vestibular nuclei. Afferents to the cerebellum are blue, cerebellar efferents are red, and other neurons are black.

SPINOCEREBELLUM

The following four afferent systems project to the spinocerebellar cortex.

1. **Somatic sensory systems.** The dorsal and ventral spinocerebellar tracts convey data from proprioceptive endings and from touch and pressure receptors (Fig. 10-14). The dorsal tract, consisting of the axons of the neurons constituting the nucleus thoracicus in spinal segments T1 to L3 or L4, conveys information from the trunk and leg. The ventral tract, which arises in various parts of the lumbosacral gray matter (see Chapter 5), is mainly involved in conduction from the leg. Cuneocerebellar fibers from the acces-

sory cuneate nucleus (see Chapter 7) are equivalent, for the arm and neck, to those of the dorsal spinocerebellar tract. Most of the fibers afferent to the cells of origin of the spinocerebellar and cuneocerebellar tracts have ascended into the dorsal funiculi of the spinal cord. All three trigeminal sensory nuclei (see Chapter 8) contain some neurons that project to the spinocerebellum. These are functionally equivalent to the spinocerebellar and cuneocerebellar projections, except for the head.

2. **Precerebellar reticular nuclei.** Modified data from cutaneous receptors are carried by spinoreticular fibers to the lateral and paramedian reticular nuclei (see Figs. 9-1

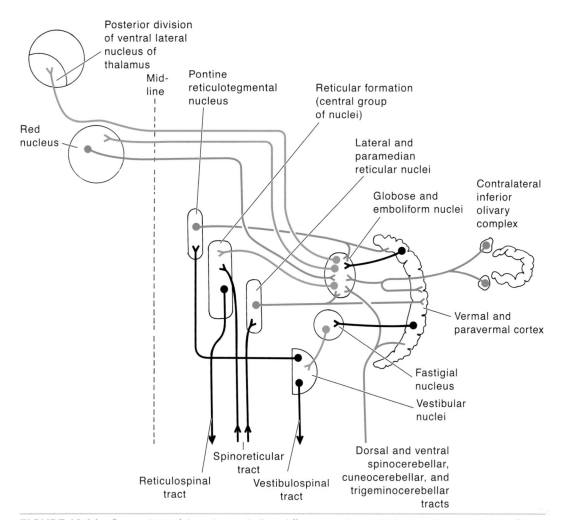

FIGURE 10-14 Connections of the spinocerebellum. Afferents to the cerebellum are blue, cerebellar efferents are red, and other neurons are black.

and 9-2), which project to the cerebellum. These two precerebellar reticular
nuclei also receive afferent fibers from
primary motor and sensory areas of the
cerebral cortex. Another precerebellar reticular nucleus that projects to the vermis
and medial parts of the hemispheres is
the reticulotegmental nucleus in the pons
(see Fig. 9-1). This nucleus receives afferents from the cerebral cortex and from
the vestibular nuclei (see Fig. 10-13).

3. **Inferior olivary complex.** The accessory
   olivary nuclei (in which spino-olivary
   tracts terminate) project to the spinocerebellum. The olivocerebellar fibers end as
   climbing fibers in the cortex.

4. **Special senses.** Tectocerebellar fibers
   arise in the superior and inferior colliculi
   of the midbrain, which are parts of the visual and auditory pathways, respectively.

    Collateral branches of the axons from
    all the various afferent sources terminate
    in the interposed nuclei, which also re-
    ceive a small contingent of fibers from the
    red nucleus.

Each half of the body is represented in the
ipsilateral cerebellar cortex; if afferent fibers
have crossed the midline from cells of origin
at lower levels, they cross again in the white
matter of the cerebellum. In monkeys and
probably also in humans, the half-body is represented in two areas. One is upside down, in
and alongside the vermis of the anterior lobe.
The other is the right way up, in the medial
part of the hemisphere on the inferior surface
of the posterior lobe. The two "head areas" are
in the vermis and adjacent cortex of the posterior lobe, and they are separated by an area
that receives auditory and visual input from
the tectum, both directly and by way of a tecto-
ponto-cerebellar circuit. Somatotopic representation in the spinocerebellum is less clearly
defined than in some areas of the cerebral cortex; there is overlap of different inputs, so that
trains of impulses from various sources may
reach the same Purkinje cell.

The spinocerebellar cortex projects to the fastigial nucleus (from the vermis) and to the interposed (globose and emboliform) nuclei (from the
paravermal zones of the hemispheres). Synergy of
muscle action and control of muscle tone are effected in part through fastigiobulbar connections,
as described for the vestibulocerebellum. Axons
from the interposed nuclei traverse the superior
cerebellar peduncle and terminate in the central
group of reticular nuclei. Thus, the spinocerebellum may influence motor neurons through reticulospinal fibers and a similar projection to motor
nuclei of cranial nerves. Alpha and gamma motor
neurons are involved in cerebellar control of muscle action, and the influence of the spinocerebellum on the skeletal musculature is ipsilateral.

Some axons from the interposed nuclei
traverse the superior cerebellar peduncle and
end in the red nucleus, which, in turn, projects to the inferior olivary nucleus. Others pass
through or around the red nucleus and continue to the ventral lateral nucleus of the thalamus, which projects to the primary motor area
of the cerebral cortex.

In summary, the spinocerebellum receives
information from proprioceptive and exterocep-
tive sensory endings and, indirectly, from the
cerebral cortex. Visual and auditory input to
areas of the spino- and pontocerebellar cortex
also takes place. These data are processed in the
circuitry of the cerebellar cortex, which modifies and refines the discharge of signals from the
central nuclei. Motor neurons are influenced
mainly through relays in the vestibular nuclei,
the reticular formation, and the primary motor
area of the cerebral cortex. The end result is control of muscle tone and synergy of collaborat-
ing muscles, as appropriate at any moment for
the adjustment of posture and in many types of
movement, including those of locomotion.

PONTOCEREBELLUM

Pontocerebellar fibers constitute the whole of the
middle cerebellar peduncle. They originate in the
pontine nuclei (nuclei pontis) of the opposite
side. Pontocerebellar axons have branches that
synapse with neurons in the dentate nucleus, and
they are distributed throughout the cortex of the
cerebellar hemispheres and the superior vermis
of the posterior lobe. The corticopontine tracts
originate in widespread areas of the contralateral
cerebral cortex (especially that of the frontal and
parietal lobes but also temporal and occipital)
and end in the pontine nuclei. Through the corticopontine and pontocerebellar projections, the
cortex of a cerebellar hemisphere receives infor-

mation concerning volitional movements that are anticipated or in progress. Some of the pontine nuclei receive afferents from the superior colliculus and relay data used by the cerebellum in the control of visually guided movements.

In addition to pontine afferents, the superior vermis of the posterior lobe, similar to the spinocerebellar cortex, receives tectocerebellar fibers from the superior and inferior colliculi. There are also olivary afferents, the axons of cells in the contralateral inferior olivary nucleus.

Purkinje cell axons from the pontocerebellar cortex terminate in the dentate nucleus, the efferent fibers of which compose most of the superior cerebellar peduncle. After traversing the decussation of the peduncles, some dentatothalamic fibers give off branches to the red nucleus, but the majority passes through or around the red

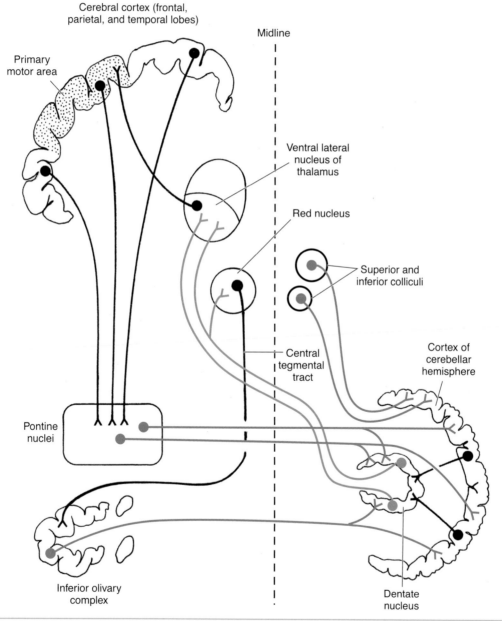

FIGURE 10-15   Connections of the pontocerebellum. Afferents to the cerebellum are blue, cerebellar efferents are red, and other neurons are black.

nucleus and end in the ventral lateral nucleus of the thalamus. In turn, this thalamic nucleus projects to the primary motor area of cerebral cortex in the frontal lobe. Through these connections, the pontocerebellum can modify activity in corticospinal, corticoreticular, and reticulospinal pathways (Fig. 10-15).

The output of the dentate nucleus, similar to that of the other cerebellar nuclei, fluctuates according to the excitatory input from extracerebellar sources and the refinement of discharge by the inhibitory action of Purkinje cells. Mainly through its influence on the cerebral motor cortex, the pontocerebellum en-

---

CLINICAL NOTE

Cerebellum Disorders

Pathological conditions are broadly classified into those that affect the vermis and flocculonodular lobe (the vestibulocerebellum and spinocerebellum) and those that affect the hemispheres (pontocerebellum).

MIDLINE LESIONS

The midline portions of the cerebellum may be the site of a tumor, typically, a malignant "medulloblastoma" that occurs in childhood. In adults, a similar syndrome may be seen in chronic alcoholism, which causes degeneration of the vermis. The patient has an unsteady, staggering **ataxic gait**, walks on a wide base, and sways from side to side. **Cerebellar nystagmus** is usually in the horizontal plane and is most pronounced when the eyes are looking to one side. It is attributed to interruption of connections of the vermis with the ocular motor nuclei by way of the vestibular nuclei and the reticular formation. At first, the signs are limited to a disturbance of equilibrium; additional cerebellar signs appear when a tumor invades other parts of the cerebellum.

NEOCEREBELLAR SYNDROME

With respect to the cerebellar hemispheres, signs of dysfunction accompany lesions that interrupt afferent pathways, cause destruction of the cortex and white matter, or involve the central nuclei or the efferent pathways in the superior cerebellar peduncle. The motor disorder is more severe and more enduring when a lesion involves the central nuclei or the superior cerebellar peduncle. When the lesion is unilateral, the signs of motor dysfunction are on the same side of the body.

The following signs, in varying degrees of severity, are those of a neocerebellar syndrome:

1. Movements are **ataxic** (intermittent or jerky). **Dysmetria** is present; for example, when the patient reaches out with the finger to an object, the finger overshoots the mark or deviates from it (known as **"past pointing"**).
2. Rapidly alternating movements, such as flexion and extension of the fingers or pronation and supination of the forearm, are performed in a clumsy manner **(adiadochokinesis)**.
3. **Asynergy** is separation of smoothly flowing voluntary movements into successions of mechanical or puppetlike movements **(decomposition of movement)**.
4. **Hypotonia** of muscles may be present, and muscles may tire easily.
5. Cerebellar **tremor**, which occurs most frequently with demyelinating lesions in the cerebellar peduncles, usually occurs at the end of a particular movement **(intention tremor)**.
6. **Dysarthria** is evident if asynergy involves muscles used in speech, which is then thick and monotonous (slurring; scanning speech).
7. Nystagmus may be present if the lesion encroaches on the vermis.

The deficits noted are superimposed on volitional movements that are otherwise intact.

A **cerebellar cognitive affective syndrome** can result from damage to the posterior but not the anterior lobe of the cerebellum. In addition to the motor changes of a neocerebellar syndrome, there are effects more usually attributable to destructive lesions in the cerebral cortex. These include uninhibited behavior and impairment of planning, reasoning, and verbal fluency, which are functions of the anterior part of the frontal lobe. Testing also reveals blunting of affect, poor visuospatial organization and memory, loss of the vocal cadence that normally puts feeling and expression into speech, and failure to connect words in a grammatically correct way. These disorders are otherwise seen in patients with lesions in various parts of the temporal and parietal lobes (see Chapters 15 and 18).

sures a smooth and orderly sequence of muscle contractions and the intended precision in the force, direction, and extent of volitional movements. These functions are particularly important for the upper limbs. A cerebellar hemisphere influences the musculature of the same side of the body because of the compensating decussations of the superior cerebellar peduncles and of the descending motor pathways.

ADDITIONAL CEREBELLAR CONNECTIONS AND FUNCTIONS

The climbing fibers from the inferior olivary complex are believed to carry instructions relating to movements that have not yet been performed. The patterns or programs concerned are stored in the cerebellum, probably as structural or functional modifications of synapses. It has been suggested that activity of the climbing fibers excites the Purkinje cell dendrites but also lowers their sensitivity to excitatory input from the much more numerous parallel fibers. Protracted but reversible changes in synaptic efficiency constitute a proposed mechanism of memory. The execution and coordination of learned movements are mediated by the mossy fiber afferents, of which those from the pontine nuclei are the most numerous in primates. When a monkey makes an intended movement, the neurons in the dentate nucleus (which receives its excitatory afferents from the pontine nuclei) are active several milliseconds before those in the primary motor area (which receives signals from the cerebellum by way of the dentato-thalamo-cortical projection).

The movements coordinated by the ponto-cerebellum are usually guided by input from the special senses, especially vision. The vermis receives visual and auditory input by way of tectocerebellar and tecto-ponto-cerebellar projections. Stimuli perceived by the eyes and ears can also influence the cerebellum through corticopontine fibers that originate in visual and auditory areas of the cerebral cortex.

Results of animal experiments have shown that the cerebellum also has a role in visceral functions. Under certain conditions, electrical stimulation of the spinocerebellar cortex produces respiratory, cardiovascular, pupillary, and urinary bladder responses. These responses are sympathetic in nature when the anterior lobe is stimulated and parasympathetic when the tonsils (see Fig. 10-3) of the posterior lobe are stimulated. The postulated pathway includes the interposed nuclei, reticular formation, and hypothalamus.

NONMOTOR FUNCTIONS OF THE CEREBELLUM

The human cerebellar hemispheres are large, and they receive afferents (by way of the pontine nuclei) from all the lobes of the cerebral cortex. This anatomy suggests involvement of the cerebellum in more activities of the brain than just the coordination of movements. Functional imaging techniques such as positron emission tomography (PET) and functional nuclear magnetic resonance imaging (fMRI) (see Chapter 4) reveal increased activity in the cerebellum in a variety of sensory and cognitive tasks in addition to the expected activation seen in specific areas of the cerebral cortex. For example, there is a four times greater increase of oxygen use in the cerebllar cortex, dentate nucleus, and red nucleus in response to passive touching of the skin (with no movement) than in response to moving the skin across a stationery surface. Heightened cerebellar activity is also seen in association with recognition of words and faces. These are cognitive functions of the parietal and temporal lobes.

Suggested Reading

Decety J, Sjööholm H, Ryding E, et al. The cerebellum participates in mental activity: tomographic measurements of regional cerebral blood flow. *Brain Res* 1990;535:313–317.

Glickstein M, Gerrits N, Kraljhans I, et al. Visual pontocerebellar projections in the macaque. *J Comp Neurol* 1994;349:51–72.

Ito M. Cerebellar circuitry as a neuronal machine. *Prog Neurobiol* 2006;78:272–303.

Kim JJ, Andreasen NC, O'Leary DS, et al. Direct comparison of the neural substrates of recognition memory for words and faces. *Brain* 1999;122:1069–1083.

Leiner HC, Leiner AL, Dow RS. Cognitive and language functions of the human cerebellum. *Trends Neurosci* 1993;16:444–447.

Liu YJ, Pu YL, Gao JH, et al. The human red nucleus and lateral cerebellum in supporting roles for sensory information processing. *Hum Brain Mapp* 2000;10:147–159.

Llinás RR, Walton KD, Lang EJ. Cerebellum. In: Shepherd GM, ed. *The Synaptic Organization of the Brain*, 5th ed. New York: Oxford University Press, 2004:271–310.

Nitschke MF, Kleinschmidt A, Wessel K, et al. Somatotopic motor representation in the human anterior cerebellum: a high-resolution functional MRI study. *Brain* 1996;119:1023–1029.

Ohtsuka K, Enoki T. Transcranial magnetic stimulation over the posterior cerebellum during smooth pursuit eye movements in man. *Brain* 1998;121:429–435.

Robinson FR, Fuchs AF. The role of the cerebellum in voluntary eye movements. *Annu Rev Neurosci* 2001;24:981–1004.

Schmahmann JD, Sherman JC. The cerebellar cognitive affective syndrome. *Brain* 1998;121:561–579.

Tredici G, Barajon I, Pizzini G, et al. The organization of corticopontine fibres in man. *Acta Anat* 1990;137:320–323.

Young PA, Young PH. The cerebellum: Ataxia. In: *Basic Clinical Neuroanatomy*. Baltimore: Williams & Wilkins, 1997:99–115.

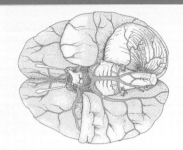

Chapter 11

DIENCEPHALON

Important Facts

- The thalamus, epithalamus, and hypothalamus form the walls and floor of the third ventricle. The thalamus also forms the floor of the lateral ventricle.

- The reticular nucleus of the thalamus modulates the exchange of signals between other thalamic nuclei and the cerebral cortex.

- Neurons in the thalamus are reciprocally connected with the cerebral cortex. Most thalamic nuclei also receive subcortical afferents.

- The ventral group of thalamic nuclei includes the medial and lateral geniculate bodies, which are parts of the auditory and visual systems and the somatosensory ventral posterior nucleus. The ventral lateral and ventral anterior nuclei are parts of pathways to the motor areas of the cerebral cortex.

- The intralaminar nuclei of the thalamus receive afferents from many sources, including the spinal cord and the brain stem reticular formation. They project to the whole neocortex and to the striatum. Involvement in arousal, awareness, and motor control is suspected as their function.

- The anterior and lateral dorsal nuclei of the thalamus are parts of the limbic system (which consists of the hippocampus, amygdala, and other parts of the brain connected with these components of the temporal lobe).

- The mediodorsal thalamic nucleus receives afferents from the amygdala, entorhinal area, spinal cord, and corpus striatum. It projects to the prefrontal cortex. The lateral posterior nucleus and the pulvinar receive input from the visual system and project to the cortex of the parietal and frontal lobes and the cingulate gyrus.

- The subthalamus contains various bundles of fibers connected with the thalamus, rostral parts of some midbrain nuclei, and the subthalamic nucleus. The subthalamic nucleus is connected with the pallidum; a destructive lesion causes contralateral hemiballismus.

- The epithalamus consists of the stria medullaris thalami, habenular nuclei, posterior commissure, and pineal gland.

- The hypothalamus contains several nuclei. Afferents include fibers from the limbic forebrain and the brain stem. Some hypothalamic neurons directly sense changes in hormone concentrations, osmotic pressure, and temperature of the blood.

- Hypothalamic efferent fibers go to the brain stem and spinal cord for control of autonomic and other involuntary functions.

- Some hypothalamic neurons secrete hormones, including those of the posterior lobe of the pituitary gland. Releasing hormones enter the hypophysial portal vessels and control the secretion of anterior pituitary hormones.

The diencephalon and telencephalon together constitute the cerebrum, of which the diencephalon forms the central core, and the telencephalon, the cerebral hemispheres. Because it is almost entirely surrounded by the hemispheres, only the ventral surface of the diencephalon is exposed to view, in an area that contains hypothalamic structures (Fig. 11-1). This area is bounded by the optic chiasma and tracts and the region where the internal capsule becomes the basis pedunculi of the midbrain. The diencephalon is divided into symmetrical halves by the slit-like third ventricle. As seen in a median section (Fig. 11-2), the junction of the midbrain and diencephalon is represented by a line that passes through the posterior commissure and is immediately caudal to the mamillary body. The boundary between the diencephalon and the telencephalon is represented by a line that traverses the interventricular foramen (foramen of Monro) and the optic chiasma.

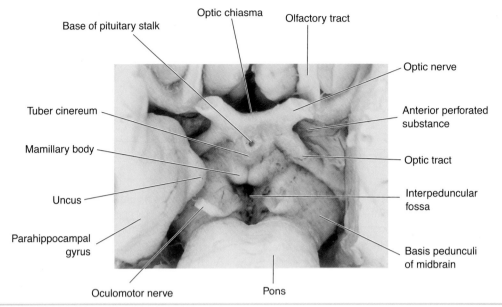

FIGURE 11-1   Landmarks of the diencephalon on the ventral surface of the brain. Part of the left temporal lobe (right side of picture) has been cut away.

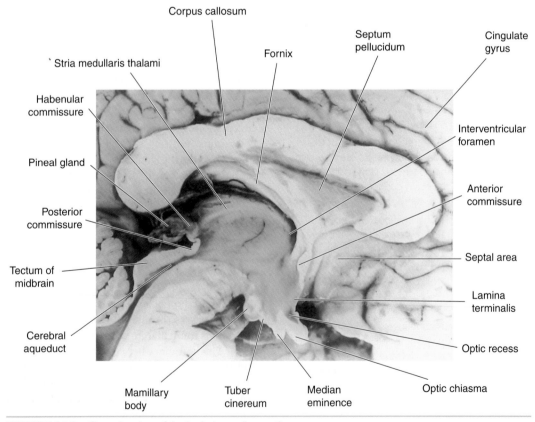

FIGURE 11-2   Central region of the brain in median section.

Gross Features

SURFACES

Each half of the diencephalon has the following landmarks and relations. The medial surface of the diencephalon forms the **wall of the third ventricle** (see Fig. 11-2). In about 70% of brains, a bridge of gray matter, the **interthalamic adhesion** or massa intermedia, joins the left and right thalami. A bundle of nerve fibers called the **stria medullaris thalami** forms a prominent ridge along the junction of the medial and dorsal surfaces. The ependymal lining of third ventricle is reflected from one side to the other along the striae medullares, forming the **roof of the third ventricle**, from which a small choroid plexus is suspended.

The dorsal surface is largely concealed by the **fornix** (Fig. 11-3), which is a robust bundle of fibers that originates in the hippocampal formation of the temporal lobe, curves over the thalamus, and ends mainly in the mamillary body. Between the left and right fornices, vascular connective tissue known as the **tela choroidea** is continuous with the vascular core of the choroid plexuses of the lateral and third ventricles. Lateral to the fornix, the dorsal surface of the thalamus forms the **floor of the central part of the lateral ventricle**, much of which is concealed by the choroid plexus (see Fig. 11-3).

Laterally, the diencephalon is bounded by the **internal capsule**, which is a thick band of fibers connecting the cerebral cortex with the thalamus and other parts of the central nervous system. The ventral surface of the diencephalon presents to the surface of the brain, as previously noted.

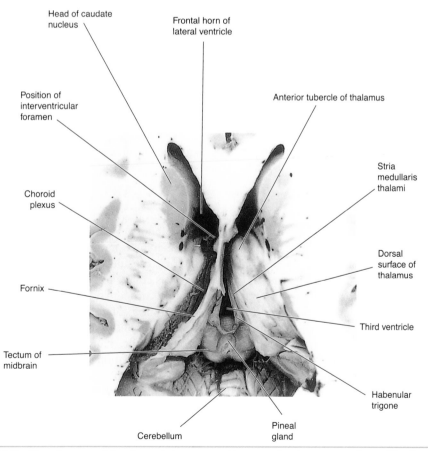

FIGURE 11-3 Dorsal aspect of the diencephalon, exposed by removing the corpus callosum. The fornix and the choroid plexus of the lateral ventricle have been removed on the right side.

MAJOR COMPONENTS

The diencephalon has four parts on each side: the thalamus, subthalamus, epithalamus, and hypothalamus. The **thalamus**, by far the largest component, is subdivided into nuclei that have different afferent and efferent connections. Certain thalamic nuclei receive input from the pathways for all the senses except smell; these nuclei project to corresponding sensory areas of the cerebral cortex. Other thalamic nuclei are connected with motor and association areas of the cortex, and yet others participate in memory, sleep, and mental activities. The **subthalamus** is a complex region ventral to the thalamus; it includes a nucleus with motor functions (the subthalamic nucleus) and tracts from the brain stem, cerebellum, and corpus striatum, which terminate in the thalamus. The **epithalamus**, situated dorsomedially to the thalamus and adjacent to the roof of the third ventricle, includes the pineal gland as well as nuclei and tracts concerned with autonomic and behavioral responses to emotional changes. The **hypothalamus** occupies the region between the third ventricle and the subthalamus; it is the part of the forebrain that integrates and controls the activities of the autonomic nervous system and of several endocrine glands. The **neurohypophysis**, which includes the posterior lobe of the **pituitary gland**, is an outgrowth of the hypothalamus. (The anterior lobe of the pituitary gland arises from the embryonic pharynx and is not a part of the brain.)

Thalamus

The thalamus is a roughly egg-shaped structure, about 3 cm anteroposteriorly and 1.5 cm in the other two directions. Its narrower end, the **anterior tubercle**, forms the posterior wall of the interventricular foramen, and its wide posterior end, the **pulvinar**, faces the subarachnoid space below the fornix and the splenium of the corpus callosum and above the pineal gland and tectum. Thin laminae of white matter partly outline the thalamus, the **stratum zonale** on the dorsal surface (see Fig. 11-12), and the **external medullary lamina** (see Fig. 11-9) laterally. The external medullary lamina is separated from the internal capsule by a thin layer

of gray matter that constitutes the **reticular nucleus** of the thalamus. The **internal medullary lamina** (Figs. 11-4B and 11-9) divides the thalamus into groups of nuclei.

SCHEME OF THALAMIC ORGANIZATION

Every nucleus of the thalamus except the reticular nucleus sends axons to the cerebral cortex, either to a sharply defined area or diffusely to a large area. Every part of the cortex receives afferent fibers from the thalamus, probably from at least two nuclei. Every thalamocortical projection is faithfully copied by a reciprocal corticothalamic connection. Thalamic nuclei receive other afferent fibers from subcortical regions. Probably only one noncortical structure, the striatum (see Chapter 12), receives afferent fibers from the thalamus.

The thalamocortical and corticothalamic axons give collateral branches to neurons in the reticular nucleus, whose neurons project to and inhibit the other nuclei of the thalamus (Fig. 11-5). Contrary to earlier beliefs, no connections exist between the various nuclei of the main mass of the thalamus, although each individual nucleus contains interneurons. The synapses of the interneurons are inhibitory, and most are dendrodendritic. Other synapses in the thalamus are excitatory, with glutamate as the transmitter, and so are thalamocortical projections (see Fig. 11-5).

RETICULAR NUCLEUS

As noted, the reticular nucleus is a thin sheet of inhibitory (γ-aminobutyrate-ergic) neurons between the external medullary lamina and the internal capsule (see Fig. 11-9). The nucleus receives collateral branches of some of the excitatory corticothalamic and thalamocortical fibers. Some excitatory afferents ascend from the pedunculopontine nucleus, which is a cluster of cholinergic neurons in the rostral pontine reticular formation.

The axons of cells in the reticular nucleus project into the deeper parts of the thalamus to end in the same nuclei that gave rise to afferents to those cells (see Fig. 11-5). All the other thalamic nuclei and all areas of the cerebral cortex are associated with corresponding regions in the reticular nucleus. Certain features of the electro-

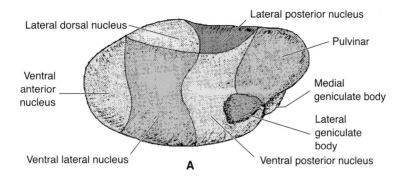

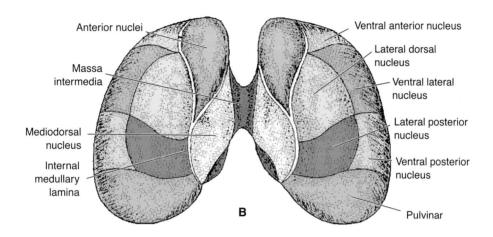

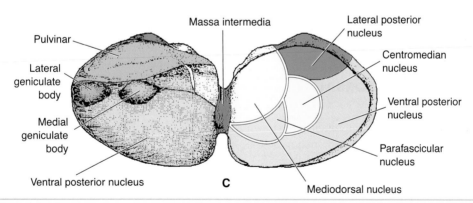

FIGURE 11-4 The thalami, showing positions of the larger nuclei. **(A)** Lateral view. **(B)** Dorsal view. **(C)** Posterior view, with the posterior half of the right thalamus cut away. Nuclei of the ventral group are colored in shades of blue to violet, the lateral group green to yellow, the medial group pink to red, and the midline and intralaminar nuclei bluish green. The internal medullary lamina is white. (From a model made by Dr. D. G. Montemurro.)

encephalogram in normal sleep depend on the activity of neurons in the reticular nucleus of the thalamus, which can suppress the transmission of signals through the thalamic nuclei of the ascending sensory pathways (see Chapter 9).

Despite its name, the reticular nucleus is not connected with the reticular formation of the brain stem; the alternative name of **perithalamus** is more appropriate but seldom used. The reticular nucleus, together with a few small

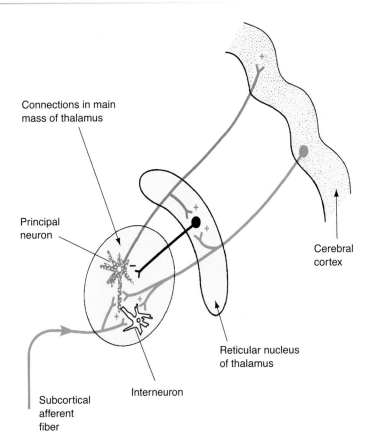

Connections in main mass of thalamus

Principal neuron

Cerebral cortex

Reticular nucleus of thalamus

Interneuron

Subcortical afferent fiber

FIGURE 11-5 Scheme of neuronal connections of the thalamus. Excitatory and inhibitory synapses are marked + and −, respectively. The dendrodendritic synapses of the interneurons also inhibit the principal cells.

thalamic nuclei not discussed here, is sometimes called the **ventral thalamus**. The other thalamic nuclei are then said to constitute the **dorsal thalamus**.

NUCLEI OF THE DORSAL THALAMUS

The positions of the thalamic nuclei are shown in Figures 11-6 to 11-12. Their major neural connections are summarized in Table 11-1, which also indicates the functional systems associated with the various nuclei. The cortical areas named in this table are shown in Figure 11-13. (For a complete account, refer to the recommended reading at the end of this chapter.)

Subthalamus

The subthalamus contains sensory fasciculi, fiber bundles from the cerebellum and the globus pallidus, rostral extensions of midbrain nuclei, and the subthalamic nucleus.

The **sensory fasciculi** are the medial lemniscus, spinothalamic tract, and trigeminothalamic tracts. They are spread out immediately beneath the ventral posterior nucleus of the thalamus, in which the fibers terminate (see Figs. 11-7 and 11-8). **Cerebellothalamic fibers** from the dentate and interposed nuclei have crossed the midline in the decussation of the superior cerebellar peduncles (see Fig. 7-13). They pass through and around the red nucleus and then form the prerubral area, or **field H of Forel** (*H* is from the German *Haube*; see Figs. 11-8 and 11-9). The cerebellothalamic fibers end in the posterior division (VLp) of the ventral lateral nucleus of the thalamus. Efferent fibers of the globus pallidus pass through the **lenticular fasciculus** and the **ansa lenticularis** (see Figs. 11-9, 11-10, and 12-5) and terminate in the VLa and VA nuclei of the thalamus (see Table 11-1). Beneath the thalamus, the pallidothalamic and cerebellothalamic fibers together constitute the **thalamic fasciculus** (see Fig. 11-9). A small contingent of axons from the globus pallidus turns caudally and ends in the pedunculopontine nucleus, which is one of the cholinergic nuclei

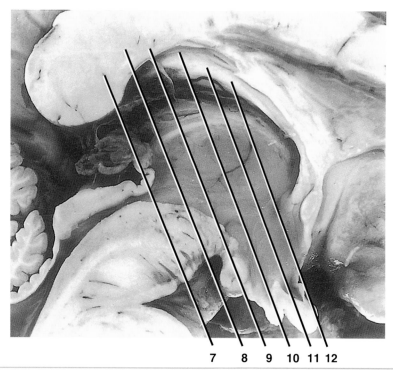

FIGURE 11-6   Key to levels for Figures 11-7 to 11-12. See Figures 11-2 and 11-3 for names of gross anatomical landmarks. (Anterior is to the right.)

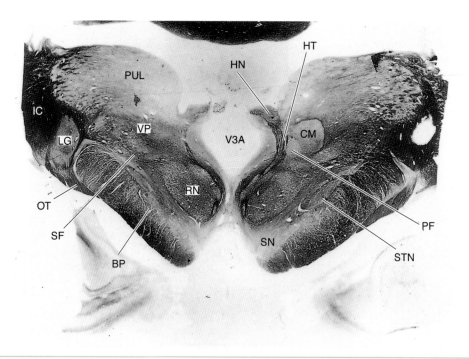

FIGURE 11-7   Transverse section at the transition between the midbrain and the diencephalon, immediately caudal to the mamillary bodies (Weigert stain for myelin). For abbreviations used in this chapter, see inside front cover of book.

Thalamic Syndrome and Central Neurogenic Pain

The thalamic syndrome (Dejerine-Roussy syndrome) is a disturbance of the somatosensory aspects of thalamic function subsequent to a lesion (usually vascular in origin) that involves the ventral posterior parts of the thalamus. Adjacent structures, including the internal capsule, are also involved in these lesions. The symptoms vary according to the location and extent of the damage. Proprioception and the sensations of touch, pain, and temperature are typically impaired on the opposite side of the body. When a threshold is reached, the sensation is exaggerated, painful, perverted, and exceptionally disagreeable. For example, the prick of a pin may be felt as a severe burning sensation, and even music that is ordinarily pleasing may be disagreeable. Spontaneous pain may develop in some instances, which may become intractable to analgesics. Emotional instability may also be present, with spontaneous or forced laughing and crying. These symptoms are not correlated with destruction of individual thalamic nuclei.

Pain may also result from destructive lesions in parts of the CNS other than the thalamus, including the spinal cord, brain stem, and the cortex and white matter of the parietal lobe. In all these conditions, there is impairment of the perception of real sensory stimuli, attributable to damage to the somatosensory pathways (see Chapter 19). The physiology of pain of central origin is poorly understood, but it has been hypothesized that the condition is caused by abnormal activity in thalamic and cortical neurons that have been deprived of their normal afferents.

OTHER THALAMIC DISORDERS

A rare disease that first affects the thalamus is **fatal familial insomnia.** This is a prion disease. (**Prions** are protein molecules, or abnormal variants of normal animal proteins, that behave as infectious agents. Prions are similar to viruses but slower in their actions. Prion molecules may be transferred among individuals by ingestion or transplantation of infected tissue. The gene encoding a prion protein can move vertically from one generation to the next.) The destructive lesions of fatal familial insomnia occur in the mediodorsal nucleus and in the anterior ventral nucleus, a member of the anterior nuclear group. With progression of the disease, dementia and other neurological symptoms develop. Degenerative changes are present in the cerebral cortex and in the inferior olivary nuclei of the medulla. The relationship of the lesions to the neural circuitry involved in sleep is not obvious.

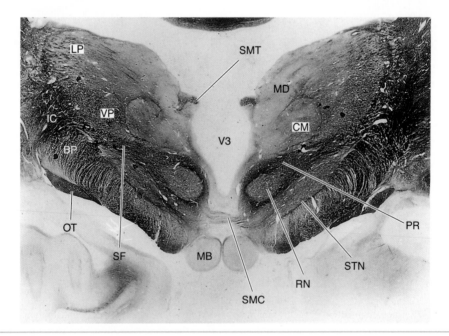

FIGURE 11-8 Diencephalon at the level of the mamillary bodies (Weigert stain).

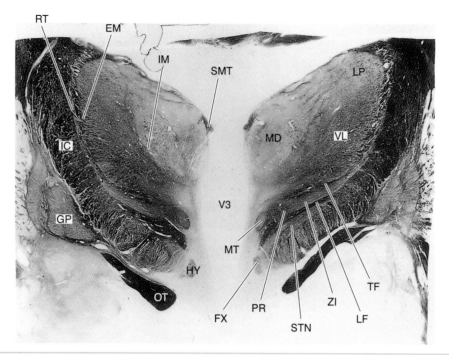

FIGURE 11-9   Diencephalon at the level of the middle of the tuber cinereum (Weigert stain).

in the reticular formation of the brain stem (see Chapters 9 and 23).

The **substantia nigra** and **red nucleus** extend from the midbrain part way into the subthalamus (see Figs. 11-7 and 11-8). The mesencephalic reticular formation also extends into the subthalamus, where it appears as the **zona incerta** between the lenticular and thalamic fasciculi (see

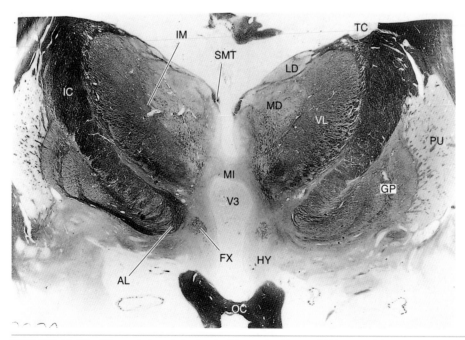

FIGURE 11-10   Diencephalon at the level of the optic chiasma (Weigert stain).

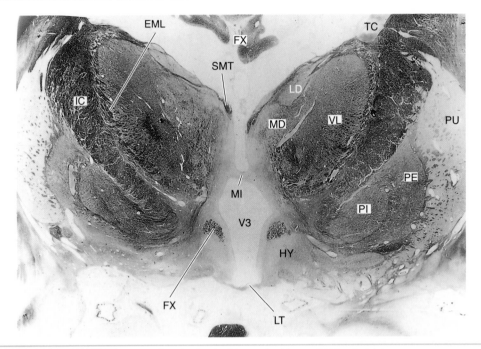

FIGURE 11-11   Diencephalon rostral to the level of the optic chiasma (Weigert stain).

Fig. 11-9). The zona incerta is part of a circuit that recognizes thirst and stimulates drinking.

The biconvex **subthalamic nucleus** (body of Luys) lies against the medial side of the internal capsule (see Figs. 11-7 to 11-9). The subthalamic nucleus has reciprocal connections with the globus pallidus, which are described in more detail in Chapters 12 and 23. These fibers

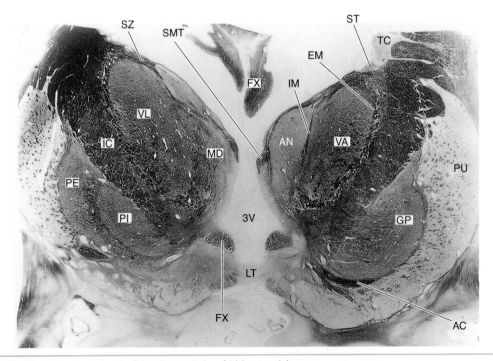

FIGURE 11-12   Rostral end of the diencephalon (Weigert stain).

TABLE 11-1 **Connections of Thalamic Nuclei and Associated Functions**

Nucleus	Afferents	Efferents	Functions
Reticular nucleus	Collateral branches of thalamocortical and corticothalamic axons	To each thalamic nucleus that sends afferents to the reticular nucleus	Inhibitory modulation of thalamocortical transmission
Intralaminar nuclei (the centromedian, parafascicular, and central lateral nuclei are the members of this group)	Cholinergic and central nuclei of reticular formation, locus coeruleus, collateral branches from spinothalamic and trigeminothalamic tracts, parabrachial nuclei, cerebellar nuclei, pallidum	Extensive cortical projections, especially to frontal and parietal lobes; striatum (see Chapter 12)	Stimulation of cerebral cortex in waking state and arousal from sleep; somatic sensation, especially pain (from contralateral sides of body and head); control of movement
Ventral group of nuclei:			
Medial geniculate body (MGB)	Inferior colliculus	Primary auditory cortex (transverse temporal gyri)	Auditory pathway (from both ears)
Lateral geniculate body (LGB)	Ipsilateral halves of both retinas	Primary visual cortex	Visual pathway (from contralateral visual fields)
Ventral posterior lateral (VPl)	Contralateral gracile and cuneate nuclei; contralateral dorsal horn of spinal cord	Primary somatosensory area (postcentral gyrus)	Somatic sensation (principal pathway, from contralateral side of body below head)
Ventral posterior medial (VPm)	Contralateral trigeminal sensory nuclei	Primary somatosensory area (postcentral gyrus)	Somatic sensation (principal pathway, from contralateral side of head: face, mouth, larynx, pharynx, dura mater)
Ventral lateral, posterior division (VLp)	Contralateral cerebellar nuclei	Primary motor area (precentral gyrus)	Cerebellar modulation of commands sent to motor neurons
Ventral lateral, anterior division (VLa)	Pallidum	Premotor and supplementary motor areas (see Chapter 15)	Planning commands to be sent to motor neurons

(continued)

CLINICAL NOTE

Hemiballismus

A lesion in the subthalamic nucleus is typically caused by local vascular occlusion. The resulting motor disturbance on the opposite side of the body is known as **ballism** or **hemiballismus**. The condition is characterized by involuntary movements that come on suddenly with great force and rapidity. The movements are purposeless and usually of a throwing or flailing type. The spontaneous movements occur most severely at proximal joints of the limbs, especially the arms. The muscles of the face and neck are sometimes also involved.

TABLE 11-1 **Connections of Thalamic Nuclei and Associated Functions** *(continued)*

Nucleus	Afferents	Efferents	Functions
Ventral anterior (VA)	Pallidum	Frontal lobe, including premotor and supplementary motor areas	Motor planning and more complex behavior
Posterior group of nuclei	Spinothalamic and trigeminothalamic tracts	Insula and nearby temporal and parietal cortex, including second somatosensory area	Visceral and other responses to somatic sensory stimuli
Lateral group of nuclei:			
Lateral dorsal (LD)	Hippocampal formation; pretectal area, and superior colliculus	Cingulate gyrus; visual association cortex (occipital, posterior parietal, and temporal lobes)	Memory; interpretation of visual stimuli
Lateral posterior (LP)	Superior colliculus	Parietal, temporal, and occipital association cortex	Interpretation of visual and other sensory stimuli, formulation of complex behavioral responses
Pulvinar	Pretectal area; primary and all association cortex for vision; retinas	Parietal lobe, anterior frontal cortex, cingulate gyrus, amygdala	Interpretation of visual and other sensory stimuli, formulation of complex behavioral responses
Medial group of nuclei:			
Mediodorsal (MD)	Entorhinal cortex, amygdala, collaterals from spinothalamic tract, pallidum (ventral parts and substantia nigra pars reticulata)	Prefrontal cortex	Behavioral responses that involve decisions based on prediction and incentives
Medioventral (MV, "midline nuclei")	Amygdala, hypothalamus	Hippocampal formation and parahippocampal gyrus	Behavior, including visceral and "emotional" responses
Anterior group of nuclei	Mamillary body	Cingulate gyrus	Memory

For simplicity, some groups (e.g., intralaminar, anterior, mediodorsal) are treated as if they were individual nuclei. The functions are those of the larger circuits in which the nuclei of the thalamus participate.

constitute the **subthalamic fasciculus**, which cuts across the internal capsule.

Epithalamus

The epithalamus consists of the habenular nuclei and their connections and the pineal gland.

HABENULAR NUCLEI

A slight swelling in the habenular trigone marks the position of the medial and lateral habenular nuclei (see Figs. 11-3 and 11-7). Afferent fibers are received through the **stria medullaris thalami**, which runs along the dorsomedial border of the thalamus (see Figs. 11-2, 11-3, and 11-9) and is also considered part of the epithalamus.

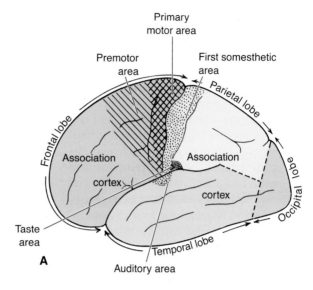

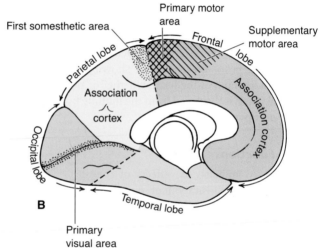

FIGURE 11-13 Cortical areas connected with the thalamic nuclei described in Table 11-1. **(A)** Lateral surface of left cerebral hemisphere. **(B)** Medial surface of left cerebral hemisphere.

Most of the cells of origin of the stria are situated in the septal area. This area is located on the medial surface of the frontal lobe beneath the rostral end of the corpus callosum (see Fig. 11-2) and is part of the limbic system of the brain, considered in Chapter 18.

The habenular nuclei give rise to a well-defined bundle of fibers known as the **habenulointerpeduncular tract** (fasciculus retroflexus of Meynert; see Fig. 11-7). The main destination of the fasciculus is the interpeduncular nucleus in the midline of the roof of the interpeduncular fossa of the midbrain. Through relays in the reticular formation of the midbrain, the interpeduncular nucleus influences neurons in the hypothalamus and preganglionic autonomic neurons. No clearly defined function is attributed to the habenular nuclei.

PINEAL GLAND

The pineal gland or body, also called the epiphysis, has the shape of a pine cone. It is attached to the diencephalon by the pineal stalk, into which the third ventricle extends as the pineal recess (see Figs. 11-2 and 11-3). The pineal gland and its stalk develop as an outgrowth from the ependymal roof of the third ventricle. The habenular commissure in the dorsal wall of the stalk includes fibers of the stria medullaris thalami that terminate in the opposite habenular nuclei. The ventral wall of the pineal stalk is attached to the posterior commissure, which carries axons involved in pupillary reflexes and eye movements (see Chapter 8).

Pineal Anatomy

In mammals, the pineal organ has the structural organization of an endocrine gland. It receives an afferent nerve supply from the superior cervical ganglion of the sympathetic trunk through the **nervus conarii**, which runs subendothelially in the straight sinus (within the tentorium cerebelli) before penetrating the dura and distributing its branches to the pineal parenchyma. The characteristic cells of the gland (**pinealocytes**) have granular cytoplasm and processes that end in bulbous expansions close to blood vessels. The pineal gland is one of the four **circumventricular organs** associated with the third ventricle because its capillary blood vessels have endothelial fenestrations and are permeable to large molecules. The other circumventricular organs are reviewed in the last section of this chapter. After about age 16 years, granules of calcium and magnesium salts appear in the gland and later coalesce to form larger particles (**brain sand**). The deposits are useful for showing, in a simple radiograph of the head, whether or not the pineal gland is displaced from the midline by a space-occupying lesion.

Pineal Functions

In laboratory animals, the effects of pinealectomy and of administration of pineal extracts indicate an antigonadotrophic action of pineal secretions. Chemical extraction of pineal glands has produced several possible active principles, most notably **melatonin**, an indoleamine related to serotonin. In humans, the circulating level of melatonin decreases sharply with the onset of puberty. Women of reproductive age experience cyclic variations, with the melatonin levels reaching minimum values at the time of ovulation.

Clinical observations support the notion of an antigonadotrophic function for the human pineal gland. A pineal tumor developing around the time of puberty may alter the age of onset of pubertal changes. Puberty may be precocious if the tumor is of a type that destroys the pinealocytes, or puberty may be delayed if the tumor is derived from the pinealocytes. A pineal tumor can also impair vertical eye movements by pressing on the tectum (Parinaud's syndrome; see Chapter 8).

Pineal secretion of melatonin is influenced by ambient light. Some axons from the retina leave the optic tract near the optic chiasma and terminate in the nearby suprachiasmatic nucleus of the hypothalamus. This projects to other hypothalamic nuclei, which send axons caudally to the preganglionic neurons of the sympathetic nervous system in the thoracic segments of the spinal cord. The suprachiasmatic nucleus serves as a clock that regulates rhythmic activities of the brain and endocrine system. Melatonin can change the speed of the clock, and knowledge of this has led to popular use of the hormone as a treatment for jet lag and other sleep disorders. In principle, a dose of the hormone is taken before lying down and attempting to sleep. The popularity of melatonin (which can be taken by mouth and apparently has no toxic effects) was enhanced by claims in the 1980s that its administration to mice resulted in increased life span.

Hypothalamus

The hypothalamus has a functional importance that is quite out of proportion to its size. Input from the limbic system has a special behavioral significance, and afferents from the brain stem convey information that is largely of visceral origin. The hypothalamus is not influenced solely by neuronal systems; some of its neurons respond directly to properties of the circulating blood, including temperature, osmotic pressure, and the levels of various hormones. Hypothalamic function becomes manifest through efferent pathways to autonomic nuclei in the brain stem and spinal cord and through an intimate relationship with the pituitary gland by means of **neurosecretory cells**. These cells elaborate the hormones of the posterior lobe of the gland and produce releasing hormones that control the anterior lobe. By these means, the hypothalamus has a major role in producing responses to emotional changes and to needs signaled by hunger and thirst. It is instrumental in maintaining a constant internal environment (homeostasis) and is essential for reproductive function.

ANATOMY AND TERMINOLOGY

The hypothalamus surrounds the third ventricle ventral to the hypothalamic sulci (see Fig. 11-2). The mamillary bodies are distinct swellings on the ventral surface (see Fig. 11-1). The region bounded by the mamillary bodies, optic chiasma, and beginning of the optic tracts is known as the **tuber cinereum**. The **pituitary stalk** arises from the **median eminence** just behind the optic chiasma and expands to form the neural or posterior lobe of the **pituitary gland**. The median eminence and the neural components of the pituitary stalk and gland have similar cytological and functional characteristics; together they constitute the **neurohypophysis**. For reference, these and some other names applied to the hypothalamohypophysial system are summarized in Table 11-2. The neuro-

TABLE 11-2 **Terminology of the Hypothalamohypophysial System***

Name	Definition
Adenohypophysis	The structures derived from the ectoderm of Rathke's pouch: pars distalis (i.e., anterior lobe), pars intermedia, and pars tuberalis
Anterior lobe	The largest part of the adenohypophysis, excluding the pars intermedia and pars tuberalis
Anterior pituitary	A term commonly applied to the anterior lobe and its hormones
Hypophysis	All the parts of the adenohypophysis and neurohypophysis (full name is hypophysis cerebri)
Infundibular process	The neural lobe of the pituitary gland
Infundibular stem	The nervous tissue joining the median eminence to the neural lobe; the major component of the pituitary stalk
Infundibulum	The most ventral part of the hypothalamus, with the third ventricle extending into the median eminence; in some animals, the infundibular recess of the ventricle continues through the infundibular stem into the neural lobe
Median eminence	The part of the neurohypophysis that is a small lump in the midline of the tuber cinereum of the hypothalamus; it contains the primary capillaries of the hypophysial portal system
Neural lobe	The larger part of the posterior lobe, excluding the pars intermedia
Neurohypophysis	The parts of the pituitary gland derived from the infundibulum of the embryonic diencephalon: median eminence, infundibular stem, and neural lobe (i.e., infundibular process or pars nervosa)
Neurosecretion	An activity of certain neurons that have synapse-like contacts with blood vessels and release physiologically important substances (hormones) into the blood
Pars distalis	The anterior lobe of the pituitary gland
Pars intermedia	The part of the adenohypophysis that intervenes between the anterior lobe and the neural lobe; it is smaller in humans than in most other animals and consists of several tiny cystic structures
Pars nervosa	The neural lobe of the pituitary gland
Pars tuberalis	A part of the adenohypophysis consisting of a thin layer of cells on the surface of the median eminence and pituitary stalk
Pituitary gland	The hypophysis cerebri, consisting of the neurohypophysis and adenohypophysis
Pituitary stalk	The infundibular stem, together with the adjacent parts of the pars tuberalis and the hypophysial portal veins
Posterior lobe	The part of the pituitary gland posterior (in humans) or dorsal (in most other animals) to the anterior lobe, from which it is separated by the pars intermedia
Posterior pituitary	A term commonly applied to the neural lobe and its hormones

*This list includes several terms that are not used in this textbook but that students may encounter when studying clinical endocrinology or neuroscience.

hypophysis contains permeable blood vessels and is therefore one of the circumventricular organs associated with the third ventricle.

The **lamina terminalis** limits the third ventricle anteriorly (see Figs. 11-2 and 11-14), extending in the midline from the optic chiasma to the anterior commissure. Embedded in the lamina is another of the four circumventricular organs associated with the third ventricle. This is the **organum vasculosum laminae terminalis (OVLT)**. It has been implicated in mechanisms of fever and also in the regulation of sodium metabolism by way of appetite for salt. The lamina terminalis and anterior commissure are telencephalic structures and so is the **preoptic area**, which is the gray matter within and immediately lateral to and behind the lamina terminalis. The connections and functions of the preoptic area are inseparable from those of the anterior (rostral) part of the medial zone of the hypothalamus. One group of intensely staining cells in this area is notable for containing more than twice as many neurons in men as in women.

The columns of the fornix traverse the hypothalamus to reach the mamillary bodies and serve as points of reference for sagittal planes that divide each half of the hypothalamus into a medial and a lateral zone. The **medial zone** is subdivided into **suprachiasmatic**, **tuberal**, and **mamillary regions**, with ventral structures as landmarks. It contains several distinct nuclei and a thin layer of fine myelinated and unmyelinated axons beneath the ependymal lining of the third ventricle. The **lateral zone** contains fewer neuronal cell bodies, but there are many fibers, with most of them running longitudinally.

HYPOTHALAMIC NUCLEI AND CONNECTIONS

Several hypothalamic nuclei are recognized on the basis of cellular characteristics and connections. For reference, Figure 11-14 shows the positions of the major nuclei of the medial zone. The lateral zone of the hypothalamus contains the cells of the **lateral nucleus**, which are interspersed among the abundant myelinated axons

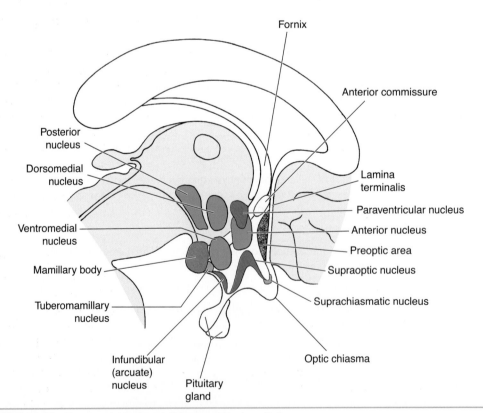

FIGURE 11-14   Some nuclei in the medial zone of the hypothalamus.

of the region and the **lateral tuberal nucleus**, which consists of small groups of neurons near the surface of the tuber cinereum.

Some hypothalamic nuclei have distinct functions; some of these functions are discussed here. For physiological discussion, it is therefore convenient to consider the hypothalamus as a unit or "black box," with functions localized to regions larger than individual nuclei. As the main integrator of the autonomic and endocrine systems and of many involuntary actions of skeletal muscles, the hypothalamus receives signals from diverse sources, including data of somatic and visceral origin and the special senses of taste and smell. Fibers from the amygdala and hippocampus provide input derived from the activities of the temporal and prefrontal cortex, which are concerned with emotional drives and memory. The output of the hypothalamus is directed caudally to the brain stem and spinal cord and rostrally to the thalamus and cerebral cortex. Some of these afferent and efferent connections are summarized in Figure 11-15.

Afferent fibers reach the hypothalamus by way of the anterior limb of the **internal capsule** (see Figs. 11-15 and 16-7), the **fornix** (see Figs. 11-10 to 11-12, 11-16, and 16-7), the **stria terminalis** (see Figs. 11-12 and 16-9), the **diagonal band** (within the anterior perforated substance), the medial forebrain bundle, and the dorsal longitudinal fasciculus. The **medial forebrain bundle** consists of ascending and descending myelinated axons of different lengths extending from the septal area and anterior perforated substance of the forebrain into the lateral zone of the hypothalamus. The **dorsal longitudinal fasciculus** is formed from unmyelinated periventricular axons in the medial zone of the hypothalamus; these converge into a distinct bundle in the periaqueductal gray matter of the midbrain, continuing caudally in the medial part of the floor of the fourth ventricle. Efferent fibers ascend from the hypothalamus to the thalamus in the **mamillothalamic fasciculus** (bundle of Vicq d'Azyr; Fig. 11-16) and to the basal cholinergic forebrain nuclei (see Chapter 12) in the diagonal band. Descending efferents are carried in the medial forebrain bundle and dorsal longitudinal fasciculus and in the **mamillotegmental tract**, which is a branch of the mamillothalamic fasciculus.

The other major output of the hypothalamus consists of hormones secreted into blood vessels by neurosecretory cells. This is explained in connection with the hypothalamic control of the pituitary gland.

AUTONOMIC AND RELATED FUNCTIONS OF THE HYPOTHALAMUS

Knowledge of hypothalamic function has been derived partly from human clinicopathological correlations but largely from experimentation in animals. In interpreting the effects of electrical stimulation or of destructive lesions, it is necessary to appreciate that the axons of neurons in the anterior parts of the medial zone of the hypothalamus pass through the posterior parts of the medial zone and through the lateral zone on their way to the brain stem. It is therefore difficult to infer the localization of functions from abnormalities that follow stimulation or ablation of individual hypothalamic nuclei.

The responses most regularly elicited by **stimulation of the anterior hypothalamus** (preoptic area and anterior nucleus) include slowing of the heart rate, vasodilation, lowering of blood pressure (BP), salivation, increased peristalsis in the gastrointestinal (GI) tract, contraction of the urinary bladder, and sweating. These effects are mediated peripherally by cholinergic neurons, including those of the parasympathetic system (see Chapter 24). **Stimulation in the region of the posterior and lateral nuclei** elicits noradrenergic sympathetic responses; these include cardiac acceleration, elevation of BP, cessation of peristalsis in the GI tract, dilation of the pupils, and hyperglycemia.

Regulation of body temperature is an instructive example of the role of the hypothalamus in maintaining homeostasis. Certain hypothalamic cells monitor the temperature of blood and initiate physiological changes necessary to maintain a normal body temperature. Thermosensitive neurons in the anterior hypothalamus respond to an increase in temperature of the blood and activate mechanisms that promote heat loss, such as cutaneous vasodilation and sweating. A lesion in the anterior hypothalamus may therefore result in hyperthermia.

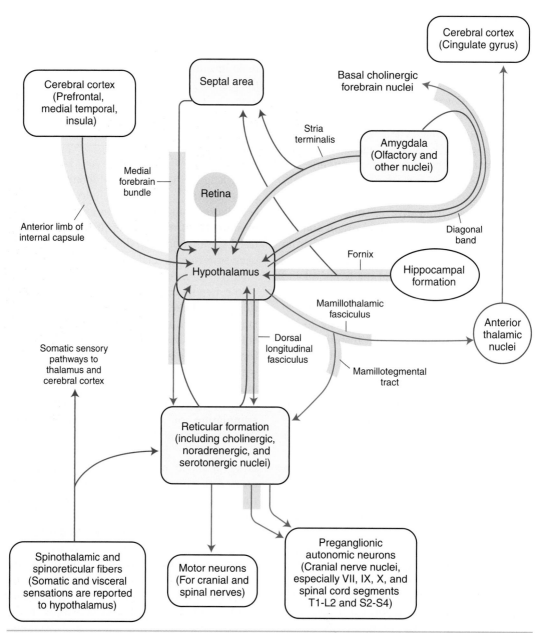

FIGURE 11-15 Diagram showing direct and indirect neural connections of the hypothalamus with other parts of the brain and spinal cord.

Cells in the posterior hypothalamic nucleus (see Fig. 11-14) respond to lowering of blood temperature, triggering such responses as cutaneous vasoconstriction and shivering, for conservation and production of heat, respectively. A lesion in the posterior part of the hypothalamus destroys cells involved in conservation and production of heat, and it also interrupts fibers running caudally from the heat-dissipating region. This results in a serious impairment of temperature regulation in either a cold or hot environment.

An abnormally high body temperature (**fever**) is typically associated with infectious disease. Products of bacterial decomposition (pyrogens) enter the circulation and pass into the preoptic area by way of the permeable blood vessels of the OVLT. Contact of pyrogens with the dendrites of anterior hypothalamic neurons results in inhibition of the mechanisms that cause loss of heat.

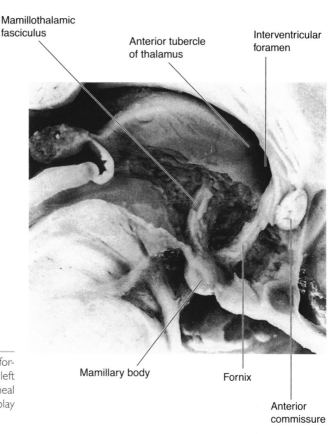

Mamillothalamic
fasciculus

Anterior tubercle
of thalamus

Interventricular
foramen

Mamillary body

Fornix

Anterior
commissure

FIGURE 11-16 Dissection showing the fornix and mamillothalamic fasciculus on the left side. Gray matter has been removed piecemeal from the wall of the third ventricle to display the bundles of myelinated fibers.

Hypothalamic **regulation of food and water intake** has been demonstrated by electrical stimulation and by placing small electrolytic lesions in the hypothalamus. Feeding is also regulated by various hypothalamic afferents, including those from visceral sensory neurons and the olfactory and limbic systems as well as by the level of glucose in the blood. **Leptin**, a hormone secreted by adipose tissue, acts on hypothalamic neurons and causes reduction of food intake. A hunger or feeding "center" located in the lateral zone of the hypothalamus is now known to include **orexin-secreting neurons**. In animals, intraventricular injection of orexin causes increased eating. A "satiety center" (inhibiting food intake) has been demonstrated in the region of the ventromedial hypothalamic nucleus. Destruction of the ventromedial nucleus in a laboratory animal results in excessive food intake and obesity.

The zona incerta of the subthalamus, the lateral and ventromedial hypothalamic nuclei, and the subfornical organ are interconnected to control **water intake**. (See also under "Third Ventricle" near the end of this chapter.) The volume of water excreted in the urine is controlled by one of the posterior pituitary hormones (see under "Hypothalamic Control of the Pituitary Gland").

CLINICAL NOTE

Naturally occurring anterior hypothalamic lesions in humans can also result in obesity. The cell bodies or axons of cells that regulate the output of gonadotrophic hormones by the anterior lobe of the pituitary gland may be destroyed at the same time. The combination of obesity and deficiency of secondary sex characteristics is known as the **adiposogenital** or **Fröhlich's syndrome**.

THE HYPOTHALAMUS AND SLEEP

Two nuclei in the posterior hypothalamus are active in the wakeful state, and one nucleus in the preoptic area is active in sleep. (For more about sleep and consciousness, see Chapter 9.)

The tuberomamillary nucleus (see Fig. 11-14) contains the brain's only **histaminergic neurons**, which have long, branched axons that extend caudally to the reticular formation of the brain stem and rostrally to the thalamus and all parts of the cerebral cortex. These neurons are active in the awake state and quiescent during sleep. They form part of the ascending arousal system described in Chapter 9. In the posterior part of the lateral hypothalamic area, neurons are present that use peptides known as *orexins* or *hypocretins* as excitatory transmitters. **Orexin neurons** are active in the waking state. They have axons that ramify extensively in the thalamus, basal cholinergic nuclei of the forebrain, and cerebral cortex, and they also stimulate tuberomamillary histaminergic neurons and the cholinergic and adrenergic neurons of the rostral pontine reticular formation.

The **ventrolateral preoptic area** includes a nucleus of neurons that produce γ-aminobuty-rate and the peptide galanin. These neurons are most active during deep sleep. Their axons extend caudally to the tuberomamillary nucleus, where they inhibit the histaminergic neurons and to the cholinergic neurons of the reticular formation, which they also inhibit.

HYPOTHALAMIC CONTROL OF THE PITUITARY GLAND

Neurohypophysial hormones are synthesized in the hypothalamus, and hormone production by the anterior lobe of the pituitary gland is controlled by hormones of hypothalamic origin. Some of the anterior lobe hormones act on and interact with other endocrine organs. Consequently, through the neurosecretory function of hypothalamic cells, the brain controls much of the endocrine system. Only the major features of the hypothalamohypophysial system are discussed here; the subject is a large one, constituting much of the science of **neuroendocrinology**. The anatomical nomenclature special to this system is explained in Table 11-2 and illustrated in Figure 11-17. Some of the clinical and endocrinological terminology is explained in the Glossary at the end of the book.

CLINICAL NOTE

Encephalitis Lethargica

As the First World War was ending, a pandemic of an exceptionally severe influenza killed even more people than those who died from hostile action. A second pandemic soon followed. This was a neurological disorder, now generally guessed to have been a viral infection, that was given the name **encephalitis lethargica**. The infection usually caused excessive sleepiness. Some patients experienced a wide variety of other neurological symptoms, with some persisting for decades after the acute phase of the illness had subsided. In a minority of patients, the principal symptom was insomnia rather than somnolence. Many of the people afflicted with encephalitis lethargica died, and associations were made between the clinical manifestations and the sites of damage seen postmortem in the brain. Extensive studies of this kind were made by von Economo, who associated insomnia with lesions in the preoptic area and de-

duced that the posterior hypothalamus contained neurons needed for wakefulness.

A frequent long-term consequence of encephalitis lethargica was parkinsonism (see Chapters 7 and 23) caused by lesions in the substantia nigra.

NARCOLEPSY

Narcolepsy is a troublesome disorder in which the patient frequently passes from a wakeful state into REM sleep (see Chapter 9) for brief periods. The condition can also occur in dogs and several other mammals and is present in genetically modified mice that are unable to produce either orexin or one of its two receptor proteins. The brains of people and dogs with narcolepsy have been shown to have greatly reduced numbers of orexin-containing neurons in the hypothalamus. The presence of gliosis suggests that the cells have died as a result of a degenerative or autoimmune disease process.

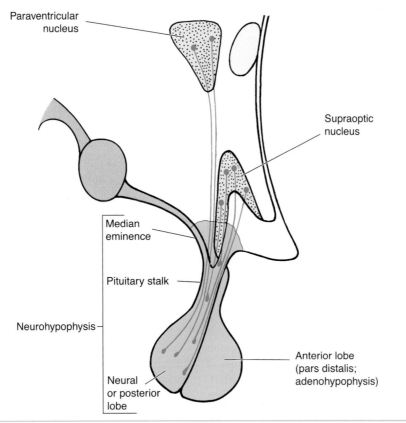

FIGURE 11-17   Hypothalamohypophysial tract and the parts of the neurohypophysis.

Neurohypophysis

As noted previously, the neurohypophysis consists of structures of diencephalic origin in the embryo: the median eminence, pituitary stalk, and the posterior or neural lobe of the pituitary gland (see Fig. 11-17). It contains axons, which end around blood vessels and atypical neuroglial cells. In the median eminence, **tanycytes** are present (see Chapter 2), and in the pituitary stalk and posterior lobe, atypical astrocytes known as **pituicytes** are present. Hormones released from the neural lobe of the pituitary gland enter the general circulation and act on cells in the kidney, mammary gland, and uterus. Hormones released from the median eminence act on cells in the anterior lobe of the pituitary gland.

Posterior Lobe Hormones

The two hormones of the posterior lobe of the pituitary gland are **vasopressin** (also called **antidiuretic hormone [ADH]**) and **oxytocin**. They are synthesized in the cell bodies of large neurosecretory cells in the supraoptic and paraventricular nuclei. Vasopressin-producing neurons are most abundant in the supraoptic nucleus, and oxytocin-producing neurons are most abundant in the paraventricular nucleus. The unmyelinated axons of the cells in these nuclei constitute the **hypothalamohypophysial tract**, and they terminate as expansions in contact with capillaries in the neurohypophysis (see Fig. 11-17). The hormones are stored in the expansions, which are known as **Herring bodies**. A Herring body has the physiological properties of a presynaptic terminal, and the arrival of an action potential results in the release of some of its contents. The hormone diffuses through the permeable endothelium of a nearby capillary and enters the general circulation.

Vasopressin Secretion and Action

A slight elevation of osmotic pressure of the blood causes the osmoreceptive cells of the supraoptic nucleus to propagate impulses with greater fre-

Disordered Vasopressin Secretion

Destruction of the supraoptic nuclei, the hypothalamohypophysial tract, and the neurohypophysis results in **neurogenic diabetes insipidus**, which is characterized by excretion of large quantities of dilute urine (polyuria) and excessive thirst and water intake (polydipsia) to compensate. A destructive lesion restricted to the posterior lobe of the pituitary gland is not, as a rule, followed by diabetes insipidus because some ADH enters the blood from the median eminence and pituitary stalk. Diabetes insipidus is not necessarily caused by failure of ADH secretion. **Nephrogenic diabetes insipidus** can result from renal disease,

with the kidneys failing to respond to the hormone.

Excessive secretion of ADH can result from disease processes that irritate the hypothalamus, such as meningitis or head injury. It occurs also as an occasional adverse effect of several commonly used drugs and in several nonneurological disorders. For example, a tumor in the lung, pancreas, or thymus may secrete ADH or a similar peptide. **SIADH** (syndrome of inappropriate secretion of antidiuretic hormone) consists of elevated plasma vasopressin in the absence of appropriate physiological stimuli. The resulting hyponatremia causes weakness and confusion followed by coma and seizures if untreated.

---

quency. The arrival of impulses at the axonal terminals causes the release of ADH into the capillary blood of the neurohypophysis. Resorption of water from the distal and collecting tubules of the kidney is accelerated by the action of ADH, and the osmolarity of the blood plasma returns to normal. A delicate mechanism is thereby provided to ensure homeostasis with respect to water balance. Other endocrine mechanisms, outside the scope of this book, determine the renal excretion of sodium ions, which also contribute to the osmolarity of plasma and the volume of urine produced. ADH acting alone tends to lower the circulating level of Na^+ (hyponatremia) by diluting the plasma with conserved water.

Oxytocin Secretion and Action

Oxytocin has a physiological role in parturition. It is secreted as a reflex response to dilatation of the uterine cervix, and it causes contraction of the uterus. Secretion of the hormone is induced also when the nipple is stimulated by a suckling infant. Oxytocin causes contraction of the myo-

epithelial cells of the mammary glands, with ejection of milk into the duct system and out of the ducts' openings at the tip of the nipple. Simultaneous contraction of the uterus contributes to the postpartum shrinkage (involution) of this organ for several hours after delivery. Involution of the uterus prevents the hemorrhage that can follow delivery of the placenta.

Pituitary Portal System

Secretion of hormones by the anterior lobe is under the control of the hypothalamus, by a vascular route rather than nervous connections.

Anterior Pituitary Hormones

The following hormones are produced in the anterior lobe:

1. **Follicle-stimulating hormone (FSH)** stimulates the growth of ovarian follicles and

Posterior Pituitary Hormones as Drugs

Vasopressin is used as replacement therapy for neurogenic diabetes insipidus. Larger doses are sometimes used to produce vasoconstriction to

control some types of hemorrhage, such as bleeding esophageal varices. Oxytocin is used as a drug to induce labor. Both hormones are octapeptides. These were the first peptide hormones to be sequenced and synthesized, by Du Vigneaud in the 1950s. This achievement led to a Nobel Prize.

induces their cells to secrete estradiol and other estrogens. In men, FSH makes cells of the seminiferous tubules respond to testosterone; this effect is necessary for the production of spermatozoa.

2. **Luteinizing hormone (LH)** stimulates the formation of a corpus luteum in the ovary after ovulation and induces the luteal cells to secrete progesterone. FSH and LH act together to induce ovulation. LH is also known as *interstitial cell-stimulating hormone* in men because it induces the interstitial cells (Leydig cells) of the testis to secrete testosterone and other androgens.

3. **Prolactin** stimulates development of the mammary glands and lactation. Its action, if any, in men is unknown.

4. **Thyrotrophic** or **thyroid-stimulating hormone (TSH)** stimulates the thyroid gland to synthesize and release thyroxine and triiodothyronine.

5. **Adrenocorticotrophic hormone (ACTH)** stimulates the cortex of the adrenal gland to produce and secrete cortisol (hydrocortisone) and other steroids (glucocorticoids) that modulate carbohydrate metabolism and protect against many effects of stress. (Secretion of aldosterone, the corticosteroid that limits sodium excretion and is necessary for life, is not under pituitary control.)

6. **Growth hormone (GH)** or **somatotrophic hormone (STH)** stimulates growth at the epiphyses of the long bones and elsewhere. Its actions are largely mediated by another protein hormone, **insulin-like growth factor 1 (ILGF-1)**, which is secreted by cells acted on by STH. The largest production of ILGF-1 is in the liver.

The pituitary portal system begins with the superior hypophysial arteries, which arise from the internal carotid arteries at the base of the brain and break up into capillary tufts and loops in the median eminence (Fig. 11-18). The capillaries are drained by veins that pass along the pituitary stalk and then enter the anterior lobe of the gland, where they empty into large capillaries or sinusoids among the hormone-producing cells. The preoptic area and hypothalamus contain neurons that produce releasing hormones, which are peptides and at least two release-inhibiting hormones (a peptide called *somatostatin* for STH and the catecholamine dopamine for prolactin). There is a separate hypothalamic-releasing hormone for each hormone of the anterior lobe, with the exception of FSH, which is secreted in response to the LH-releasing hormone, which is known as either LHRH or GnRH (gonadotrophin-releasing hormone). The releasing and inhibiting hormones pass distally by axoplasmic transport in the axons of the cells that produce them, enter the capillaries of the portal system in the median eminence, and are then delivered in locally high concentrations to cells of the anterior lobe. There they modulate the synthesis of the adenohypophysial hormones and their release into the general circulation.

The neurosecretory cells that produce releasing and release-inhibiting hormones are influenced by the various afferent fiber connections of the hypothalamus. Their activity is more directly regulated, however, by hormones of the target organs of pituitary hormones. For example, when the concentration of triiodothyronine in the blood is high, hypothalamic cells that produce thyrotrophin-releasing hormone (TRH) are suppressed. Conversely, if the circu-

---

Kallman's Syndrome

The neurons that produce LHRH (GnRH) have an unusual embryonic origin. They are generated in the olfactory placode, an area of ectoderm that gives rise to the olfactory epithelium of the nose, the glial cells of the olfactory nerves, and the tiny nervus terminalis (see Chapter 17). Neurons that synthesize LHRH migrate centrally along the nervus terminalis to the region of the lamina termina-

lis and enter the preoptic and anterior hypothalamic areas. Because they stimulate secretion of gonadotrophins, these neurons are essential for the functions of the testes and ovaries. Kallman's syndrome is a rare disorder in which defective development of the olfactory placode causes anosmia and nonfunctional gonads. The condition is associated with absence of hypothalamic LHRH-containing neurons.

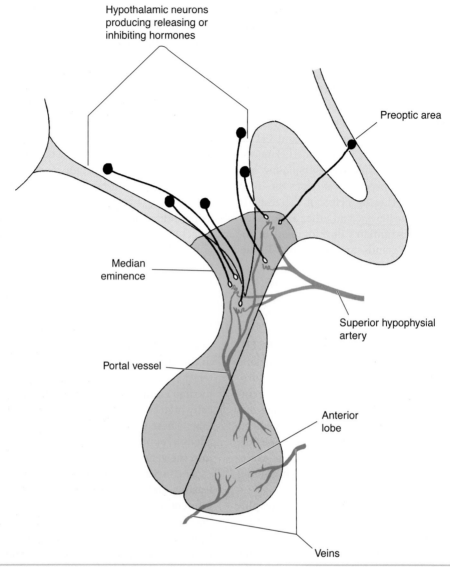

Hypothalamic neurons
producing releasing or
inhibiting hormones

Preoptic area

Median
eminence

Superior hypophysial
artery

Portal vessel

Anterior
lobe

Veins

FIGURE 11-18   The pituitary portal system. Arteries are red, veins are blue, and neurons that secrete releasing hormones are black.

lating levels of thyroid hormones are low, the hypothalamic cells produce more TRH. This stimulates increased output of TSH, and the thyroid gland, in its turn, is induced to synthesize and release more of its hormones.

Third Ventricle

The diencephalic part of the ventricular system consists of the narrow third ventricle (see Fig. 11-2). The anterior wall of this ventricle is formed by the **lamina terminalis**; the **anterior**

commissure crosses the midline in the dorsal part of the lamina terminalis. The rather extensive lateral wall is marked by the **hypothalamic sulcus**, which runs from the interventricular foramen to the opening of the cerebral aqueduct and divides the wall of the third ventricle into thalamic and hypothalamic regions. An **interthalamic adhesion** (massa intermedia) bridges the ventricle in 70% of human brains. The floor of the third ventricle is indented by the **optic chiasma**. An **optic recess** is located in front of the chiasma; behind the chiasma, the **infundibular recess** extends into the median eminence and the proximal part of the pituitary stalk. The floor then slopes upward to the cerebral aqueduct of the midbrain, with the **posterior commissure** forming a slight prominence above the entrance to the aqueduct. A **pineal recess** extends into the stalk of the pineal gland, and the dorsal wall of the pineal stalk accommodates the small **habenular commissure**. Immediately ventral to the body of the fornix, the membranous **roof of the third ventricle** is attached along the **striae medullares thalami**. A small choroid plexus is suspended from the roof. The body of the **fornix** (see Figs. 11-11 and 11-12) is located immediately above the membranous roof.

Cerebrospinal fluid enters the third ventricle from each lateral ventricle through the **interventricular foramen** (foramen of Monro). The crescent-shaped foramen is bounded by the fornix and by the anterior tubercle of the thalamus and is closed posteriorly by a reflection of ependyma between the fornix and the thalamus. The **subfornical organ**, mentioned earlier in this chapter, is a small eminence on the medial side of the column of the fornix, above the interventricular foramen. It is one of the circumventricular organs—a nucleus of neurons containing blood vessels that are permeable to circulating macromolecules, unlike the vessels of most parts of the brain. In laboratory animals, the nucleus responds to circulating levels of angiotensin II, a peptide whose concentration in plasma varies with circulating levels of sodium and potassium ions and with changes in blood volume. The neurons of the subfornical organ project to the zona incerta and hypothalamus, and their activity influences drinking.

Cerebrospinal fluid leaves the third ventricle by way of the **cerebral aqueduct** of the midbrain, through which it reaches the fourth ventricle and then the subarachnoid space surrounding the brain and spinal cord.

Suggested Reading

Braak H, Braak E. Anatomy of the human hypothalamus (chiasmatic and tuberal region). *Prog Brain Res* 1992;93: 3–16.

Caldani M, Antoine M, Batailler M, et al. Ontogeny of GnRH systems. *J Reprod Fertil* 1995;49(suppl):147–162.

Casanova C, Nordmann JP, Molotchnikoff S. Le complexe noyau latéral postérieur-pulvinar des mammifères et la fonction visuelle. *J Physiol* (Paris) 1991;85:44–57.

Dai J, Swaab DF, Van Der Vliet J, et al. Postmortem tracing reveals the organization of hypothalamic projections of the suprachiasmatic nucleus in the human brain. *J Comp Neurol* 1998;400:87–102.

Dermon CR, Barbas H. Contralateral thalamic projections predominantly reach transitional cortices in the rhesus monkey. *J Comp Neurol* 1994;344:508–531.

Grieve KL, Acuna C, Cudeiro J. The primate pulvinar nu-clei: vision and action. *Trends Neurosci* 2000;23: 35–39.

Groenewegen HJ, Berendse HW. The specificity of the nonspecific midline and intralaminar thalamic nuclei. *Trends Neurosci* 1994;17:52–57.

Gross PM, ed. *Circumventricular Organs and Body Fluids.* Boca Raton, FL: CRC Press, 1987.

Guilleminault C, Lugaresi E, Montagna P, et al, eds. *Fatal Familial Insomnia.* New York: Raven Press, 1994:27–31.

Guillery RW. Anatomical evidence concerning the role of the thalamus in corticocortical communication: a brief review. *J Anat* 1995;187:583–592.

Gutierrez C, Cola MG, Seltzer B, et al. Neurochemical and connectional organization of the dorsal pulvinar complex in monkeys. *J Comp Neurol* 2000;419:61–86.

Hirai T, Jones EG. A new parcellation of the human thalamus on the basis of histochemical staining. *Brain Res Rev* 1989;14:1–34.

Hofman MA, Swaab DF. The sexually dimorphic nucleus of the preoptic area in the human brain: a comparative morphometric study. *J Anat* 1989;164:55–72.

Ikeda H, Suzuki J, Sasani N, et al. The development and morphogenesis of the human pituitary gland. *Anat Embryol* 1988;178:327–336.

Jones EG. *The Thalamus.* New York: Plenum Press, 1985.

Karasek M. Melatonin, human aging, and age-related diseases. *Exp Gerontol* 2004;39:1723–1729.

Mark MH, Farmer PM. The human subfornical organ: an anatomic and ultrastructural study. *Ann Clin Lab Sci* 1984;14:427–442.

McCormick DA, Bal T. Sleep and arousal: thalamocortical mechanisms. *Annu Rev Physiol* 1997;20:185–215.

McEntree WJ, Mair RG. The Korsakoff syndrome: a neuro-chemical perspective. *Trends Neurosci* 1990;13: 340–344.

Moltz H. Fever: causes and consequences. *Neurosci Biobehav Rev* 1993;17:237–269.

Morel A, Magnin M, Jeanmonod D. Multiarchitectonic and stereotactic atlas of the human thalamus. *J Comp Neurol* 1997;387:588–630.

Parent A, Smith Y. Organization of efferent projections of the subthalamic nucleus in the squirrel monkey as revealed by retrograde labeling methods. *Brain Res* 1987;436:296–310.

Percheron G. Thalamus. In: Paxinos G, Mai JK, eds. *The Human Nervous System,* 2nd ed. Amsterdam: Elsevier Academic Press, 2004:592–675.

Raisman G. An urge to explain the incomprehensible: Geoffrey Harris and the discovery of the neural control of the pituitary gland. *Annu Rev Neurosci* 1997;20: 533–566.

Scheithauer BW, Horvath E, Kovacs K. Ultrastructure of the neurohypophysis. *Microsc Res Tech* 1992;20: 177–186.

Sherman SM, Guillery RW. Thalamus. In: Shepherd GM, ed. *The Synaptic Organization of the Brain*, 5th ed. New York: Oxford University Press, 2004:311–359.

Swaab DF, Hofman MA, Lucassen PJ, et al. Functional neuroanatomy and neuropathology of the human hypothalamus. *Anat Embryol* 1993;187:317–330.

Thannickal TC, Siegel JM, Nienhuis R, et al. Pattern of hypocretin (orexin) soma and axon loss, and gliosis, in human narcolepsy. *Brain Pathol* 2003;13:340–351.

Willie JT, Chemelli RM, Sinton CM, et al. To eat or to sleep? Orexin in the regulation of feeding and wakefulness. *Annu Rev Neurosci* 2001;24:429–458.

Willis WD. Central neurogenic pain: Possible mechanisms. In: Nashold BS, Ovelmen-Levitt J, eds. *Deafferentation Pain Syndromes: Pathophysiology and Treatment*. New York: Raven Press, 1991:81–102.

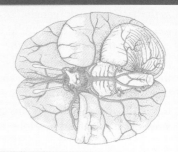

Chapter 12

CORPUS STRIATUM

Important Facts

- The corpus striatum is the telencephalic gray matter associated with the lateral ventricle. It is composed of the striatum (caudate nucleus, nucleus accumbens, and putamen) and the pallidum (globus pallidus), which is composed of external and internal divisions.

- In clinical and physiological usage, *basal ganglia* refers collectively to the corpus striatum, subthalamic nucleus, and substantia nigra. The best-understood functions of the basal ganglia are in the production of movements, but extensive connections with the temporal and anterior frontal cortex indicate involvement in memory, emotion, and other cognitive functions.

- The striatum, subthalamic nucleus, and substantia nigra receive excitatory afferents from the cerebral cortex. Dopaminergic neurons in the substantia nigra and ventral tegmental area excite some striatal neurons and inhibit others.

- The major output of the striatum is to the pallidum, and it is inhibitory. Excitatory input to the pallidum comes from the subthalamic nucleus.

- The output of the pallidum, which is also inhibitory, is to various thalamic nuclei. The thalamic nuclei project to and excite the premotor and supplementary motor areas of the cerebral cortex, cortical areas concerned with eye movements, and parts of the prefrontal and temporal cortex.

- Other pallidal efferents inhibit the subthalamic nucleus, superior colliculus, and pedunculopontine nucleus. The pedunculopontine nucleus, which is located in the reticular formation, has extensive projections that influence descending motor pathways, the waking state, and (by way of the basal cholinergic forebrain nuclei) neuronal activity throughout the cerebral cortex.

- At rest, neurons in the striatum are quiescent, and those in the pallidum are active, thereby inhibiting the thalamic excitation of the motor cortex. Before and during a movement, the striatum becomes active and inhibits the pallidum, allowing more excitation of the motor thalamic nuclei and cortex.

- The corpus striatum may normally be the site in which instructions for parts of learned movements are remembered and from which they are transmitted to the motor cortex for assembly and eventual execution by corticospinal and reticulospinal pathways to the motor neurons. Comparable circuitry exists for the control of movements of the eyes.

- The nucleus accumbens and the most ventral parts of the pallidum are active in behavioral responses to a wide variety of rewarding or pleasurable stimuli. Conditioned reflexes passing through these nuclei and their associated cortical areas have been implicated in drug addiction.

- Disorders of the motor circuitry of the basal ganglia (dyskinesias) include Parkinson's disease (degeneration of nigral dopaminergic neurons), Huntington's chorea (degeneration in the striatum), and ballism (damage to subthalamic nucleus). Some features of these disorders can be explained from knowledge of the disrupted neuronal pathways.

- The basal cholinergic nuclei of the forebrain are ventral to the corpus striatum, within the anterior perforated substance. Their axons are distributed to the whole cerebral cortex. Afferents to the basal nuclei are from the amygdala, the pallidum, and the reticular formation of the brain stem. Subcortical cholinergic neurons degenerate in patients with Alzheimer's disease and some other forms of dementia.

The corpus striatum is a substantial region of gray matter near the base of each cerebral hemisphere. It consists of the **caudate nucleus** and the **lentiform nucleus**, with the latter divided into the **putamen** and the **globus pallidus**. Traditionally, the corpus striatum, claustrum, and amygdaloid body were referred to by anatomists as the basal nuclei or "ganglia" of the telencephalon. The caudate nucleus and putamen together constitute the **striatum**, and the globus pallidus is referred to as the **pallidum**. Nearby structures include the **claustrum** (a thin sheet of gray matter situated between the putamen and the cortex of the insula) and the **amygdaloid body** or **amygdala** in the temporal lobe, which is a component of the olfactory and limbic systems (see Chapters 17 and 18).

Clinically, the term **basal ganglia** is usually applied to the corpus striatum (Fig. 12-1), subthalamic nucleus, and substantia nigra. These neuronal populations are grouped under this common heading because they are interconnected to form a functional unit, and destructive lesions in any of the components result in disorders of motor control characterized by akinesia (i.e., a poverty of voluntary movement), rigidity, or dyskinesias (in which purposeless involuntary movements take place).

Terminology

The following correlations may be helpful in understanding the terminology of the corpus striatum and "basal ganglia":

- Corpus striatum: Lentiform and caudate nuclei, including the nucleus accumbens
- Lentiform nucleus: Putamen and globus pallidus (the latter has external and internal divisions)
- Striatum: Putamen, caudate nucleus, and nucleus accumbens
- Pallidum: Globus pallidus (It is composed of external and internal divisions; the substantia nigra pars reticulata belongs functionally with the internal pallidum.)
- Basal ganglia (clinical and physiological usage): Corpus striatum, substantia nigra, and subthalamic nucleus

Lentiform and Caudate Nuclei

The configuration and relations of the lentiform and caudate nuclei contribute to the topography of the lateral ventricle and the cerebral white matter, which are described in Chapter 16. This anatomy is best appreciated by dissection. For understanding the afferent and efferent connections, the pallidum and striatum are the more functionally relevant divisions of the corpus striatum.

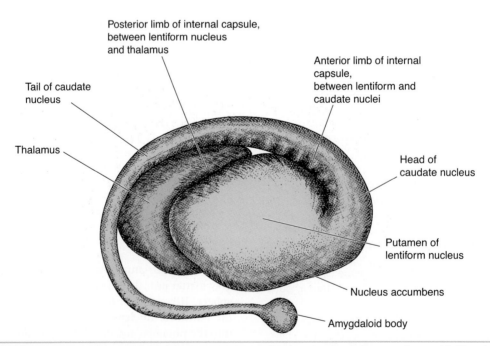

Posterior limb of internal capsule, between lentiform nucleus and thalamus

Anterior limb of internal capsule, between lentiform and caudate nuclei

Tail of caudate nucleus

Thalamus

Head of caudate nucleus

Putamen of lentiform nucleus

Nucleus accumbens

Amygdaloid body

FIGURE 12-1   Lateral aspect of the right corpus striatum, showing also the thalamus and amygdala. The globus pallidus is concealed by the larger putamen.

LENTIFORM NUCLEUS

The lentiform nucleus is wedge shaped and has been described as having the approximate size and form of a Brazil nut (Figs. 12-2 and 12-3). The narrow part of the wedge, facing medially, is occupied by the **globus pallidus**, which is divided into external and internal parts by a lamina of white matter. The **putamen** is the lateral part of the lentiform nucleus, and it extends beyond the globus pallidus in all directions except at the base of the nucleus. The external pallidum is separated from the putamen by another lamina of white matter.

The lentiform nucleus is bounded laterally by a thin layer of white matter that constitutes the **external capsule** (see Figs. 12-2 and 12-3). This is followed by the **claustrum**, which is a thin sheet of gray matter coextensive with the lateral surface of the putamen. The best-documented connections of the claustrum are reciprocal connections with the cortices of the frontal, parietal, and temporal lobes, but their functional significance is unknown. The **extreme capsule** separates the claustrum from the **insula** (island

of Reil), an area of cortex buried in the depths of the lateral sulcus of the cerebral hemisphere. The medial surface of the lentiform nucleus lies against the internal capsule. The ventral surface is close to structures at the base of the hemisphere, such as the anterior perforated substance, optic tract, and amygdaloid body (see Fig. 12-3).

CAUDATE NUCLEUS

The caudate nucleus consists of an anterior portion or **head**, which tapers into a slender **tail**. The tail extends backward and then forward into the temporal lobe (see Fig. 12-1), where it terminates at the amygdaloid body.

The head of the caudate nucleus bulges into the frontal horn of the lateral ventricle, and the first part of the tail lies along the lateral margin of the central part of the ventricle (see Figs. 12-2 and 12-3). The tail follows the contour of the lateral ventricle into the roof of its temporal horn. Two structures lie along the medial side of the tail of the caudate nucleus. These are the **stria terminalis**, a bundle of axons that originates in the amygdaloid body and the

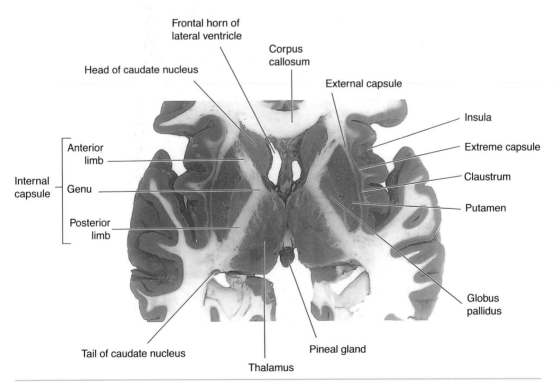

FIGURE 12-2 Horizontal section of the cerebrum stained to differentiate gray matter (dark) from white matter (light), showing the components and relations of the corpus striatum and internal capsule.

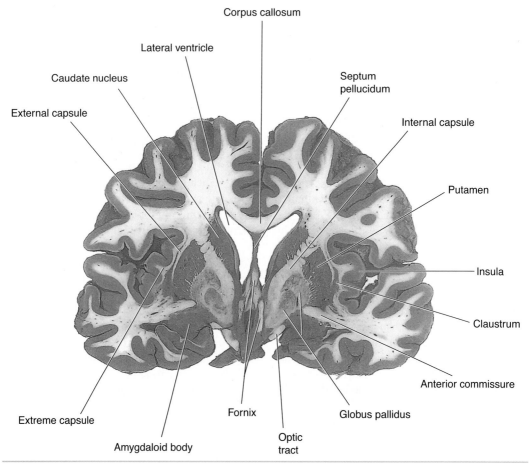

Corpus callosum

Lateral ventricle

Caudate nucleus

Septum
pellucidum

External capsule

Internal capsule

Putamen

Insula

Claustrum

Anterior commissure

Extreme capsule

Fornix

Globus pallidus

Amygdaloid body

Optic
tract

FIGURE 12-3 Coronal section of the cerebrum anterior (rostral) to the thalamus, stained to differentiate gray matter (dark) from white matter (light), showing the components and relations of the corpus striatum.

thalamostriate vein (vena terminalis), which drains the caudate nucleus, thalamus, internal capsule, and nearby structures (see Fig. 11-12). Groups of neuronal cell bodies within the stria terminalis constitute the **bed nucleus of the stria terminalis**, which belongs functionally with certain nuclei of the amygdala.

The anterior limb of the internal capsule intervenes between the head of the caudate nucleus and the lentiform nucleus. The tail of the caudate nucleus is medial to the internal capsule as the latter merges with the central white matter of the hemisphere. The cortical afferent and efferent fibers that constitute the internal capsule do not completely separate the two components of the striatum. The head of the caudate nucleus and the putamen are continuous with each other through a bridge of gray matter beneath the anterior limb of the internal capsule

(see Fig. 12-1). In addition, numerous strands of gray matter join the caudate nucleus with the putamen by cutting across the internal capsule (see Fig. 12-3). The most ventral part of the striatum in this region is called the **nucleus accumbens**, also known as the **ventral striatum**.

Ventral to the nucleus accumbens is the **substantia innominata**, which contains the most ventral part of the globus pallidus (the ventral pallidum) and the **basal cholinergic nuclei of the forebrain**, which are described at the end of this chapter.

CONNECTIONS

The major neuronal connections of the parts of the corpus striatum are summarized in Figures 12-4 and 12-5 and explained in the following paragraphs.

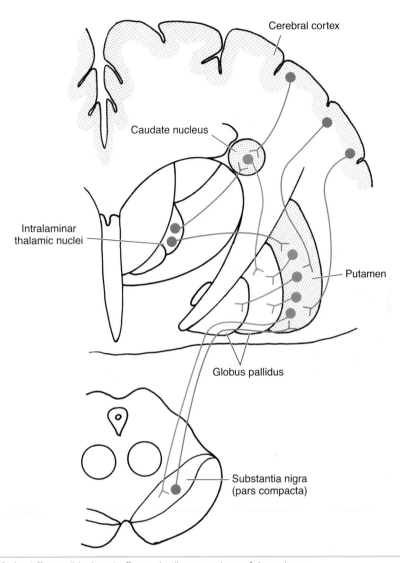

Cerebral cortex

Caudate nucleus

Intralaminar
thalamic nuclei

Putamen

Globus pallidus

Substantia nigra
(pars compacta)

FIGURE 12-4 Afferent (blue) and efferent (red) connections of the striatum.

STRIATUM

The striatum receives afferent fibers from the cerebral cortex, thalamus, and substantia nigra (see Fig. 12-4). **Corticostriate fibers**, which are excitatory, originate in the cortex of all four lobes, but especially the frontal and parietal lobes. The corticostriate fibers are topographically organized. The somatosensory and motor areas project to the putamen; the cingulate gyrus and temporal lobe cortex (including the parahippocampal gyrus) project to the nucleus accumbens or ventral striatum, and other cortical areas project mainly to the caudate nucleus. Most of these fibers enter the striatum from the internal capsule, although a sub-

stantial number enter the putamen from the external capsule. The **amygdala** (see also Chapter 18) is a source of afferents to the nucleus accumbens and the caudate nucleus. Some of the amygdalostriate fibers pass through the substantia innominata; others arrive by way of the stria terminalis. **Thalamostriate** fibers, also excitatory, originate in the intralaminar nuclei of the thalamus, especially the centromedian nucleus. **Nigrostriate** fibers from the pars compacta of the substantia nigra use dopamine as a transmitter; they excite some striatal neurons and inhibit others. In Parkinson's disease, discussed later in this chapter, degeneration of neurons in the pars compacta deprives the striatum of its dopaminergic input. Dopaminergic

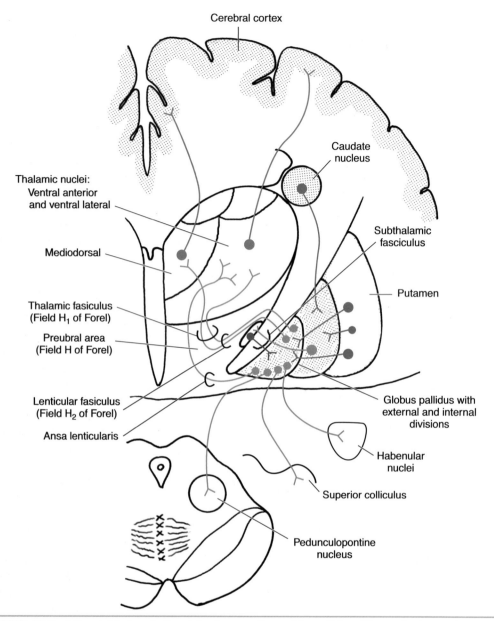

FIGURE 12-5   Afferent (blue) and efferent (red) connections of the pallidum. (The projection to the superior colliculus is not included in the diagram.)

afferents of the nucleus accumbens arise from the **ventral tegmental area**, which is medial to the substantia nigra (see Fig. 7-15).

The axons that leave the striatum are **striopallidal**, bringing both segments of the globus pallidus under the influence and control of the striatum and **strionigral**, which pass through the globus pallidus before entering the midbrain and terminating in both parts of the substantia nigra. (The pars reticulata of the substantia nigra, which is ventral to the pars compacta,

has connections similar to those of the internal division of the globus pallidus.)

Striatal efferent projections are all inhibitory, with γ-aminobutyric acid (GABA) as their transmitter. Different populations of striatal principal cells contain various peptides and calcium-binding proteins in addition to GABA. The striatum also contains many interneurons, which use GABA, acetylcholine, and several peptides as their neuro-transmitters. Histochemical studies reveal "patches" or "striosomes," separated by a "matrix."

Corticostriate and nigrostriate fibers terminate throughout the striatum, but afferents from the intralaminar thalamic nuclei end only in the matrix.

PALLIDUM

The globus pallidus contains the myelinated axons of its own neurons together with great numbers of myelinated striopallidal and strionigral fibers. The abundance of myelin accounts for the somewhat pale appearance of the region in fresh sections and for the name "globus pallidus." The pallidum is notable in that it receives GABA-ergic inhibitory input from the striatum and its own principal neurons are also GABA-ergic and inhibitory. The **substantia nigra pars reticulata** in the midbrain has connections similar to those of the globus pallidus and is best thought of as a caudally displaced part of the pallidum.

The inhibitory GABA-ergic **striopallidal** fibers noted previously are the principal afferents to the globus pallidus (see Fig. 12-5). They end in the external and internal segments. In the following discussion, the word "pallidofugal" applies to efferents of the globus pallidus, ventral pallidum, and substantia nigra pars reticulata.

Fibers leaving the globus pallidus initially take either of two routes (see Fig. 12-5). Some cross the internal capsule and appear as the **lenticular fasciculus** (field H$_2$ of Forel) in the subthalamus, dorsal to the subthalamic nucleus. Other pallidofugal fibers curve around the medial edge of the internal capsule, forming the **ansa lenticularis**. These two fasciculi (shown in Figs. 11-9 and 11-10) consist mainly of **pallidothalamic** fibers, which originate in the internal segment of the globus pallidus. They enter the prerubral area of the subthalamus (field H of Forel), turn laterally into the **thalamic fasciculus** (field H$_1$ of Forel), and terminate in at least three thalamic nuclei. The anterior division of the **ventral lateral nucleus (VLa)** projects to the premotor area of cortex in the frontal lobe and to the contiguous part of the medial surface of the hemisphere that is designated the supplementary motor area (see Chapters 15 and 24). The **ventral anterior nucleus** projects to these motor areas as well as to the frontal eye field and parts of the prefrontal cortex, which covers the frontal pole and the orbital surface of the frontal lobe. The **mediodorsal nucleus** consists of subnuclei; most of these project to the prefrontal cortex and anterior end of the cingulate gyrus, but one contains neurons connected with the frontal eye field. The regions of the VL thalamic nucleus that receive pallidal afferents (VLa) are largely separate from those that receive input from the cerebellum (VLp), although some overlap exists.

A few pallidofugal fibers accompany the main outflow to the thalamus but continue into the stria medullaris thalami and terminate in the habenular nuclei. Through this connection, the corpus striatum is potentially able to modify the descending output of the limbic system, which exerts control over autonomic and other involuntary activities.

Other pallidofugal fibers (mostly from the substantia nigra pars reticulata) go to the superior colliculus, which has numerous connections with other nuclei involved in the control of eye movements.

Although the efferent fasciculi of the internal (medial) segment of the globus pallidus project principally to the VLa, ventral anterior (VA), and mediodorsal (MD) nuclei of the thalamus, some pallidofugal fibers turn caudally and end in the **pedunculopontine nucleus**, which is one of the cholinergic groups of reticular nuclei (see Chapter 9) in the brain stem. Fibers from the pedunculopontine nucleus proceed caudally to the central nuclei of the reticular formation and rostrally to the substantia nigra pars compacta, subthalamic nucleus, intralaminar thalamic nuclei, pallidum, striatum, and basal cholinergic forebrain nuclei.

The external segment of the globus pallidus has an inhibitory projection to the subthalamic nucleus, consisting of axons that pass across the internal capsule in the **subthalamic fasciculus** (see Fig. 12-5). This bundle also contains the axons of neurons of the subthalamic nucleus, which end in the internal segment of the globus pallidus and in the closely related pars reticulata of the substantia nigra.

Physiology and Neurochemistry of the Basal Ganglia

THE DIRECT AND INDIRECT LOOPS

Knowledge of the excitatory and inhibitory synapses in the basal ganglia may explain some clinical features of disorders of the system and has provided indications for therapy with drugs that mimic or inhibit the neurotransmitters. Figure 12-6 shows some of the connections with their actins and the known or suspected transmitters.

Fibers from motor and other areas of the cerebral cortex end in the striatum (corticostriate fibers), subthalamic nucleus (corticosubthalamic fibers), and pars compacta of the substantia nigra (corticonigral fibers). These cortical projections are excitatory, with glutamate as the neurotransmitter.

Pallidal neurons are spontaneously active. The medial segment of the globus pallidus and the substantia nigra pars reticulata receive additional excitatory drive from the glutamatergic neurons of the subthalamic nucleus. Thus, increased activity in the subthalamic nucleus results in reduced activity of thalamocortical neurons.

The striatum inhibits both divisions of the pallidum, and pallidofugal neurons inhibit thalamocortical neurons. In both cases, the inhibitory transmitter is GABA. The different connections of the external and internal divisions of the globus pallidus provide two loops of connected neurons that have opposite effects on the cerebral cortex. The **direct loop** begins with neurons in the striatum that contain GABA and substance P (SP). Increased activity of these striatal neurons leads to disinhibition of thalamic neurons and, consequently, increased stimulation of the cerebral cortex. Different striatal neurons, containing

GABA and enkephalin (ENK), participate in the **indirect loop**, which includes the subthalamic nucleus. Activity of the striatal GABA-ENK neurons results in inhibition of the thalamus and reduced stimulation of the cortex. The nigrostriate input excites the GABA-ENK neurons and inhibits the GABA-SP neurons because of different types of dopamine receptors on the surfaces of the cells. Both these actions of dopamine lead to increased activity of thalamocortical neurons.

MOTOR FUNCTIONS

The best-understood functions of the corpus striatum are those related to movement. The neurons of the striatum are quiescent, and those of the pallidum are active when no movements are being made. Shortly before and during a movement, the situation is reversed. Removal of pallidal inhibition allows the VLa and VA thalamic nuclei to be stimulated by other afferent fibers, most of which come from the premotor and supplementary motor areas of the cerebral cortex. The thalamocortical neurons are excitatory to the same motor cortical areas.

Nigrostriatal dopaminergic neurons are active all the time; their rates of firing increase with activity of the contralateral musculature.

Clinical observations and animal experiments indicate that the corpus striatum is probably a

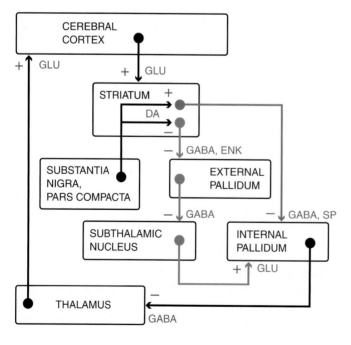

FIGURE 12-6 General plan of the neuronal circuitry of the basal ganglia showing neurotransmitters and their actions. Neurons in the direct loop are blue and those of the indirect loop are green. (+ indicates excitation; −, inhibition; DA, dopamine; ENK, enkephalin; GABA, γ-aminobutyrate; GLU, glutamate; SP, substance P.)

repository of instructions for fragments of learned movements. When a movement is to be carried out, the instructions encoded by the corpus striatum are presumably transmitted from the pallidum to the thalamus (VLa and VA) and then sent on to the supplementary motor area and the premotor cortex. Corticospinal, corticoreticular, and reticulospinal projections then modulate the motor neurons. The pallidal projection to the pedunculopontine nucleus provides another functional connection with the central nuclei of the reticular formation, which are the source of the reticulospinal tracts. Degenerative diseases of the basal ganglia result in unwanted movements, and it has been suggested that the circuitry of the corpus striatum normally allows choices to be made in the types of motor responses rather than making stereotyped movements in response to stimuli.

OTHER FUNCTIONS OF THE CORPUS STRIATUM

The topographical projections of different cortical areas with parts of the striatum are associated with parallel but separate channels through the pallidum and thalamus. Four such channels are usually recognized; these are summarized in Table 12-1.

The great size of the human corpus striatum indicates collaboration with the cerebral cortex in aspects of memory and thought that are more complex than formulation of the component parts of movements. These higher functions probably involve the connections of the striatum and pallidum with the mediodorsal thalamic nucleus and with the prefrontal, cingulate, and temporal cortex. Despite the numerous known connections of the basal ganglia, it is not possible to ascribe simple functions to the four channels summarized in Table 12-1. Diseases that affect the basal ganglia result principally in the motor disorders described later in this chapter.

An animal with an electrode implanted in either the ventral tegmental area or the lateral hypothalamus derives gratification from delivering small electrical stimuli to these regions and will press the switch repeatedly to the exclusion of such activities as eating and drinking. The ventral tegmental area is the source of dopaminergic axons that pass through the lateral hypothalamic area (medial forebrain bundle) en route to the nucleus accumbens. Numerous other experiments implicate the dopaminergic

TABLE 12-1   Parallel Circuits ("Channels") Involving the Corpus Striatum

Channel	Sources of Cortical Input to Striatum	Striatal Nuclei	Pallidal Nuclei	Thalamic Nuclei Relaying Pallidal Input to Cortex	Cortical Areas Receiving Thalamic Input
Motor	Primary somatic sensory and motor areas; premotor area	Putamen	Globus pallidus	Ventral lateral and ventral anterior nuclei	Supplementary and primary motor areas and premotor area
Ocular motor	Prefrontal and posterior parietal cortex	Caudate nucleus (tail)	Globus pallidus; substantia nigra pars reticulata	Ventral anterior and mediodorsal nuclei	Frontal eye fields
Prefrontal	Premotor area and posterior parietal cortex	Caudate nucleus (head)	Globus pallidus	Ventral anterior and mediodorsal nuclei	Prefrontal cortex
Limbic	Temporal lobe; hippocampal formation; amygdala	Nucleus accumbens	Ventral pallidum	Mediodorsal nucleus	Cingulate gyrus and orbital prefrontal cortex

Dyskinesias and the Corpus Striatum

Despite the central position of the corpus striatum in the neural circuitry of motor control (see Chapter 23), lesions in the basal ganglia do not cause paralysis. They result in unwanted involuntary movements.

TYPES OF DYSKINESIA

The involuntary movements seen in the dyskinesias related to the corpus striatum take various forms. **Choreiform** movements involve multiple muscles. They are brisk, jerky, and purposeless, resembling isolated fragments of movements that might be useful. They are irregularly timed, most pronounced in the upper limbs and face, and cannot be voluntarily inhibited. Hypotonia of the affected muscles may present when the muscles are not contracting.

Dystonic movements are sustained contractions that lead to abnormal posture or twisting of the neck, trunk, or limbs. **Dystonia musculorum deformans** (also called **generalized dystonia**) is a particularly disabling motor disturbance in which slow, writhing, involuntary movements of the axial and limb musculature are sustained, leading in rare cases to permanent contractures. The symptoms first appear in older children and young adults. Lesions may be present in the corpus striatum and elsewhere, but the pathology is poorly understood. The most common dystonia is **spasmodic torticollis**, with rotation and lateral flexion of the neck. **Athetosis** is a type of dystonia in which slow and sinuous movements occur involving the proximal and distal musculature of the limbs. The movements blend together in a continuous mobile spasm and are usually associated with varying degrees of paresis and spasticity. The muscles of the face, neck, and tongue may be affected, with grimacing, protrusion, and writhing of the tongue as well as difficulty in speaking and swallowing. The term **choreoathetosis** is applied to involuntary movements with both choreiform and athetoid features.

Myoclonus consists of sudden, strong contractions that may be isolated, repetitive, or rhythmic. Regularly alternating movements of small amplitude constitute **tremor**. Whereas stereotyped purposeless movements that occur at random are called **tics** or habit spasms, a generalized inability to be still, with constant motion

of the limbs, is sometimes called **akathisia**. The largest involuntary movements are those of **ballism**, an exaggerated form of chorea in which the limbs make large, irregular flinging and rotational movements caused by contractions of muscles acting on the shoulder or hip joints.

The lesions responsible for dyskinesias are poorly understood. In chorea, extensive damage is present in the striatum. Some cases of dystonia are attributable to a tumor or a vascular lesion in the contralateral putamen, and myoclonus has been associated with lesions in the ventral part of the thalamus. More often than not, no pathology can be identified by clinical imaging in patients with dystonias. Ballism is usually attributed to a small destructive lesion in the contralateral subthalamic nucleus. The uncontrolled movements may be attributable to a loss of excitatory input to the internal division of the globus pallidus, which then fails to inhibit the VLa and VA nuclei of the thalamus. Excessive activity in these thalamic nuclei stimulates the premotor area of the cerebral cortex, causing excessive movement at the proximal joints of the limbs. The most common type of ballism is **hemiballismus**, described in Chapter 11. Lesions in the pars compacta of the substantia nigra are responsible for the tremor, bradykinesia, and other features of **Parkinson's disease**, described in Chapter 7.

DISEASES

Choreiform movements are a cardinal sign in numerous conditions. **Huntington's chorea** is a dominant hereditary disorder with onset of clinical signs in middle life. Patients have atrophy of the striatum, most conspicuous in the caudate nucleus. The choreiform movements become more severe with time, and progressive mental deterioration is also present, attributed partly to degeneration of the nonmotor parts of the striatum and partly to concurrent loss of neurons in the cerebral cortex. **Sydenham's chorea** (or St. Vitus' dance) is now a rare disorder. It typically occurred in childhood after an infectious disease caused by hemolytic streptococci. Because the disease was seldom fatal, the pathology of Sydenham's chorea is poorly understood. The most common findings were microscopic hemorrhages and emboli in the corpus striatum.

Athetosis and choreoathetosis often form part of a complex of neurological signs that result from metabolic disorders of the developing brain or

(continued)

from birth injury. Athetoid movements are most frequently associated with pathological changes in the striatum and the cerebral cortex, although lesions are sometimes also present in the globus pallidus and the thalamus. The term **cerebral palsy** refers to movement disorders caused by brain injury incurred near or at the time of birth. Spastic paresis or paralysis (caused by loss of function of descending motor pathways; see Chapter 23) is another common type of cerebral palsy.

    Wilson's disease (hepatolenticular degeneration) is caused by a genetically determined error in copper metabolism. The signs of Wilson's disease usually appear between the ages of 10 and 25 years and include muscle rigidity, dystonia, tremor, impairment of voluntary movements (including those of speech), and loss of facial expression. Uncontrollable laughing or crying may be present without apparent cause, and dementia ensues if the condition is left untreated. The degenerative changes are most pronounced in the putamen and progress to cavitation of the lentiform nucleus. Cellular degeneration may take place in the cerebral cortex, thalamus, red nucleus,

and cerebellum. In addition to these neurological abnormalities, affected patients have cirrhosis of the liver. The neurological and hepatic changes of Wilson's disease respond to treatment with drugs that enhance the urinary excretion of copper.

    Some drugs used in psychiatry inhibit the action of dopamine in the striatum. When given for a long time, in high doses, or to unusually susceptible patients, these drugs can cause a variety of acute parkinsonian or dystonic reactions or dyskinesias. The most common of these iatrogenic disorders is known as **tardive dyskinesia**.

    The connections of the corpus striatum indicate that the control of movement is only one of the functions of this large part of the cerebral hemisphere, but disorders other than dyskinesias are not well documented. A condition known as **abulia**, in which patients have a loss of willpower and initiative with long delays in answering questions, has been reported in patients with small lesions confined to the caudate nucleus. Abulia, however, is more commonly seen in patients with large bilateral frontal lobe lesions.

projection to the nucleus accumbens in behavioral responses to stimuli that are perceived as rewards. Drugs of addiction activate the system. Thus, amphetamines enhance dopamine release from presynaptic terminals, cocaine potentiates the action of dopamine by blocking its reuptake by presynaptic terminals, and opiates act on neurons in the ventral tegmental area and the striatum. Nicotine and ethanol have also been shown to induce elevated levels of dopamine in the nucleus accumbens.

SUBSTANTIA INNOMINATA AND BASAL CHOLINERGIC NUCLEI

The substantia innominata is the territory ventral to the internal capsule, nucleus accumbens, and anterior commissure; dorsal to the anterior perforated substance; medial to the amygdala; and lateral to the hypothalamus. The region contains axons passing in all directions, including a large contingent on their way from the amygdala to the ventral striatum and hypothalamus. The substantia innominata also con-

tains the ventral pallidum, small numbers of dopamine-synthesizing neurons, and the **basal forebrain nuclei**. The latter comprise three groups of large cholinergic neurons: the largest cholinergic cell group is the **nucleus basalis of Meynert**; the others are the **nucleus of the diagonal band** and part of the **septal area**. These groups of cells receive afferent fibers from the amygdala; the cortex of the temporal lobe; the insula; the orbital surface of the frontal lobe; the hypothalamus; and the central, cholinergic, and noradrenergic nuclei of the reticular formation. The cholinergic neurons in the basal forebrain nuclei have branching axons that end in all areas of the cerebral cortex as well as in the hippocampus and all components of the basal ganglia. They constitute the sole source of cholinergic innervation of the cortex, perhaps providing an important link between the limbic system and the neocortex. Amnesia can occur after surgical damage that interrupts the cholinergic projection from the basal forebrain nuclei to the hippocampal formation, indicating an involvement of this connection in learning and recall. The basal cholinergic nuclei also

Alzheimer's Disease

The magnocellular basal forebrain nuclei are among several parts of the brain that degenerate in **Alzheimer's disease**. This disorder, the first manifestation of which is the failure of memory for recent events, is a common cause of mental deterioration (dementia) in elderly people. The large cholinergic neurons at the base of the forebrain degenerate, and the cortex loses its cholinergic afferent fibers. Severe degenerative changes are also seen in the entorhinal cortex, hippocam-

pus, and locus coeruleus. In advanced Alzheimer's disease, considerable neuronal loss is also present, with shrinkage of gyri, throughout the cerebral cortex but most prominently in the temporal and parietal lobes. Fibrillary tangles in neuronal somata are present in all affected parts of the brain, together with large extracellular deposits of fibrillary material known as *senile plaques*. Similar pathological changes are found in several other diseases that cause dementia.

receive input from nuclei in the brain stem (see Chapter 9) and are implicated in arousal and the wakeful state.

Suggested Reading

Albin RL, Young AB, Penney JB. The functional anatomy of basal ganglia disorders. *Trends Neurosci* 1989;12: 366–375.

Bhatia KP, Marsden CD. The behavioural and motor consequences of focal lesions of the basal ganglia in man. *Brain* 1994;117:859–876.

Hedreen JC, Struble RG, Whitehouse PJ, et al. Topography of the magnocellular basal forebrain system in the human brain. *J Neuropathol Exp Neurol* 1984;43:1–21.

Heimer L. Basal forebrain in the context of schizophrenia. *Brain Res Rev* 2000;31:205–235.

Heimer L. A new anatomical framework for neuropsychiatric disorders and drug abuse. *Am J Psychiat* 2003;160: 1726–1739.

Holt DJ, Graybiel AM, Saper CB: Neurochemical architecture of the human striatum. *J Comp Neurol* 1997;384:1–25.

Ikemoto K, Nagatsu 1, Kitahama K, et al. A dopamine-synthesizing cell group demonstrated in the human basal forebrain by dual labeling immunohistochemical technique of tyrosine hydroxylase and aromatic L-amino acid decarboxylase. *Neurosci Lett* 1998;243:129–132.

Inase M, Tanji J. Thalamic distribution of projection neurons to the primary motor cortex relative to afferent terminal fields from the globus pallidus in the macaque monkey. *J Comp Neurol* 1995;353:415–426.

Lehericy S, Vidailhet M, Dormont D, et al. Striatopallidal and thalamic dystonia: a magnetic resonance imaging anatomoclinical study. *Arch Neurol* 1996;53: 241–250.

Ma TP. The basal ganglia. In: Haines DE, ed. *Fundamental Neuroscience*. New York: Churchill Livingstone, 1997: 363–378.

Mesulam M-M, Geula C. Nucleus basalis and cortical cholinergic innervation in the human brain: observations based on the distribution of acetylcholinesterase and choline acetyltransferase. *J Comp Neurol* 1988;275: 216–240.

Morris MK, Bowers D, Chatterjee A, et al. Amnesia following a discrete basal forebrain lesion. *Brain* 1992;115: 1827–1847.

Parent A, Hazrati LN. Functional anatomy of the basal ganglia, 1: the cortico- basal ganglia-thalamo-cortical loop. *Brain Res Rev* 1995;20:91–127.

Parent A, Hazrati LN. Functional anatomy of the basal ganglia, 2: the place of subthalamic nucleus and external pallidum in basal ganglia circuitry. *Brain Res Rev* 1995;20:128–154.

Perry RH, Candy JM, Perry EK, et al. The substantia innominata and adjacent regions in the human brain: histochemical and biochemical observations. *J Anat* 1984;138:713–732.

Sakai ST, Inase M, Tanji J. Comparison of cerebellothalamic and pallidothalamic projections in the monkey (Macaca fuscata): a double anterograde labeling study. *J Comp Neurol* 1996;368:215–228.

Shindo K, Shima K, Tanji J. Spatial distribution of thalamic projections to the supplementary motor area and the primary motor cortex: a retrograde multiple labeling study in the macaque monkey. *J Comp Neurol* 1995;357:98–116.

Ulfig N. Configuration of the magnocellular nuclei in the basal forebrain of the human adult. *Acta Anat* 1989;134:100–105.

Wilson CJ. Basal ganglia. In: Shepherd GM, ed. *The Synaptic Organization of the Brain*, 5th ed. New York: Oxford University Press, 2004:361–413.

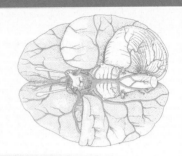

Chapter 13

TOPOGRAPHY OF THE CEREBRAL HEMISPHERES

Important Facts

- The large surface area of the human cerebral cortex results in a pattern of gyri and sulci. Some of these convolutions are important anatomical landmarks or functional areas.
- Five lobes (including the insula) are recognized in each cerebral hemisphere.
- On the medial surface of the hemisphere, the parieto-occipital sulcus separates the parietal from the occipital lobe.
- In the occipital lobe, the calcarine sulcus is the site of the primary visual cortex.
- In the parietal lobe, the postcentral gyrus corresponds to the first general somatic sensory area. The supramarginal and angular gyri are association cortex and include parts of the receptive language area, which extends from the posterior part of the superior temporal gyrus to adjacent parts of the parietal lobe.
- The central sulcus is located between the parietal and frontal lobes, separating the first somesthetic area from the primary motor area.
- In the frontal lobe, the precentral gyrus corresponds to the primary motor area. The olfactory bulb and tract are applied to the orbital surface of the frontal lobe.
- The lateral sulcus (sylvian fissure) separates the frontal and parietal lobes from the temporal lobe.
- The insula (insular lobe), located in the floor of the lateral sulcus, is a landmark for part of the corpus striatum. Its cortex has visceral functions.
- The superior surface of the superior temporal gyrus includes the primary auditory area.
- The parahippocampal gyrus includes the uncus (a primary olfactory area) and the entorhinal area, which is involved in olfaction and memory.
- The limbic lobe includes the parahippocampal and cingulate gyri, parts of the limbic system.

The complicated folding of the surface of the cerebral hemispheres substantially increases the surface area and therefore the volume of the cerebral cortex. The folds or convolutions are called **gyri**, and the intervening grooves are called **sulci**. About two thirds of the cortex forms the walls of the sulci and is therefore hidden from surface view. Although some gyri are constant features of the cerebral surface, others vary from one brain to another and even between the two hemispheres of the same brain. Subtler depressions in the cerebral cortex are grooves and notches unrelated to the pattern of gyri and sulci. They are made by extracerebral structures such as the bones of the skull and the venous sinuses of the dura mater.

Whereas a sulcus is a groove that indents the surface of a cerebral hemisphere, a **fissure** is a cleft that separates different components of the brain. Despite the different definitions of sulci and fissures, the two terms are frequently used interchangeably for the deepest sulci.

At an early stage in studying human neuroanatomy, students should be able to delineate the lobes of the cerebral hemispheres and to recognize the major sulci, fissures, and gyri that are commonly referred to as landmarks. Of the smaller sulci and gyri, some are of great functional importance, but others have no known significance.

Major Sulci and Fissures

The lateral and parieto-occipital sulci appear early in fetal development and are especially deep in the mature brain. These, together with the central and circular sulci, are the boundaries for division of the cerebral hemisphere into the frontal, parietal, insular, temporal, and occipital lobes (Figs. 13-1 and 13-2).

The **lateral sulcus** (fissure of Sylvius or sylvian fissure) begins as a deep furrow on the inferior

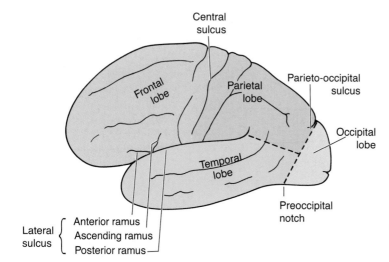

FIGURE 13-1   Lobes of the cerebral hemisphere (lateral surface).

surface of the hemisphere. This is the **stem** of the sulcus, which extends laterally between the frontal and temporal lobes and divides into three rami when reaching the lateral surface. Whereas the **posterior ramus** is the main part of the sulcus on the lateral surface of the hemisphere, the **anterior** and **ascending rami** project for only a short distance into the frontal lobe. An area of the cortex called the **insular lobe** or **insula** (island of Reil) lies at the bottom of the lateral sulcus and is hidden from surface view. This cortex appears to have been bound to the underlying corpus striatum during late embryonic and early fetal development; growth of the surrounding cortex would then produce the deep lateral sulcus.

The **central sulcus** (sulcus of Rolando; rolandic sulcus) is an important landmark for the sensorimotor cortex because the first somatic sensory area is immediately behind the sulcus, and the primary motor area is immediately in front of it. The central sulcus indents the superior border of the hemisphere about 1 cm behind the midpoint between the frontal and occipital poles. The sulcus slopes downward and forward, stopping just short of the lateral sulcus, and there are usually two bends along its course. The central sulcus is about 2 cm deep; its walls therefore constitute much of the sensorimotor cortex.

The **calcarine sulcus** on the medial surface of the hemisphere begins under the posterior end of the corpus callosum and follows an arched course to the occipital pole. In some brains, the sulcus continues over the pole for

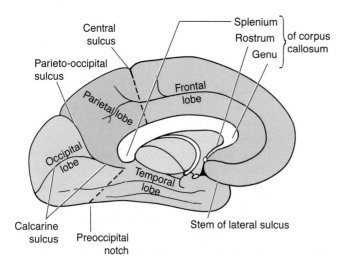

FIGURE 13-2   Lobes of the cerebral hemisphere (medial and inferior surfaces).

a short distance on the lateral surface. The calcarine sulcus is an important landmark for the visual cortex, most of which lies in the walls of the sulcus.

The **parieto-occipital sulcus** extends from the calcarine sulcus to the superior border of the hemisphere, which it intersects about 4 cm from the occipital pole.

The longitudinal and transverse cerebral fissures are external to the hemispheres and are therefore in a different category from the foregoing surface markings. The **longitudinal cerebral fissure** separates the hemispheres. A dural partition called the *falx cerebri* extends into the fissure. The corpus callosum, which constitutes the main cerebral commissure, crosses from one hemisphere to the other at the bottom of the longitudinal fissure. The **transverse cerebral fissure** intervenes between the cerebral hemispheres above and the cerebellum, midbrain, and diencephalon below. The posterior part of this fissure is located between the cerebral hemispheres and the cerebellum; it contains a dural partition known as the *tentorium cerebelli*. The anterior part of the transverse fissure intervenes between the corpus callosum and the diencephalon. It is triangular in outline, tapering anteriorly, and contains the **tela choroidea**, which consists of vascular connective tissue derived from the pia mater that covers the brain. The tela choroidea is continuous with the connective tissue core of the choroid plexuses of the lateral ventricles and the third ventricle, and the plexuses are completed by choroid epithelium derived from the ependymal lining of the ventricles. Choroid plexuses secrete cerebrospinal fluid (see Chapter 26).

Lobes of the Cerebral Hemispheres

Each cerebral hemisphere has lateral, medial, and inferior surfaces on which the extent of the lobes of the hemisphere are now defined (see Figs. 13-1 and 13-2).

The **frontal lobe** occupies the entire area in front of the central sulcus and above the lateral sulcus on the lateral surface. The medial surface of the frontal lobe envelops the anterior part of the corpus callosum and is bounded

posteriorly by a line drawn between the central sulcus and the corpus callosum. The inferior surface of the frontal lobe rests on the orbital plate of the frontal bone.

The natural boundaries of the **parietal lobe** on the lateral surface are the central and lateral sulci. The other boundaries consist of two lines; the first of these is drawn between the parieto-occipital sulcus and the preoccipital notch, and the second line runs from the middle of the one just established to the lateral sulcus. (The **preoccipital notch**, indicated in Figs. 13-1 and 13-2, is an inconspicuous indentation of the brain formed by the petrous part of the temporal bone.) On the medial surface, the parietal lobe is bounded by the frontal lobe, corpus callosum, calcarine sulcus, and parieto-occipital sulcus.

The **temporal lobe** is outlined on the lateral surface by the lateral sulcus and the lines previously noted. The inferior surface of the temporal lobe extends to the temporal pole from a line drawn between the anterior end of the calcarine sulcus and the preoccipital notch. Most of the **occipital lobe** appears on the medial surface of the hemisphere, where it is separated from the temporal lobe, as already described, and from the parietal lobe by the parieto-occipital sulcus. On the lateral surface, the occipital lobe consists of the small area posterior to the line that joins the parieto-occipital sulcus and preoccipital notch.

The portion of the great cerebral commissure in and near the midline is known as the **trunk of the corpus callosum**, and the fibers of the commissure that spread out within the centers of the hemispheres constitute the **radiations of the corpus callosum**. Names are assigned to certain regions of the trunk of the commissure (see Fig. 13-2); these regions are used as reference points further on. The enlarged posterior portion of the trunk is called the **splenium**. The anterior portion, or **genu**, curves ventrally and thins out to form the **rostrum**. This is continuous with the lamina terminalis, which limits the third ventricle anteriorly.

Gyri and Sulci

Some surface markings of the hemisphere are landmarks for important functional areas; the central sulcus for the sensorimotor cortex and the calcarine sulcus for the visual cortex are examples. For the most part, the sulci and gyri serve only as a rough frame of reference for cortical areas whose functions may or may not be known. The markings can be identified according to lobes for the lateral surface, but this is not practicable for the medial and inferior surfaces.

The text and illustrations that follow apply to sulci and gyri of varying functional significance. Students may need to refer to this material when studying the localization of functions in the cerebral cortex (see Chapter 15).

LATERAL SURFACE

Frontal Lobe

The **precentral sulcus** (often broken into two or more parts) runs parallel to the central sulcus; these sulci outline the **precentral gyrus**, which

is a landmark for the primary motor area of the cerebral cortex (Fig. 13-3). The remainder of the lateral surface of the frontal lobe is divided into **superior**, **middle**, and **inferior frontal gyri** by the **superior** and **inferior frontal sulci**. The anterior and ascending rami of the lateral sulcus divide the inferior frontal gyrus into **opercular**, **triangular**, and **orbital portions**. In the left hemisphere, the opercular and triangular portions consist of cortex of Broca's expressive or motor speech area. In the frontal lobe, as in the other lobes of the hemisphere, secondary gyri and sulci contribute to the variable topography of different brains.

Parietal Lobe

The **postcentral sulcus** runs parallel to the central sulcus; these sulci bound the **postcentral gyrus**, which is the landmark for the first somatic sensory

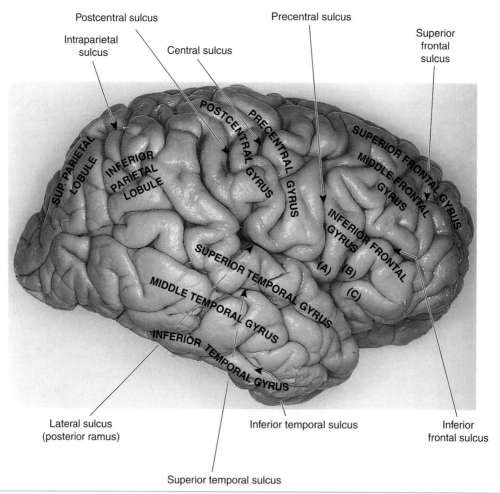

FIGURE 13-3   Gyri and sulci on the lateral surface of the right cerebral hemisphere. **(A), (B),** and **(C)** indicate the opercular, triangular, and orbital parts of the inferior frontal gyrus, respectively.

(somesthetic) area of the cortex. The **intraparietal sulcus** extends posteriorly from the postcentral sulcus and divides that part of the surface not occupied by the postcentral gyrus into **superior** and **inferior parietal lobules**. The portions of the inferior parietal lobule that surround the upturned ends of the lateral sulcus and superior temporal sulcus are called the **supramarginal gyrus** and the **angular gyrus**, respectively. In the left hemisphere, these gyri are included in the receptive language area, which is necessary for perception and interpretation of spoken and written language.

Insular Lobe (Insula)

The regions that conceal the insula are known as the **frontal**, **parietal**, and **temporal opercula**; they must be spread apart or cut away to expose the insula (Fig. 13-4). The insula is outlined by a **circular sulcus** and is divided into two regions by a central sulcus. Several short gyri lie in front of the central sulcus, and one or two long gyri lie behind it. The inferior part of the insula in the region of the stem of the lateral sulcus is known as the **limen insulae**. The cortex of the insula is involved in involuntary activities such as the control of viscera by the autonomic nervous system. Cortical areas for the special visceral sensations of taste and smell also extend onto the insula.

The insula is an important landmark for certain structures inside the cerebral hemisphere. The lentiform nucleus, a component of the corpus striatum, is separated from the insula by two layers of white matter (the extreme and external capsules) and an intervening layer of gray matter (the claustrum).

Temporal Lobe

Superior and **inferior temporal sulci** divide the lateral surface of the temporal lobe into **superior**, **middle**, and **inferior temporal gyri**. Among variations in the temporal lobe, the inferior temporal sulcus may be discontinuous, making it difficult to identify. The inferior temporal gyrus is called the *lateral occipitotemporal gyrus* when viewed from the inferior aspect of the temporal lobe. The superior temporal gyrus has a large surface that forms the floor of the lateral sulcus. On the anterior part of this surface, **transverse temporal gyri** (also known as *Heschl's convolutions*) extend to the bottom of the lateral sulcus and mark the location of the primary auditory area of the cortex. The posterior part of the superior temporal gyrus is the **planum temporale**, which is larger on the left side in males but not in females. The planum temporale includes part of the receptive language area, which extends onto the parietal lobe.

Occipital Lobe

In the brains of primates other than humans and in some human brains, the calcarine sulcus continues for a short distance over the occipital pole. There is then a curved **lunate sulcus** around the end of the calcarine sulcus. Except for this inconstant marking, the small area of the occipital lobe on the lateral surface has minor grooves and folds of no special significance.

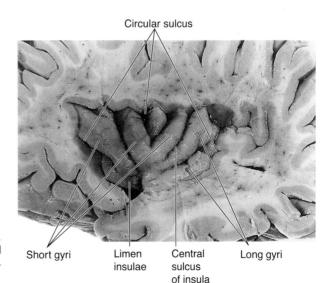

Circular sulcus

Short gyri   Limen insulae   Central sulcus of insula   Long gyri

FIGURE 13-4 The insula of the left cerebral hemisphere, exposed by cutting away the frontal, parietal, and temporal opercula.

The primary visual cortex occupies and surrounds the calcarine sulcus. The remainder of the occipital lobe consists of association cortex for interpretation of visual stimuli. The visual association cortex extends onto the parietal and temporal lobes (see also Chapters 15 and 20).

Medial and Inferior Surfaces

The **cingulate gyrus** begins beneath the genu of the corpus callosum and continues above the corpus callosum as far back as the splenium

(Fig. 13-5). The **cingulate sulcus** intervenes between the cingulate gyrus and the **medial frontal gyrus**, which is continuous with the superior frontal gyrus on the lateral surface of the hemisphere. The cingulate sulcus gives off a **paracentral sulcus** and then divides into **marginal** and **subparietal sulci** in the parietal lobe. The region bounded by the paracentral and marginal sulci, which surrounds the indentation made by the central sulcus on the superior border, is called the **paracentral lobule**. The anterior and posterior parts of the paracentral lobule are, respectively, extensions of the precentral and postcentral gyri of the lateral surface of the hemisphere. The area above the

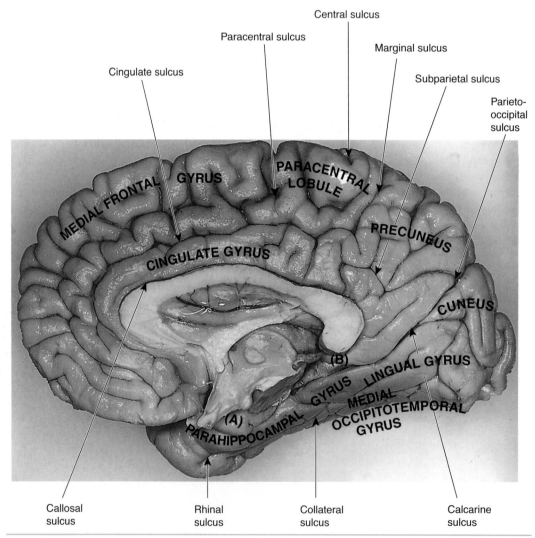

FIGURE 13-5   Gyri and sulci on the medial and inferior surfaces of the right cerebral hemisphere. **(A)** Uncus. **(B)** Isthmus (retrosplenial cortex) connecting the cingulate and parahippocampal gyri.

subparietal sulcus is called the **precuneus** and is continuous with the superior parietal lobule on the lateral surface. The parieto-occipital and calcarine sulci bound the **cuneus** of the occipital lobe.

On the medial surface of the frontal lobe, underneath the rostrum of the corpus callosum, is the **subcallosal gyrus**, also known as the *parolfactory area*. This is part of the **septal area**, a component of the limbic system (see Chapter 18).

On the inferior surface of the hemisphere (see Figs. 13-5 and 13-6), a convolution extends from the occipital pole almost to the temporal pole. The posterior part of the convolution consists of the **lingual gyrus**. The anterior part forms the **parahippocampal gyrus**, which hooks sharply backward on its medial aspect as the **uncus**, a region where fibers of the olfactory tract end. The **collateral sulcus** defines the lateral margin of the lingual and parahippocampal gyri. The short **rhinal sulcus**, at the lateral edge of the parahippocampal gyrus anteriorly, delimits the **entorhinal area**, which belongs to the olfactory and limbic systems. The **medial occipitotemporal gyrus**, also commonly called the **fusiform gyrus**, lies along the lateral side of the collateral sulcus. It is broken up by several small, variable sulci. The **occipitotemporal sulcus** intervenes between the medial occipitotemporal gyrus and the **lateral occipitotemporal gyrus**. The latter is continuous with the inferior temporal gyrus of the lateral surface of the hemisphere.

The inferior surface of the frontal lobe is commonly known as the **orbitofrontal cortex**. The **olfactory bulb** and **olfactory tract** (see Fig. 13-6) conceal most of the **olfactory sulcus**. The **gyrus rectus** is located medially to the olfactory sulcus. The large area lateral to the olfactory sulcus typically consists of four irregular **orbital gyri** (medial, anterior, posterior, and lateral) separated by an H-shaped arrangement of sulci.

Limbic Lobe

The cingulate and parahippocampal gyri are connected by a narrow **isthmus** (more often called **retrosplenial cortex**) behind and beneath the splenium of the corpus callosum. The connected

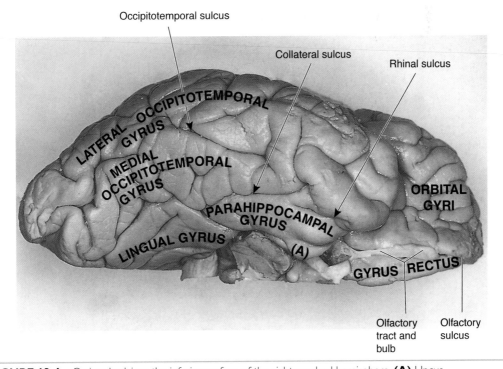

FIGURE 13-6   Gyri and sulci on the inferior surface of the right cerebral hemisphere. **(A)** Uncus.

gyri form the limbic lobe. This is part of the **limbic system** of the brain, which incorporates several additional structures, most prominently the hippocampus, the dentate gyrus and the amygdaloid body (in the temporal lobe), the hypothalamus, the septal area, and some nuclei of the thalamus (see Chapter 18). The term *limbic system* is still in use but may soon become obsolete. It embraces neural circuitry involved in such diverse functions as learning, remembering, defensive and reproductive behavior, and responses to subjective feelings.

Suggested Reading

Chiavaras MM, Petrides M. Orbitofrontal sulci of the human and macaque monkey brain. *J Comp Neurol* 2000;422:35–54.

Haines DE. Neuroanatomy. *An Atlas of Structures, Sections and Systems*, 7th ed. Baltimore: Williams & Wilkins, 2007.

Hanke J. Sulcal pattern of the anterior parahippocampal gyrus in the human adult. *Ann Anat* 1997;179:335–339.

Kulynych JJ, Vladar K, Jones DW, et al. Gender differences in the normal lateralization of the supratemporal cortex: MRI surface-rendering morphometry of Heschl's gyrus and the planum temporale. *Cereb Cortex* 1994;4: 107–118.

Montemurro DG, Bruni JE. *The Human Brain in Dissection*, 2nd ed. New York: Oxford University Press, 1988.

Naidich TP, Valavanis AG, Kubik S. Anatomic relationships along the low-middle convexity, 1: normal specimens and magnetic resonance imaging. *Neurosurgery* 1995;36: 517–532.

Nieuwenhuys R, Voogd J, van Huijzen C. *The Human Central Nervous System. A Synopsis and Atlas*, 3rd ed. Berlin: Springer-Verlag, 1988.

Nolte J, Angevine JB. *The Human Brain in Photographs and Diagrams*, 3rd ed. St. Louis: Mosby, 2007.

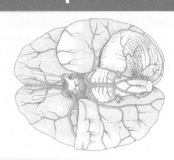

Chapter 14

HISTOLOGY OF THE CEREBRAL CORTEX

Important Facts

- The surface of the cerebral hemisphere consists of the archicortex (hippocampal formation); paleocortex (olfactory and some limbic areas); and neocortex, which has six layers and, in the human brain, contains approximately 10^{10} neurons.

- The cortex contains principal (pyramidal) cells, which are most conspicuous in layers 3 and 5 and several types of interneurons. Brodmann's numbered areas are based on regional variations in microscopic appearance of the cortex.

- The six layers are most distinct in association areas. In the primary sensory areas, stellate cells are prominent in layer 4. These interneurons are rarely seen in motor areas. The primary motor area contains giant pyramidal (Betz) cells.

- Afferent fibers are from other cortical areas, the thalamus, the basal forebrain cholinergic nuclei, the noradrenergic and serotonergic neurons of the brain stem, and histaminergic and certain peptidergic (orexin) neurons of the hypothalamus. Corticocortical, thalamocortical, cholinergic, and peptidergic afferents excite the pyramidal cells. Some aminergic fibers are excitatory and others are inhibitory.

- The cortex is composed of vertical strings of neurons, known as mini-columns, which are grouped into larger columns or modules. Each module responds only to a specific type of signal. Maturation of the columnar organization requires exposure to sensory experiences early in postnatal life.

- The electroencephalogram shows summated differences of membrane potentials between the proximal and distal ends of the apical dendrites of pyramidal cells. These potentials fluctuate as a result of changes in activity of thalamocortical and corticocortical neurons.

Each cerebral hemisphere has a mantle of gray matter, the **cortex** or **pallium**, with a characteristic structure that consists of neuronal cell bodies and axons arranged in layers.

Histology is the study of tissues, as distinct from the study of individual cells, by microscopy. Three types of cortical tissue are recognized by microscopic examination of sections cut in a plane perpendicular to the surface of the brain. The names of the types of cortex are based on phylogeny, which is the graded variation of similar structures across different groups of organisms. The **paleocortex** is that of the olfactory system, and the **archicortex** is that of the hippocampal formation. Their locations in the temporal lobe are described in Chapters 17 and 18. The remainder of the cerebral cortex is of the type known as **neocortex**.

The number of layers evident histologically in the paleocortex and archicortex varies according to region. There may be as many as five layers in the paleocortex, although the more superficial ones are indistinct. The largest number of layers in the archicortex is three. In the neocortex, which is the subject of this chapter, six layers are always recognizable at some stage of embryonic or fetal development. In some areas of the adult brain, however, the typical six layers cannot all be discerned.

Cortical Neurons

Values obtained for the number of neurons in the human cerebral cortex vary widely because of the technical difficulties in their enumeration. They range from 2.6×10^9 to 1.6×10^{10}, and the number of cortical neurons is therefore enormous.

The principal cells (neurons with long axons) are known as **pyramidal cells**. Their cell bodies range in height from 10 to 50 μm for most cells. Giant pyramidal cells, also known as **Betz cells**, have cell bodies up to 100 μm

219

high. These are present only in the primary motor area of the frontal lobe, where they are conspicuous but not numerous. Each pyramidal cell (Fig. 14-1) has conspicuous apical and lateral dendrites, with branches that are covered with dendritic spines. The axon emerges from the base of the pyramid or from one of the larger dendrites and gives off many collateral branches before it enters the subcortical white matter. About two thirds of cortical neurons are pyramidal cells, but the proportion is higher in motor areas of the frontal lobe and lower in the primary sensory areas. The axons of pyramidal neurons are excitatory at their synapses and are thought to use glutamate as their neurotransmitter. **Fusiform cells**, which are located in the deepest layer of the cortex, are atypical principal cells with irregularly elliptical cell bodies.

In addition to their local intracortical branches, the axons of the principal cells connect with other neurons in three ways. **Projection neurons** transmit impulses to subcortical locations such as the corpus striatum, brain stem, spinal cord, or thalamus (which receives the axons of the fusiform cells). **Association neurons** establish connections with cortical neurons elsewhere in the same hemisphere. The axons of **commissural neurons** proceed to the cortex of the opposite hemisphere. Most of the commissural fibers constitute the corpus callosum; smaller numbers connect cortical areas of the temporal lobes through the anterior commissure.

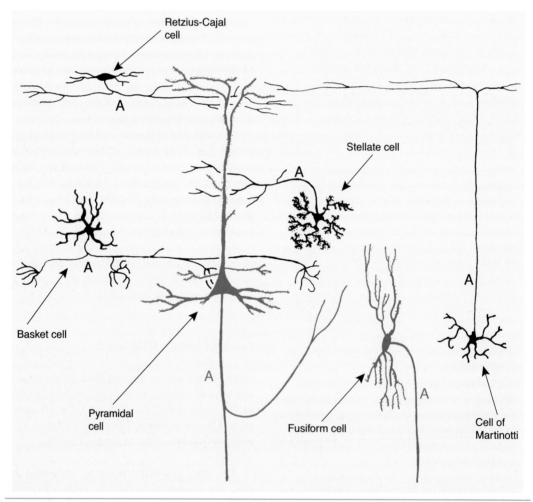

FIGURE 14-1   Cortical neurons: principal cells in red, interneurons in black. In reality, the dendrites are more numerous and more richly branched than shown in this drawing. (The letter A indicates the axon of each type of neuron.)

About 30 types of cortical interneurons are recognized, on the basis of dendritic architecture, by researchers who study Golgi preparations. A few of the major cell types are shown schematically in Figure 14-1. **Stellate cells**, which have dendritic spines, occur only in the fourth cortical layer (see the next section of this chapter). They are excitatory, and the transmitter is probably glutamate. All the other types of interneurons are inhibitory and probably all secrete gamma-aminobutyric acid at their synapses. **Basket cells** have axons that branch laterally and embrace the cell bodies of pyramidal cells. The **Retzius-Cajal cells** are confined to the most superficial layer of the cortex, and the **cells of Martinotti** are more deeply placed, with axons that project toward the pial surface.

Cortical Layers

The thickness of the neocortex varies from 4.5 mm in the primary motor area of the frontal lobe to 1.5 mm in the visual area of the occipi-

tal lobe. The cortex is thicker over the crest of a gyrus than in the depths of a sulcus. The cerebral cortex has its full complement of neurons by the 18th week of intrauterine life, and six layers, which differ in the density of cell population and in the size and shape of constituent neurons, can be recognized by about the 7th month. The layers, starting at the surface and omitting regional differences for the present, are as follows (Fig. 14-2A):

1. **Molecular layer.** The superficial layer predominantly consists of terminal branches of dendrites and axons, which give a punctate or "molecular" appearance in sections stained for nerve fibers. Most of the dendritic branches come from pyramidal cells. The axons originate in cortex elsewhere in the same hemisphere, in that of the opposite hemisphere, and in the thalamus. Cells of Martinotti in any deeper layer also contribute axons to layer 1. The infrequent horizontal Retzius-Cajal cells intervene between some axons

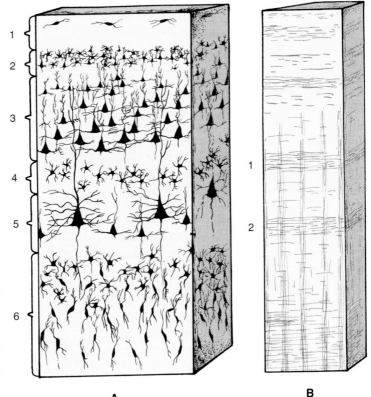

FIGURE 14-2 Cortical histology, as revealed by two staining methods. **(A)** Golgi method: **1.** Molecular layer. **2.** External granular layer. **3.** External pyramidal layer. **4.** Internal granular layer. **5.** Internal pyramidal layer. **6.** Multiform layer. **(B)** Weigert's method for myelin: **1.** Outer line of Baillarger. **2.** Inner line of Baillarger.

A

B

and dendrites. The molecular layer is essentially a synaptic field of the cortex.

2. **External granular layer**. This layer contains many small pyramidal cells and interneurons.

3. **External pyramidal layer**. The neurons are typical pyramidal cells that increase in size from the external to the internal borders of the layer. Their axons project to other cortical areas as association and projection fibers.

4. **Internal granular layer**. This layer is dominated by stellate cells, although smaller numbers of other interneurons and pyramidal cells are also present.

5. **Internal pyramidal layer**. This layer contains pyramidal cells, which are larger than those of layer 3, intermingled with interneurons. The giant pyramidal cells (of Betz) in the primary motor area of cortex in the frontal lobe are located in layer 5. Neurons in layer 5 project to subcortical targets such as the striatum, brain stem, and spinal cord.

6. **Multiform layer**. Although fusiform cells are typical of this layer, pyramidal cells and interneurons of various shapes are also present. Efferent fibers that end in the thalamus and claustrum arise from layer 6.

The layers described are evident in sections stained by the Nissl or Golgi techniques (see Chapter 4). With silver staining methods for axons or the Weigert method for myelin sheaths, axons within the neocortex are seen in radial bundles and in tangential bands (see Fig. 14-2B). The radial bundles include axons entering and leaving the cortex. The tangential bands consist largely of collateral and terminal branches of afferent fibers. They leave the radial bundles and run parallel to the surface for some distance, branching again and making synaptic contacts with large numbers of cortical neurons. The most prominent tangential bands are the **outer** and **inner lines of Baillarger**, in layers 4 and 5, respectively. Axons originating in the thalamic sensory nuclei contribute heavily to the lines of Baillarger, especially the outer one, and they are therefore prominent in the primary sensory areas. In the primary visual area in the walls of the calcarine sulcus,

the outer line of Baillarger on the cut surface is just visible to the unaided eye and is known as the **line of Gennari** (Fig. 14-3). Because of the presence of the line of Gennari, the primary visual cortex is known alternatively as the **striate area**.

Variations in Cytoarchitecture

Six layers can be identified in most areas of the neocortex. Exceptions are the primary visual area and parts of the primary auditory and primary somatic sensory areas, where layers 2 to 5 merge into a single layer of numerous small interneurons. The opposite extreme is found in the primary motor and premotor areas of the frontal lobe, where pyramidal cells are much more numerous than interneurons, and layers 2 to 6 appear as a single zone consisting almost entirely of pyramidal cells of different sizes, with the larger ones more deeply located.

The cerebral cortex has been divided into cytoarchitectural areas based on differences

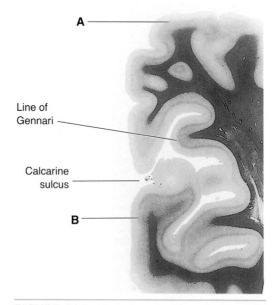

FIGURE 14-3 Vertical section through the medial surface of the occipital lobe at the site of the calcarine sulcus. The line of Gennari, extending from **A** to **B**, identifies the primary visual area: the striate cortex (Weigert stain).

in the thickness of individual layers, neuronal morphology in the layers, and the distribution of axonal bundles. Different investigators have divided the cortex into 20 to 200 areas, depending on the criteria used. Brodmann's numbered map, which was published in 1909 and consists of 52 areas, provides the most widely used scheme of cortical cytoarchitectural areas. Some areas of Brodmann's map referred to later in the text are shown in Figures 15-1 and 15-2.

Some of the cortical areas recognized histologically correspond closely with areas whose functions are known from clinical and experimental investigations (see Chapter 15). These areas are summarized in Table 14-1.

Intracortical Circuits

Investigations of cortical neurons using the Golgi technique, electron microscopy, and immunohistochemical methods, combined with electrical recording from microelectrodes placed in the cortex, have yielded much information concerning intrinsic circuits. These are summarized in simplified form in Figure 14-4.

Afferent and Efferent Fibers

The major sources of afferent fibers entering the cortex are as follows:

1. **Other cortical areas** in the same and the opposite hemisphere; corticocortical fibers are the most numerous afferents. They are excitatory and are the axons of glutamatergic (or possibly aspartatergic) cortical pyramidal cells.
2. **The thalamus**, which is the best understood source of subcortical afferents. These are also excitatory, but the transmitter is excitatory, probably glutamate.
3. **The claustrum** (see Chapter 12), about which little is known. It has reciprocal connections, especially with the cortex of the parietal and occipital lobes.
4. **The basal cholinergic forebrain nuclei** of the substantia innominata (see Chapters 9 and 12), which send their much-branched axons to all areas of the neocortex, where they have excitatory effects.
5. **Noradrenergic axons** from neurons in the locus coeruleus (see Chapter 9), which inhibit cortical neurons.
6. **Serotonergic axons** from the more rostral of the raphe nuclei of the brain stem (see Chapter 9), which are also inhibitory and are even more abundant than the noradrenergic afferents.
7. **Histaminergic axons** and **peptidergic axons** (which have orexin as their transmitter) from certain hypothalamic nuclei (see Chapters 9 and 11), which are involved in sleep and arousal.
8. **Cortical efferent fibers**, which are axons of the larger neurons, notably pyramidal

TABLE 14-1 **Some Cytoarchitectonic Areas and Associated Functions**

Brodmann's Numbers (Cytoarchitecture)	Area Defined by Functional Studies
1, 2, 3	Primary somatic sensory cortex (see Chapters 15 and 19)
4	Primary motor area (see Chapters 15 and 23)
6	Premotor and supplementary motor areas (see Chapters 15 and 23)
8	Frontal eye field (see Chapters 15 and 8)
17	Primary visual area (see Chapters 15 and 20)
28, 34	Olfactory cortex (see Chapters 15 and 17)
42	Primary auditory area (see Chapters 15 and 21)
43	Gustatory cortex (see Chapters 15 and 8)
44, 45	Broca's expressive speech area (see Chapters 15 and 25)

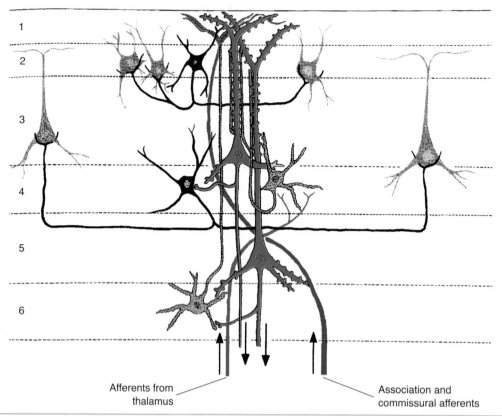

FIGURE 14-4   Some intracortical connections. Axons of neurons in other cortical areas (magenta) excite the apical dendrites of pyramidal cells. Afferents from specific thalamic nuclei (blue) excite basal dendrites of pyramidal cells in layers 3, 5, and 6 and the stellate cells (green) in layer 4, which, in turn, excite pyramidal cells (red) in the same column. Also in layer 4, branches of thalamic afferent and pyramidal cell axons excite basket cells (black), which inhibit pyramidal cells in adjacent columns (pink). (Reprinted with permission from Martin JH. In: Kandel ER, Schwartz JH, Jessell TM, eds. *Principles of Neural Science*, 3rd ed. New York: Elsevier, 1991:781.)

and fusiform cells, enter the white matter for distribution as projection, association, or commissural fibers (see Chapter 16).

Columnar Organization

Recordings from microelectrodes inserted into the cortex have shown that it is organized functionally as minute vertical units, known as *columns* or *modules*, that include neurons of all layers. This has been demonstrated best in sensory areas. All the neurons in a module are selectively activated by the same peripheral stimulus, whether it originates in a particular type of cutaneous receptor at a particular location or in a specific point on the retina. Each module is 200 to 500 μm in diameter and is composed of about 100 mini-columns. A mini-column is a string of neurons formed by outward migration during development.

Vertically organized functional modules corresponding to those detected with microelectrodes can also be defined by autoradiography (see Chapter 4). To do this, a labeled amino acid is injected into the appropriate thalamic nucleus, or labeled 2-deoxyglucose is given systemically while a sensory system is receiving stimuli. Columns with increased metabolic activity can also be made visible by staining histochemically for the activity of cytochrome oxidase, the enzyme that enables cells to use oxygen.

The columnar organization of the neocortex is established in fetal life, but the synaptic connections increase in number postnatally in

Clinical Uses of Electroencephalography

Electroencephalography (EEG) is informative in the clinical investigation of **epilepsy**, a group of maladies in which abnormal spread of neuronal excitation occurs through the brain, typically leading to loss of consciousness and convulsions. Abnormalities in the EEG characterize the different types of epilepsy and can help to localize the epileptogenic focus in which the abnormal discharges begin. The EEG is also useful in the study of sleep (see Chapter 9). A technique known as **magnetoencephalography** records the magnetic fields associated with intracortical electric currents. This procedure can localize activity in smaller areas of the cortex than can EEG.

A "flat" EEG 2 days or more after cardiac arrest and resuscitation is associated with halving of the cortical oxygen consumption and is an almost certain indicator of permanent loss of function of the cerebral cortex. The diagnosis of **brain death** in comatose patients is made on the basis of absence of functions of the brain stem: failure of spontaneous respiration and absence of reflexes mediated by any of the cranial nerves. This must not be confused with **vegetative states**, in which no communication exists between the brain stem and the cerebrum, although breathing, swallowing, chewing, and cranial nerve reflexes are largely preserved. Recovery from a vegetative state of long duration can occur, but there is no reliable way to distinguish the patients who will recover from the majority in whom the condition is permanent.

---

response to external sensory stimuli. This maturation occurs in an **early critical period** in response to adequate sensory stimulation. If sensory stimuli are lacking in number and variety during the first year of life, the functions of the cerebral cortex fail to develop normally. For example, if refractive errors or misalignment (strabismus) of the eyes is not corrected early in childhood, visual acuity is permanently impaired because of inadequate development of neuronal circuitry in the primary visual cortex of the occipital lobe.

Visual stimuli are easily controlled in the laboratory, so the organization of cortical neurons has been most intensively studied in the primary visual cortex. There, distinct columns of cells respond to neural input associated with one or both eyes (ocular dominance columns) and to meaningful features in the observed image, such as edges, horizontal lines, and right angles. Populations of the different kinds of cell columns form stripes that extend across the surface of the calcarine cortex.

Electroencephalography

Changes in electrical potential recorded from a point on the surface of the scalp are caused by summed membrane potentials in the apical dendrites of thousands of underlying pyramidal cells. Whereas activity in thalamic affer-

ents to the cortex stimulates (depolarizes) the pyramidal cell dendrites in layer 4, input from association and commissural fibers causes depolarization in layer 1 (see Fig. 14-4). The magnitude and direction of flow of electric current across the thickness of the cortex depend on the differences in membrane potential of the proximal and distal ends of the apical dendrites.

Suggested Reading

Braak H. *Architectonics of the Human Telencephalic Cortex.* Berlin: Springer-Verlag, 1980.

Dinopoulos A, Dori I, Parnevelas JG. Immunohistochemical localization of aspartate in corticofugal pathways. *Neurosci Lett* 1991;121:25–28.

Douglas R, Markram H, Martin K. Neocortex. In: Shepherd GM, ed. *The Synaptic Organization of the Brain*, 5th ed. New York: Oxford University Press, 2004:499–558.

Hubel TH, Wiesel TN. Functional architecture of macaque monkey visual cortex. *Proc R Soc Lond [Biol]* 1977;198: 1–59.

Jones EG. Neurotransmitters in the cerebral cortex. *J Neurosurg* 1986;65:135–153.

Jones EG, Friedman DP, Endry SHC. Thalamic basis of place- and modality-specific columns in monkey somatosensory cortex: a correlative anatomical and physiological study. *J Neurophysiol* 1982;48:545–568.

Mountcastle VB. The columnar organization of the neocortex. *Brain* 1997;120:701–722.

Nieuwenhuys R. The neocortex: an overview of its evolutionary development, structural organization and synaptology. *Anat Embryol* 1994;190:307–337.

Ong WY, Garey LJ. Neuronal architecture of the human temporal cortex. *Anat Embryol* 1990;181:351–364.

Pakkenberg B, Gundersen HJG. Neocortical neuron number in humans: effect of sex and age. *J Comp Neurol* 1997;384:312–320.

Young B, Blume W, Lynch A. Brain death and the persistent vegetative state: similarities and contrasts. *Can J Neurol Sci* 1989;16:388–393.

Zilles K. Architecture of the Human Cerebral Cortex. Regional and Laminar Organization. In: Pakinos G, Mai JK, eds. *The Human Nervous System*, 2nd ed. Amsterdam: Elsevier, 2004:997–1055.

Chapter 15

FUNCTIONAL LOCALIZATION IN THE CEREBRAL CORTEX

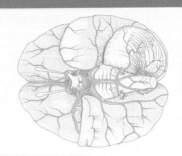

- Stimulation and ablation, electrophysiological recording, and observations of regional blood flow and associated metabolic changes have all contributed to knowledge of the localization of functions in different parts of the cerebral cortex.

- Primary sensory areas, which are topographically organized, are necessary for conscious recognition and localization of sensory stimuli. Each main primary sensory area is surrounded by a larger zone of association cortex, which interprets the incoming signals and is appropriately connected to other parts of the cerebral cortex. Various types of agnosia and apraxia result from damage to sensory association cortex.

- General somatic sensory pathways go to the postcentral gyrus. The visual pathway ends in the cortex around the calcarine sulcus. The primary auditory cortex is located on the superior surface of the superior temporal gyrus. The cortex for taste is in the anterior, inferior part of the parietal lobe and an adjacent region of the insula. The primary olfactory area is the uncus and nearby parts of the insula and frontal operculum.

- The supplementary and cingulate motor areas are involved in the planning and initiation of movements. The premotor cortex controls movements at proximal joints. The primary motor area (precentral gyrus) receives input from the other three motor areas and is topographically organized in relation to groups of muscles, with a large proportion of its extent being devoted to the hand and face. All the motor areas give rise to descending tracts that end in the brain stem and spinal cord.

- The frontal eye field controls conjugate saccadic eye movements. The parieto-occipital eye field controls slower, involuntary movements of the eyes. Activity in the ocular motor cortical areas directs the gaze toward the opposite side.

- In most people, an expressive or motor speech area is located in the left frontal lobe, and a receptive or sensory language area is located in the left temporo-parietal cortex. Various types of aphasia result from lesions that damage the language areas.

- The right cerebral cortex contains (in most people) areas necessary for awareness of the positions and conditions of parts of the body, appreciation of three-dimensional shapes, prosody (i.e., properties of the voice other than its verbal content), and musical ability.

- The rostral parts of the frontal lobes are involved in some higher mental functions, including judgment, foresight, and socially proper behavior. The anterior part of the cingulate gyrus is active in the perception of pain. Other functions of the temporal lobe and cingulate gyrus, including memory, are discussed in the context of the limbic system in Chapter 18.

Results of clinicopathological studies and animal experiments conducted over more than a century have provided information concerning functional specialization in different regions of the cerebral cortex. For example, large **primary sensory areas** are recognized for general somatic sensation, smell, vision, and hearing. Smaller areas exist for taste and vestibular sensation (i.e., awareness of position and movement of the head). **Motor** areas are also present from which contraction of skeletal muscles can be elicited by electrical stimulation. The remainder of the neocortex, accounting for most of its area, is usually referred to as **association cortex**, which may be closely related functionally to the sensory areas or to more complex levels of behavior, communication, and the intellect.

In certain surgical procedures, it is essential to identify the motor area, a sensory area, or even a particular region within these areas. Identification of sensory areas requires operating on a conscious patient under local anesthesia. This is possible because the brain does not perceive pain when injured in ways that would be painful else-where in the body. Electrical stimulation of the human cerebral cortex has provided information more detailed than that obtainable by observing the effects of destructive wounds and diseases.

Since 1980, the classical studies of functional localization have been largely confirmed and ex-tended by means of modern noninvasive tech-niques (see Chapter 4). The cortex can be electri-cally stimulated by an externally applied magnetic field, for example, or electrodes on the scalp can record potentials evoked by transcutaneous stimu-lation of peripheral nerves. Magnetoencephalogra-phy (see Chapter 4), although available in only a few centers, can also provide accurate localization of cortical function, expecially in the walls of sulci. Single-photon emission computed tomography (SPECT) and positron emission tomography (PET) are used to map regional cerebral blood flow or oxygen or glucose uptake, to provide information about cortical activity in the normal brain, and to detect abnormal function. Functional nuclear mag-netic resonance imaging (fMRI) provides similar information with superior anatomical resolution.

Parietal, Occipital, and Temporal Cortex

The parietal, occipital, and temporal lobes con-tain primary sensory areas, which are the des-tinations of pathways that begin in the various sensory organs. Adjacent to each primary sen-sory area is a larger region of association cortex, which interprets and uses the incoming data. Much of the frontal lobe is also considered to be association cortex; it receives input from the sensory lobes, instructs the motor areas, and is also involved in subjective feelings, thought, judgment, and the planning of activities.

GENERAL SOMATIC SENSATION

The **first somesthetic area** (primary somatic sensory area) occupies the postcentral gyrus on the lateral surface of the hemisphere and the posterior part of the paracentral lobule on the medial surface (Figs. 15-1 and 15-2). It consists of areas 3, 1, and 2 of the Brodmann cytoarchi-

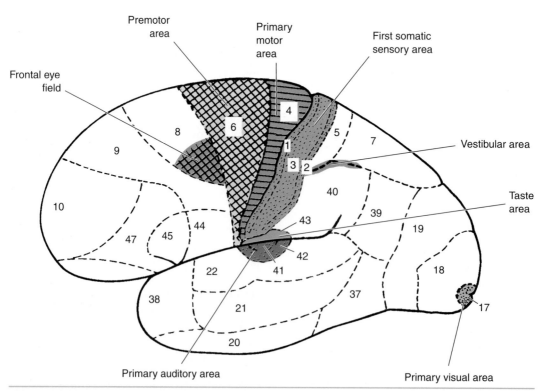

FIGURE 15-1   Motor and primary sensory areas on the lateral surface of the left cerebral hemisphere. Some of Brodmann's numbered areas, based on cytoarchitecture, are also shown.

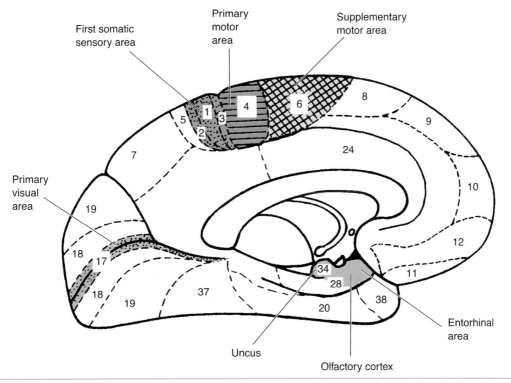

FIGURE 15-2 Motor and primary sensory areas on the medial surface of the left cerebral hemisphere. Some of Brodmann's numbered areas, based on cytoarchitecture, are also shown.

tectural map. Electrical stimulation of the first somesthetic area elicits modified forms of the tactile sense such as a tingling sensation. It is possible to elicit motor responses by stimulating the first somesthetic area, as well as eliciting sensory responses from the motor area in the precentral gyrus. The functions of the two areas overlap to some extent, and they are often considered as a **sensorimotor strip** that surrounds the central sulcus. The overlap is greater in laboratory animals than in humans. The postcentral gyrus and its extension in the paracentral lobule are designated as the first somatic sensory area because they have the highest density of points that produce localized sensations on electrical stimulation.

The ventral posterior nucleus of the thalamus is the main source of afferent fibers for the first somatic sensory area. This thalamic nucleus is the site of termination of all the fibers of the medial lemniscus and of most of the fibers of the spinothalamic and trigeminothalamic tracts. The thalamocortical projection traverses the internal capsule and cerebral white matter, conveying data for the various modalities

of somatic sensation. Thalamocortical fibers for cutaneous sensibility end preferentially in the anterior part of the first somatosensory area, and those for deep sensibility, including proprioception, end in the posterior part.

The contralateral half of the body is represented as inverted. The pharyngeal region, tongue, and jaws are represented in the most ventral part of the somesthetic area, followed by the face, hands, arms, trunk, and thighs. The area for the remainder of the legs and the perineum is in the extension of the somesthetic cortex on the medial surface of the hemisphere. The size of the cortical area for a particular part of the body is determined by the functional importance of the part and its need for sensitivity. The area for the face, especially the lips, is disproportionately large, and a large area is assigned to the hand, particularly the thumb and index finger. A picture of the body with the proportions of its cortical map is known as a **homunculus** (Fig. 15-3).

A crude form of awareness persists for pain, heat, and cold sensations on the affected opposite side of the body if the first somesthetic

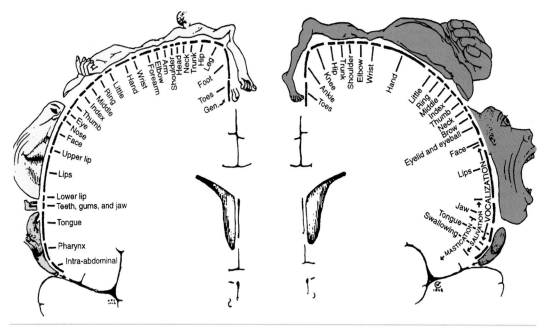

FIGURE 15-3   Homunculi of the primary somatosensory area (*left*) and primary motor area (*right*).

area has been destroyed. There is poor localization of the stimulus, for which qualitative and quantitative interpretations are diminished or absent. The somesthetic cortex must be intact for any appreciation of the more discriminative sensations of fine touch, position, and movement of the parts of the body.

An additional or **second somesthetic area** has been demonstrated in primates, including humans. This small area is located in the dorsal wall of the lateral sulcus in line with the postcentral gyrus and may extend onto the insula. The parts of the body are represented bilaterally, although contralateral representation predominates. The second sensory area receives input from the intralaminar nuclei and from the posterior group of nuclei of the thalamus. The afferent fibers to these nuclei come,

---

CLINICAL NOTE

Parietal Lobe Lesions

A destructive lesion in the somesthetic association cortex may leave the somesthetic area itself intact. Then, a defect in understanding the significance of sensory information, called **agnosia**, is present. In this disorder, awareness of the general senses persists, but the significance of the information received on the basis of previous experience is elusive. There are several types of agnosia, depending on the sense that is most affected. A lesion that destroys a large portion of the somesthetic association cortex causes **tactile agnosia** and **astereognosis**, which are closely related. They combine when a person is unable to identify a common object, such as a pair of scissors, held in the hand while the eyes are closed. It is impossible to correlate the surface texture, shape,

size, and weight of the object or to compare the sensations with previous experiences. Astereognosis includes a loss of awareness of the spatial relations of parts of the contralateral side of the body. The most extreme form of the condition is **cortical neglect**, in which the patient ignores and even denies the existence of one side of the body and of the corresponding visual field. The condition most often is caused by large lesions in the superior part of the right parietal lobe.

Association fibers connect the somesthetic association cortex with the motor areas of the frontal lobe, providing interpreted proprioceptive and other sensory input needed for the accurate execution of movements. Consequently, damage to the parietal lobe can cause **apraxia**, which is discussed also in connection with the premotor cortex.

respectively, from the reticular formation and from the spinothalamic and trigeminothalamic tracts. Consequently, the area is mainly involved in the less discriminative aspects of sensation. An intact second somesthetic area may explain such residual sensibility as exists after destruction of the first somatic sensory area. No clinical disorder has been ascribed to a lesion in the second somesthetic area.

The **somesthetic association cortex** is located mainly in the superior parietal lobule on the lateral surface of the hemisphere and in the precuneus on the medial surface. Much of it coincides with Brodmann's areas 5 and 7. This association cortex receives fibers from the first somesthetic area, and its thalamic connections are with the lateral posterior nucleus and the pulvinar. Data pertaining to the general senses are integrated in this association area, permitting, for example, assessment of the characteristics of an object held in the hand and its identification without visual aid.

VISION

The **primary visual area** surrounds the calcarine sulcus on the medial surface of the occipital lobe, extending over the occipital pole in some brains (see Fig. 15-2). The area is more extensive than Figure 15-2 suggests because most of it is located in the walls of the deep calcarine sulcus, in which secondary folds are also present. The primary visual cortex, which corresponds to area 17 of Brodmann's map, is called the **striate area** because it contains the line of Gennari (see Chapter 14), which is just visible to the unaided eye. The chief source of afferent fibers to area 17 is the lateral geniculate body of the thalamus by way of the geniculocalcarine tract.

The primary visual cortex, through a synaptic relay in the lateral geniculate body, receives data from the lateral (temporal) half of the ipsilateral retina and the medial (nasal) half of the contralateral retina. The left half of the field of vision is, therefore, represented in the visual area of the right hemisphere and vice versa (see also Chapter 20). Spatial patterns are also present within the striate area. The lower retinal quadrants (upper field of vision) project onto the lower wall of the calcarine sulcus, and the upper retinal quadrants (lower field of vision) project onto the upper wall of the sulcus. Another pattern is related to central and peripheral vision. The center of the retina, which is responsible for central vision of maximal discrimination, is represented at the occipital pole in the posterior part of area 17; the peripheral retina is represented more anteriorly. Thus, the part of area 17 that receives signals for central vision accounts for a disproportionately large amount (i.e., one third) of the primary visual cortex.

The extensive **visual association cortex** surrounds the primary visual area on the medial, lateral, and inferior surfaces of the hemisphere (see Figs. 15-1 and 15-2), extending from areas 18 and 19 (occipital lobe) to the posterior part of the parietal lobe and the lateral and inferior parts of the temporal lobe. These areas receive fibers from area 17 and have reciprocal connections with other cortical areas and with the

CLINICAL NOTE

Visual Cortex Lesions

A destructive lesion that involves the striate cortex of a hemisphere causes an area of blindness in the opposite visual field. The size and location of the defect are determined by the extent and location of the lesion. With a large unilateral lesion in the occipital lobe (e.g., an infarction caused by a thrombus in the posterior cerebral artery), central vision may be spared. This clinical observation is known as **macular sparing**. (The macula lutea is the central part of the retina that is opposite the pupil.) The relatively large area of cortex devoted to central vision may be partly spared by the lesion. It has also been suggested that anastomoses between branches of the middle and posterior cerebral arteries partly maintain the posterior part of area 17 after occlusion of the posterior cerebral artery. The occipital cortex and adjacent posterior parietal cortex are necessary for certain types of eye movement (see Chapter 8), and it has been suggested that in some cases, macular sparing is an artifact of testing caused by uncontrollable slight movements of the patient's eyes during examination of the visual fields.

pulvinar of the thalamus. The role of this association cortex includes, among other complex aspects of vision, the relating of present to past visual experiences, recognition of what is seen, and appreciation of its significance. Different parts of the visual association cortex have different functions. These have been determined experimentally in monkeys and have been inferred from the deficits that follow destructive lesions in the human brain. The cortex of the superior part of the occipital lobe and posterior part of the parietal lobe is functionally distinct from that of the inferior parts of the occipital and temporal lobes. These two large regions of visual association cortex are known, respectively, as the **"where?"** and the **"what?"** streams of visual processing. Whereas the dorsal "where?" stream analyzes motion and spatial relations, the ventral "what?" stream identifies colors and familiar shapes such as faces and letters. Lesions that involve the visual association cortex result in various types of **visual agnosia**.

Corticotectal fibers connect the visual cortex, the visual association cortex, and the posterior part of the parietal lobe with the superior colliculus of the midbrain. Through indirect connections, the superior colliculus controls the oculomotor, trochlear, and abducens nuclei (see Chapter 8). This is part of a pathway for fixation of gaze and for tracking of a moving object in the field of vision. It also participates in the accommodation–convergence reaction when looking at a near object. These motor aspects of the occipital and parietal cortex are related to those of the frontal eye field, which are described later in this chapter.

HEARING

The **primary auditory area** (acoustic area) is concealed because it is located in the ventral wall of the lateral sulcus (Fig. 15-4; see also Fig. 15-1). The superior surface of the superior temporal gyrus, forming the floor of the sulcus, is marked by transverse temporal gyri. The two most ante-

---

CLINICAL NOTE

Visual Agnosias

Destructive lesions in visual association cortex cause disorders attributable to malfunction of the "where?" and "what?" streams of visual data processing. Bilateral lesions that involve the superior parts of area 19 cause **visual disorientation**, with an inability to recognize the extent of the visual field and to perceive moving objects. A lesion in the superior part of the occipital lobe commonly extends onto the adjacent visual association cortex of the parietal lobe, causing **ocular apraxia**, which is the inability to direct the gaze at a consciously selected target in the visual field because rapid eye movements (i.e., saccades; see Chapter 8) are inaccurate. Ocular apraxia is associated with **optic ataxia**, which is a loss of the ability to carry out visually guided movements of the hands. The combination of visual disorientation, ocular apraxia, and optic ataxia is known as **Balint's syndrome**.

A lesion in the inferior surface of the occipital cortex anterior to the primary visual area causes **acquired achromatopsia**, which is loss of color vision in the contralateral halves of the visual fields of both eyes, indicating the normal involvement of this cortex in color vision.

The inferolateral surface of the temporal lobe (inferior temporal and the lateral and medial occipitotemporal gyri) is also visual association cortex. Electrical stimulation of this region evokes vivid hallucinations of scenes from the past, indicating a role of this cortex in the storage or recall of **visual memories**. Destruction of the inferior surfaces of the occipital and temporal lobes associated with damage to the superior part of the visual association cortex causes **apperceptive visual agnosia**, which can take various forms. The lesions are usually bilateral but are sometimes present only on the right side. The condition is called **prosopagnosia** when the patient has an impaired recognition of previously known familiar faces. This is part of a more general failure to appreciate shapes, and patients are also unable to make simple pictures by putting together a few pieces. Other types of apperceptive agnosia include an inability to recognize buildings or familiar objects viewed from unusual angles. The posterior part of the medial occipitotemporal gyrus (fusiform gyrus) is particularly associated with recognition of faces and is known as the **fusiform face area**.

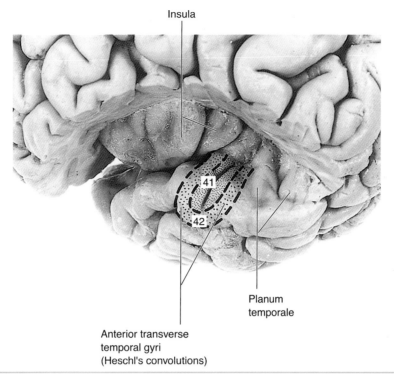

Insula

41

42

Planum
temporale

Anterior transverse
temporal gyri
(Heschl's convolutions)

FIGURE 15-4   Primary auditory cortex on the superior surface of the left temporal lobe, exposed by removing the frontal and parietal opercula.

rior of these, called **Heschl's convolutions**, are the classical landmarks for the auditory area, which corresponds to Brodmann's areas 41 and 42. Recordings made from neurosurgical patients indicate that only the posteromedial part of this region is primary auditory cortex.

The medial geniculate body of the thalamus is the principal source of axons that end in the primary auditory cortex, with these fibers constituting the auditory radiation in the cerebral white matter. A spatial representation is present in the auditory area with respect to the pitch of sounds.

Impulses for low frequencies impinge on the anterolateral part of the area, and impulses for high frequencies impinge on the posteromedial part. The medial geniculate body receives signals that originate in both ears, ensuring bilateral cortical representation (see Chapter 21).

TASTE

The **taste area** (gustatory area) is adjacent to the general sensory area for the tongue at the inferior end of the postcentral gyrus (area 43,

---

CLINICAL NOTE

Auditory Cortex Lesions

An epileptic seizure that originates in the primary auditory area typically begins with perception of a roaring sound, apparently originating from somewhere contralateral to the affected temporal lobe. With other types of temporal lobe epilepsy, auditory hallucinations are usually not localized by the patient to either of the ears.

Sometimes a unilateral destructive lesion involving the auditory area results in difficulty with the interpretation of complex combinations of sounds, but it causes almost no impairment of hearing in the contralateral ear. Large bilateral lesions in the temporal lobes are rare, but they can cause bilateral deafness, among other symptoms.

Auditory Agnosias

The **auditory association cortex** for more elaborate perception of acoustic information occupies the floor of the lateral sulcus behind the auditory area (the region labeled *planum temporale* in Fig. 15-4) and the posterior part of Brodmann's area 22 on the lateral surface of the superior temporal gyrus. In the left cerebral hemisphere of most people, the region of cortex thus defined is also known as **Wernicke's area** and is of major importance in language functions. Bilateral

destruction of the auditory association cortices causes **auditory agnosia,** in which patients fail to identify and respond appropriately to complex sounds. In severe cases, speech cannot be distinguished from other auditory stimuli. If the lesion is located in the hemisphere (usually the left) that is dominant for linguistic functions, the patient has receptive aphasia, a condition discussed later in this chapter. A lesion on the right side can cause **amusia**, which is loss of the ability to recognize previously familiar voices and music.

Fig. 15-1) and extends onto the insula and then anteriorly to the frontal operculum. Nerve impulses from taste buds reach the gustatory nucleus in the brain stem (i.e., the rostral part of the solitary nucleus; see Chapters 7 and 8). Fibers from the gustatory nucleus travel in the ipsilateral central tegmental tract to the most medial part of the medial division of the ventral posterior nucleus of the thalamus. The pathway is completed by thalamocortical fibers.

OLFACTION

Most of the fibers of the olfactory tract (see Chapter 17) end in the region of the limen insulae and the uncus (area 34) and the underlying amygdaloid body. Some end in the entorhinal cortex (area 28), which is also a major component of the limbic system (see Chapter 18) used for acquiring and recalling memories. The proximity of olfactory and gustatory areas in the region of the insula suggests that this may be a site of integration of the two special senses that are functionally related to feeding. Insular cortex is also involved in the control of visceral functions. The lateral part of the orbital surface of the frontal lobe receives projections from the primary olfactory areas and is presumed to be involved in behavioral reactions to recognized odors.

VESTIBULAR REPRESENTATION

Neuroanatomical tracing studies in animals reveal ascending fibers from the vestibular nuclei that are almost entirely crossed, travel near the medial lemniscus, and end in and near the

medial division of the ventral posterior nucleus (VPm) of the thalamus. The VPm also receives fibers for somatic sensation from the head. In studies of monkeys, electrical stimulation of the vestibular nerve evokes potentials in the anterior end of the intraparietal sulcus, in the nearby somatosensory cortex, and in the posterior part of the insula. These areas are strategically placed for the integration of vestibular input with proprioceptive signals from muscles that act on the head. Similar areas have been identified by PET and fMRI scans after stimulation of the human vestibular nerve. No cortical area is known that is activated exclusively by the vestibular system. The cortical projection of the vestibular system presumably contributes to motor regulation, awareness of spatial orientation, and sensations of vertigo and nausea associated with excessive vestibular stimulation.

OTHER ASSOCIATION CORTEX

Areas of association cortex adjacent to the main sensory areas and closely related functionally to them have already been described. Additional association cortex is located in the parietal lobe and in the posterior part of the temporal lobe. Data reaching the sensory areas and analyzed in the adjacent association cortex are correlated in this intervening region to yield a comprehensive assessment of the immediate environment. The association cortex of the three "sensory" lobes has abundant connections with cortex of the frontal lobe through long fasciculi in the white matter of the cerebral hemisphere (see Chapter 16). Complex and flexible behavioral patterns are formulated on the basis of experience, emotional tones are added, and overt expression may follow through the motor system.

The anterior part of the temporal lobe, similar to the area for visual memory on its inferolateral surface, appears to have special properties related to thought and memory. Electrical stimulation of this region in conscious subjects may elicit recall of objects seen, music heard, or other experiences in the recent or distant past. Patients with a temporal lobe tumor may have auditory or visual hallucinations that reproduce earlier events. The connections and functions of the medial parts of the temporal lobe, along with those of the cingulate gyrus, are discussed in more detail in Chapter 18.

The total expanse of parieto-occipitotemporal and frontal association cortex is responsible for many of the unique qualities of the human brain. **Engrams**, or long-term memory traces, are laid down over the years, possibly as macromolecular changes in neurons and structural changes in synapses throughout the cerebral cortex. These form the basis of learning at an intellectual level and of skills acquired through practice. The complex neuronal circuitry of the cortex permits the coalescence of memory traces in the form of ideas and conceptual, abstract thinking. Recently acquired information is not consolidated into long-term memory if bilateral lesions are present in the limbic system (see Chapter 18). There is no localized disease that causes loss of established memories, indicating that the engram is contained in many parts of the brain. Rare instances of permanent amnesia that occur after head injury are probably caused by failure of the recalling mechanisms because most amnesic patients eventually recover their memories. The eventual failure of all intellectual function in advanced cases of Alzheimer's disease and other types of dementia is attributed to the loss of enormous numbers of neurons throughout the cerebral cortex and in various subcortical nuclei. For more information about memory, see Chapter 18.

Frontal Cortex

The neocortex of the frontal lobe has a special role in motor activities, in the attributes of judgment and foresight, and in determining mood or affect.

PRIMARY MOTOR AREA

The **primary motor area** has been identified on the basis of elicitation of motor responses at a low threshold of electrical stimulation. The area is located in the precentral gyrus, including the anterior wall of the central sulcus, and in the anterior part of the paracentral lobule on the medial surface of the hemisphere (see Figs. 15-1 and 15-2). Neurons other than pyramidal cells are not easily recognized in this cortex, and the six layers are difficult to define. Giant pyramidal cells (Betz cells), present in small numbers in layer 5, occur only in the primary motor area.

The main sources of input to area 4 are the other motor areas of the cortex, the somesthetic cortex, and the posterior division of the ventral lateral thalamic nucleus (VLp), which, in turn, receives input from the cerebellum. Although area 4 contributes fibers to several motor pathways, the efferents that give it a special significance are those included in the **pyramidal system**, which comprises the corticospinal and corticobulbar tracts. In monkeys, 30% of these fibers arise in area 4; another 30% come from area 6; and about 40% arise in the parietal lobe, notably the first somatic sensory area. The Betz cells contribute some 30,000 large, thickly myelinated axons to the corticospinal tract of each side, accounting for about 3% of the tract's axons. The rapidly conducting axons of Betz cells probably have some terminal branches that synapse directly with motor neurons. Other neurons in the primary motor cortex have axons that end in the motor regions of the reticular formation (see also Chapter 23).

Electrical or magnetic stimulation of the primary motor area elicits contraction of muscles that are mainly on the opposite side of the body. Although cortical control of the skeletal musculature is predominantly contralateral, there is some ipsilateral control of most of the muscles of the head and of the axial muscles of the body. The body is represented in the motor area as inverted, with the pattern or homunculus (see Fig. 15-3) being similar to that of the somesthetic cortex. The sequence, from below upward, begins with the pharynx, larynx, tongue, and face; the region for muscles of the head comprises about one third of area 4. Continuing dorsally, there is a small region for muscles of the neck, followed by a large area for muscles of the hand; this is consistent with the functional importance of manual dexterity. Next in order are small areas for the arm, shoulder, trunk, and thigh, continuing with an area on the medial surface of the hemisphere for the remainder of the leg and the foot.

The primary motor area has a lower threshold of excitability than other areas from which contraction of skeletal muscles can be elicited by electrical stimulation. Contractions are usually of contralateral muscles, as has been noted, and the muscles responding depend on the part of area 4 that is stimulated. The response typically involves muscles that make up a functional group, although contraction of a single muscle occasionally occurs. Studies with microelectrodes in laboratory animals indicate that small clusters of columns of cortical neurons control individual muscles.

SUPPLEMENTARY AND CINGULATE MOTOR AREAS

A **supplementary motor area** and a **cingulate motor area** have been identified by cortical stimulation in primates, including humans. The supplementary motor area is located in the part of area 6 that lies on the medial surface of the hemisphere (see Fig. 15-2), and the cingulate motor area is located in the adjoining cortex of the anterior half of the cingulate sulcus. Both of these cortical areas receive input from many other cortical areas and from the ventral anterior (VA) and the anterior division of the ventral lateral (VLa) nucleus of the thalamus. Efferent axons go into the corticospinal and corticobulbar tracts, to motor regions of the reticular formation, and to the primary motor area (Fig. 15-5).

Electrical stimulation in humans indicates a somatotopic organization of the supplementary motor area, with the face represented rostrally and the lower limbs in the caudal part of the region. The effects of stimulation are predominantly contralateral and are preceded by a conscious urge to make the movements. Increased regional blood flow in the supplementary motor area can be demonstrated during the mental processes that precede the execution of a movement. The anterior cingulate area exhibits increased activity during anticipation of motor and purely cognitive tasks.

Results of experiments in monkeys indicate that loss of function of the supplementary mo-

CLINICAL NOTE

Motor Cortex Lesions

The primary motor area may be abnormally irritated by, for example, a small tumor or a splinter of bone from a fracture of the skull. The resulting scarring of cortical tissue causes episodes of abnormal excitation of the neurons, with involuntary twitching movements of the corresponding part of the body. Most frequently, this is the mouth, tongue, or thumb, regions that account for much of the area of the precentral gyrus. Typically, these movements are the beginning of a **jacksonian seizure**. As the abnormal cortical activity spreads across the precentral gyrus, a progression of jerking movements to other muscles takes place, leading eventually to generalized convulsions. The study of this type of epilepsy by John Hughlings Jackson (1835–1911, English clinical neurologist) provided early evidence for the representation of the opposite side of the body in the precentral and postcentral gyri. For more about epilepsy, see Chapters 9 and 18.

Damage in the primary motor area, without involvement of adjacent cortex or underlying white matter, is seldom encountered clinically. Deficits resulting from such damage are inferred from results of experiments on nonhuman primates and from isolated human cases in which part of area 4 was removed as a therapeutic procedure, as in the treatment of jacksonian epilepsy.

A destructive lesion in area 4 results in paresis (weakness) of the affected part of the opposite side of the body. The muscles involved are flaccid if the damage is restricted to the precentral gyrus. The much more common condition of spastic paralysis is characteristically caused by lesions that spread beyond area 4 or that interrupt fibers in the subcortical white matter or internal capsule. Considerable recovery occurs with time, with the residual deficit being most evident as weakness in the distal parts of the limbs.

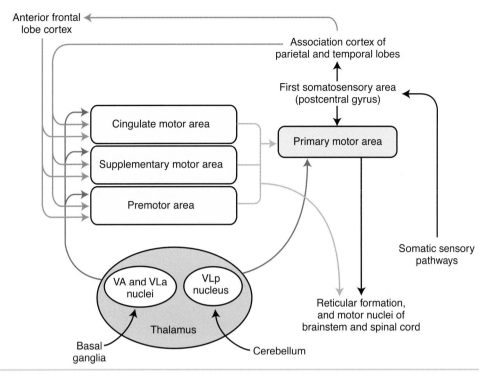

FIGURE 15-5   Connections of the motor areas of the cerebral cortex. The primary motor area is influenced by many other cortical areas, but descending motor projections from all cortical motor areas are also present. The interactions of the cerebellum and basal ganglia with the cerebral cortex are discussed in Chapters 10, 12, and 23. VA, ventral anterior; VLa, ventral lateral anterior; VLp, ventral lateral posterior.

tor area may cause the spasticity of muscles paralyzed as the result of an "upper motor neuron" lesion. Infarctions involving the human supplementary and cingulate motor areas of either side cause loss of most volitional movements and loss of the power of speech. Evidently, patients with this condition, known as **akinetic mutism**, have no motivation or will to move or speak. These patients often recover completely after a few weeks. Akinetic mutism is more severe and longer lasting if bilateral lesions are present. A clinically similar condition, also called akinetic mutism, can follow infarction of the medial part of the reticular formation in the rostral pons or midbrain (see Chapter 23).

PREMOTOR AREA

The premotor area is situated in Brodmann's area 6 anterior to the primary motor area on the lateral surface of the hemisphere (see Fig. 15-1). In addition to connections with other cortical areas, the premotor cortex receives fibers from the VA and the anterior division of the VLa nu-

cleus of the thalamus, which, in turn, receive input from the pallidum of the corpus striatum (Chapter 12).

The premotor area contributes to motor function as one of the sources of the pyramidal and other descending motor pathways and by its influence on the primary motor cortex (see Fig. 15-5 and Chapter 23). The premotor and supplementary motor areas generate programs for motor routines necessary for skilled voluntary action, both when a new program is established and when a previously learned program is altered. In general, the primary motor area is the cortex through which commands are channeled for the *execution* of movements. In contrast, the premotor and supplementary motor areas program skilled motor activity and thus *direct* the primary motor area in its execution. Connections of the premotor area with the posterior part of the parietal lobe provide an integrated system for the use of visual, proprioceptive, and other sensory information in the preparation of movements.

Apraxia

The term **apraxia** refers to the result of a cerebral lesion characterized by impairment in the performance of learned movements in the absence of paralysis. One form of apraxia follows a lesion that involves the premotor area. The disability includes functional impairment of muscles that work on the proximal joints of the limbs, especially the shoulder. The ability to carry out tasks at arm's length is then severely impaired. Other forms of apraxia are caused by lesions that involve the somesthetic association cortex of the parietal lobe because proprioception is a necessary background for motor proficiency. When the disability affects writing, it is called **agraphia**. Agraphia without impairment of speech typically results from damage to the left angular gyrus, which is located in the inferior part of the parietal lobe, a site strategically placed between the visual association cortex and the cortical language areas, which are discussed later.

Frontal Eye Field

The **frontal eye field** is located in the lower part of area 8 on the lateral surface of the hemisphere. It controls voluntary conjugate saccadic movements of the eyes. Electrical stimulation of the frontal eye field causes deviation of the eyes to the opposite side. The cortex of the frontal eye field is also active during pursuit movements, but this and convergence of the eyes are principally directed by the cortex of the occipital lobe and adjacent parts of the parietal lobe. Convergence is another ocular movement that is not controlled by the frontal eye fields. The connections of the cortical eye fields are explained in connection with eye movements in Chapter 8.

Destruction of the frontal eye field causes conjugate deviation of the eyes toward the side of the lesion. This condition is frequently seen as part of a larger syndrome dominated by hemiplegia and is attributable to a large vascular lesion that puts the motor areas of the cortex out of action. The deviated eyes are directed (as if in horror) away from the paralyzed side of the body. The patient, if conscious, cannot voluntarily move his or her eyes in the opposite direction, but this movement does occur when the eyes follow an object moving across the field of vision.

PREFRONTAL CORTEX

The large expanse of cortex in the frontal lobe from which motor responses are not elicited on stimulation falls under the heading of association cortex. This region envelops the frontal pole and is called the **prefrontal cortex**. Corresponding to Brodmann's areas 9, 10, 11, and 12, it is well developed only in primates, especially in humans. The prefrontal cortex has extensive connections through association fasciculi (see Chapter 16) with the cortex of the parietal, temporal, and occipital lobes, thus gaining access to contemporary sensory experience and to the repository of data derived from past experiences. Reciprocal connections are also present with the amygdaloid body in the temporal lobe and with the mediodorsal thalamic nucleus, forming a system that determines affective reactions to present situations on the basis of past experiences. The prefrontal cortex also monitors behavior and exercises control based on such higher mental faculties as judgment and foresight. The lateral part of the orbital surface of the frontal lobe has already been mentioned as association cortex for olfaction. This is a sense that can evoke a wide range of mental and visceral feelings, such as pleasurable anticipation, nostalgia, disgust, nausea, and so on.

FUNCTIONAL AREAS WITHIN THE PREFRONTAL CORTEX

Language Areas

The use of language is a peculiarly human accomplishment, requiring special neural mechanisms in association areas of the cerebral cortex. Areas of the cortex that have particular roles with respect to language have been known for more than a century from the study of patients with cortical damage caused by occlusion of blood vessels. The infarcted regions of the brain were first identified postmortem.

Prefrontal Lobe Disorders

Knowledge of the functions of the prefrontal cortex is derived largely from the effects of diseases and injuries. Some diseases affect the frontal lobes more than other parts of the brain. Examples include **general paralysis of the insane** (one of many effects of syphilis, a bacterial infection) and **Pick's disease** (in which neurons degenerate for no known reason, leading to dementia). The prefrontal cortex can also be damaged by appropriately placed tumors and by penetrating injuries.

The classical case of prefrontal lobe damage was that of Phineas Gage, an American railroad construction worker injured in 1848 by the premature explosion of a blasting charge. This drove an iron-tamping rod (105 cm long and 3 cm in diameter) through his head. The missile entered through Gage's left cheek and emerged from his right frontal bone, anterior to the coronal suture, having passed through the left orbit and the anterior parts of both frontal lobes of the brain. Gage's motor and speech areas were spared by the injury, and the most conspicuous abnormalities were in his changed personality, with loss of his former industriousness, self-restraint, patience, and consideration for others. These changes persisted until his death nearly 20 years later.

The operation of **prefrontal leukotomy** (or lobotomy) was introduced by de Egas Moniz in 1935. This simple surgical procedure, which interrupts the connections between the thalami and the cortices of the orbital surfaces of the frontal lobes, was formerly performed as treatment for various mental disorders.

A person with bilateral loss of function of the prefrontal cortex typically becomes rude, inconsiderate to others, incapable of accepting advice, and unable to anticipate the consequences of rash or reckless words or actions. The patient no longer suffers from anxiety or depression or even from severe pain, although there is no loss of awareness of pain. Despite the profoundly changed personality, memory and intellect are spared. The awarding of a share of the Nobel Prize for medicine and physiology to de Egas Moniz in 1949 recognized prefrontal leukotomy as a major advance in the relief of suffering but perhaps without due concern for the importance of the accompanying personality changes. By the 1960s, the operation was reserved for patients with severe affective disorders who did not respond to drugs and psychotherapy. Since the 1970s, the operation has seldom been deemed justifiable. Stereotactic lesions beneath the heads of the caudate nuclei may relieve affective disorders with fewer adverse effects than complete prefrontal leukotomy, but the consequences of the operation are still permanent.

Behavioral and Affective Disorders

The ventral and medial parts of the prefrontal cortex are those most associated with acceptable social interactions. **Acquired sociopathy** is a name given to the abnormal behavioral state that follows bilateral damage to this region. Lesions in the right ventral prefrontal cortex can cause **anosognosia**, in which the patient does not acknowledge that there is anything wrong with a paralyzed limb or other severe disability or loss of cognitive powers. Causative lesions include tumors, surgical damage, and hemorrhage from an aneurysm of the anterior communicating artery. Slowly developing bilateral degeneration of extensive areas of prefrontal cortex occurs in **general paralysis of the insane**, which is a manifestation of syphilis of the central nervous system, and in **Pick's disease**, the cause of which is unknown. The same areas degenerate in some cases of **Alzheimer's disease** (see also Chapter 12). These are diseases in which **dementia** or generalized deterioration of the memory and intellect are present, but the involvement of the prefrontal cortex causes additional behavioral abnormalities similar to those that occur after prefrontal leukotomy.

Depression can occur with many diseases that affect the cerebral cortex, although detectable lesions are absent from the majority of people with this disabling symptom. A single cortical lesion in a depressed patient is more likely to be located in the inferior part of the prefrontal cortex than elsewhere, but the causal relationship, if any, is not understood.

More accurate information was obtained with the availability of computed tomography and nuclear magnetic resonance imaging (MRI) to scan the brains of living patients. With PET and, more recently, fMRI, it is possible to localize parts of the normal brain that are selectively activated in such activities as listening, reading, speaking, and writing. (These imaging techniques are reviewed in Chapter 4.)

Two cortical areas have specialized language functions (Fig. 15-6). The **receptive language area** (also called the *sensory language area* or *posterior speech area*) consists of the auditory association cortex (Wernicke's area) in the posterior part of the superior temporal gyrus. Reading involves visual association cortex in the inferior parts of the occipital and temporal lobes, which is connected with Wernicke's area (for interpretation of words) and with the cortex of the angular gyrus (for formulation of commands that can be sent to the motor cortex for writing). The **expressive speech area** (Broca's area, motor speech area, or anterior speech area) occupies the opercular and triangular parts of the inferior frontal gyrus, corresponding to Brodmann's areas 44 and 45, together with the adjacent anterior part of the insula. The integrity of the **supplementary motor area** on the medial surface of the hemisphere is also necessary for normal speech. The language areas are situated in the left hemisphere with few exceptions, and this is, therefore, the dominant hemisphere as a rule with respect to language. The receptive and expressive language areas are in communication with each other through the **superior longitudinal (arcuate) fasciculus** in the white matter of the hemisphere (Chapter 16).

fMRI investigations reveal activation in the posterior part of the right superior temporal gyrus associated with speaking. This area may send instructions to the primary motor cortical areas for the muscles of articulation and respiration, which are bilateral.

Hemispheral Dominance

Memory traces established in one hemisphere (e.g., in the cortex of the left hemisphere as a result of some particular activity involving the right hand) are transferred to the cortex of the other hemisphere through the corpus callosum. Therefore, bilateral cortical memory patterns exist for previous experiences.

LEFT HEMISPHERE FUNCTIONS

In right-handed people and in most left-handed people, language is a function of the left hemisphere. The "talking" hemisphere is said to be

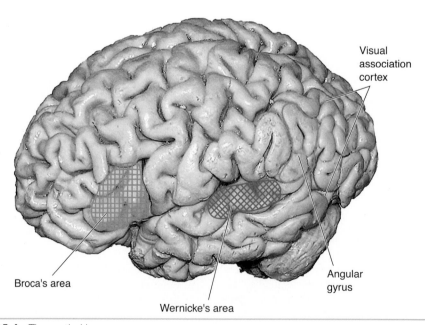

Visual association cortex

Broca's area

Wernicke's area

Angular gyrus

FIGURE 15-6 The cortical language areas.

Aphasia

Damage to the language areas or their connections results in aphasia; there are several types, depending on the location of the lesion (see Table 15-1). **Receptive aphasia** (Wernicke's aphasia), in which auditory and visual comprehension of language, naming of objects, and repetition of a sentence spoken by the examiner are all defective, is caused by a lesion in the receptive language area, notably in Wernicke's area. Infarcts that isolate the sensory language area from surrounding parietal and temporal cortex may cause **anomic aphasia** (isolation syndrome), characterized by fluent but circumlocutory speech caused by word-finding difficulties. Some authorities doubt the existence of anomic aphasia as a distinct clinical entity because most patients with lesions in the left parietal lobe have difficulty with naming. Some patients cannot understand words and sentences or produce intelligible speech, but they can correctly repeat what the examiner says. This disorder is called **transcortical aphasia** of the receptive (or sensory) type, and it is associated with destruction of cortex in the middle temporal gyrus, inferior and posterior to Wernicke's receptive language area.

Alexia refers to loss of the ability to read and is a common accompaniment of aphasia caused by temporal or parietal lobe lesions. In most cases, alexia is accompanied by **agraphia**, the inability to write. **Pure alexia** (without agraphia and with normal comprehension of spoken words) may result either from a single lesion lateral to the occipital horn of the left lateral ventricle or from a combination of two lesions, one in the left occipital lobe and the other in the splenium of the corpus callosum. Such lesions sever connections between both visual cortices and the unilaterally located language areas. **Dyslexia** is incomplete alexia and is characterized by an inability to read more than a few lines with understanding. **Developmental dyslexia** is a common condition in children of normal intelligence who have difficulty learning to read. MRI examination reveals that some such children lack the usual anatomical asymmetry in the size of the planum temporale on the left and right sides.

Expressive aphasia (Broca's aphasia), which is caused by a lesion in Broca's area of the frontal lobe, is characterized by hesitant and distorted speech with relatively good comprehension. Whereas a patient with Broca's aphasia can hear that he or she is talking nonsense, one with receptive aphasia talks fluently without being aware of the failure to produce meaningful words. A cortical lesion anterior to Broca's expressive speech area causes **transcortical aphasia** of the expressive (or motor) type. The impairment of spontaneous speech is similar to Broca's aphasia, but the patient can accurately repeat words or phrases spoken by someone else. The term **global aphasia** refers to a virtually complete loss of the ability to communicate after destruction of the cortex on both sides of the lateral sulcus. This is one of the consequences of occlusion of the left middle cerebral artery (see Chapter 25).

Interruption of the arcuate fasciculus connecting Wernicke's and Broca's areas causes **conduction aphasia**, in which the patient has poor repetition of a sentence spoken by the examiner but relatively good comprehension and spontaneous speech. Aphasia can also result from lesions in the subcortical gray matter of the hemisphere that is dominant for speech. In **subcortical aphasia**, the patient has impairment of language production and comprehension associated with **dysarthria** (attributable to faulty control of the muscles of the larynx and mouth) and contralateral hemiparesis. The lesion is most commonly either laterally located in the left thalamus or involves the head of the left caudate nucleus.

Patients usually have some recovery of function, even in severe cases of aphasia. This is attributed to assumption of linguistic functions by the intact contralateral cerebral hemisphere.

dominant relative to the "nontalking" hemisphere. A left-sided cerebral lesion is therefore more serious than one in the right hemisphere because aphasia may be added to other neurological deficits. The reverse is true for the few whose right hemisphere is dominant for linguistic functions.

Although factors that determine hemispheral dominance for speech are not well known, heredity is almost certainly involved to some extent. The **planum temporale** posterior to the auditory area on the dorsal (superior) surface of the superior temporal gyrus (see Fig. 15-4) is larger in the left than in the right hemisphere in 65% of human brains and larger on the right side in only 11% of brains. This indicates that the dominance with respect to language may be

TABLE 15-1 **Agnosias, Aphasias, and Other Disorders of the Association Cortex**

Disorder	Site of Lesion
Agnosias	
Tactile agnosia (including astereognosis)	Left or right anterior parietal lobe posterior to primary somesthetic area
Cortical neglect	Right (usually) superior parietal lobe; may extend to occipital lobe

Apperceptive visual agnosia
    Acquired achromatopsia
    Prosopagnosia
	Left and right inferior occipital cortex
	Right (usually also left) inferior occipital and posterolateral temporal cortex

Associative visual agnosia	Occipitotemporal cortex, bilaterally

Balint syndrome—combination of:
    Visual disorientation
    Ocular apraxia
    Optic ataxia
	
	Left and right superior occipital cortex
	Posterior parietal cortex
	Posterior parietal cortex

Auditory agnosia	Posterior, superior temporal cortex, bilaterally
Amusia	Right posterior, superior temporal cortex
Disordered control of movement	
Akinetic mutism	Left and right supplementary and cingulate motor areas
Apraxia	Left or right premotor area (positioning of limb) or anterior, inferior parietal cortex (caused by astereognosis)
Agraphia (without aphasia)	Left angular gyrus
Behavioral and affective changes	
Acquired sociopathy	Ventromedial prefrontal cortex, usually bilaterally
Anosognosia (and anosodiaphoria)	Either right inferior parietal cortex or right inferior medial prefrontal cortex
Depression	Left prefrontal cortex more often than other localized lesions
Speech and language disorders	
Receptive (Wernicke's) aphasia	Left posterior, superior temporal cortex (Wernicke's area)
Anomic aphasia	Left parietal lobe posterior to Wernicke's area

Transcortical aphasia:
    Receptive type
    Expressive type
	
	Left middle temporal gyrus inferior to Wernicke's area
	Left frontal lobe anterior to Broca's area

Alexia with agraphia	Wernicke's area and left angular gyrus
Pure alexia (without agraphia):	Left occipital lobe and associated commissural fibers either in the underlying white matter or in the splenium of the corpus callosum
Expressive (Broca's) aphasia	Left frontal operculum (Broca's area)
Global aphasia	Whole left perisylvian area (frontal, parietal, and temporal opercula)
Conduction aphasia	Left inferior parietal lobe (supramarginal gyrus) and underlying arcuate fasciculus
Subcortical aphasia	Head of left caudate nucleus; left thalamus
Aprosodia	Right perisylvian area (frontal, parietal, and temporal opercula)

It is assumed that the language areas are in the left cerebral hemisphere.

reflected in structural asymmetry because the left planum temporale constitutes a large part of Wernicke's receptive language area. Functional MRI shows that the left planum temporale is less active than the adjacent cortical areas (i.e., superior temporal sulcus, middle temporal gyrus, angular gyrus) in subjects listening to words. This observation indicates that the planum temporale may be involved in stages of auditory processing that precede the paying of attention to formed elements of language.

About 75% of the population is right-handed, preferring the right hand for skilled tasks. In these people, the right hand is controlled by the left cerebral hemisphere, which is also the dominant hemisphere for language. Handedness is not always correlated with linguistic dominance because 70% of those who are left-handed have their language areas in the left hemisphere rather than in the one that controls the left hand.

RIGHT HEMISPHERE FUNCTIONS

For some activities, the right hemisphere is the dominant one in most people. The most notable faculty residing in the right hemisphere is three-dimensional, or spatial, perception. The evidence is derived partly from studies of patients with right-sided lesions and partly from investigation of those in whom the corpus callosum has been transected as a therapeutic measure in severe epilepsy. After commissurotomy, these patients were able to copy drawings and arrange blocks in a desired position more efficiently with the left hand than with the right hand. The right hemisphere is therefore better equipped to direct such acts.

Spatial awareness extends to the whole body and its surroundings, and this awareness is lost contralaterally in the condition of cortical neglect discussed in connection with the somesthetic association cortex. Severe cortical neglect most often occurs after development of a right-sided lesion. The condition of **anosognosia**, discussed in connection with the prefrontal cortex, is also caused by right-sided damage. Anosognosia can also develop after injury to the right parietal lobe.

Although it is not essential for verbal communication, the right cerebral cortex, on both sides of the lateral sulcus (sylvian fissure), is necessary for **prosody**, which is the combination of tones, cadences, and emphasis on particular words and syllables that normally contribute to the thoughts being conveyed. Loss of function of the right perisylvian cortex leads to **aprosodia**, in which the voice is monotonous and the speech apparently has no emotional content. Related abilities for which the right hemisphere dominates are singing, the playing of musical instruments, and the recognition and appreciation of music. Musical skills and comprehension are commonly lost (**amusia**) after the development of vascular occlusions that cause infarction of the posterior part of the right superior temporal gyrus. Patients severely aphasic from lesions in the left hemisphere sometimes retain the ability to sing.

Suggested Reading

Allison T, McCarthy G, Wood CC, et al. Human cortical potentials evoked by stimulation of the median nerve: I and II. *J Neurophysiol* 1989;62:694–722.

Asanuma H. *The Motor Cortex.* New York: Raven Press, 1989.

Augustine JR. Circuitry and functional aspects of the insular lobe in primates including humans. *Brain Res Rev* 1996;22:229–244.

Binder JR, Frost JA, Hammeke TA, et al. Function of the left planum temporale in auditory and linguistic processing. *Brain* 1996;119:1239–1247.

Bisulli F, Tinuper P, Avoni P, et al. Idiopathic partial epilepsy with auditory features (IPEAF): a clinical and genetic study of 53 sporadic cases. *Brain* 2004;127:1343–1352.

Blumenfeld H. *Neuroanatomy through Clinical Cases.* Sunderland, MS: Sinauer, 2002.

Damasio AR, Tranel D, Damasio H. Face agnosia and the neural substrate of memory. *Annu Rev Neurosci* 1990;13:89–109.

DaSilva AFM, Becerra L, Makis N, et al. Somatotopic activation in the human trigeminal pain pathway. *J Neurosci* 2002;22:8183–8192.

Devinsky O, Morrell MJ, Vogt BA. Contributions of anterior cingulate cortex to behaviour. *Brain* 1995;118:279–306.

de Waele C, Baudonniere PM, Lepecq JC, et al. Vestibular projections in the human cortex. *Exp Brain Res* 2001;141:541–551.

Frith CD, Friston K, Liddle PF, et al. Willed action and the prefrontal cortex in man: a study with PET. *Proc R Soc Lond [Biol]* 1991;244:241–246.

Grefkes C, Fink GR. The functional organization of the intraparietal sulcus in humans and monkeys. *J Anat* 2005;207:3–17.

Iannetti GD, Porro CA, Pantano P, et al. Representation of different trigeminal divisions within the primary and secondary human somatosensory cortex. *Neuroimage* 2003;19:906–912.

James TW, Culham J, Humphrey GK, et al. Ventral occipital lesions impair object recognition but not object-directed grasping: an fMRI study. *Brain* 2003;126:2463–2475.

Kertesz A, Polk M, Black SE, et al. Anatomical asymmetries and functional laterality. *Brain* 1992;115:589–605.

Kurata K. Somatotopy in the human supplementary motor area. *Trends Neurosci* 1992;15:159–160.

Leventhal AG, Ault SJ, Vitek DJ. The nasotemporal division in primate retina: the neural bases of macular sparing and splitting. *Science* 1988;240:66–67.

Liegeois-Chauvel C, Musolino A, Chauvel P. Localization of the primary auditory area in man. *Brain* 1991;114:139–153.

Lobel E, Kleine JF, Le Bihan D, et al. Functional MRI of galvanic vestibular stimulation. *J Neurophysiol* 1998;80:2699–2709.

MacKinnon CD, Kapur S, Hussey D, et al. Contributions of the mesial frontal cortex to the premovement potentials associated with intermittent hand movements in humans. *Hum Brain Mapp* 1996;4:1–22.

Miyashita Y. Inferior temporal cortex: where visual perception meets memory. *Annu Rev Neurosci* 1993;16:245–263.

Muri RM, Ibazizen MT, Derosier C, et al. Location of the human posterior eye field with functional magnetic resonance imaging. *J Neurol Neurosurg Psychiatry* 1996;60:445–448.

Murtha S, Chertkow H, Beauregard M, et al. Anticipation causes increased blood flow to the anterior cingulate cortex. *Hum Brain Mapp* 1996;4:103–112.

Penfield W, Rasmussen T. *The Cerebral Cortex of Man: A Clinical Study of Localization of Function.* New York: Macmillan, 1950.

Polk M, Kertesz A. Music and language in degenerative disease of the brain. *Brain Cogn* 1993;22:98–117.

Price CJ. The anatomy of language: contributions from functional neuroimaging. *J Anat* 2000;197:335–359.

Tehovnik EJ, Sommer MA, Chou IH, et al. Eye fields in the frontal lobes of primates. *Brain Res Rev* 2000;32:413–448.

Tranel D. Higher brain functions. In: Conn PM, ed. *Neuroscience in Medicine.* Philadelphia: Lippincott, 1995:555–580.

Chapter 16

CEREBRAL WHITE MATTER AND LATERAL VENTRICLES

Important Facts

- The white matter of the cerebral hemisphere consists of association, commissural, and projection fibers.

- Most named association bundles (superior longitudinal, arcuate, inferior longitudinal, inferior occipitofrontal, uncinate, and superior occipitofrontal fasciculi) interconnect lobes.

- The cingulum, fornix, and stria terminalis are association bundles of the limbic system.

- The corpus callosum and anterior commissure, which interconnect symmetrical cortical regions, exchange information between the left and right sides.

- After transection of the commissures, a task that is newly learned with one hand cannot be performed by the other. Sensory data that enter only the right hemisphere cannot be put into words because of disconnection from the language areas in the left hemisphere.

- Most projection fibers pass through the internal capsule.

- All parts of the internal capsule contain thalamocortical and corticothalamic fibers.

- Motor fibers, including those of the pyramidal system, descend in the posterior limb of the internal capsule. A small infarct in this area can cause contralateral hemiplegia.

- The geniculocalcarine tract is located in the retrolentiform part of the internal capsule. Some of its fibers loop into the temporal lobe.

- The frontal and central parts of the lateral ventricle have the corpus callosum for the roof, the thalamus and fornix as the floor, the caudate nucleus in the lateral wall, and the septum pellucidum in the medial wall.

- The temporal horn is indented by the amygdala and hippocampus. The occipital horn is indented by the calcarine sulcus.

- The interventricular foramen is bounded by the column of the fornix and the anterior tubercle of the thalamus.

Each cerebral hemisphere includes a large volume of white matter, sometimes called the **medullary center**, that accommodates vast numbers of axons running to and from all parts of the cortex. Axons that establish connections between the cortex and subcortical gray matter continue into the internal capsule. The lateral ventricles, one in each hemisphere, are the largest of the four ventricles of the brain and are important in the dynamics of the cerebrospinal fluid (CSF) system.

Cerebral White Matter

Three types of axons are present in the cerebral white matter (Fig. 16-1). **Association fibers** are confined to a hemisphere and connect one cortical area with another. Many of these fibers accumulate in named longitudinally running bundles that can be displayed by dissection. **Commissural fibers** connect the cortices of the two hemispheres; most are located in the corpus callosum, and the remainder are located in the anterior commissure. **Projection fibers** establish connections between the cortex and such subcortical structures as the corpus striatum, thalamus, brain stem, and spinal cord. They are afferent (corticopetal) or efferent (corticofugal) with respect to the cortex. Most corticopetal projection fibers originate in the thalamus; some ascend from nuclei in the hypothalamus and brain stem (see Chapters 9 and 11).

ASSOCIATION FASCICULI

Association fibers are the most numerous of the three types of fiber noted. Operative procedures, vascular accidents, and lesions that transect the fasciculi may lead to dysfunction

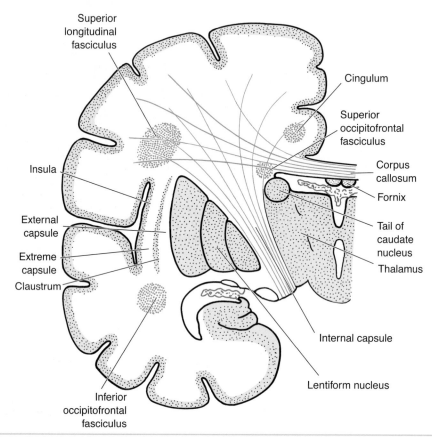

FIGURE 16-1   Coronal section through a cerebral hemisphere, indicating the major bodies of gray matter (yellow) and positions of the larger bundles of association, commissural, and projection fibers (blue). The choroid plexus of the lateral and third ventricles is outlined in red.

by disconnecting functionally related regions of the cerebral cortex.

The **cingulum**, which is most easily displayed by dissection in the cingulate gyrus (Figs. 16-2 and 16-3), is an association fasciculus of the limbic lobe. The axons in this longitudinal bundle run in both directions and interconnect the cingulate gyrus, parahippocampal gyrus of the temporal lobe, and septal area below the genu of the corpus callosum.

The **superior longitudinal fasciculus** (see Figs. 16-2 and 16-3), also known as the **arcuate fasciculus,** runs in an anteroposterior direction above the insula, and many of the fibers turn downward into the temporal lobe. This, similar to the other large association bundles, consists of axons of various lengths that enter or leave the fasciculus at any point along its course. The superior longitudinal fasciculus provides important communications between cortices of the parietal, temporal, and occipital lobes and the cortex of the

frontal lobe. These provide a pathway whereby interpreted sensory signals (especially visual and proprioceptive) from the parietal cortex influence the formulation in the frontal lobe of neuronal programs for appropriate movements. The arcuate fasciculus also includes fibers that connect the receptive (sensory) and expressive (motor) language areas (see Chapter 15). An **inferior longitudinal fasciculus,** beneath the lateral and ventral surfaces of the occipital and temporal lobes, is difficult to demonstrate by dissection.

The **inferior occipitofrontal fasciculus** and **uncinate fasciculus** are components of a single association system (Figs. 16-4 and 16-5). The fibers are compressed into a well-defined bundle below the insula and lentiform nucleus. The longer part of the fiber system, extending the length of the hemisphere, is the inferior occipitofrontal fasciculus. The uncinate fasciculus is the part that hooks around the stem of the lateral sulcus to connect the frontal lobe, espe-

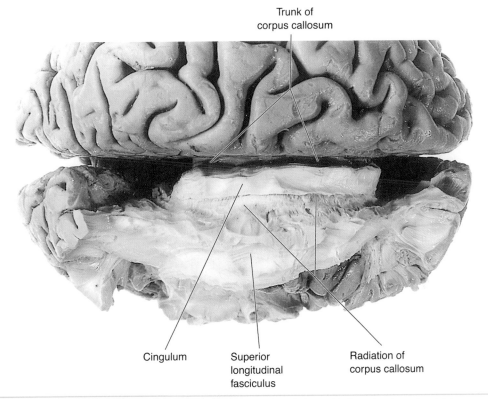

FIGURE 16-2   Dissection of the right cerebral hemisphere: dorsal view with frontal pole at the right.

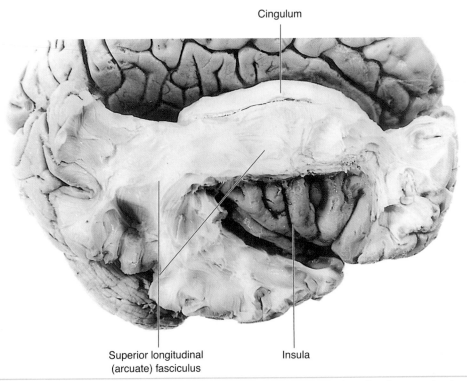

FIGURE 16-3   Dissection of the right cerebral hemisphere: dorsal view with frontal and temporal poles at the right.

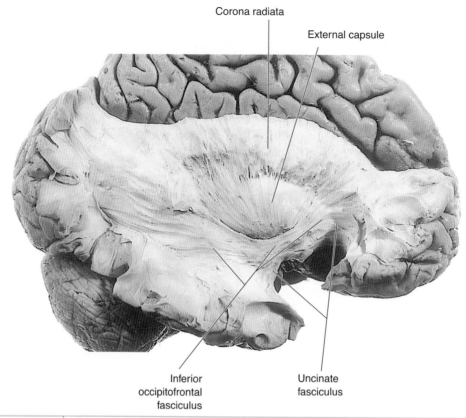

Corona radiata

External capsule

Inferior
occipitofrontal
fasciculus

Uncinate
fasciculus

FIGURE 16-4   White matter of the right cerebral hemisphere after removal of the superior longitudinal fasciculus, insula, and underlying structures down to the external capsule.

cially cortex on its orbital surface, with cortex in the region of the temporal pole.

The **superior occipitofrontal fasciculus**, also called the **subcallosal bundle**, is located deep in the hemisphere (see Fig. 16-1). Its fibers spread out to cortex of the frontal lobe and to cortex in the posterior part of the hemisphere.

Large numbers of **arcuate fibers** connect adjacent gyri. These short subcortical association fibers are oriented at right angles to the gyri and bend sharply under the intervening sulci. Spread of activity along a gyrus or sulcus is provided by other subcortical association fibers and by axons within the cortex.

COMMISSURES

Corpus Callosum

Most of the neocortical commissural fibers constitute the **corpus callosum**; the remainder are included in the anterior commissure, along with fibers of other than neocortical origin. The corpus callosum varies considerably in size and shape. The sectional area of the corpus callosum in the midline may be, on average, slightly larger in right- than in left-handed people, although this observation has been disputed. In laboratory animals, commissural fibers from an area of cortex in one hemisphere have been shown to terminate in the corresponding area and in cortex closely related functionally with that area, in the other hemisphere. The hand areas of the primary somatosensory cortices and large parts of the primary visual areas are notable in that they are not directly connected by commissural fibers. They communicate functionally, however, through callosal fibers that connect the adjacent association areas. Much of the cortex of the temporal lobe makes its commissural connections by way of the anterior commissure rather than the corpus callosum.

The **trunk** of the corpus callosum is the compact part of the commissure in and near the midline (see Fig. 16-2). As they pass laterally,

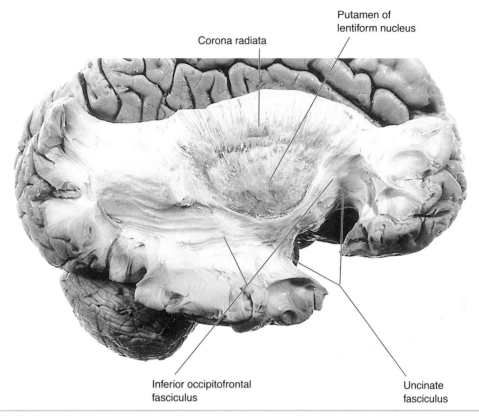

Corona radiata

Putamen of
lentiform nucleus

Inferior occipitofrontal
fasciculus

Uncinate
fasciculus

FIGURE 16-5   The dissection shown in Figure 16-4 has been continued by removal of the external capsule to expose the lentiform nucleus.

the callosal fibers intersect association bundles and projection fibers. The trunk of the corpus callosum is considerably shorter than the hemispheres; this accounts for the enlargements of the ends, which are the **splenium** posteriorly and the **genu** anteriorly (see Fig. 13-2). The splenium and the radiations that connect the occipital lobes constitute the **forceps occipitalis** (forceps major) (Fig. 16-6), and the genu and the radiations that connect the frontal lobes form the **forceps frontalis** (forceps minor). The genu tapers into the **rostrum** of the corpus callosum, which is continuous with the lamina terminalis forming the anterior wall of the third ventricle. Callosal fibers that form a thin sheet over the temporal horn of the lateral ventricle constitute the **tapetum** (see Fig. 16-6), which provides some of the communication between the cortices of the temporal lobes.

The ventral surface of the corpus callosum forms the roof of the lateral ventricles and has relations with the fornix and septum pellucidum in the midline. The **fornix**, consisting of symmetrical halves, is a robust fiber system that connects the hippocampal formation of each temporal lobe with the hypothalamus (see Fig. 18-2) and the septal area of the forebrain. The **crura** of the fornix begin at the posterior end of each hippocampus; they curve forward and merge to form the **body** of the fornix, which is in contact with the undersurface of the trunk of the corpus callosum. The body of the fornix divides into two **columns** that turn ventrally away from the corpus callosum; they form the anterior boundaries of the interventricular foramina and continue to the hypothalamus. The resulting interval between the fornix and corpus callosum is bridged by the **septum pellucidum** (see Fig. 11-2), a thin sheet of neuroglial tissue that contains scattered groups of neurons at its anterior end and is covered on each side by ependyma. The septum pellucidum separates the frontal horns of the lateral ventricles; it is a double membrane containing a slit-like cavity, the **cavum septi pellucidi**, which does not communicate with the ventricular system or with the subarachnoid space.

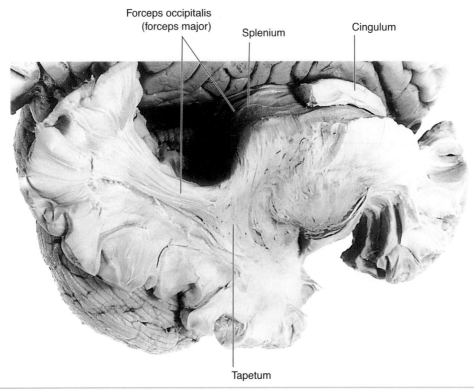

Forceps occipitalis (forceps major)   Splenium   Cingulum

Tapetum

FIGURE 16-6   Dissection of parts of the corpus callosum in the right hemisphere. The posterior half of the cingulum has been removed, and the longitudinal striae are visible on the upper surface of the exposed corpus callosum.

ANTERIOR COMMISSURE

The **anterior commissure** is a bundle of axons that crosses the midline in the lamina terminalis; it traverses the anterior parts of the corpora striata and provides for additional communication between the temporal lobes (Fig. 16-7). The anterior commissure includes fibers that connect the middle and inferior temporal gyri of the two sides; this is a neocortical component similar to the corpus callosum. Other fibers run between the olfactory cortex of the temporal lobes (the lateral olfactory areas), for which the uncus is a landmark. Also present are axons that interconnect the olfactory bulbs, but these are a minor component of the human anterior commissure.

FUNCTIONS OF THE CEREBRAL COMMISSURES

The interhemispheric connections provided by the corpus callosum and anterior commissure contribute to the bilaterality of memory traces. All knowledge that arrives from the senses is

Traumatic Encephalopathy

A large hole in the septum pellucidum is often present in the brains of professional boxers. No functional disability is known to result from this perforation, but boxers commonly have numerous other small lesions that transect axons in cerebral white matter. The resulting generalized reduction in the number of cortical connections leads to the condition known as **chronic trauma-** **tic encephalopathy** or **dementia pugilistica**, popularly called "punch-drunkenness." Whereas deterioration of the personality, impairment of memory, and possibly some features of parkinsonism are attributable to functional disconnections in the cerebrum, dysarthria and ataxia may be caused by similar multiple interruptions of cerebellar connections.

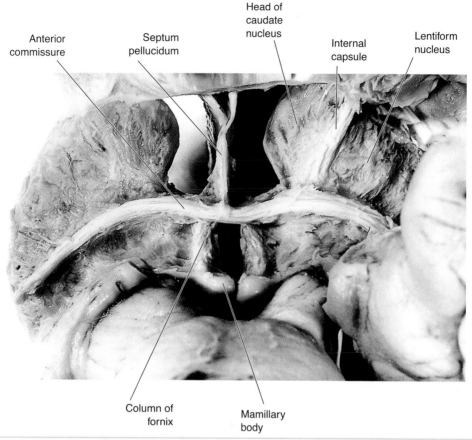

Anterior commissure — Septum pellucidum — Head of caudate nucleus — Internal capsule — Lentiform nucleus

Column of fornix — Mamillary body

FIGURE 16-7 Dissection exposing the anterior commissure, photographed by a camera anterior to the left frontal pole of the dissected brain.

collected by both cerebral hemispheres. In some people with severe epilepsy, the corpus callosum has been transected to confine the epileptic discharge to one hemisphere and the seizures to one side of the body. This operation leads to no significant changes in intellect, behavior, or emotional responses that can be attributed to commissurotomy. A task that has been newly learned with one hand, however, is no longer transferable to the other hand.

A particularly significant result of commissurotomy is related to language. In most people, the linguistic faculties reside in the left hemisphere. After recovering from the operation, the patient is unable to describe an object held in the left hand (with the eyes closed) or seen only in the left visual field, although the nature of the object is understood. There is no such difficulty when the sensory data reach the left hemisphere. After commissurotomy, the right hemisphere is rendered mute and

agraphic because it has no access to memory for language in the left hemisphere. The hemisphere that is subordinate with respect to language is superior in certain other activities, however. These include copying drawings that include perspective and arranging blocks in a prescribed manner. The nonlinguistic hemisphere is therefore the more proficient side of the brain in functions that require special competence in three-dimensional perspective. Interhemispheric differences are discussed in more detail in Chapter 15.

INTERNAL CAPSULE AND PROJECTION FIBERS

The projection fibers are concentrated in the internal capsule and fan out as the **corona radiata** in the cerebral white matter (see Fig. 16-5). The internal capsule consists of **an anterior limb**, a **genu**, a **posterior limb**, a **retrolentiform**

part, and a **sublentiform part**, all of which have topographic relations with adjacent gray masses. The anterior limb is bounded by the lentiform nucleus and by the head of the caudate nucleus. The genu is located medially to the apex of the lentiform nucleus, and the posterior limb intervenes between the lentiform nucleus and the thalamus. The retrolentiform part of the internal capsule occupies the region behind the lentiform nucleus, and the sublentiform part consists of fibers that pass beneath the posterior part of the lentiform nucleus. The anatomical relations of the internal capsule are best appreciated in a horizontal section at the level of the insula (Fig. 16-8).

THALAMIC RADIATIONS

Many of the projection fibers establish reciprocal connections between the thalamus and the cerebral cortex. The **anterior thalamic radiation**, located in the anterior limb of the internal capsule, consists mainly of fibers connecting the mediodorsal thalamic nucleus and prefron-

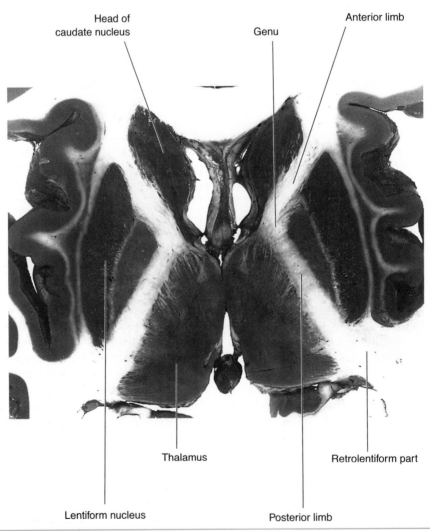

FIGURE 16-8 Horizontal section of the cerebrum at the level of the insula, stained to distinguish gray matter (*dark*) from white matter (light). The genu and limbs of the internal capsule are labeled. The sublentiform part of the internal capsule is ventral to the plane of this section below the posterior part of the lentiform nucleus. For other structures seen in a section at this level, see Figure 12-2.

tal cortex. The **middle thalamic radiation** is a component of the posterior limb of the internal capsule. This radiation includes the somatosensory projection from the ventral posterior thalamic nucleus to the somesthetic area in the parietal lobe; these fibers run in the posterior part of the posterior limb, where they are partly intermingled with motor projection fibers. Other fibers of the middle thalamic radiation establish reciprocal connections between the thalamus and the association cortex of the parietal lobe. Fibers from the ventral anterior and ventral lateral nucleus of the thalamus reach the motor, premotor, supplementary motor, and cingulate motor areas of the frontal lobe by traversing the genu and adjacent region of the posterior limb of the internal capsule.

The **posterior thalamic radiation** establishes connections between the thalamus and cortex of the occipital lobe. The **geniculocalcarine tract** that ends in the visual cortex is a particularly important component of this radiation. Originating in the lateral geniculate body, the geniculocalcarine tract first traverses the sublentiform and retrolentiform parts of the internal capsule. The constituent fibers then spread out into a broad band bordering the lateral ventricle and turn backward into the occipital lobe. Some of the fibers, constituting **Meyer's loop**, proceed forward for a considerable distance into the temporal lobe above the temporal horn of the lateral ventricle before turning back into the occipital lobe (see Fig. 20-7). The posterior thalamic radiation also contains fibers that establish reciprocal connections between the pulvinar of the thalamus and the cortex of the occipital lobe. The **inferior thalamic radiation** consists of fibers directed horizontally in the sublentiform part of the internal capsule that connect thalamic nuclei with cortex of the temporal lobe. Most of the fibers are included in the **auditory radiation**, which originates in the medial geniculate body and terminates in the primary auditory area, on the superior surface of the superior temporal gyrus.

MOTOR PROJECTION FIBERS

The remaining projection fibers are corticofugal, and many of them have motor functions. The **corticobulbar** (**corticonuclear**) and **corticospinal tracts**, which together constitute the pyramidal motor system, originate in the motor, premotor, supplementary motor, and cingulate motor areas in the frontal lobe and in the rostral (anterior) parts of the parietal lobe. These axons are probably accompanied by motor corticoreticular fibers (see below). The descending axons converge as they traverse the corona radiata and enter the anterior half of the posterior limb. In their passage caudally through the internal capsule, the motor fibers are shifted into the posterior half of the posterior limb by frontopontine fibers that have already traversed the anterior limb. Corticobulbar fibers are most anterior, followed in sequence by corticospinal fibers related to the upper limb, trunk, and lower limb. There is considerable overlap of the territories occupied by fibers for the major regions of the body, so a small destructive lesion in the internal capsule has serious effects.

Corticopontine fibers originate in all four lobes of the cerebral cortex but in greatest numbers in the frontal and parietal lobes. They terminate in the pontine nuclei (nuclei pontis) in the basal part of the pons. Fibers of the **frontopontine tract** traverse the anterior limb of the internal capsule and the anterior part of the posterior limb. Most of the fibers of the **parietotemporopontine tract** originate in the parietal lobe and traverse the retrolentiform part of the internal capsule.

Corticostriate fibers originate in all parts of the neocortex and end in the striatum. The caudate nucleus and putamen receive these fibers from the internal capsule; the putamen receives some from the external capsule as well.

Other projection fibers pass caudally to nuclei in the brain stem. **Corticorubral fibers** arise from the motor areas of the frontal lobe and end in the red nucleus. The **corticoreticular fibers** begin in the motor cortex and in the cortex of the parietal lobe, especially the primary somesthetic area. They terminate mainly in the central group of reticular nuclei. **Cortico-olivary fibers**, also mostly from the motor areas, go to the inferior olivary complex of nuclei. These descending pathways accompany the axons of the pyramidal system through the internal capsule and basis pedunculi into the pons and medulla. Along with the corticospinal and corticobulbar tracts, they are severed by destructive lesions in the internal capsule.

Internal Capsule Lesions

An infarction in the posterior part of the internal capsule results in serious neurological deficits. These include the effects of an "upper motor neuron lesion" (see Chapter 23) caused mainly by interruption of pyramidal and corticoreticular fibers. **Hemiparesis** is weakness of all the muscles of the opposite side of the body, and **hemiplegia** is complete paralysis of the affected side. A lesion in the internal capsule may also cause general sensory deficits by involvement of the thalamocortical projection to the somesthetic area and a visual field defect by interruption of geniculocalcarine fibers.

The composition of the **external capsule** is incompletely understood, but it is known that this thin layer of white matter between the putamen and claustrum consists mainly of projection fibers. These include some of the corticostriate fibers that end in the putamen and some of the corticoreticular fibers.

Such lesions also involve the thalamocortical fibers from the ventral lateral and ventral anterior thalamic nuclei to the motor areas of the cortex.

Lateral Ventricles

The lateral ventricles, one in each cerebral hemisphere, are roughly C-shaped cavities lined by ependyma and filled with CSF. Each lateral ventricle consists of a central part in the region of the parietal lobe from which horns extend into the frontal, occipital, and temporal lobes. The principal features of the ventricular walls are shown in Figures 16-9 and 16-10. The configuration of the entire ventricular system of the brain is shown in Figure 16-11.

The **central part** of the lateral ventricle has a flat roof formed by the corpus callosum. The floor includes part of the dorsal surface of the thalamus, of which the anterior tubercle is a boundary of the interventricular foramen (foramen of Monro) that leads to the third ventricle. The tail of the caudate nucleus forms a ridge along the lateral border of the floor. The **stria terminalis**, a slender bundle of fibers originating in the amygdaloid body in the temporal lobe, lies in the groove between the tail of the caudate nucleus and the thalamus along with the thalamostriate vein (vena terminalis). The fornix completes the floor medially, and the choroid plexus is attached to the margins of the **choroid fissure**, which intervenes between the fornix and thalamus. The stria terminalis and fornix are association fasciculi of the limbic system.

Temporal Horn

Within the temporal lobe, the temporal horn is normally too small to show on a CT scan. It becomes visible if the ventricle is enlarged. Dilatation of the lateral ventricle may be caused by obstructed flow of CSF or by atrophy of the surrounding brain tissue.

The floor of the temporal horn includes an important structure, the **hippocampus** (see Fig. 16-10). The hippocampus may be visualized as an extension of the parahippocampal gyrus on the external surface that has been "rolled into" the floor of the temporal horn. The slightly enlarged anterior end of the hippocampus is known as the **pes hippocampi** because it resembles an animal's paw. Efferent fibers from the hippocampus form a ridge, the **fimbria**, along its medial border. The fimbria continues as the **crus of the fornix** at the posterior end of the hippocampus beneath the splenium of the corpus callosum. The choroid plexus of the central part of the ventricle continues into the temporal horn, where it is attached to the margins of the choroid fissure above the fimbria of the hippocampus.

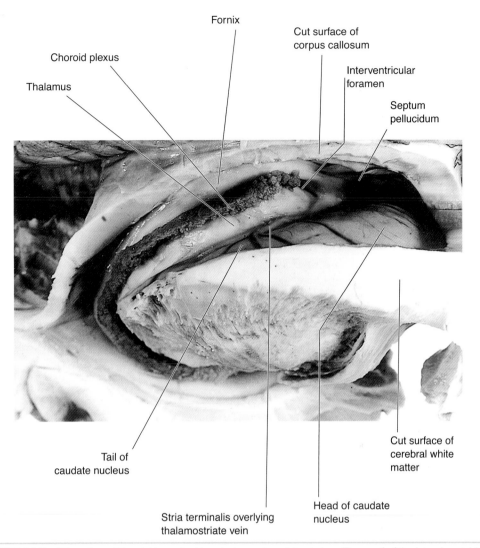

Fornix

Cut surface of
corpus callosum

Choroid plexus

Interventricular
foramen

Thalamus

Septum
pellucidum

Tail of
caudate nucleus

Cut surface of
cerebral white
matter

Stria terminalis overlying
thalamostriate vein

Head of caudate
nucleus

FIGURE 16-9   Dissection of the right cerebral hemisphere: dorsolateral view. The roof of the lateral ventricle has been removed.

The **frontal horn** of the ventricle extends forward from the region of the interventricular foramen. The corpus callosum continues as the roof, and the genu of the corpus callosum limits the frontal horn in front. The septum pellucidum bridges the interval between the fornix and corpus callosum in the midline, separating the frontal horns of the two lateral ventricles. The **occipital horn**, which is of variable length, is surrounded by cerebral white matter (Fig. 16-10). Two elevations on the medial wall of the occipital horn are the **bulb of the occipital horn**, raised by the forceps occipitalis, and the **calcar avis**, which corresponds to the calcarine sulcus.

The slender **temporal horn** extends to within about 3 cm of the temporal pole. A triangular area, called the **collateral trigone**, is found in the floor of the ventricle where the occipital and temporal horns diverge from the central part of the ventricle. A substantial part of the choroid plexus of the lateral ventricle rests on the trigone and can be seen in computed tomography scans of the brain because it contains small amounts of calcified material. The collateral sulcus on the external surface of the hemisphere is located immediately below the trigone and may produce a **collateral eminence** there. The tail of the caudate nucleus, now considerably attenuated, extends forward in the roof of the temporal horn as

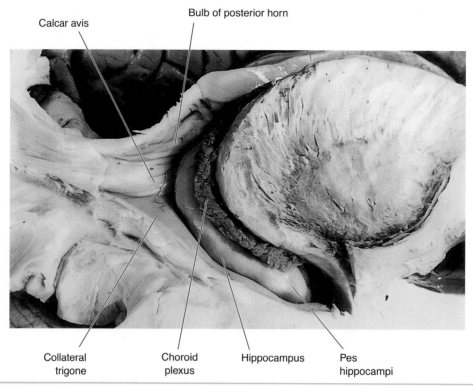

FIGURE 16-10   Dissection of the right cerebral hemisphere: lateral view showing the occipital and temporal horns of the lateral ventricle.

far as the amygdaloid body. This latter is a group of nuclei above the anterior end of the temporal horn, close to the uncus on the external surface.

The stria terminalis and thalamostriate vein run along the medial side of the tail of the caudate nucleus.

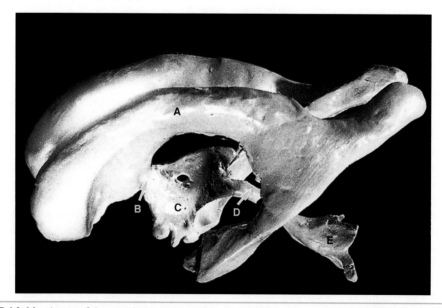

FIGURE 16-11   A cast of the ventricular system of the brain. **(A)** Left lateral ventricle. **(B)** Interventricular foramen. **(C)** Third ventricle. **(D)** Cerebral aqueduct. **(E)** Fourth ventricle. (Prepared by Dr. D. G. Montemurro.)

Suggested Reading

Driesen NR, Raz N. The influence of sex, age, and handedness on corpus callosum morphology: a meta-analysis. *Psychobiology* 1995;23:240–247.

Gazzaniga MS, Sperry RW. Language after section of the cerebral commissures. *Brain* 1967;90:131–148.

Kretschmann H-J. Localization of the corticospinal fibres in the internal capsule in man. *J Anat* 1988;160:219–225.

Mitchell TN, Free SL, Merschemke M, et al. Reliable callosal measurement: population normative data confirm sex-related differences. *ANJR Am J Neuroradiol* 2003;24:410–418.

Montemurro DG, Bruni JE. *The Human Brain in Dissection*, 2nd ed. New York: Oxford University Press, 1988.

Nolte J, Angevine JB. *The Human Brain in Photographs and Diagrams with CD-ROM*, 3rd ed. New York: Elsevier, 2007.

Seymour SE, Reuter-Lorenz PA, Gazzaniga MS. The disconnection syndrome: basic findings reaffirmed. *Brain* 1994;117:105–115.

Tredici G, Pizzini G, Bogliun G, et al. The site of motor corticospinal fibres in man: a computerized tomographic study of restricted lesions. *J Anat* 1982;134:199–208.

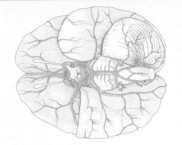

Chapter 17

OLFACTORY SYSTEM

- The olfactory receptor cells are unique neurons located in an epithelium and are regularly replaced from a population of precursor cells.

- The unmyelinated axons of the olfactory neurosensory cells constitute about 20 olfactory nerves on each side. These nerves pass through the cribriform plate of the ethmoid bone and end in the overlying olfactory bulb.

- A fracture of the cribriform plate is likely to be followed by anosmia and cerebrospinal fluid rhinorrhea.

- The principal neurons of the olfactory bulb have axons that form the olfactory tract. This follows the ventral surface of the frontal lobe and ends in the olfactory trigone, anterior (rostral) to the anterior perforated substance.

- Most of the axons of the olfactory tract follow the lateral olfactory stria and end in the lateral olfactory area, which comprises the cortex of the uncus, limen insulae, entorhinal area, and corticomedial nuclei of the amygdaloid body.

- Smaller numbers of olfactory tract fibers end in the anterior olfactory nucleus and in various nuclei in the region of the anterior perforated substance. Some of these cell groups give rise to fibers that pass centrifugally in the olfactory tracts and terminate in the olfactory bulbs of both sides, providing a mechanism for modulation of the input from the olfactory apparatus.

- The regions in which fibers of the olfactory tract terminate are connected, directly and indirectly, with the prefrontal cortex, limbic system, hypothalamus, and reticular formation of the brain stem. These connections provide for visceral and behavioral responses to different odors.

The olfactory system consists of the olfactory epithelium, olfactory nerves, olfactory bulbs, and olfactory tracts, together with function-ally associated cerebral cortex and subcortical structures. The parts of the brain that process olfactory signals are sometimes collectively called the **rhinencephalon**.

Olfaction is a significant sense that conjures up memories and arouses emotions. Smell also contributes to alimentary pleasures. Those who have lost their sense of smell complain of impairment of taste, stating that everything is bland and tastes alike, and they may be unaware of their inability to smell. Much of our enjoyment of taste is, in fact, an appreciation of aromas through the olfactory system. Some chemical stimuli, notably those from foods with "hot" flavors, excite general sensory fibers of the trigeminal nerve in the nose and mouth. The olfactory, gustatory, and general sensory responses to chemical stimuli in the nose may be integrated in the insula, where the primary cortical areas for the three systems are in proximity.

Olfactory Epithelium and Olfactory Nerves

The olfactory epithelium is derived from an ectodermal thickening, the **olfactory placode**, at the rostral end of the embryonic head. The cells of this placode give rise to the cells of the epithelium, the glial cells of the olfactory nerves, and some of the glial cells of the most superficial layer of the olfactory bulb. In adults, the olfactory epithelium (Fig. 17-1) covers an area of 2.5 cm^2 in the roof of each nasal cavity and extends for a short distance on the lateral wall of the cavity and the nasal septum. The olfactory sensory cells are contained in a pseudostratified columnar epithelium, which is thicker than that lining the respiratory passages elsewhere. Olfactory glands (Bowman's glands)

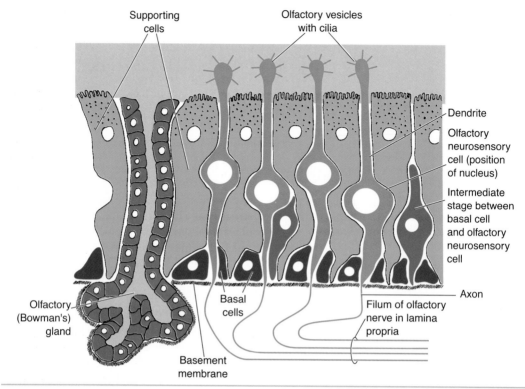

FIGURE 17-1 Olfactory epithelium.

beneath the epithelium bathe the surface with a layer of mucous fluid, in which odoriferous substances dissolve. The **olfactory neurosensory cells** (also known as *primary olfactory neurons* or simply as *olfactory cells*) are bipolar neurons that serve as sensory receptors as well as conductors of impulses. The major modification consists of specialization of the dendrite; this process extends to the surface of the epithelium, where it ends as an exposed bulbous enlargement known as an *olfactory vesicle*, bearing unusually long ($\leq$100 μm) cilia.

Unmyelinated axons of the olfactory cells are gathered into about 20 bundles on each side, which are the **olfactory nerves**. These enter the cranial cavity by passing through the foramina of the cribriform plate of the ethmoid bone and then enter the **olfactory bulb**. The axons form a superficial fibrous layer in the olfactory bulb; continue more deeply; and terminate in specialized synaptic configurations, the **glomeruli**. The olfactory axon terminals release an excitatory neurotransmitter; in rodents, it is glutamate.

The few neurosensory cells shown in Figure 17-1 represent approximately 25 million of

such cells in the olfactory epithelium of each side of the nose. The olfactory cells are continuously produced by mitosis and differentiation of some of the basal cells of the olfactory epithelium, and the cells are lost by desquamation. Observations in animals indicate that olfactory neurons probably are lost by wear and tear rather than because of an innately short life span. In healthy human noses, each receptor neuron probably survives for about 3 months. Consequently, new axons are always growing along the olfactory nerves and into the olfactory bulbs.

The olfactory system is exquisitely sensitive to minute amounts of excitants in the air. Direct stimulation of the receptors, convergence of many neurosensory cells on the principal neurons of the olfactory bulb, and facilitation by neuronal circuits in the bulb are among the factors responsible for the low threshold. Smell is a chemical sense, as is taste. For a substance to be smelled, it must enter the nasal cavity as a gas or as an aerosol and then dissolve in the fluid that covers the olfactory epithelium. The secretory product of Bowman's glands contains glycoproteins that can bind odoriferous substances that are not otherwise soluble in water for presentation to receptor molecules on the surfaces of the sensory cilia.

A large range of odors can be appreciated because of the existence of approximately 3,000 different receptor proteins, each with a different chemical specificity, embedded in the surface membranes of the cilia of the olfactory neurosensory cells. Combination of an odorant with its specific receptor initiates changes that tend to depolarize the cell membrane. Individual olfactory neurons have receptors for several odorants but in different combinations, and the olfactory epithelium is a mosaic of overlapping sets of neurons whose activities encode different odors. Experiments with animals reveal that the projection from the epithelium to the olfactory bulb is topographically organized, with the specific sites of termination of the axons of neurons that possess particular combinations of odorant receptor molecules. This mode of organization is comparable to the topographic distribution of neuronal circuitry in the other sensory systems.

The olfactory system adapts rather quickly to continuous stimuli, so that the odor becomes unnoticed. The mechanisms of adaptation involve the receptor cells themselves and neuronal circuitry in the olfactory bulb. A physiological mechanism that allows the receptors to recover from continuous exposure to odors is a cyclic alternation of mucosal blood flow in the left and right sides of the nose. At any instant, the side with the higher flow of blood presents greater resistance to the flow of air because of swelling of the mucosa. The nasal cavity with lower air flow consequently receives smaller amounts of the ambient odorants. Most older people have a reduced acuity of smell, caused by a progressive reduction (about 10% per decade between 30 and 90 years of age) in the populations of olfactory neurosensory cells and of neurons in the olfactory bulb.

Olfactory Bulb, Tract, and Striae

The olfactory bulb is ventral to the orbital surface of the frontal lobe. It is connected by the olfactory tract to a central point of attachment in front of the anterior perforated substance. The bulb contains two types of glutamatergic principal cells (**mitral** and **tufted cells**) and at least two types of interneurons (Fig. 17-2). The five layers are irregular and indistinct in the adult human olfactory bulb, although they are obvious in the fetal stages of development. The nerve fiber layer is of interest because it continuously

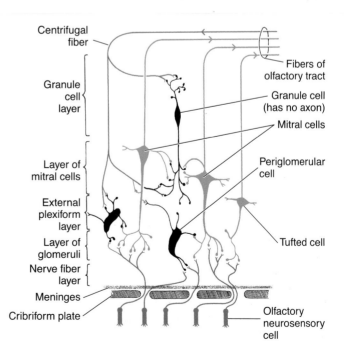

FIGURE 17-2 Neuronal circuitry of the olfactory bulb. Principal cells are red, interneurons are black, and afferents to the olfactory bulb are blue.

admits newly growing axons from the olfactory nerves into the central nervous system (CNS). A mixture of neuroglial cells (i.e., astrocytes from the neural tube and **olfactory ensheathing cells** of placodal origin that surround bundles of primary olfactory axons) may account for this unique circumstance of axonal growth into the adult mammalian CNS. Olfactory ensheathing cells encourage axonal growth not only in the olfactory nerves and bulb but also in laboratory animals after transplantation to sites of injury elsewhere in the CNS, including the spinal cord.

Deep to the nerve fiber layer, the 25 million axons of the olfactory receptors terminate in some 8,000 spherical masses of neuropil known as **glomeruli**. Each glomerulus receives many afferent axons, which synapse with dendrites of about 5 of the 40,000 principal cells. The activity of the principal cells is modified by the predominantly inhibitory (dopaminergic and γ-aminobutyrate-ergic) interneurons of the olfactory bulb, especially the extremely numerous granule cells. The complex circuitry (see Fig. 17-2) is believed to be largely responsible for identifying different odors.

Three small groups of neurons make up the **anterior olfactory nucleus**. One is situated at the transition between the olfactory bulb and olfactory tract; the others are deep to the lateral and medial olfactory striae described in the next paragraph. Collateral branches of axons of mitral and tufted cells terminate in this nucleus. Fibers that originate in the anterior olfactory nucleus pass through the anterior commissure to the contralateral olfactory bulb. This is only one of the populations of centrifugal fibers that project to the olfactory bulb. Centrifugal fibers synapse principally with the dendrites of the interneurons. This arrangement probably sets the sensitivity or indifference of the olfactory system to specific odors.

The principal cells of the olfactory bulb have axons that pass through the olfactory tract and end as excitatory (glutamatergic) presynaptic terminals in primary olfactory areas for subjective appreciation of smells. The primary olfactory areas establish connections with other parts of the brain for emotional and visceral responses to olfactory stimuli. The olfactory tract expands into the **olfactory trigone** at the rostral margin of the anterior perforated sub-

stance. Most of the axons of the tract pass into the **lateral olfactory stria** (Fig. 17-3), which passes to the lateral olfactory area. Other axons of the olfactory tract leave the olfactory trigone to enter the anterior perforated substance. The name *medial olfactory stria* was applied to a ridge once thought to carry olfactory fibers to the septal area. It is now known that no such connection exists.

Olfactory Areas of the Cerebral Hemisphere

RHINENCEPHALON

The "nose brain" was once thought to include more parts of the forebrain than those currently believed to be devoted to the sense of smell. The term is now restricted to the regions that receive afferent fibers from the olfactory bulbs. The **primary olfactory area**, believed to be the region for conscious awareness of olfactory stimuli, receives afferents through the lateral olfactory stria (Fig. 17-4; see also Fig. 17-3). The area consists of the paleocortex (see Chapter 14) of the **uncus** (periamygdaloid cortex) together with adjacent parts of the **entorhinal area**, in the anterior part of the parahippocampal gyrus, and the **limen insulae** (Fig. 17-3). The uncus, entorhinal area, and limen insulae are collectively known as the **pyriform cortex** (or lobe) because the homologous area has a pear-shaped outline in some animals. Part of the **amygdaloid body** (amygdala) is also included in the lateral olfactory area; the uncus is its landmark on the medial surface of the temporal lobe. The dorsomedial part of the amygdala, consisting of the **corticomedial group of nuclei**, receives olfactory fibers. The larger ventrolateral portion, a component of the limbic system, is considered in Chapter 18. The lateral olfactory area, believed to be the principal region for conscious awareness of olfactory stimuli, is also called the **primary olfactory area**.

Axons of the olfactory tract also connect with neurons in the **anterior perforated substance**. In the human brain, this region blends into the ventral pallidum and the nucleus accumbens of the striatum (see Chapter 12).

Neuroanatomical tracing experiments in nonhuman primates and functional imaging stud-

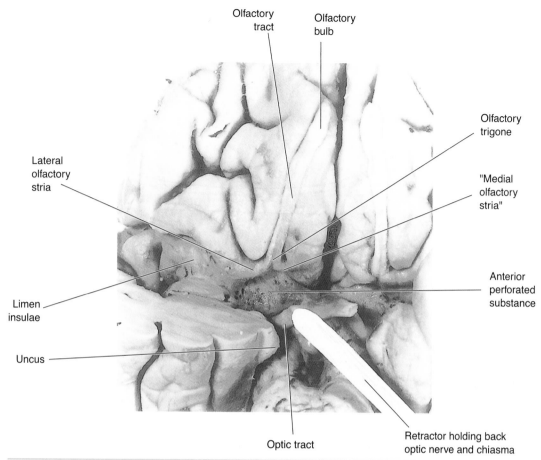

FIGURE 17-3   Some components of the olfactory system seen on the ventral surface of the brain. The right temporal pole has been cut away to give a clear view of the olfactory trigone, anterior perforated substance, and limen insulae.

ies in humans indicate that the lateral part of the orbital surface of the frontal lobe is the **olfactory association cortex**, receiving afferents from the primary olfactory area. Positron emission tomography (PET) studies of the human brain show increased blood flow in the right orbitofrontal cortex when olfactory stimuli are presented to both sides of the nose. The orbital cortex is otherwise better known for its essential roles in foresight, decision making, and social interactions with other people (see Chapter 15). Subtle ipsilateral impairment of odor identification occurs after surgical removal of parts of the temporal lobe that are not otherwise known to be connected with the olfactory system. The olfactory association cortex may prove to extend beyond the currently recognized areas.

Another group of neurons in the anterior perforated substance, the **nucleus of the diagonal band**, is a major source of centrifugal fibers to the olfactory bulb; the other source is the contralateral anterior olfactory nucleus.

Olfactory stimuli induce visceral responses by modulating the activities of the autonomic nervous system. Examples are salivation when pleasing aromas from the preparation of food are present and nausea or even vomiting evoked by an offensive stench. The olfactory system shares the entorhinal cortex with the limbic system, and the limbic system has extensive connections with the septal area and the hypothalamus. Most of the fibers that connect the septal area and hypothalamus with autonomic nuclei are situated in the **medial forebrain bundle**. This bundle, which

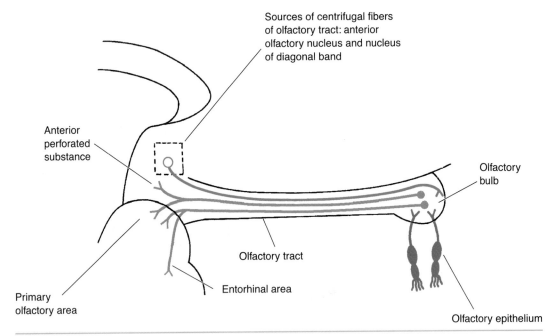

Sources of centrifugal fibers
of olfactory tract: anterior
olfactory nucleus and nucleus
of diagonal band

Anterior
perforated
substance

Olfactory
bulb

Olfactory tract

Entorhinal area

Primary
olfactory area

Olfactory epithelium

FIGURE 17-4   Components of the olfactory tract.

contains fibers projecting rostrally as well as caudally, traverses the lateral part of the hypothalamus. Descending fibers from the hypothalamus proceed to autonomic nuclei in the brain stem and spinal cord. Other descending fibers of the medial forebrain bundle end in raphe reticular nuclei and in the solitary nucleus.

Terminal and Vomeronasal Nerves

Two small cranial nerves associated with the olfactory system were discovered after the 12 main cranial nerves were given their numbers. The terminal nerve (nervus terminalis) is pres-

Olfactory Symptoms

Deterioration of the sense of smell often occurs with normal aging. It can also be an early symptom of degenerative disorders, including Parkinson's (Chapter 7) and Alzheimer's diseases (Chapter 12). The olfactory deficit is associated with neuronal loss in the corticomedial nuclei of the amygdala.

Fractures of the floor of the anterior fossa of the skull often involve the cribriform plate of the ethmoid bone, damaging the olfactory nerves and causing **anosmia**. The same injury may result in leakage of cerebrospinal fluid (CSF) from the subarachnoid space into the nasal cavity, so that the fluid runs from the nose (**CSF rhinorrhea**). This abnormal communication with the external environment is dangerous because it provides a route whereby bacteria may enter and attack the meninges and the brain.

A tumor, usually a meningioma, in the floor of the anterior cranial fossa may interfere with the sense of smell because of pressure on the olfactory bulb or olfactory tract. It is necessary to test each nostril separately because the olfactory loss is likely to be unilateral.

An irritating lesion that affects the lateral olfactory area may cause **uncinate fits**, characterized by an imaginary disagreeable odor, by involuntary movements of the lips and tongue, and often by other features of disturbed function of the temporal lobe (see Chapter 18). Ipsilateral olfactory impairment follows destructive lesions of the temporal lobe but is detectable only by careful testing. Such impairment can occur even when the damage is outside the recognized olfactory areas.

ent, although of microscopic size, in the adult human brain. Sometimes it is called *cranial nerve zero* because it is located medially (and therefore perhaps rostrally) to the olfactory nerves. The terminal nerve is mentioned in Chapter 11 as the conduit through which certain neurons migrate from the olfactory placode into the preoptic area and hypothalamus.

The vomeronasal system appears only transiently in human embryonic development, but in most other terrestrial vertebrates, it has important functions in adult life.

The fibers of the tiny **terminal nerve** lie along the medial side of the olfactory bulb and olfactory tract. Bipolar neuronal cell bodies are present in small ganglia along the course of the nerve. Their distal processes pass through the cribriform plate and are distributed to the nasal septum. In animals, the proximal processes have been traced experimentally to the septal and preoptic areas.

The vomeronasal nerve is part of an accessory olfactory system present in most terrestrial vertebrate animals other than humans. It is used for detection of pheromones that serve for sexual attraction and territorial marking. The human vomeronasal receptor organ and nerve are present only from the 8th to the 14th weeks of intrauterine life.

Suggested Reading

Boyd JG, Doucette R, Kawaja MD. Defining the role of olfactory ensheathing cells in facilitating remyelination following damage to the spinal cord. *FASEB J* 2005;19: 694–703.

Buck LB. Information coding in the vertebrate olfactory system. *Annu Rev Neurosci* 1996;19:517–544.

Carmichael ST, Clugnet MC, Price JL. Central olfactory connections in the macaque monkey. *J Comp Neurol* 1994;346:403–434.

Doucette R. PNS-CNS transitional zone of the first cranial nerve. *J Comp Neurol* 1991;312:451–466.

Eccles R, Jawad MSM, Morris S. Olfactory and trigeminal thresholds and nasal resistance to airflow. *Acta Otolaryngol (Stockh)* 1989;108:268–273.

Eisthen HL. Phylogeny of the vomeronasal system and of receptor cell types in the olfactory and vomeronasal epithelia of vertebrates. *Microsc Res Tech* 1992;23:1–21.

Feron F, Perry C, Cochrane J, et al. Autologous olfactory ensheathing cell transplantation in human spinal cord injury. *Brain* 2005;128:2951–2960.

Graziadei PPC, Karlan MS, Monti Graziadei GA, et al. Neurogenesis of sensory neurons in the primate olfactory system after section of the fila olfactoria. *Brain Res* 1980;186:289–300.

Harding AJ, Stimson E, Henderson JM, et al. Clinical correlates of selective pathology in the amygdala of patients with Parkinson's disease. *Brain* 2002;125: 2431–2445.

Hinds JW, Hinds PL, McNelly NA. An autoradiographic study of the mouse olfactory epithelium: evidence for long-lived receptors. *Anat Rec* 1984;210:375–383.

Ichikawa M. Neuronal development, differentiation, and plasticity in the mammalian vomeronasal system. *Zoolog Sci* 1996;13:627–639.

Jones-Gotman M, Zatorre RJ, Cendes F, et al. Contribution of medial versus lateral temporal-lobe structures to human odour identification. *Brain* 1997;120:1845–1856.

Mackay-Sim A, Kittel W. On the life span of olfactory receptor neurons. *Eur J Neurosci* 1991;3:209–215.

Meisami E, Mikhail L, Baim D, et al. Human olfactory bulb: aging of glomeruli and mitral cells and a search for the accessory olfactory bulb. *Ann N Y Acad Sci* 1998;855:708–715.

Mesholam RI, Moberg PJ, Mahr RN, et al. Olfaction in neurodegenerative disease: a meta-analysis of olfactory functioning in Alzheimer's and Parkinson's diseases. *Arch Neurol* 1998;55:84–90.

Mombaerts P, Wang F, Dulac C, et al. Visualizing an olfactory sensory map. *Cell* 1996;87:675–686.

Morrison EE, Costanzo RM. Morphology of olfactory epithelium in humans and other vertebrates. *Microsc Res Tech* 1992;23:49–61.

Price JL. Olfaction. In: Paxinos G, Mai JK, eds. *The Human Nervous System*, 2nd ed. Amsterdam: Elsevier, 2004: 1197–1211.

Smith TD, Bhatnagar KP. The human vomeronasal organ, Part II: prenatal development. *J Anat* 2000;197:421–436.

Strotmann J, Beck A, Kubick S, et al. Topographic patterns of odorant receptor expression in mammals: a comparative study. *J Comp Physiol A—Sensory Neural and Behavioral Physiology* 1995;177: 659–666.

Zatorre RJ, Jones-Gotman M, Evans AC, et al. Functional localization and lateralization of human olfactory cortex. *Nature* 1992;360:339–340.

Chapter 18

LIMBIC SYSTEM: THE HIPPOCAMPUS AND THE AMYGDALA

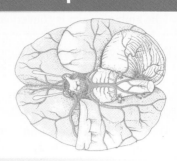

Important Facts

- The limbic system comprises the limbic lobe (parahippocampal and cingulate gyri and septal area), hippocampal formation (subiculum, hippocampus, and dentate gyrus), amygdaloid body, and many other parts of the brain that are connected with these structures.

- Hippocampal afferents include fibers from the entorhinal area of the parahippocampal gyrus, cholinergic fibers from the septal area and basal forebrain nuclei, dopaminergic fibers from the ventral tegmental area, noradrenergic fibers from the locus coeruleus, and serotonergic fibers from the raphe nuclei.

- Hippocampal efferent fibers enter the circuit of Papez, which includes the subiculum, fornix, mamillary body, anterior thalamic nuclei, and cingulate and parahippocampal gyri. Association fibers connect the parahippocampal and cingulate gyri with association areas of the neocortex.

- The remembering of new facts and events (i.e., declarative memory) may occur through synaptic modifications within the hippocampus. It also requires the integrity of the circuit of Papez in at least one cerebral hemisphere. Intact hippocampal connections are not essential for recall of memories, which are probably stored as synaptic modifications in extensive areas of the cerebral cortex.

- The amygdala receives input from the temporal and prefrontal neocortex and from the cholinergic and catecholaminergic nuclei that also project to the hippocampal formation.

- The amygdala sends fibers to the nucleus accumbens (ventral striatum), the mediodorsal thalamic nucleus, and, through the stria terminalis and the diagonal band, to the hypothalamus and septal area. The nucleus accumbens and ventral pallidum modulate the activity of the prefrontal and anterior cingulate cortex.

- The septal area projects through the stria medullaris thalami to the habenular nuclei, through the fornix to the hippocampus, and through the medial forebrain bundle to the hypothalamus.

- The major descending pathways from the limbic system and hypothalamus are the mamillotegmental fasciculus, fasciculus retroflexus, medial forebrain bundle, and dorsal longitudinal fasciculus.

- Stimulation of the amygdala results in fear, generalized irritability, and increased activity of the sympathetic nervous system. Destructive lesions in both temporal lobes can lead to docility, abnormal sexual behavior, and loss of short-term memory.

- Anxiolytic drugs mimic the inhibitory action of γ-aminobutyrate in the amygdala. Antidepressive drugs enhance the actions of noradrenaline and serotonin. Drugs used to treat schizophrenia antagonize the action of dopamine in the limbic system and in the nucleus accumbens.

- Certain components of the cerebral hemispheres and diencephalon are brought together under the heading of the limbic system of the brain. The notion of such a system developed from comparative neuroanatomical and neurophysiological investigations, but the terminology is rather vague and not used consistently by all authors. The **limbic lobe** is a ring of gray matter on the medial aspect of each hemisphere that is composed of the parahippocampal and cingulate gyri and the septal area. The term **limbic system** is less precise. The broadest interpretation, which is probably the most useful, includes the aforementioned structures together with the hippocampus, dentate gyrus, amygdaloid body, septal area, hypothalamus (especially the mamillary bodies), and the anterior and some other nuclei of the thalamus. Bundles of myelinated axons that interconnect these regions (fornix, mamillothalamic fasciculus, stria terminalis, diagonal band, and others) are also parts of the system, as are the ventral parts of the corpus striatum and certain nuclei in the midbrain that connect with the hippocampal formation and the amygdala.

The limbic system is concerned with memory and with visceral and motor responses involved in defense and reproduction.

Hippocampal Formation

The hippocampal formation consists of the hippocampus, the dentate gyrus, and most of the parahippocampal gyrus.

ANATOMY

The **hippocampus** develops in the fetal brain by a process of continuing expansion of the medial edge of the temporal lobe in such a way that the hippocampus comes to occupy the floor of the temporal horn of the lateral ventricle (Figs. 18-1 and 18-2; see also Fig. 16-10). In the mature brain, therefore, the parahippocampal gyrus on the external surface is continuous with the concealed hippocampus. The hippocampus is C-shaped in coronal section. Because its outline bears some resemblance to a ram's horn, the hippocampus is also called the **cornu ammonis**; Ammon is an early Egyptian deity with a ram's head. The ventricular surface of the hippocampus is a thin layer of white matter called the **alveus**, which consists of axons that enter and leave the hippocampal formation. These fibers form the **fimbria** of the hippocampus along its medial border and then continue as the **crus of the fornix** after the hippocampus ends beneath the splenium of the corpus callosum (Fig. 18-3).

Continued growth of the cortical tissue composing the hippocampus is responsible for the **dentate gyrus** (see Figs. 18-1 and 18-2). This gyrus occupies the interval between the fimbria of the hippocampus and the parahippocampal gyrus; its surface is toothed or beaded, hence the name.

Although the parahippocampal gyrus is included in the limbic lobe as defined anatomically, most of its cortex is of the six-layered type or nearly so. In the region of the gyrus known as the **subiculum** (see Figs. 18-1 and 18-2), there is a transition between neocortex and the three-layered archicortex of the hippocampus. The anterior end of the parahippocampal gyrus, medial to the rhinal sulcus (see Fig. 13-5), is the **entorhinal area**.

INTRINSIC ORGANIZATION AND CIRCUITRY

The hippocampus, as seen in transverse (coronal) section has three areas or sectors: **CA1**, **CA2**, and **CA3**. (CA stands for cornu ammonis.) Area CA1 is adjacent to the subiculum, and CA3 is nearest to the dentate gyrus (Fig. 18-4). Three layers are recognized in the hippocampal cortex.

1. The **molecular layer** consists of interacting axons and dendrites. It is located in the center of the hippocampal formation, surrounding the hippocampal sulcus. This synaptic layer is continuous with the molecular layers of the dentate gyrus and neocortex.
2. The prominent **pyramidal cell layer** (stratum pyramidale) is composed of large neu-

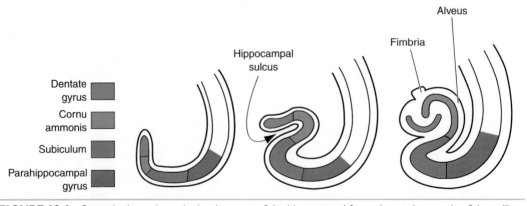

FIGURE 18-1   Stages in the embryonic development of the hippocampal formation at the margin of the pallium, showing how the external surfaces of the dentate gyrus and cornu ammonis become fused as a result of growth and folding.

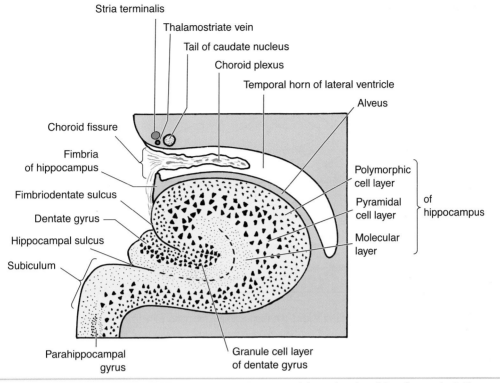

FIGURE 18-2   Simplified coronal section through the hippocampal formation (medial surface at the left).

rons, many of them pyramidal in shape, which are the principal cells of the hippocampus. The dendrites of these cells extend into the molecular layer, and their axons traverse the alveus and fimbria on their way to the fornix. Branches, called **Schaffer col-**

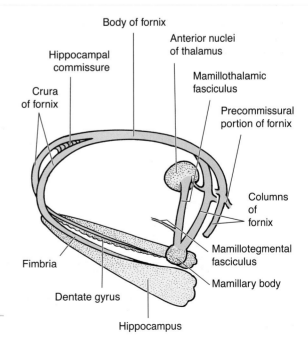

FIGURE 18-3   Fornix and related structures.

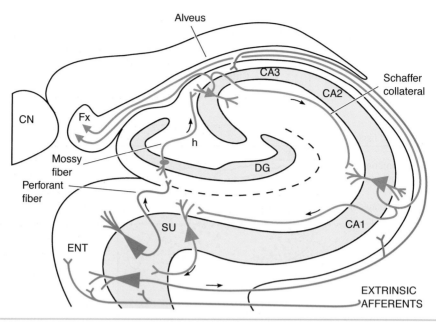

FIGURE 18-4 Some neuronal circuits within the hippocampal formation. The zone occupied by principal cells is shaded. Neurons of the hippocampus and dentate gyrus are red, and the axons of afferent neurons are blue. Small black arrows indicate a loop of connections formed by mossy fibers and Schaffer collaterals. CA1, CA2, and CA3 indicate sectors of the hippocampus; CN, tail of caudate nucleus; DG, dentate gyrus; Ent, entorhinal cortex; Fx, fimbria; h, hilus of dentate gyrus; Su, subiculum.

laterals, pass through the polymorphic and pyramidal cell layers to synapse in the molecular layer with the dendrites of other pyramidal neurons. The pyramidal cell layer is continuous with layer 5 (internal pyramidal) of the neocortex.

3. The **polymorphic layer** (or stratum oriens) is similar to the innermost layer (layer six) of the neocortex. This layer, which is located beneath the alveus, contains axons, dendrites, and interneurons.

The dentate gyrus also has three layers. The cytoarchitecture differs from that of the hippocampus in that the pyramidal cell layer is replaced by a **granule cell layer** of small neurons, which are the principal cells of the region. Efferent fibers from the dentate gyrus are known as **mossy fibers**. They have many branches that synapse with the principal cells of sectors CA3 and CA2.

OXYGEN DEPRIVATION

The large pyramidal cells in area CA1 are exceptionally sensitive to oxygen deprivation and die after only a few minutes without a supply of fresh arterial blood. Pathologists call area CA1 **Sommer's sector**. The hippocampal pyramidal cells are among the first to be affected in a variety of conditions that lead to loss of memory and intellectual functions, including Alzheimer's disease (see also Chapter 12).

LONG-TERM POTENTIATION

The neuronal circuitry is essentially the same in all mammals, and it has been studied in great detail by neuroscientists attempting to identify cellular events involved in the formation of new memories. One postulated mechanism is long-term potentiation (**LTP**), which is a property of certain synapses, including those of the Schaffer collaterals and the mossy fibers of the hippocampus. LTP is an increase in synaptic efficacy that follows a few seconds of high-frequency activity of a presynaptic terminal. Increased synaptic efficacy can be attributable to a change on either side of the synapse. The presynaptic terminal may release an increased amount of transmitter with the arrival of an action potential; this happens at synapses of the mossy fibers. Insertion of an increased number of receptor molecules into the postsynaptic membrane occurs at the synapses of Schaffer collaterals in area CA1. Fewer afferent impulses are then needed to depolarize the postsynaptic cell because more of the transmitter molecules released into the synaptic cleft can bind to postsynaptic receptors. LTP, which lasts for several days, leads to increased activity of affected postsynaptic neurons. A suitable pattern of activity in axons afferent to the hippocampal formation may lead to LTP in certain connected pyramidal and granule cells. These then continue to transmit impulses more frequently than before, even though the original external stimulus has ceased.

AFFERENT CONNECTIONS

The hippocampal formation has four main sources of afferents: the cerebral neocortex, septal area, contralateral hippocampus, and various nuclei in the reticular formation of the brain stem.

The largest contingent of fibers is from the **entorhinal area**. These fibers follow two routes to the hippocampus (see Fig. 18-4). The axons of the **perforant path** from the entorhinal area pass through the subiculum and across the base of the hippocampal sulcus to end in the dentate gyrus. The **alvear path** traverses the subcortical white matter and the alveus to end in the hippocampus. The entorhinal area is part of the primary olfactory area, and it also receives association fibers from the neocortex of the temporal lobe, which, in turn, communicates with widespread areas of neocortex, including the sensory association areas. Through these connections, as well as through others that involve the parahippocampal cortex generally, the perforant and alvear paths keep the hippocampal formation informed of all forms of sensation and of the higher activities of the brain.

Afferent fibers for the hippocampal formation are also present in the fornix and fimbria. They come from the **contralateral hippocampus** and from the **septal area** and the closely related **basal forebrain cholinergic nuclei** of the substantia innominata (see Chapter 12). Commissural fibers cross the midline in the hippocampal commissure, which is described in the next section of this chapter. Other hippocampal afferent fibers in the fornix are from

various **thalamic and hypothalamic nuclei**, the **ventral tegmental area** (dopaminergic), the **locus coeruleus** (noradrenergic), and the serotonergic **raphe nuclei** (see Chapter 9).

EFFERENT CONNECTIONS

The connections through which the hippocampal formation receives information from the entorhinal area and neocortex are paralleled by connections that provide for spread of activity from the hippocampal formation to the same cortex, and descending projections to the diencephalon and brain stem are also present. The fornix contains numerous afferent fibers, as described in the previous section of this chapter, but it also is the largest efferent pathway of the hippocampal formation.

The human **fornix** contains more than 1 million myelinated axons. Most of these axons originate in the subiculum. The rest of the axons originate in the hippocampus or are afferent to the hippocampal formation. The efferent fibers first traverse the alveus on the ventricular surface of the hippocampus on their way to the fimbria. The fimbria continues as the **crus** of the fornix, which begins at the posterior limit of the hippocampus beneath the splenium of the corpus callosum (see Fig. 18-3). The crus curves around the posterior end of the thalamus and joins its partner to form the **body** of the fornix beneath the corpus callosum. Here the **dorsal hippocampal commissure**, which is attached to the ventral surface of the splenium of the corpus callosum, carries fibers from the parahippocampal gyrus of one hemisphere to the hippocampal formation of the opposite hemisphere. (The human brain has only a vestigial ventral hippocampal commissure.)

Above the third ventricle, the body of the fornix separates into **columns**, each of which curves ventrally in front of the interventricular foramen. Here the anterior commissure lies immediately in front of the column of the fornix (see Fig. 16-7). Some fibers separate from the column just above the anterior commissure; these are distributed to the **septal area**, anterior part of the **hypothalamus**, and **substantia innominata**. The branch of the column of the fornix posterior to the anterior commissure is much larger. It gives off some fibers that end in the **lateral dorsal thalamic nucleus** and then continues through the hypothalamus, where most of the axons terminate in the **mamillary body**.

The mamillary body projects to the anterior nuclei of the thalamus through the **mamillothalamic fasciculus** (bundle of Vicq d'Azyr), which is readily demonstrable by dissection (see Fig. 11-15). The anterior and lateral dorsal thalamic nuclei are in reciprocal communication with the cingulate gyrus through fibers that travel around the lateral side of the lateral ventricle. The cingulate gyrus is also in reciprocal communication with the parahippocampal gyrus through the cingulum, a prominent association bundle in the limbic lobe (see Chapter 16). The anterior end of the cingulate gyrus and sulcus are connected by association fibers with much of the cortex of the frontal and temporal lobes, and a motor area (see Chapter 15) is also located in this region. There is increased activity in the anterior cingulate cortex when anticipating a movement or a purely cognitive task and also in association with pain and other unpleasant emotional experiences.

HIPPOCAMPAL CIRCUITS

The largest components of the limbic system contain a ring of interconnected neurons. It is named after Papez (the circuit of Papez), who postulated in 1937 that these parts of the brain "constitute a harmonious mechanism, which may elaborate functions of central emotion, as well as participate in emotional expression." These functions are now believed to be associated more with the amygdala than with the hippocampus. The sequence of components of Papez' circuit, with the names of fiber tracts italicized, is as follows: entorhinal area of parahippocampal gyrus, *perforant and alvear paths*, hippocampal formation, *fimbria and fornix*, mamillary body, *mamillothalamic fasciculus*, anterior thalamic nuclei, *internal capsule*, cingulate gyrus, *cingulum*, entorhinal area (Fig. 18-5).

The input to the circuit of Papez (see Fig. 18-5) is from the neocortex, thalamus, septal area, raphe nuclei, ventral tegmental area, and catecholamine nuclei of the reticular formation.

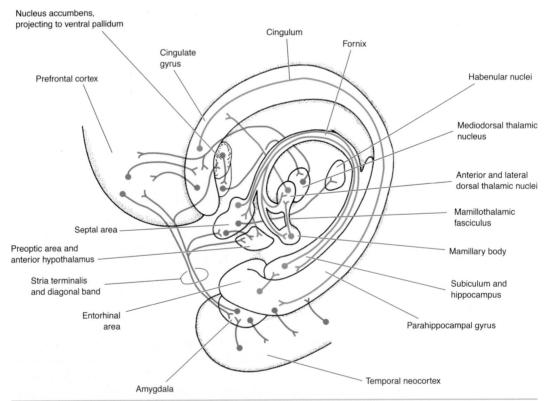

FIGURE 18-5   Connections of the hippocampal formation and amygdala in the forebrain and diencephalon, including the circuit of Papez (*red*) and other connections (*blue*).

The output is partly to the neocortex but also to regions of the reticular formation that have extensive connections with many parts of the central nervous system. The largest descending pathway is the **mamillotegmental fasciculus**, which consists of collateral branches of axons in the mamillothalamic fasciculus. These descending fibers terminate in the raphe nuclei of the reticular formation of the midbrain (Fig. 18-6). When thinking of the circuit of Papez, with its inputs and outputs, it is important to remember that ring-like circuits of neurons also exist within the hippocampal formation itself (see Fig. 18-4).

HIPPOCAMPAL FUNCTION: MEMORY

Psychologists and behavioral scientists recognize different types of long-term memory that are processed differently in the brain. **Declarative** (or **explicit**) **memory** is the knowledge and recall of facts or events that can be recalled to consciousness. The acquisition of an item into declarative memory typically occurs on a single occasion. Any fact or event is initially held in **short-term memory**. It may be forgotten during the course of the next hour or so; if not, it is moved into long-term storage. If declarative memories are not recalled from time to time, the process of recall will require mental effort or the memories may be forgotten. **Procedural** (or **implicit**) **memory** is for learned skills, including regularly performed motor tasks and mental activities such as using the common vocabulary and grammatical rules of a language. The learning occurs gradually, and recall is improved with repetition and practice. The best understood functions of the hippocampal formation are the retention of information in short-term memory and its transfer into long-term declarative memory.

The consolidation of recent memories may occur during sleep when the serotonergic raphe neurons that project to the hippocampal formation are active (see Chapter 9). In deep sleep, when the electroencephalogram (EEG) recorded over the neocortex shows regular, synchronized rhythms, the hippocampal EEG (recorded with a needle electrode) is desynchronized. In the waking state, the neocortical record is desynchronized, and the hippocampus generates a slow, regular rhythm.

Synaptic long-term potentiation was mentioned earlier as a postulated mechanism for the storage of recent memories by the hippocampus. The formation of permanent memory traces may involve the synthesis of new proteins and the formation of new synapses. The neuronal changes (sometimes called *en-*

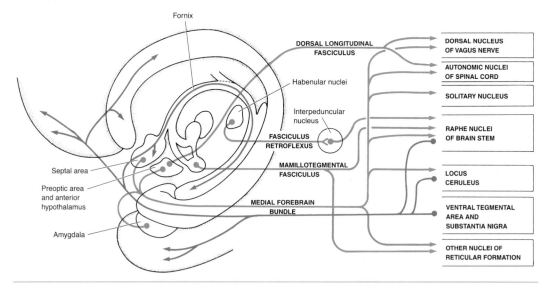

FIGURE 18-6 Pathways leading into (*blue*) and out of (*red*) the telencephalic and diencephalic components of the limbic system.

Memory Disorders

Impairment of memory is evident after bilateral temporal lobectomy (described later in this chapter) or lesser degrees of injury that bilaterally affect the hippocampal formation or its associated pathways. The hippocampus and its connections are necessary for the consolidation of new or short-term memories. The evidence for this function comes from many clinical observations, which generally agree with experimental results obtained in animals.

Loss of hippocampal function can occur if an arterial occlusion has caused an infarction in the hippocampal formation of one side and is followed at a later time by a similar infarction in the other hemisphere. More commonly, the intact hippocampus is deprived of oxygen for only a short time, after which the patient suddenly becomes unaware of the events of the preceding few hours and is temporarily unable to form new memories. The condition is known as **transient global amnesia**. Cerebral anoxia from any cause can, as mentioned earlier, cause death of the principal neurons of Sommer's sector (i.e., CA1) of the hippocampus bilaterally. Many patients resuscitated after cardiac arrest of more than a few minutes' duration are left with defective memory for this reason.

Concussion is loss of consciousness and retrograde amnesia for events immediately preceding a head injury. It is not caused by permanent brain damage. The hippocampi can be damaged by hemorrhage when a head injury causes the temporal poles to strike the greater wings of the sphenoid bone, which form the anterior wall of the middle cranial fossa. Anterograde amnesia, with impaired consolidation of new declarative memories, is a common consequence of more severe head injuries.

Bilateral hippocampal lesions interrupt the major circuit of the limbic system. Interruption of the same pathway outside the hippocampal formation, such as occurs when both mamillary bodies are involved in a destructive lesion, also results in a memory defect. Amnesia may also occur after development of bilateral lesions in the medio-dorsal nuclei of the thalamus. The mediodorsal nuclei are connected with the prefrontal cortices, and these are involved in higher mental functions, although not specifically with memory. Medial thalamic lesions are likely to interrupt the mamillothalamic fibers as well, however. Bilateral surgical transection of the fornix, performed in attempts to limit the spread of epileptic discharges or in the course of removing tumors from the region of the third ventricle, has caused severe amnesia.

Animal experiments indicate that the cholinergic neurons of the substantia innominata in the basal forebrain (see Chapter 12), which project to the hippocampus and all parts of the cerebral cortex, are involved in memory. The inability to form new memories in **Alzheimer's disease** may be caused partly by loss of these cholinergic projections (see Chapter 12), but degenerative changes in the entorhinal cortex and hippocampus also occur early in the course of this disorder, and in the late stages, extensive neocortical atrophy occurs.

Patients with any of these lesions forget information obtained recently but retain the ability to recall old memories. When the hippocampi or the circuits of Papez are no longer functional, memories of earlier events are retained because these have already been established, presumably as macromolecular changes throughout the cerebral cortex. These patients have amnesia for events that occurred more recently than the lesion because the mechanism for retention or consolidation of new or short-term memory is no longer operating. Most lesions in the diencephalon (thalamus and mamillary bodies) are attributable to metabolic disturbances caused by alcoholism. In the resulting syndrome (**Korsakoff's psychosis**), the patient inserts remembered events from the remote past into fluent but blatantly untrue stories, attempting to compensate for the absence of more recent memories.

Localized lesions do not affect old memories, although these are eventually lost along with other mental capabilities when advanced dementia caused by severe and widespread degeneration of the cerebral cortex is present.

grams) representing long-term memory, both declarative and procedural, are believed to be present throughout the parieto-occipito-temporal and frontal association cortex, and some investigators suspect that the corpus striatum, thalamus, and cerebellum are also involved.

Amygdaloid Body (Amygdala)

The amygdaloid body consists of several groups of neurons situated between the anterior end of the temporal horn of the lateral ventricle and the ventral surface of the lentiform nucleus (Fig. 18-7). The dorsomedial division of the amygdaloid body, known as the **corticomedial group** of nuclei, blends with the cortex of the uncus. Its afferent fibers come from the olfactory bulb, and it is part of the lateral olfactory area (see Chapter 17). The larger ventrolateral division consists of the **basolateral** and **central groups** of nuclei, which have no direct input from the olfactory bulb, although they connect with the corticomedial nuclei and with the cortex of the entorhinal area. The central and basolateral groups are included in the limbic system on the basis of the results of experiments that involve stimulation and ablation in laboratory animals and clinical observations in humans.

CONNECTIONS OF THE AMYGDALA

The basolateral group has widespread connections, most of which are not in the form of well-defined fiber bundles. Using the shortest routes, **reciprocal connections with cortex** of the frontal and temporal lobes and the cingulate gyrus are present. Subcortical afferent fibers come from the **thalamus** (intralaminar nuclei) and the **catecholamine nuclei, raphe nuclei,** and **parabrachial nuclei** of the reticular formation. Some of these afferents carry signals relating to painful stimuli. Also present are dopaminergic afferents, mostly from the **ventral tegmental area** and some from the substantia nigra, and cholinergic fibers from the **basal forebrain nuclei** in the substantia innominata.

The **central nuclei** of the amygdala receive afferent fibers from both the olfactory corticomedial and the nonolfactory basolateral nuclei. The projections of the central nuclei are similar to those of the basolateral group, described in the following paragraphs.

The principal connections of the basolateral and central groups of nuclei of the amygdala are shown in Figures 18-5 and 18-6. Reciprocal connections with neocortical areas (prefrontal and temporal lobes and anterior cingulate gyrus) are prominent. The projections to the

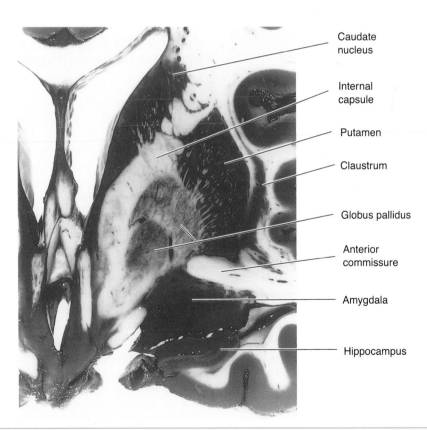

Caudate nucleus

Internal capsule

Putamen

Claustrum

Globus pallidus

Anterior commissure

Amygdala

Hippocampus

FIGURE 18-7   Coronal section through the amygdaloid body and neighboring parts of the brain, stained by a method that differentiates gray matter (*dark*) from white matter (*light*).

prefrontal cortex are modulated by circuitry involving the nucleus accumbens and ventral pallidum, explained in Chapter 12.

The most conspicuous efferent bundle of the amygdala is the **stria terminalis**. This slender bundle of axons (see Fig. 16-9) follows the curvature of the tail of the caudate nucleus, continuing along the groove between the caudate nucleus and thalamus in the floor of the central part of the lateral ventricle. Most of the constituent fibers terminate in the **septal area** and in the **preoptic area** and **anterior hypothalamus**. Other axons in the stria terminalis enter the **medial forebrain bundle** and go to various parts of the brain stem, including the dorsal nucleus of the vagus nerve and the solitary nucleus, which have visceral functions (see Chapters 8 and 24).

The stria terminalis is a long tract because it follows the curve of the lateral ventricle. Other efferent fibers of the amygdala form a shorter **ventral amygdalofugal pathway**, which passes through the **diagonal band of Broca**, a body of white matter within the anterior perforated substance. The ventral amygdalofugal pathway carries axons from the amygdala to the septal area; to the **nucleus accumbens** (ventral striatum); and to the **dorsomedial nucleus of the thalamus**, which projects to the prefrontal cortex. There are also direct connections between the amygdala and the prefrontal cortex (Fig. 18-5).

The septal area is a major target of projections from the amygdala. The septal area sends fibers in the **stria medullaris thalami** to the **habenular nuclei**. These project through the **fasciculus retroflexus** (habenulointerpeduncular tract) to the **interpeduncular nucleus**, and the pathway continues through the reticular formation to autonomic nuclei. The habenular nuclei also receive some afferent fibers from the globus pallidus, providing a pathway through which the neocortex and the corpus striatum can influence autonomic functions. Direct hypothalamospinal fibers in the **dorsal longitudinal fasciculus** provide another pathway whereby the limbic system is able to influence preganglionic autonomic neurons.

FUNCTIONS OF THE AMYGDALA

The behavioral and emotional functions of the limbic system are chiefly associated with the central and basolateral nuclei of the amygdala.

In ordinary speech, the word *emotion* refers to subjective feelings that are difficult to define. Neuroscientists also use this word for activities of the brain evoked by incentives for survival. Emotional responses, therefore, include running away from a potential predator, drinking when thirsty, sweating when hot, and responses to the presence of a potential mate or rival.

Functional nuclear magnetic resonance imaging (fMRI) studies show variation in activity of the amygdala when a person is looking at pictures that evoke different emotional feelings. Electrical stimulation of the amygdala in conscious humans evokes feelings of fear and sometimes of general irritability or even anger. Injury or disease of the amygdala is usually combined with damage to the hippocampal formation and sometimes also the visual association cortex of the temporal lobe, thereby causing a mixture of behavioral and cognitive disturbances.

Temporal Lobe Disorders

EFFECTS OF DESTRUCTIVE LESIONS IN BOTH TEMPORAL LOBES

In monkeys, complete removal of both temporal lobes leads to the **Klüver-Bucy syndrome**, consisting of docility, loss of the ability to learn, excessive exploratory behavior using the mouth more than the hands, visual agnosia, and (in males) abnormal sexual activity. Smaller lesions have less bizarre consequences, with dysfunction partly attributable to the loss of individual parts of the limbic system.

Bilateral removal of the temporal pole, including the amygdaloid body and much of the hippocampal formation, is followed by docility and lack of emotional responses such as fear or anger to situations that normally arouse those responses. Male animals exhibit increased sexual activity, and the sexual drive may be perverted, being directed toward either gender, a member of another species, or even inanimate objects. Lesions confined to the amygdaloid bodies produce similar changes, with sexual behavior less affected. With lesions that also include the

Human Bilateral Lesions

In humans, removal or destructive disease of both temporal lobes sometimes results in a voracious appetite, increased (sometimes perverse) sexual activity, and flattened affect. These abnormalities, together with visual agnosia, can occur also after head injury, in viral infections of the brain, and in some patients with Alzheimer's disease. An intensively studied individual case is "H.M.," who underwent removal of the medial parts of both temporal lobes as treatment for epilepsy in 1953 at age 27 years. Since the operation, H.M. has been unable to remember any new fact or event for more than 5 minutes. Despite the large sizes of his temporal lobe lesions, H.M. does not have other features of the Klüver-Bucy syndrome.

TEMPORAL LOBE EPILEPSY

Epilepsy is a condition in which abnormal synaptic excitation causes uncontrolled propagation of action potentials in the brain. Such an episode (variously called an *attack*, *fit*, or *seizure*) may begin with sensory symptoms or a subjective feeling of strangeness, known as an **aura**. The nature of the aura may provide a clue to the location of the **epileptogenic focus** in which the abnormal activity is initiated. During the attack, a loss of consciousness or at least of full awareness of the surroundings occurs, and generalized convulsions attributable to stimulation of motor neurons commonly occur. Jacksonian epilepsy, arising from a focus in the primary motor cortex, was mentioned in Chapter 15. *Petit mal* is a type of childhood epilepsy that causes frequent episodes of loss of consciousness, each lasting less than 1 second, known as *absence seizures*. It is associated with a characteristic spike-and-wave appearance in the EEG, and it may arise from a focus in the thalamus. The term *grand mal* is applied to forms of epilepsy associated with convulsions. Between attacks, the EEG includes bursts of high-voltage spikes and large low-frequency waves.

The most frequent site of an epileptogenic focus is the medial surface of the temporal lobe, which can be damaged by the nearby tentorium cerebelli (see Chapter 25) when the head is squeezed during birth. Neurons near the resulting scar constitute the focus, which is often in the amygdala, the anterior end of the hippocampus, or the entorhinal area. In many cases, the seizure activity does not spread to the whole brain, and the diagnosis may be overlooked because of the absence of convulsions. An attack often begins with a hallucination of a nasty but unidentifiable smell caused by stimulation of the cortex of uncus and corticomedial nuclei of amygdala. The aura commonly includes déjà vu, which is an unnatural feeling of familiarity with the surroundings and circumstances, attributed to activity in the hippocampal formation, amygdala, and sensory association cortex of the temporal lobe. As the attack continues, there are feelings of fear and anxiety (stimulation of central and basolateral nuclei of the amygdala) and autonomic manifestations such as sweating, tachycardia (fast heart rate), and peculiar abdominal sensations (stimulation of amygdala, insular cortex, hypothalamus, and preganglionic sympathetic neurons). Rarely, there may be irrational speech and behavior that the patient does not remember afterward.

Antiepileptic drugs act by various mechanisms, including partial blockade of sodium and other ion channels and potentiation of the action of GABA, the transmitter at most inhibitory synapses (see Chapter 2). The drugs reduce the frequency and severity of attacks. It is sometimes feasible to cure the condition by locating the epileptogenic focus and removing it surgically. The anterior part of one temporal lobe may be removed for this purpose, but the surgeon must first ensure that the other temporal lobe is intact. It is also necessary to avoid damage to Wernicke's receptive speech area (see Chapter 15), which is located in the temporal lobe of the cerebral hemisphere that is dominant for language.

hippocampi, the animals can no longer be trained to perform tricks or carry out tasks, having evidently lost the ability to learn anything new.

When bilateral ablations extend to the posterior parts of the temporal lobes, the animal has all the abnormalities mentioned previously and is also unable to recognize things that it

sees. It compensates by exploring objects with its mouth. This **visual agnosia**, termed "psychic blindness" by Klüver and Bucy in 1937, is now attributed to loss of visual association cortex concerned with formed images in the posterior part of the inferior temporal gyrus (see Chapters 15 and 20). The excessive oral exploration leads to excessive eating.

Anxiety States

Inappropriate activity of the amygdala may occur in abnormal mental states with excessive symptoms of anxiety. Patients may experience severe episodes (panic attacks) of excessive activity of the sympathetic nervous system or a generalized condition dominated by subjective feelings of worry with motor manifestations such as muscle tension and jitteriness. Anxiolytic drugs (useful for the treatment of anxiety states) include the benzodiazepines such as chlordiazepoxide, diazepam, and several others with names ending in -azepam. These drugs enhance the action of the inhibitory neurotransmitter GABA by binding to a subtype of its postsynaptic receptor that occurs abundantly on the surfaces of neurons in the amygdala and other parts of the limbic system.

DEPRESSION

In several psychiatric disorders, great suffering results from depression, which is an abnormal condition quite different from the sadness anyone can experience in appropriate circumstances. Drugs that relieve depression enhance the synaptic actions of noradrenaline and serotonin, either by blocking the reuptake of the amines into presynaptic terminals (tricyclic antidepressants such as amitriptyline and imipramine) or by inhibiting monoamine oxidase, an enzyme that catalyzes the oxidative degradation of noradrenaline and serotonin. Other antidepressive drugs selectively inhibit serotonin reuptake (SSRIs such as fluoxetine and paroxetine). Most of the neurons that use amines as transmitters are located in the brain stem (see Chapter 9). Their greatly branched axons end in gray matter throughout the forebrain, including all parts of the limbic system.

EMOTIONAL AND VISCERAL RESPONSES

Experimental and clinical studies have led to the view that the normal limbic system, especially the amygdala, is responsible for such strong affective reactions as fear and anger and the emotions associated with sexual behavior. Changes in visceral and somatic motor function accompany these emotions, and electrical stimulation of the amygdala has been shown to produce similar responses. These include increased heart rate, suppression of salivation, increased gastrointestinal movements, and pupillary dilatation. Respiratory and facial movements also are changed, and patients have generalized irritability, typically manifested as sudden movements (startle reaction) in re-

Schizophrenia

Abnormalities of the limbic system have also been found in **schizophrenia**. In this disease, the processes of thinking are profoundly disturbed, with delusions, auditory hallucinations, inability to make associations between ideas, and reduced emotional expression. Careful anatomical measurements show that the hippocampal formation, amygdala, and parahippocampal gyrus are smaller than normal in the brains of schizophrenic patients, possibly as a result of abnormal growth of these parts of the brain.

Drugs that alleviate the clinical features of schizophrenia (antipsychotic agents) antagonize the actions of dopamine, which is the principal neurotransmitter of the neurons in the ventral tegmental area that project to the amygdala, nucleus accumbens, hippocampal formation, and prefrontal cortex. None of these drugs are entirely selective in their actions on dopamine receptors; they also block noradrenaline and serotonin receptors. Antipsychotics of one group, the dibenzodiazepines typified by clozapine, antagonize the actions of noradrenaline and serotonin more strongly than those of serotonin. Not surprisingly (see Chapter 7), the drugs that strongly antagonize dopamine (especially the butyrophenones, typified by haloperidol) can cause parkinsonism as a side effect. Prolonged treatment may also lead to a movement disorder called **tardive dyskinesia** in which choreiform movements (see Chapter 12) of the lips and tongue are prominent. Unlike the parkinsonian side effect, tardive dyskinesia quite frequently persists after withdrawal of the drug.

sponse to a slight sensory stimulus. Electrical stimulation of the amygdala in humans induces feelings of fear or anger. These observations may indicate that activity in the amygdala gives rise to the autonomic and somatic accompaniments of fear and anxiety.

Suggested Reading

Bancaud J, Brunet-Bourgin F, Chauvel P, et al. Anatomical origin of deja vu and vivid "memories" in human temporal lobe epilepsy. *Brain* 1994;117:71–90.

Corkin S. What's new with the amnesic patient H.M.? *Nature Rev Neurosci* 2002;3:153–160.

Corkin S, Amaral DG, Gonzalez RG, et al. H.M.'s medial temporal lesion: findings from magnetic resonance imaging. *J Neurosci* 1997;17:3964–3979.

Davis M. The role of the amygdala in fear and anxiety. *Annu Rev Neurosci* 1992;15:333–375.

Delacalle S, Lim C, Sobreviela T, et al. Cholinergic innervation in the human hippocampal formation including the entorhinal cortex. *J Comp Neurol* 1994;345:321–344.

Devinsky O, Morrell MJ, Vogt BA. Contributions of anterior cingulate cortex to behaviour. *Brain* 1995;118:279–306.

Gaffan D, Gaffan EA. Amnesia in man following transection of the fornix: a review. *Brain* 1991;114:2611–2618.

Gloor P, Salanova V, Olivier A, et al. The human dorsal hippocampal commissure: an anatomically identifiable and functional pathway. *Brain* 1993;116:1249–1273.

Irwin W, Davidson RJ, Lowe MJ, et al. Human amygdala activation detected with echo-planar functional magnetic resonance imaging. *NeuroReport* 1996;7:1765–1769.

Kier EL, Fulbright RK, Bronen RA. Limbic lobe embryology and anatomy: dissection and MR of the medial surface of the fetal cerebral hemisphere. *Am J Neuroradiol* 1995;16:1847–1853.

Kier EL, Kim JH, Fulbright RK, et al. Embryology of the human fetal hippocampus: MR imaging, anatomy, and histology. *Am J Neuroradiol* 1997;18:525–532.

Klüver H, Bucy PC. "Psychic blindness" and other symptoms following bilateral temporal lobectomy in rhesus monkeys. *Am J Physiol* 1937;119:352–353.

LeDoux JE. Emotion circuits of the brain. *Annu Rev Neurosci* 2000;23:155–184.

Lilly R, Cummings JL, Benson F, et al. The human Klüver-Bucy syndrome. *Neurology* 1983;33:1141–1145.

Milner B, Squire LR, Kandel ER. Cognitive neuroscience and the study of memory. *Neuron* 1998;20:445–468.

Murtha S, Chertkow H, Beauregard M, et al. Anticipation causes increased blood flow to the anterior cingulate cortex. *Hum Brain Mapp* 1996;4:103–112.

Müller F, O'Rahilly R. The amygdaloid complex and the medial and lateral ventricular eminences in staged human embryos. *J Anat* 2006;208:547–564.

O'Rahilly R, Müller F. *The Embryonic Human Brain. An Atlas of Developmental Stages,* 3rd ed. New York: Wiley-Liss, 2006.

Papez JW. A proposed mechanism for emotion. *Arch Neurol Psychiatry* 1937;38:725–734.

Penfield W, Milner B. Memory deficit produced by bilateral lesions in the hippocampal zone. *Arch Neurol Psychiatry* 1958;79:475–497.

Vanderwolf CH, Cain DP. The behavioral neurobiology of learning and memory: a conceptual reorientation. *Brain Res Rev* 1994;19:264–297.

Van Hoesen GW, Hyman BT, Damasio AR. Entorhinal cortex pathology in Alzheimer's disease. *Hippocampus* 1991;1:1–8.

von Cramon DY, Hebel N, Schuri U. A contribution to the anatomical basis of thalamic amnesia. *Brain* 1985;108:993–1008.

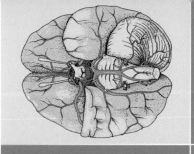

PART III

Review of the Major Systems

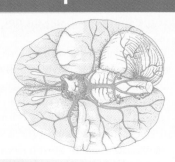

Chapter 19

GENERAL SENSORY SYSTEMS

Important Facts

- Neuronal signals from skin and deeper structures are segregated in the spinal cord. Transmission to the thalamus and cerebral cortex may occur through the spinothalamic tract or through the dorsal funiculus (posterior column) and medial lemniscus.

- For pain, temperature, and the less discriminative aspects of touch, neurons in the dorsal horn have axons that cross the midline in the spinal cord and ascend as the spinothalamic tract, which is laterally situated in the spinal cord and brain stem.

- For discriminative touch and conscious proprioception, the axons of primary sensory neurons ascend ipsilaterally in the dorsal funiculus and end in the gracile or cuneate nucleus. Lateral inhibition in these nuclei provides a mechanism for enhancing sensory discrimination between adjacent parts of the peripheral fields. Fibers arising in the gracile and cuneate nuclei cross in the medulla and ascend in the medial lemniscus, which is located near the midline in the medulla and shifts to a lateral location in the midbrain.

- For conscious proprioception from the lower limb, an additional pathway exists through the spinal cord and caudal part of the medulla. This involves the caudal part of the gracile fasciculus, the dorsal spinocerebellar tract, and nucleus Z.

- Both the spinothalamic tract and the medial lemniscus end in the ventral posterolateral (VPl) nucleus of the thalamus. This thalamic nucleus projects to the primary somesthetic cortex of the postcentral gyrus, where the contralateral half of the body is represented as an upside-down homunculus.

- The somesthetic pathways for the head include the trigeminal sensory nuclei and their projections to the contralateral ventral posteromedial (VPm) thalamic nucleus. Primary afferent axons for touch end in the pontine trigeminal nucleus. Pain and temperature fibers descend in the spinal trigeminal tract before ending in the caudal part of its nucleus.

- Lesions in the spinal cord and brain stem can affect the somesthetic pathways separately, causing dissociated sensory loss.

- The main pathways are supplemented by others, especially for pain, with relays in the reticular formation and thalamic nuclei other than the VPl or VPm. A pathway through the mediodorsal thalamic nucleus to the anterior cingulate cortex is active in the perception of pain.

- The primary somatosensory area and associated parietal association cortex are necessary for localizing the source of a painful stimulus and for recognizing objects by touch.

- Descending projections influence transmission in the ascending somatosensory pathways. These include the raphespinal tract, which inhibits the perception of stimuli that would be painful.

This chapter deals with the pathways from the general sensory receptors to the thalamus and thence to the cerebral cortex, where the sensations are appreciated subjectively. With an understanding of the anatomy of these pathways, an appraisal of sensory deficits provides information concerning the location of a lesion in the central nervous system (CNS).

Sensory axons that enter the spinal cord in dorsal roots of spinal nerves segregate in such a way that there are two main general sensory systems. The first of these includes one or more synaptic relays in the dorsal gray horn. Spinal neurons give rise to axons that cross the midline and ascend in the ventrolateral white matter to the thalamus. This, the **spinothalamic system**, carries signals that report the senses of pain; temperature; and the less discriminative tactile sensations, including light touch and firm pressure.

In the second system, primary afferent axons turn rostrally in the ipsilateral dorsal funiculus of the spinal cord and do not end until they reach certain nuclei in the lower medulla. Axons from these nuclei cross the midline and then ascend as the medial lemniscus to the thalamus. Hence, this second pathway is called the **medial lemniscus system**. It is concerned primarily with discriminative aspects of sensation, especially the awareness of position and movement of parts of the body and the tactile recognition of shapes and textures and of changes in the positions of stimuli that move across the surface of the skin. The medial lemniscus system is often called the **posterior column system**, especially in clinical usage, because it includes the dorsal funiculi ("posterior columns") of the spinal cord.

The **spinoreticulothalamic pathway**, which includes relays in the reticular formation of the brain stem, also conducts ascending signals generated by cutaneous sensation. It is therefore closely related to the spinothalamic system. The association is especially seen in central conduction for pain. In fact, the spinothalamic pathway and the less direct spinoreticulothalamic pathway, with their projections to the cerebral cortex, may be combined under the term **ventrolateral** (or **anterolateral**) **system**. The comparable term **dorsomedial system** is then used for the medial lemniscus system. The various names for the pathways for general sensation are summarized in Table 19-1. Unfortunately, all the terms are in fairly widespread use by anatomists, physiologists, and clinicians. The **trigeminothalamic** pathways serve the same functions as the spinothalamic and medial lemniscus systems, but for the head. They are also mentioned in Chapter 8 in connection with the central connections of the trigeminal, facial, glossopharyngeal, and vagus nerves.

The general sensory pathways are said to consist of primary, secondary, and tertiary neurons, with cell bodies in sensory ganglia, the spinal cord or brain stem, and the thalamus, respectively. The concept of a simple relay of three neurons is not accurate, however, because interneurons act on the secondary and tertiary neurons. In addition, the activity of the secondary neurons is influenced by descending axons from the cerebral cortex and the brain stem.

Spinothalamic System

The spinothalamic or ventrolateral system is known also as the "pathway for pain and temperature" because these modalities of sensation are transmitted to the brain in the spinothalamic tract. It is also concerned with touch, as already noted.

RECEPTORS

The **receptors for pain** (**nociceptors**) are the unencapsulated axonal endings of the thinnest group A fibers (group Aδ) and of unmyelinated (group C) fibers. Pain may be felt as two waves separated by an interval of a few tenths of a second. The first wave is sharp and localized, with conduction by group Aδ fibers. The second wave, which is rather diffuse and more disagreeable, depends on group C fibers, with a slow conduction speed. The two waves are most easily noticed in the feet (as when treading on something sharp) because of the greater lengths of the axons in the nerves of the lower limb.

The mechanism of pain perception is inseparable from that of the initiation of **inflammation**, which is the response of living tissue to any kind of injury. Injured cells release several substances known as *mediators*, which act on venules and nerve endings. The venules dilate, causing redness of the affected area and become permeable to blood plasma, which leaks out to cause swelling of the tissue. Simultaneous stimulation of the nociceptive endings results in perception of pain. Action potentials do not pass solely to the CNS; they are also propagated antidromically along other peripheral branches of the afferent axon. In the case of cutaneous group C fibers, these impulses cause a peptide neurotransmitter known as *substance P* to be released into the interstitial tissues of the dermis. This acts upon arterioles and in the dermis, which dilate. Substance P also causes degranulation of mast cells, which release more mediators, thereby enhancing the dilatation of arterioles and sometimes also causing edema in the area surrounding the injury. In the skin, the total result constitutes the **triple response** (of Lewis): a red mark and a wheal, surrounded by a flare of neurogenic

TABLE 19-1   **Names and Components of the Somatic Sensory Pathways Concerned With Parts of the Body Below the Head**

Medial Lemniscus System	Spinothalamic System
Alternative names:	
Dorsomedial system	Ventrolateral system
Posterior column system	Anterolateral system
Dorsal column system	
Includes:	
Neurons with cell bodies in the peripheral nervous system	
Dorsal root ganglia	Dorsal root ganglia
Dorsal (posterior) funiculi (also called the *dorsal* or *posterior columns*), each consisting of the gracile fasciculus and cuneate fasciculus	Dorsolateral tract of Lissauer
Neurons with decussating axons that end in the thalamus	
Gracile and cuneate nuclei (also nucleus Z*)	Dorsal horn of spinal gray matter
Decussation of the medial lemnisci	Ventral white commissure of spinal cord
Medial lemniscus	Spinothalamic tract (also spinoreticular fibers)
	Spinal lemniscus (also called *spinothalamic fibers* in the brain stem; also reticulothalamic fibers)
Thalamocortical neurons	
Ventral posterior nucleus of thalamus	Ventral posterior nucleus of thalamus and other thalamic nuclei (mediodorsal, posterior group, intralaminar group)
Internal capsule	Internal capsule
Cerebral cortex	
Primary somatosensory cortex	Primary somatosensory cortex
Parietal association cortex	Parietal association cortex
	Anterior cingulate cortex

*The pathway for conscious proprioception from the lower limb includes an additional relay in the nucleus thoracicus, with axons that ascend in the dorsal spinocerebellar tract and have branches in the medulla that synapse with neurons in nucleus Z.

arteriolar vasodilation. A neurally mediated phenomenon such as this, which does not involve any synapses, is called an **axon reflex**. The **receptors for temperature** are probably also morphologically nondescript free nerve endings. The axons are of similar caliber to those that conduct impulses for pain. The **receptors for light touch** are unencapsulated nerve endings, Merkel and peritrichial end-ings, and Meissner's corpuscles. Ruffini endings respond to firm pressure on the skin, especially when this causes the dermis to move on the underlying subcutaneous tissue. Conduction for light touch and pressure in peripheral nerves is by myelinated group A fibers of medium diameter. (Descriptions of the specialized sensory nerve endings can be found in Chapter 3.)

ASCENDING CENTRAL PATHWAY

Synapses and Interneurons in the Dorsal Horn

Cell bodies of small and intermediate size in the dorsal root ganglia have central processes that constitute the lateral divisions of the dorsal rootlets. These axons conduct impulses from pain and temperature receptors (Fig. 19-1). Afferents for light touch and pressure enter the dorsal gray horn through the medial division of the dorsal rootlets. The pain and temperature fibers enter the **dorsolateral tract** (tract of Lissauer) of the spinal cord, in which ascending and descending branches travel, in most instances, for lengths that correspond to about one segment.

The terminals and the collateral branches of the axons in the dorsolateral tract enter the dorsal horn, where they branch profusely (see Fig. 5-8). The **substantia gelatinosa**, which is located near the tip of the dorsal horn, is an important region in which patterns of incoming sensory impulses are modified. The dendrites of the gelatinosa cells are contacted not only by primary afferent axons but also by reticulospinal fibers, notably those derived from the raphe nuclei of the medulla. (The descending pathways that modulate transmission in the ascending sensory pathways are discussed later in this chapter.) The axons of the cells in the substantia gelatinosa ascend and descend in the dorsolateral tract and in the adjacent white matter, mostly for about the length of one segment. Throughout its length, the axon of a gelatinosa cell gives off branches that end by synapsing with the dendrites of **tract cells**, whose axons constitute the spinothalamic tract.

The dendrites of the tract cells are contacted by excitatory primary afferent axons for pain and temperature, by inhibitory axons of the gelatinosa cells, and by excitatory primary afferents for light touch and pressure. These connections, shown diagrammatically in Figures 5-8 and 19-2, enable a tract cell to decide whether a potentially harmful stimulus is intense enough to initiate the onward transmission of a signal of pain perception. The neuronal circuitry for pain is discussed in more detail later.

Spinothalamic Tract

Most of the tract cells have their cell bodies in the **nucleus proprius**, near the base of the dorsal horn. Large neurons at the tip of the dorsal horn also contribute a proportion of the spinothalamic fibers, notably those concerned with pain. The axons of the tract cells cross the midline in the ventral white commissure. Continuing through the ventral horn of gray matter, the axons ascend in the **spinothalamic tract**, situated in the ventral part of the lateral funiculus and in the adjoining region of the ventral funiculus (see Fig. 5-10). Proceeding rostrally, axons are continually being added to the internal aspect of the tract. At upper cervical levels, therefore, fibers from sacral segments are most superficial, followed by fibers from lumbar and thoracic segments. The fibers from cervical segments are closest to the gray matter.

The spinothalamic fibers continue into the medulla without appreciable change of position initially (see Figs. 7-2 to 7-4). At the level of the inferior olivary nucleus, the tract is close to the surface of the medulla, between the inferior olivary nucleus and the spinal trigeminal nucleus (see Figs. 7-5 to 7-7). At and above this level, the spinothalamic fibers constitute most of the **spinal lemniscus**, which also includes axons of the spinotectal (spinomesencephalic) tract destined for the superior colliculus. The spinal lemniscus continues through the ventrolateral region of the dorsal pons, and in the midbrain, it runs along the lateral edge of the medial lemniscus (see Figs. 7-8 to 7-15). In their passage through the brain stem, the spinothalamic axons give off collateral branches that terminate in the medullary and pontine reticular formation and in the periaqueductal gray matter of the midbrain. There are also **spinoreticular fibers** that go no farther rostrally than the pons.

Thalamus and Cerebral Cortex

Most of the spinothalamic axons end in the **ventral posterior nucleus of the thalamus**. This nucleus consists of two parts: the **ventral posterolateral (VPl) division**, in which spinothalamic axons and the medial lemniscus terminate and the **ventral posteromedial (VPm) division**, which receives trigeminothalamic axons. The somatotopic organization is such that the contralateral lower limb is represented

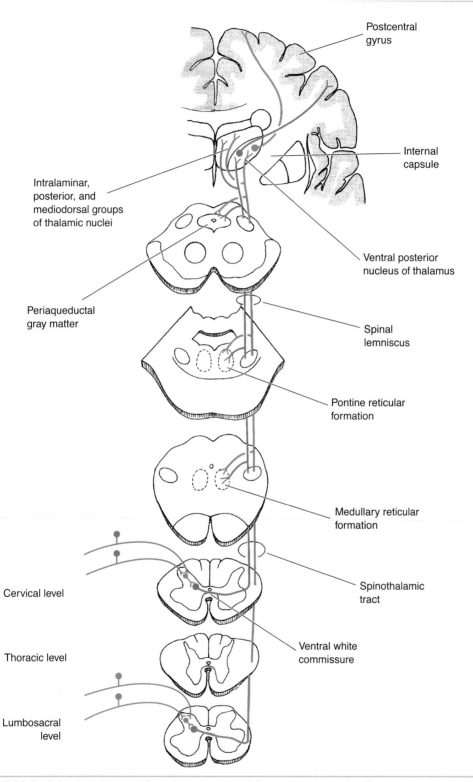

FIGURE 19-1   Spinothalamic system for pain, temperature, light touch, and pressure. The pathway from the lower limb is shown in red, and that from the upper limb is shown in blue.

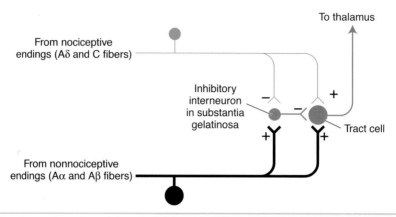

FIGURE 19-2   Simple illustration of the gate control theory of pain. Whereas nonnociceptive primary sensory neurons stimulate the inhibitory interneurons, nociceptive afferents inhibit them. An increase in nonnociceptive input reduces the rate of firing of the spinothalamic tract neuron. Compare this diagram with Figure 5-8.

dorsolaterally, and the contralateral upper limb is represented ventromedially in the VPl; the opposite side of the head is represented in the VPm.

The thalamocortical projection consists of neurons in the ventral posterior nucleus, whose axons traverse the **posterior limb of the internal capsule** and corona radiata to reach the **primary somesthetic area** in the parietal lobe. The contralateral half of the body, exclusive of the head, is represented as inverted in the dorsal two thirds of the primary somesthetic area (see Fig. 15-3). The cortical area for the hand is disproportionately large, providing for maximal sensory discrimination. The somatotopic arrangement at various levels of the sensory pathways forms the basis for recognition of the site of stimulation.

Some axons of the spinal lemniscus end in thalamic nuclei other than the VPl, notably those of the **posterior** and **intralaminar** groups and the **mediodorsal nucleus**. The posterior group projects to the insula and to the adjacent parietal cortex, including that of the second somatic sensory area, which is situated at the lower end of the postcentral gyrus. The intralaminar nuclei project diffusely to the frontal and parietal lobes of the cerebral cortex and to the striatum. They may be involved in the maintenance of a conscious, alert state (see Chapter 9). The mediodorsal nucleus is connected with the frontal lobes, especially their medial and orbital surfaces—cortical regions concerned with affect, decision making, and foresight (see

Chapter 15). A projection of the mediodorsal nucleus to the anterior part of the cingulate gyrus is activated by painful stimuli.

PAIN

Pain is a common complaint, and it is therefore necessary to become conversant with the anatomy, physiology, and pharmacology of this symptom. The mechanisms whereby peripheral nerve endings respond to injurious stimuli have already been reviewed. The central pathways concerned with pain are now discussed in further detail.

Spinal Mechanisms

Perception of pain is thought to be modified by neural mechanisms in the dorsal horn. In addition to the influence of reticulospinal and corticospinal fibers, to be discussed later, the transmission of impulses for pain to the brain is altered by dorsal root afferents for other sensory modalities. Afferent axons of larger diameter, especially those for touch and deep pressure, have branches that synapse with the dendrites of the gelatinosa cells. Trains of impulses coming through the larger axons can stimulate the gelatinosa cells, causing these interneurons to inhibit the tract cells that are concerned with nociception. The inhibitory effect can be overcome by sufficient nociceptive input to the tract cells. This postulated mechanism, known as the **gate control theory** of pain (see Fig. 19-2), enables the neurons in the spinal cord to determine, on the basis of all incoming sensory stimuli, whether a particular event should be reported to the brain as being painful. A similar mechanism is presumed to exist in the caudal part of the spinal trigeminal nucleus, which is the rostral continuation of the tip of the dorsal horn. The gate mechanism probably operates when pain arising in deep structures such as muscles and joints is relieved by stimulating sensory endings in the overlying skin (e.g., by rubbing or by applying warmth or a mild chemical irritant such as a liniment).

A simpler, direct pathway is provided by the large neurons (Waldeyer cells) at the tip of the dorsal horn. These are activated by nociceptive primary afferent fibers and have axons that travel in the spinothalamic tract to the ventral posterior and mediodorsal thalamic nuclei.

The simplest defensive reflex initiated by pain is the **flexor reflex**, which involves at least two synapses in the spinal cord (see Fig. 5-13) and causes flexion of a limb to withdraw it from the source of a sudden painful stimulus. In quadrupeds, there is also a **crossed extensor reflex** in which the withdrawal is assisted by extension of the contralateral limb. In normal humans, the crossed extensor reflex is largely suppressed as a result of activity in descending tracts of the spinal cord, but both it and the flexor reflex are conspicuous and, because of a lowered threshold, troublesome in paraplegic patients.

Ascending Pathways

Impulses that signal pain are transmitted rostrally in the spinothalamic and spinoreticular tracts (Fig. 19-3). Additional axons with this function appear to be present in the dorsolateral funiculus. Tractotomy or surgical transection of the ventrolateral region of the spinal cord, which contains the spinothalamic and spinoreticular tracts, results in almost complete loss of the ability to experience pain on the opposite side of the body below the level of the lesion. The sensibility usually returns gradually over several weeks. The recovery is probably a consequence of synaptic reorganization and increased usage of intact alternative pathways. A surgical cut in the midline of the spinal cord (commissural myelotomy) causes prolonged analgesia in the segments affected by the lesion.

Pain is still felt, although poorly localized, after destruction of the primary somesthetic area. This clinical observation led to an early assumption that painful sensations reached the level of consciousness within the thalamus. It is more likely that spinothalamic and reticulothalamic afferents to the intralaminar and mediodorsal thalamic nuclei are responsible for the persistence of sensibility to pain after destruction of the primary somesthetic area. These thalamic nuclei are connected with most of the neocortex, including the prefrontal areas and the anterior part of the cingulate gyrus. A unilateral painful stimulus is associated with increased blood flow in both cingulate gyri. The ventral posterior nucleus of the thalamus and the primary somesthetic area are undoubtedly necessary for the accurate localization of the site of the painful stimulus.

Descending Pathways

Descending pathways modify the activity of all ascending systems; they are prominent in controlling the conscious and reflex responses to noxious stimuli. Both the subjective awareness of pain and the occurrence of defensive reflexes may be suppressed under circumstances of intense emotional stress. This effect may be mediated by **corticospinal fibers** that originate in the parietal lobe and terminate in the dorsal horn (see Fig. 19-7).

Control of a subtler kind is exerted by certain reticulospinal pathways. The best understood of these is the **raphespinal tract**, which arises from neurons in the raphe nuclei of the medullary reticular formation, mainly those of the nucleus raphes magnus. The unmyelinated axons of this tract traverse the dorsal part of the lateral funiculus of the spinal cord (see Figs. 5-10 and 19-7) and use serotonin as a neurotransmitter. The highest density of serotonin-containing synaptic terminals (observable by histochemical methods) is seen in the substantia gelatinosa. The nucleus raphes magnus is itself influenced by descending fibers from the periaqueductal gray matter of the midbrain. Electrical stimulation of the nucleus raphes magnus or the periaqueductal gray matter causes profound analgesia. This is reversed either by transection of the dorsolateral funiculus or by administration of naloxone or similar drugs that antagonize the actions of morphine

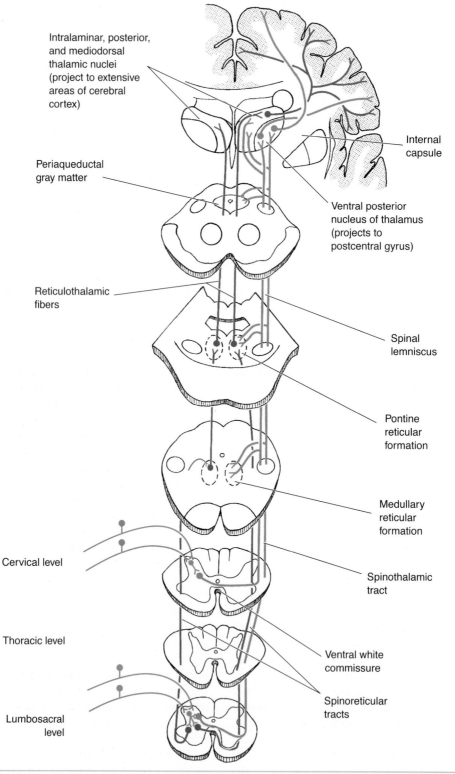

Intralaminar, posterior, and mediodorsal thalamic nuclei (project to extensive areas of cerebral cortex)

Periaqueductal gray matter

Reticulothalamic fibers

Cervical level

Thoracic level

Lumbosacral level

Internal capsule

Ventral posterior nucleus of thalamus (projects to postcentral gyrus)

Spinal lemniscus

Pontine reticular formation

Medullary reticular formation

Spinothalamic tract

Ventral white commissure

Spinoreticular tracts

FIGURE 19-3 Ascending pathways for pain. The spinothalamic system is shown in red, and the spinoreticular and reticulothalamocortical pathways are shown in blue. Interneurons in the spinal cord are green.

and related alkaloids of opium. Furthermore, the analgesic action of opiates is suppressed by transection of the dorsolateral funiculus.

The actions of the opiates and their antagonists are attributable to selective binding molecules (**opiate receptors**) on the surfaces of neurons in several parts of the brain. The normal function of the opiate receptor is to bind naturally occurring **opioid peptides**, of which the best understood are two pentapeptides, known as **enkephalins**. These serve either as neurotransmitters or as neuromodulators. The analgesic action of morphine and related opiates can be attributed to simulation of the effects of endogenously secreted enkephalins on neurons that bear opiate receptors on their surfaces. Major anatomical sites of action include the dorsal horn, nucleus raphes magnus, periaqueductal gray matter, and probably the thalamus. Many other parts of the CNS contain enkephalins, mainly in local circuit neurons. These regions may be the sites of other pharmacological actions of the opiates, such as nausea, suppression of coughing, euphoria, and the development of addiction.

Information about the descending pathways that modulate pain has led not only to increased understanding of the sites of action of the opium alkaloids but also to a technique occasionally used for the relief of chronic pain. An electrode stereotaxically implanted into the periaqueductal gray matter enables a patient to relieve pain instantly by switching on an electrical stimulator.

Medial Lemniscus System

The set of sensory pathways known as the *medial lemniscus system* is for proprioception, discriminative touch, and (although not exclusively) vibration. In contrast to the spinothalamic system, in which ascending axons cross the midline at spinal segmental levels, the pathways that constitute the medial lemniscus system ascend ipsilaterally in the cord and cross the midline in the caudal half of the medulla.

RECEPTORS

The medial lemniscus (or dorsomedial) system is especially important in humans because of

the discriminative quality of the sensations as perceived subjectively and their value in the learning process. The characteristics of fine or discriminative touch are that the subject can recognize the location of the stimulated points with precision and is aware that two points are touched simultaneously even though they are close together (two-point discrimination). These qualities accentuate recognition of textures and of moving patterns of tactile stimuli. Of the **tactile receptors**, Meissner's corpuscles, which have been found only in primates, have a special significance in discriminative touch (see also Chapter 3). These rapidly adapting receptors occur in the ridged, hairless skin of the palmar surface of the hands, which are moved over surfaces to feel texture and other small irregularities. Several additional touch receptors, noted in connection with the spinothalamic system, also produce sensations through the medial lemniscus system. Pacinian corpuscles are the principal receptors for the sense of **vibration**, although this modality, once believed to be served exclusively by the dorsal funiculi, is now known to also be carried in the lateral white matter of the spinal cord.

With respect to **proprioception**, the dorsomedial pathway provides information concerning the precise positions of parts of the body; the shape, size, and weight of an object held in the hand; and the range and direction of movement. The proprioceptors are neuromuscular spindles, neurotendinous spindles, and endings in and near to the capsules and ligaments of joints. For conscious proprioception (kinesthesia), input from muscle spindles probably is of greater significance than the input from other proprioceptors (see Chapter 3).

ASCENDING CENTRAL PATHWAYS

Identical pathways transmit discriminative touch and proprioception from the trunk and limbs. An additional pathway for proprioceptive signals from the lower limbs is also present.

Discriminative Touch

The primary sensory neurons for discriminative touch and proprioception are the largest cells in the dorsal root ganglia, having large axons with thick myelin sheaths. The central branches of these axons are medially located in each rootlet, and they bifurcate on entering the **dorsal funiculus**. Most of the ascending branches proceed ipsilaterally to the medulla (Fig. 19-4). Above the midthoracic level, the dorsal funiculus consists of a medial **gracile fasciculus** and a lateral **cuneate fasciculus**. The axons of the gracile fasciculus, which enter the spinal cord below the midthoracic level, terminate in the **gracile nucleus**; axons of the cuneate fasciculus, coming from the upper thoracic and cervical spinal nerves, end in the **cuneate nucleus**. More precisely, there is a lamination of the dorsal funiculus according to segments. Axons that enter the spinal cord in lower sacral segments are most medial, and axons from successively higher segments ascend along the lateral side of those already present.

Axons of neurons in the gracile and cuneate nuclei curve ventrally as **internal arcuate fibers**, cross the midline of the medulla in the decussation of the medial lemnisci (see Figs. 7-4 and 19-4), and continue to the thalamus as the **medial lemniscus**. This substantial tract is situated between the midline and the inferior olivary nucleus in the medulla, in the most ventral portion of the tegmentum of the pons, and lateral to the red nucleus in the tegmentum of the midbrain. The medial lemniscus and spinothalamic tract intermingle in the dorsal region of the subthalamus before entering the lateral division of the **ventral posterior nucleus of the thalamus**. The fibers of the medial lemniscus, in contrast to those of the spinothalamic tract, all terminate in the VPl nucleus.

A topographic arrangement of axons is maintained throughout the medial lemniscus. In the medulla, the larger dimension of the lemniscus is vertical as seen in cross section; fibers for the lower limb are most ventral (adjacent to the pyramid), and fibers for the upper part of the body are most dorsal. On entering the pons, the medial lemniscus twists through 90°; from there to the thalamus, fibers for the lower limb are located in the lateral part of the lemniscus, and those for the upper part of the body are located in its medial portion. This pattern conforms with the representation of the body in the VPl nucleus of the thalamus. The pathway is completed by a projection from this nucleus to the **primary somesthetic cortex** of the parietal lobe.

Proprioception

The central pathways for conscious awareness of position and movement are similar to those for discriminative touch, but for the lower limb, an additional pathway is present (Fig. 19-5). The pathway for the **upper limb** corresponds exactly with the one just described. That is, the ascending branches of primary afferent fibers terminate in the cuneate nucleus, from which the impulses are relayed through the medial lemniscus to the ventral posterior nucleus of the thalamus and thence to the first somatic sensory area of the cerebral cortex.

An equivalent pathway exists for the **lower limb**, but by way of the gracile fasciculus and gracile nucleus. The accessory pathway for conscious proprioception from the **lower limb** is different, being a series of four populations of neurons:

1. The primary afferent fibers enter the cord from the lumbar and sacral dorsal roots; they bifurcate into ascending and descending branches in the dorsal funiculus, but some of the former go only part of the way up the spinal cord. The fibers terminate in the upper lumbar and lower thoracic segments in the **nucleus thoracicus** (nucleus dorsalis; Clarke's column), which is a column of large cells on the medial side of the dorsal horn in segments C8 to L3.

2. The neurons in the caudal part of the nucleus thoracicus give rise to axons that ascend ipsilaterally as the **dorsal spinocerebellar tract** in the dorsolateral funiculus. Before entering the inferior cerebellar peduncle, some of the axons of this tract give off collateral branches, which remain in the medulla. These collaterals are concerned with conscious proprioception from the lower limb. They end in the **nucleus Z** of Brodal and Pompeiano. This is located rostrally to the gracile nucleus, of which it may be functionally an outlying part.

3. The cells of nucleus Z give rise to internal arcuate fibers that cross the midline and join the medial lemniscus. The remainder of the pathway is the same as for the upper limb, with a synapse in the VPl.

4. Thalamocortical fibers project to the leg area of the primary somatosensory cortex.

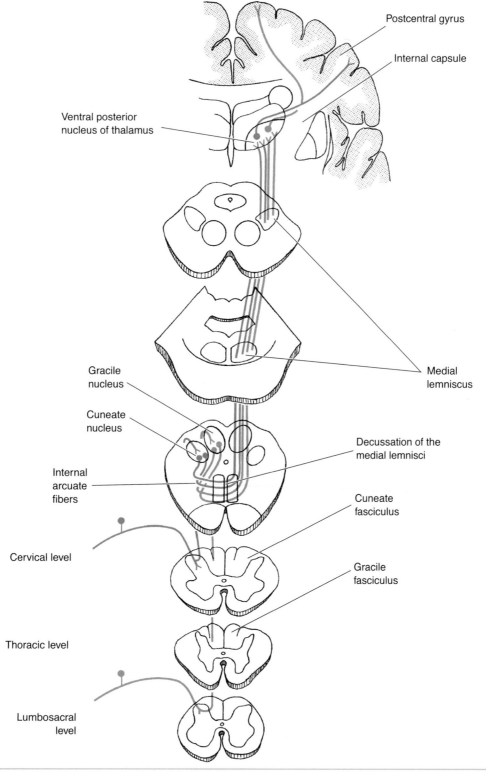

FIGURE 19-4 Medial lemniscus system for discriminative tactile sensation. The pathway from the lower limb is shown in red, and that from the upper limb is shown in blue.

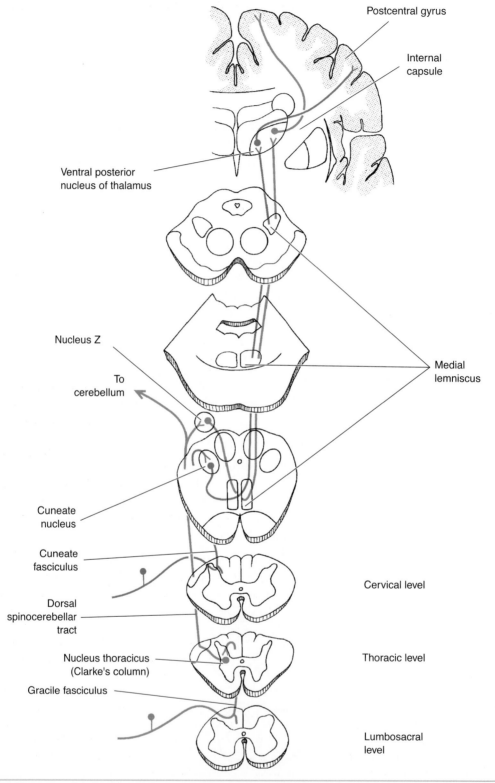

Postcentral gyrus

Internal capsule

Ventral posterior nucleus of thalamus

Nucleus Z

To cerebellum

Medial lemniscus

Cuneate nucleus

Cuneate fasciculus

Cervical level

Dorsal spinocerebellar tract

Nucleus thoracicus (Clarke's column)

Thoracic level

Gracile fasciculus

Lumbosacral level

FIGURE 19-5 Pathways for conscious proprioception. The pathway from the upper limb is shown in blue. An equivalent pathway exists for the lower limb but is not shown. The accessory pathway from the lower limb is shown in red.

CLINICAL NOTE

Dorsal Spinal Cord Lesions

The existence of an accessory pathway for proprioception from the lower limb has clinical implications. The dorsal funiculi conduct impulses concerned with proprioception in the upper and lower limbs. A lesion at a high cervical level that transects the dorsal funiculus but spares the dorsal spinocerebellar tract results in clumsiness and other symptoms of impaired position sense in the upper and lower limbs. Simple clinical testing in

such cases shows loss of awareness of position and movement of the joints of the upper limb as well as preservation of these senses in the lower limb. The patient's daily experience, however, indicates quite severe proprioceptive impairment of the leg and foot. The pathway involving the dorsal spinocerebellar tract and nucleus Z is evidently sufficient to account for conscious proprioception when this modality is specifically tested in patients with dorsal funiculus lesions.

Spinomedullary Neurons

The short descending branches of the primary sensory axons in the dorsal funiculus enter the spinal gray matter, along with collaterals of the ascending branches. Some of the axons that enter the gray matter, especially those concerned with proprioception, establish connections for spinal reflexes, and the remainder terminate on tract cells. Axons of these tract cells ascend ipsilaterally in the dorsal and dorsolateral funiculi (see Fig. 19-4). All these axons terminate in the gracile and cuneate nuclei alongside the primary ascending axons. These spinomedullary neurons, especially those sending axons into the dorsolateral funiculus, convey some information for most modalities of cutaneous and deep sensation, including vibration and pain. This relatively small population of afferents to the gracile and cuneate nuclei broadens the role of the medial lemniscus system to some extent beyond that of a pathway for discriminative touch and proprioception.

Enhancement of Discrimination in the Gracile and Cuneate Nuclei

It is convenient to think of sensory signals being "relayed" through the gracile or cuneate nucleus and the VPl nucleus of the thalamus to the cerebral cortex. Simple interruptions in the pathway would only serve to retard transmission, however. The real purpose of the nuclei is to modify the message, increasing the sensitivity of the cerebral cortex to the tiny differences in shape, texture, or movement that stimulate the peripheral receptors. The way this happens is most easily understood by considering the circuitry of the gracile or cuneate nucleus in re-

lation to stimulation of a point on the skin. This circuitry (Fig. 19-6) includes the excitatory synapses of the dorsal root ganglion neurons (*blue*) and a population of inhibitory interneurons (*black*) in the nucleus. Both are connected with the principal cells of the nucleus, whose axons (*red*) go to the thalamus.

Three principal cells (*red*) of the gracile or cuneate nucleus are shown receiving input that is strongest (highest frequency of action potentials) from the center of the area of skin represented at the bottom of the diagram. The inhibitory interneurons (*black*) that surround the principal cells receive more stimulation from the more active primary afferent (*blue*) neurons. The stimulated interneurons inhibit neighboring principal cells, thereby reducing the frequency of signals that relate to the area of skin surrounding the stimulus. Activation of inhibitory interneurons by collateral branches of afferent axons is called **feed-forward inhibition**. The same effect is also produced by recurrent collateral branches of the axons of the principal cells, also shown ending on interneurons in Figure 19-6. The action caused by recurrent collaterals is known as **feedback inhibition**. Both types of inhibition occur in the gracile and cuneate nuclei and are collectively known as **lateral inhibition**.

Lateral inhibition occurs at synaptic stations in all sensory pathways. It has been thoroughly studied in the retina (Chapter 22), and it occurs also in the thalamic "relay" nuclei (including the ventral posterior nucleus) and within the cerebral cortex.

Figure 19-6 also shows inhibitory interneurons being stimulated by a corticonuclear neuron (*green*). This arrangement provides **distal inhibi-**

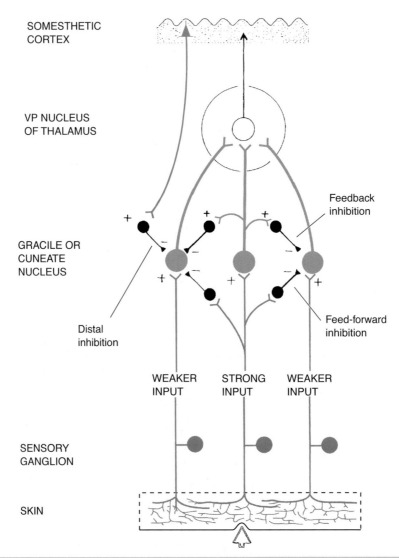

SOMESTHETIC
CORTEX

VP NUCLEUS
OF THALAMUS

Feedback
inhibition

GRACILE OR
CUNEATE
NUCLEUS

Distal
inhibition

Feed-forward
inhibition

WEAKER
INPUT

STRONG
INPUT

WEAKER
INPUT

SENSORY
GANGLION

SKIN

FIGURE 19-6   Amplification of contrast between neighboring parts of an area of skin in the overlapping territories of three primary sensory neurons (*blue*). The gracile and cuneate nuclei contain principal cells (*red*) and inhibitory interneurons (*solid black*). The activities of the principal cells that receive less excitation (*left* and *right*) are suppressed by feed-forward and feedback inhibition, mediated by the interneurons. Consequently, the thalamus receives input only from the neuron in the center, which is the one that was most strongly excited by the tactile stimulus. The diagram also shows a corticonuclear neuron (*green*), which is part of a descending system that uses distal inhibition to modulate the ascending flow of sensory signals in the medial lemniscus system.

tion (also called **remote inhibition**), with the somatosensory cortex setting the sensitivity of the principal cells of the gracile and cuneate nuclei. Other examples of distal inhibition in sensory pathways include the raphespinal tract, mentioned earlier in this chapter, and the olivocochlear projection of the auditory system (Chapter 21). Descending tracts that influence general somatic sensation are summarized in Figure 19-7.

Sensory Pathways for the Head

The back of the head and much of the external ear are supplied by branches of the second and third cervical nerves, whose central connections are with the spinothalamic and medial lemniscus systems. General sensations that

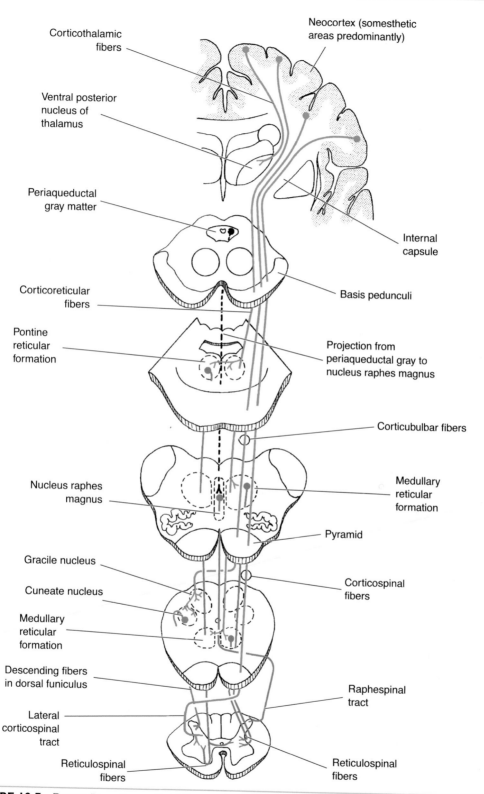

FIGURE 19-7 Descending pathways that influence the transmission of sensory information to the cerebral cortex. Reticulospinal and raphespinal projections are blue, descending axons from the periaqueductal gray matter are black, and other descending pathways are red and green.

Labels in figure:

Corticothalamic fibers

Neocortex (somesthetic areas predominantly)

Ventral posterior nucleus of thalamus

Periaqueductal gray matter

Internal capsule

Corticoreticular fibers

Basis pedunculi

Pontine reticular formation

Projection from periaqueductal gray to nucleus raphes magnus

Corticubulbar fibers

Nucleus raphes magnus

Medullary reticular formation

Pyramid

Gracile nucleus

Cuneate nucleus

Corticospinal fibers

Medullary reticular formation

Descending fibers in dorsal funiculus

Raphespinal tract

Lateral corticospinal tract

Reticulospinal fibers

Reticulospinal fibers

arise elsewhere in the head are mediated almost entirely by the trigeminal nerve. Small areas of the skin and larger areas of mucous membrane are supplied by the facial, glossopharyngeal, and vagus nerves, but the central connections of the general sensory components of these nerves are the same as for the trigeminal nerve (see Chapter 8).

The cell bodies of primary sensory neurons of the trigeminal nerve, with the exception of those in the mesencephalic nucleus, are located in the trigeminal ganglion (see Fig. 8-10). The peripheral processes have a wide distribution through the ophthalmic, maxillary, and mandibular divisions of the nerve. The central processes enter the pons in the sensory root. Some of these axons end in the pontine trigeminal nucleus; many descend in the spinal trigeminal tract and end in the associated nucleus, and still others bifurcate, with a branch ending in each nucleus.

A spatial arrangement of axons in the sensory root and spinal tract corresponds to the divisions of the trigeminal nerve. In the sensory root, ophthalmic fibers are dorsal, mandibular fibers are ventral, and maxillary fibers are in between. Because of a rotation of the axons as they enter the pons, the mandibular fibers are dorsal, and the ophthalmic fibers are ventral in the spinal trigeminal tract. The most dorsal part of this tract includes a bundle of fibers from the facial, glossopharyngeal, and vagus nerves. The cell bodies of the primary sensory neurons are located in the geniculate ganglion of the facial nerve and in the superior ganglia of the glossopharyngeal and vagus nerves. Somatic sensory axons in the facial and vagus nerves supply parts of the external ear and tympanic membrane. The glossopharyngeal and vagus nerves supply the mucosa of the back of the tongue, pharynx, esophagus, larynx, auditory (eustachian) tube, and middle ear.

PAIN AND TEMPERATURE

Primary afferent fibers for pain and temperature end in the **pars caudalis of the spinal trigeminal nucleus** (see Chapters 7 and 8); the pars caudalis is located in the lower medulla and upper two or three cervical segments of the spinal cord. (There is some evidence that the pars interpolaris receives pain afferents from the teeth.) The part of the pars caudalis in the cervical cord receives sensory data from areas of distribution of the trigeminal nerve and upper cervical spinal nerves. The cellular characteristics of the pars caudalis are similar to those of the tip of the dorsal gray horn of the spinal cord.

Neurons in the reticular formation immediately medial to the pars caudalis correspond to the nucleus proprius of the spinal gray matter. The tract cells whose axons project to the thalamus are located in both the spinal trigeminal nucleus and the adjacent reticular formation. The axons of these second-order neurons cross to the opposite side of the medulla and continue rostrally in the **ventral trigeminothalamic tract**. The tract terminates mainly in the VPm, and thalamocortical fibers complete the pathway to the inferior (ventral) one third of the **primary somesthetic area** of cortex. The axons of the tract cells associated with the pars caudalis, similar to those of the spinothalamic tract, have branches that end in the intralaminar, posterior, and mediodorsal nuclei of the thalamus, thus providing for distribution of the sensory information to areas of cortex beyond the confines of the first somatic sensory area. From the foregoing description, it is evident that the pathway for pain and temperature from the head corresponds to the spinothalamic system.

TOUCH

The central pathway for tactile sensation from the head is similar to that just described for pain and temperature, differing mainly in the sensory trigeminal nuclei involved. For light touch, the second-order neurons are located in the **pars interpolaris and pars oralis** of the spinal trigeminal nucleus and in the **pontine trigeminal nucleus**. For discriminative touch, they are located in the pontine trigeminal nucleus and the pars oralis of the spinal trigeminal nucleus. The second-order neurons project to the contralateral VPm through the ventral trigeminothalamic tract. In addition, smaller numbers of axons, crossed and uncrossed, proceed from the pontine trigeminal nucleus to the VPm in the **dorsal trigeminothalamic tract**. The two sets of trigeminothalamic fibers often are named together as the **trigeminal lemniscus**.

PROPRIOCEPTION

The primary sensory neurons for proprioception in the head are unique in that most of their cell bodies are located in a nucleus in the brain stem instead of in a sensory ganglion. Constituting the **mesencephalic trigeminal nucleus**, they are unipolar neurons similar to dorsal root ganglion cells. The peripheral branch of the single process proceeds through the trigeminal nerve without interruption; these axons supply proprioceptors in the trigeminal area of distribution, such as those related to the muscles of mastication. Central branches of the single process go to the trigeminal motor nucleus for reflex action and join the **dorsal trigeminothalamic tract**. Some neurons of the mesencephalic trigeminal nucleus send peripheral branches to receptors in the sockets of the teeth. These receptors detect **pressure on the teeth**, a sense functionally related to muscle proprioception because it participates in the reflex control of the force of biting.

The only other type of sensation perceived by a tooth is **pain**, for which the sensory pathway has already been described. Pain may originate from the dentin, the pulp, or the periodontal tissues.

CLINICAL NOTE

Clinical Considerations

SPINOTHALAMIC SYSTEM

The standard method of testing for integrity of the pain and temperature pathway is to stimulate the skin with a pin and to ask whether it feels sharp or blunt. Light touch is tested with a wisp of cotton. Temperature perception does not usually need to be tested separately; if such testing is required, the method used is to touch the skin with test tubes containing warm or cold water.

Irritation of a peripheral nerve or dorsal root by external pressure or local inflammation stimulates pain and temperature fibers, causing painful and burning sensations in the area supplied by the affected roots or nerves. An example is pressure on a dorsal root of a spinal nerve by a **herniated intervertebral disk**. An effect opposite to that of irritation is produced by **local anesthetic** drugs. These are most effective in blocking the conduction of impulses along group C fibers, so that low doses may reduce pain perception while having little or no effect on tactile sensibility. **Ischemia** of a nerve, such as that resulting from a tight tourniquet, preferentially blocks conduction in group A fibers. Pain with a burning character is the only sensation that can be perceived before the failure of conduction in an ischemic nerve becomes complete.

Degenerative changes in the region of the central canal of the spinal cord interrupt pain and temperature axons as they decussate in the ventral white commissure. The best example is **syringomyelia**, a disease in which cavities slowly develop in the center of the spinal cord. When the process is most marked in the cervical enlargement, as is frequently the case, the area of anesthesia includes the hands, arms, and shoulders (i.e., yoke-like anesthesia). A classical presenting symptom is a burn that is not painful.

A lesion that transects axons in the **ventrolateral part of the spinal cord** on one side results in loss of pain and temperature sensibility below the level of the lesion and on the opposite side of the body. If, for example, the spinothalamic and spinoreticular tracts are interrupted on the right side at the level of the first thoracic segment, the area of anesthesia includes the left leg and the left side of the trunk. Careful testing of the upper margin of sensory impairment shows that cutaneous areas supplied by the first and second thoracic nerves are spared. Some signals from these levels reach the contralateral pathways above their interruption because of the ascending branches of dorsal root axons in the dorsolateral tract. Surgical section of the pathway for pain (**tractotomy** or **chordotomy**) may be required for relief of intractable pain. Tractotomy is most likely to be considered in later stages of malignant disease of a pelvic organ; interruption of the pain pathway may be unilateral or bilateral, depending on circumstances prevailing in the particular patient. It was pointed out earlier in this chapter that mobilization of alternative ascending pathways can lead to the return of pain several weeks after a tractotomy. An alternative analgesic procedure, effective for longer periods of time, is **commissural myelotomy**, in which decussat-

(continued)

ing spinothalamic and spinoreticular axons are cut by a median incision at and a few segments above the level of the source of the pain.

The spinal lemniscus may be included in an area of infarction in the brain stem. An example is provided by Wallenberg's **lateral medullary syndrome**; the area of infarction usually includes the spinal lemniscus and the spinal trigeminal tract and nucleus. The principal sensory deficit is for pain and temperature sensibility on the side of the body opposite the lesion but on the same side for the face (see also Chapter 7). The insensitivity to normally painful stimuli is sometimes accompanied by **allodynia**, a condition in which innocuous stimuli are felt as pain. This change may be caused by reorganization of connections in the thalamus. Allodynia is more frequently caused by injury or disease affecting the dorsal horn of the spinal cord. Avulsion of dorsal rootlets can result in severe pain that feels as if it comes from the affected dermatome.

MEDIAL LEMNISCUS SYSTEM

The usual test for proprioception is to move the patient's finger or toe, asking when the movement begins and what the direction of movement is. In the **Romberg test**, any abnormal unsteadiness is noted when the patient stands with the feet together and the eyes closed, thereby evaluating proprioception in the lower limbs. Another useful test is to ask the patient to identify an object held in the hand with the eyes closed. Proprioception is especially helpful in recognizing the object on the basis of shape and size (**stereognosis**) as well as weight. This is a sensitive test that the patient may perform unsuccessfully when he or she has a lesion in the parietal association cortex even though the pathway to the somesthetic area is intact.

For testing **two-point touch discrimination**, two pointed objects are applied lightly to the skin simultaneously. A suitable test object can be devised from a paper clip. Simultaneous stimuli are normally detected in a fingertip when the points are 3 to 4 mm apart, or even less. Thorough testing of two-point discrimination is a tedious procedure. A simpler test is for the examiner to ask the subject to identify simple figures "drawn" on the skin with the finger or with some other blunt object. This test relies on the ability to recognize the distance and direction of movement of the stimulus across the surface of the skin. It is highly specific for the dorsal funiculi of

the spinal cord, provided there is no lesion in the cerebral cortex that is causing aphasia or agnosia.

Another sensory test is to ask the patient whether **vibration** as well as touch or pressure is felt when a tuning fork, preferably with a frequency of 128 Hz, is placed against a bony prominence such as an ankle or a knuckle. The sense of vibration is often reduced in elderly people, but even slight vibration should be felt in young people. For identifying the site of a lesion in the CNS, this test is less valuable than the examination of proprioception and discriminative touch. Diminished perception of vibration is often the first sign of disease affecting the largest myelinated axons in a peripheral nerve, some of which innervate pacinian corpuscles. **Peripheral neuropathy** is a term that embraces many disease processes that impair conduction in nerves, causing motor weakness or sensory deficits.

Defective proprioception and discriminative touch result from interruption of the medial lemniscus system anywhere along its course. For example, the dorsal and dorsolateral funiculi are sites of symmetrical demyelination in **subacute combined degeneration** of the spinal cord (see Chapter 5), and conduction may be interrupted at any level by trauma, infarction, or the plaques of multiple sclerosis. The **medial medullary syndrome** described in Chapter 7 is an instructive, albeit rare, example of unilateral transection of the medial lemniscus.

SENSATION FROM THE HEAD

The most common sensory abnormality affecting the face and scalp is **herpes zoster**. This disease is caused by a virus (the same one that causes chicken pox) that infects the neurons in sensory ganglia. Burning pain and itching, commonly in the field of distribution of one of the three divisions of the trigeminal nerve, is accompanied by a skin eruption. This can be a serious condition if corneal ulceration results from infection of the ganglion cells concerned with the ophthalmic division of the trigeminal nerve. Occasionally, the disability is prolonged, especially in elderly people, by **postherpetic neuralgia**. This may be particularly painful and recalcitrant to treatment. Relief can be obtained by applying capsaicin to the affected skin. Capsaicin first stimulates and then damages the terminal branches of nociceptive group C axons. Herpes zoster may also affect the geniculate ganglion or the superior vagal ganglion, causing an erup-

(continued)

tion on the tympanic membrane and parts of the external auditory canal and concha of the auricle; this is classical clinical evidence for the anatomy of the dual cutaneous innervation of this region.

A less common condition that causes episodes of severe pain in the fields of distribution of one or more divisions of the trigeminal nerve is **trigeminal neuralgia**, described in Chapter 8. The more frequent types of headache, including migraine, are not caused by anatomically discrete lesions in sensory pathways.

THALAMIC LESIONS

Surgically or pathologically produced lesions in the VP nucleus of the thalamus cause profound loss of all sensations other than pain on the op-

posite side of the body. The intralaminar and posterior groups of nuclei in the thalamus are probably almost as important as the VP nucleus in the central pathway for pain.

Central neurogenic pain, which is not caused by activity in peripheral sensory axons, can be caused by lesions that interrupt the somatosensory pathways at any level. A destructive lesion that involves the VP nucleus of the thalamus may result in the **thalamic syndrome**, characterized by exaggerated and exceptionally disagreeable responses to cutaneous stimulation. This syndrome (see Chapter 11) may include spontaneous pain and evidence of emotional instability, such as unprovoked laughing and crying.

Suggested Reading

Apkarian AV, Bushnell MC, Treede RD, et al. Human brain mechanisms of pain perception and regulation in health and disease. *Eur J Pain* 2005;9:463–484.

Apkarian AV, Hodge CJ. Primate spinothalamic pathways: I, II and III. *J Comp Neurol* 1989;288:447–511.

Brodal P. The Central Nervous System. *Structure and Function*, 3rd ed. New York: Oxford University Press, 2004.

Broman J. Neurotransmitters in subcortical somatosensory pathways. *Anat Embryol* 1994;189:181–214.

Cliffer KD, Willis WD. Distribution of the postsynaptic dorsal column projection in the cuneate nucleus of monkeys. *J Comp Neurol* 1994;345:84–93.

Cook AW, Nathan PW, Smith MC. Sensory consequences of commissural myelotomy: a challenge to traditional anatomical concepts. *Brain* 1984;107:547–568.

Craig AD. Pain mechanisms: labeled lines versus convergence in central processing. *Annu Rev Neurosci* 2003;26: 1–30.

De Broucker Th, Cesaro P, Willer JC, et al. Diffuse noxious inhibitory controls in man: involvement of the spinoreticular tract. *Brain* 1990;113:1223–1224.

Dickenson AH. Gate control theory of pain stands the test of time. *Br J Anaesth* 2002;88:755–757.

Moisset X, Bouhassira D. Brain imaging of neuropathic pain. *NeuroImage* 2007;37:S80–S88.

Nathan PW, Smith MC, Cook AW. Sensory effects in man of lesions of the posterior columns and of some other afferent pathways. *Brain* 1986;109:1003–1041.

Proske U. Kinesthesia: the role of muscle receptors. *Muscle Nerve* 2006;34:545–558.

Qi HX, Kaas JH. Organization of primary afferent projections to the gracile nucleus of the dorsal column system of primates. *J Comp Neurol* 2006;499:183–217.

Tracey I. Nociceptive processing of the human brain. *Curr Opin Neurobiol* 2005;15:478–487.

Vogt BA, Derbyshire S, Jones AKP. Pain processing in four regions of human cingulate cortex localized with co-registered PET and MR imaging. *Eur J Neurosci* 1996;8:1461–1473.

Wall PD, Noordenbos W. Sensory functions which remain after complete transection of dorsal columns. *Brain* 1977;100:505–524.

Watson CPN, Evans RJ, Watt VR. Post-herpetic neuralgia and topical capsaicin. *Pain* 1988;33:333–340.

Weiss N, Lawson HC, Greenspan JD, et al. Studies of the human ascending pain pathways. *Thalamus Relat Syst* 3:71–86, 2005.

Willis WD, Coggeshall RE. *Sensory Mechanisms of the Spinal Cord*, 3rd ed. New York: Kluwer Scientific, 1991.

Willis WD, Westlund KN. Neuroanatomy of the pain system and of the pathways that modulate pain. *J Clin Neurophysiol* 1997;14:2–31.

Zhang ML, Broman J. Cervicothalamic tract termination: a reexamination and comparison with the distribution of monoclonal antibody Cat-301 immunoreactivity in the cat. *Anat Embryol* 1998;198:451–472.

Chapter 20

VISUAL SYSTEM

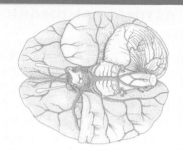

- In darkness, the retinal photoreceptors continuously release their excitatory synaptic transmitter substance. Absorption of light by the pigment in the rod or cone suppresses the release.

- Some bipolar cells are excited by illumination of the retina; others are inhibited. Other retinal interneurons modify transmission in the two synaptic layers of the retina.

- The axons of the ganglion cells of the nasal halves of the retinas cross in the optic chiasma; those from the temporal halves do not cross. Combined with the optical inversion of the retinal images, this partial decussation ensures that signals from each half of the visual field are sent to the contralateral optic tract, thalamus, and cerebral cortex.

- Most fibers of the optic tract end in the lateral geniculate body, which projects to the striate area of the occipital cortex, in and around the calcarine sulcus. There is topographical representation of the visual fields throughout this pathway, and destructive lesions cause visual field defects appropriate to the axonal or neuronal populations damaged.

- The central parts of the retinas are represented at the occipital poles; peripheral vision is served by the more anterior parts of the primary visual cortex. The visual association cortex in the occipital, parietal, and temporal lobes is necessary for recognition of colors and formed objects and for visual memory.

- Some fibers of the optic tract end in the pretectal area, which forms part of the pathway for the pupillary light reflex. Others end alongside fibers from the occipital cortex in the superior colliculus. They are involved in the control of eye movements.

The visual pathway begins with photoreceptors in the retina, and it ends in the visual cortex of the occipital lobe. The rods and cones are the two types of photoreceptor cell. Rods have a special role in peripheral vision and vision under conditions of low illumination, and cones, which function in bright light, are responsible for central discriminative vision and for the detection of colors. The responses of the photoreceptors are transmitted by bipolar cells to ganglion cells within the retina, and axons of ganglion cells reach the lateral geniculate body of the thalamus through the optic nerve and optic tract. The final relay is from the lateral geniculate body to the visual cortex by way of the geniculocalcarine tract. In addition, some fibers from the retina terminate in various parts of the midbrain, in the pulvinar of the thalamus, and in the hypothalamus.

The following account of the visual system is restricted to a discussion of the neural elements and presupposes a general understanding of the structure of the eye and the optical mechanism that projects a focused, inverted image onto the retina.

Retina

Optic vesicles evaginate from the diencephalon at an early stage of embryonic development. Each optic vesicle "caves in" to form the optic cup, which consists of two layers and is connected to the developing brain by the optic stalk. The optic cup becomes the retina, and the optic stalk becomes the optic nerve. The cornea, lens, and other parts of the eye develop from nearby ectoderm and mesoderm. The retina contains neurons and neuroglial cells and resembles the gray matter of the brain. Similarly, the optic nerve is composed of white matter and is not a peripheral nerve.

RETINAL LANDMARKS

Certain specialized regions serve as landmarks that need to be identified before the cellular components of the retina are described.

The cell layers of the retina, listed from the choroid to the vitreous body, are the pigment epithelium, rods and cones, bipolar cells, and ganglion cells (Fig. 20-1). Axons of ganglion cells run toward the posterior pole of the eye and enter the optic nerve at the **optic papilla** or **optic disk**. The papilla is slightly medial to the posterior pole, about 1.5 mm in diameter and is pale pink. The axons are heaped up as they converge at the margin of the optic papilla and then pass through the fibrous tunic (sclera) of the eyeball into the optic nerve. The optic papilla is a blind spot because it contains no photoreceptors.

The **macula lutea**, the central area of the retina in line with the visual axis, is a specialized region about 5 mm in diameter that abuts on the lateral edge of the optic papilla. The name *macula lutea* (yellow spot) is derived from the presence of a diffuse yellow pigment, which is apparent only when the retina is examined with red-free light. Consequently, the macula is not ordinarily visible with an ophthalmoscope, but its position is revealed by the absence of large blood vessels. The macula is specialized for acuity of vision. The **fovea** is a depression in the center of the macula, 1.5 mm in diameter and about 2.0 mm from the edge of the optic disk. Visual acuity is greatest at the fovea, the center of which (the **foveola**) contains only cone receptors. The capillary network present elsewhere in the retina is absent from the center of the fovea. When the retina is viewed with an ophthalmoscope, the fovea appears darker red than the surrounding parts of the retina because the black melanin pigment in the choroid and the pigment epithelium is not screened by

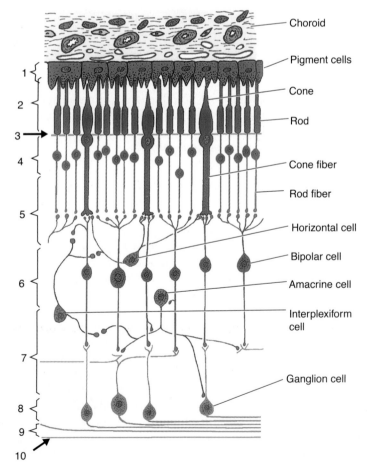

Choroid

Pigment cells

Cone

Rod

Cone fiber

Rod fiber

Horizontal cell

Bipolar cell

Amacrine cell

Interplexiform cell

Ganglion cell

FIGURE 20-1 Schematic representation of the neurons of the retina. The numbers on the left are for the 10 histological layers. (Compare with Figure 20-5.) The outer and inner limiting membranes (layers 3 and 10) are formed from horizontally extending cytoplasmic processes of neuroglial cells (Müller cells), which are not otherwise included in the diagram.

capillary blood. (The visible fovea is commonly referred to as the "macula" in ophthalmoscopic descriptions of the retina.)

The functional retina terminates anteriorly along an irregular border, the **ora serrata**. Forward of this line, the ciliary portion of the retina consists of a double layer of columnar epithelium, with the outer layer being pigmented.

PIGMENT EPITHELIUM

The pigment epithelium is a single layer of cells that reinforces the light-absorbing property of the choroid in reducing the scattering of light within the eye (see Fig. 20-1). The basal part of each cell contains the nucleus and a few pigment granules. Processes extending from the free surface of the cell interdigitate with the outer photosensitive regions of rods and cones. The processes, which are filled with granules of melanin pigment, isolate individual photoreceptors and enhance visual acuity. A second function of the pigment epithelium is the removal, by phagocytosis, of membranous disks that are shed from the outer ends of the rods and cones.

PHOTORECEPTORS

The light-sensitive part of the photoreceptor is its outer part, adjacent to the pigment epithelium. The incident light, therefore, has to pass through almost all the retina before being detected. These layers do not present a significant barrier to light because the retina is transparent and is no more than 0.4 mm thick at any point.

Rods

The human retina contains about 130 million rods, which is 20 times the number of cones.

Rods are absent from the central part of the fovea and become progressively more numerous from that point to the ora serrata. The distribution is such that rods are important for peripheral vision. There is a high density of cones along the edge of the ora serrata, possibly to provide for the recognition of objects entering the periphery of the visual field. Rods are more sensitive to dim light than cones, and the rod-free foveola is night blind. A faint point of light such as a dim star is best detected by looking slightly away from it. Each rod has three parts: the outer segment, inner segment, and rod fiber. The outer and inner segments are about 2 μm wide, and their combined lengths vary from 60 μm near the fovea to 40 μm at the periphery of the retina. The **rod fiber** is a slender filament that includes the nucleus in an expanded region and terminates as a synaptic terminal in contact with bipolar and association neurons.

In electron micrographs, most of the light-sensitive **outer segment** is seen to be occupied by about 700 double-layered membranous disks or flattened saccules (Figs. 20-2 and 20-3). These disks are continuously renewed from the inner segment of the rod and shed at the outer end of the outer segment. (Similar renewal occurs in the cones.) The disks contain the pigment **rhodopsin** (visual purple), which gives the retina a purplish-red color when removed from the eye and viewed under dim light. Rhodopsin consists of a protein, opsin, in loose chemical combination with retinal, a derivative of vitamin A. Absorption of a quantum of light changes the configuration of a rhodopsin molecule. A subsequent series of reactions results in hyperpolarization of the surface membrane of the inner segment and rod fiber, with consequent inhibition of the release of the neurotransmitter (believed to be glutamate), which is secreted continuously in darkness. It is a curious property of

---

CLINICAL NOTE

Retinal Detachment

The pigment epithelium is fixed to the choroid but is not as firmly attached to the inner layers of the retina. Detachment of the retina, which may result from a blow to the eye or occur spontaneously, consists of separation of the neural layers from the pigment epithelium. Fluid accumulates in the space thus created between the parts of the retina derived from the two layers of the optic cup. Retinal detachment can lead to blindness if left untreated.

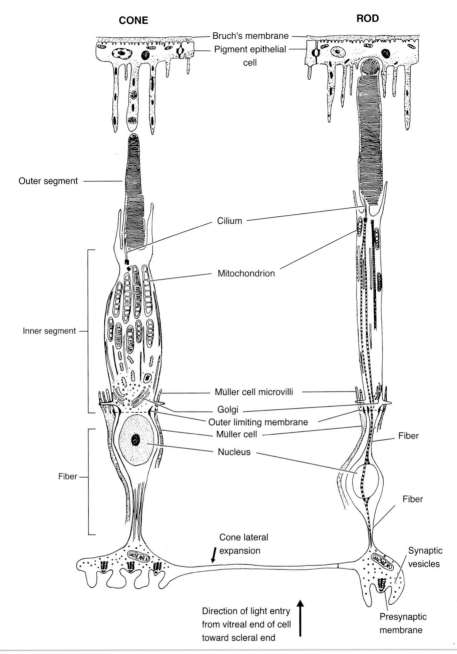

FIGURE 20-2 Ultrastructural components of rods and cones and their component parts. Named structures are described in the text. (Modified and reprinted with permission from Enoch JM, Tobey FL, eds. *Springer Series in Optical Sciences*, vol 23. Heidelberg: Springer-Verlag, 1981. Courtesy of Dr. B. Borwein.)

photoreceptors that they are inhibited by their specific stimulus.

The **inner segment** of a rod contains the organelles found in all types of cells: mitochondria, neurofilaments, vesicles, and granular endoplasmic reticulum. A cilium joins the inner to the outer segment (see Fig. 20-3).

Cones

The cone photoreceptors are especially important because of their role in visual acuity and color vision. Cones, similar to rods, consist of outer and inner segments and a cone fiber.

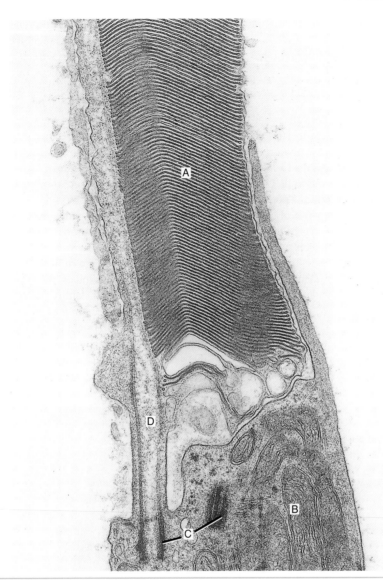

FIGURE 20-3 Electron micrograph of a rod from the human retina, showing part of the outer segment and the adjoining region of the inner segment. **(A)** Membranous disks in outer segment; **(B)** mitochondria; **(C)** centrioles; **(D)** cilium (magnification ×30,000). (Courtesy of Dr. M. Hogan.)

The tapering **outer segment** of a cone consists principally of double-layered pigment-bearing disks (see Fig. 20-2). There are three types of cone, each containing a different pigment. Each cone pigment resembles rhodopsin in consisting of retinal combined with a protein. Three proteins (**cone opsins**) are recognized, each combining with retinal in such a way as to provide maximum absorption of red, green, or blue light. The three types of cone provide for **trichromatic vision**.

The **inner segment** of a cone is similar to the inner segment of a rod, but larger.

The proportion of cones to rods is high in the macular area, but it steadily decreases from the macula to the periphery of the retina. The foveola, at the center of the fovea, contains only cones. The cone fibers and bipolar cells diverge from the center of the fovea, producing a slight concavity and reducing any slight impediment to light passing through the retina. The absence of retinal capillaries at the center of the fovea eliminates scattering of light by flowing blood. Figure 20-4 shows cone photoreceptors as they appear in a scanning electron micrograph.

BIPOLAR CELLS

There are several types of bipolar cells according to structure and physiological properties. These neurons are interposed between photoreceptor cells and ganglion cells (see Fig. 20-1). One bipolar cell is contacted by numerous rods (ranging from 10 near the macula to 100 at the periphery). Although there is some convergence of cones on bipolar cells in the peripheral parts of the retina, there is none at the fovea, at which point visual acuity is greatest. There, each cone fiber synapses with the dendrites of several bipolar cells.

GANGLION CELLS

Ganglion cells are rather large neurons with clumps of Nissl material, forming the last retinal link in the visual pathway (see Fig. 20-1). The bi-

polar cells contact both dendrites and somata of ganglion cells. The axons of ganglion cells, which form a layer adjacent to the vitreous body, converge on the optic papilla. There, bundles of axons and processes of neuroglial cells pass through foramina in the sclera, which at this point is called the **lamina cribrosa**. Behind the sclera, they constitute the optic nerve. The axons acquire myelin sheaths only after traversing the sclera, although in a few people, bundles of myelinated axons are present in the retina, where they appear ophthalmoscopically as white streaks.

A minority of retinal ganglion cells respond directly to light. These neurons contain melanopsin, a visual pigment that absorbs in the blue part of the spectrum. Their axons terminate in the pretectal area of the midbrain and in the suprachiasmatic nucleus of the hypothalamus. There is evidence that the former connection mediates sustained pupillary constriction in bright light, a function that is retained in retinitis pigmentosa, a disease in which the rods and cones degenerate. (See Chapter 8 for circuitry of the pupillary light reflex.) The retino-

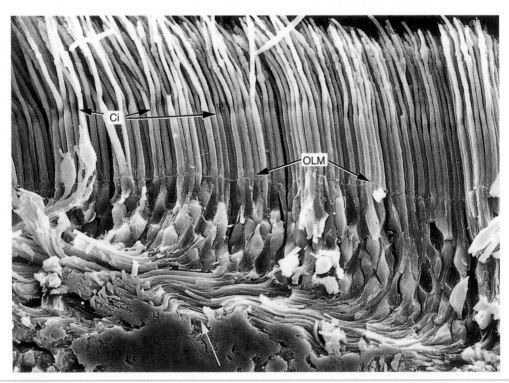

FIGURE 20-4 Scanning electron micrograph of foveal cones in a monkey. There is a constriction of each photoreceptor at the base of its cilium (Ci). The outer limiting membrane (OLM) appears as a thin line. The inner cone fibers (white arrow) turn sharply back at an angle to the photoreceptors and their nuclei. This is a feature of foveal cones. (Reprinted with permission from Enoch JM, Tobey FL, eds. *Springer Series in Optical Sciences*, vol 23. Heidelberg: Springer-Verlag, 1981. Courtesy of Dr. B. Borwein.)

Color Vision Deficiency

The three types of cones allow the visual association cortex to identify a complete range of colors on the basis of signals received from the retina. If one of the cone opsins is not produced (or is produced but has a shifted absorption spectrum), vision is **dichromatic**, and certain different colors cannot be distinguished from one another. The most common color vision deficiency is an inability to separate certain red and green hues; this is caused by a defective gene encoding the cone opsin that absorbs in the middle part of the visible spectrum. This occurs in about 8% of males and 0.5% of females because the recessive abnormal gene is located on the X chromosome in most, but not all, cases. A yellow-blue dichromatism occurs much less frequently (1% of males, 0.01% of females). **Monochromatic vision**, which is caused by defective genes encoding either two or all three of the cone opsins, is the only true color blindness, with black-and-white vision mediated either by one type of cone or by rods only. Both types of monochromatic vision occur, but they are extremely rare.

hypothalamic projection has been shown in laboratory animals to regulate physiological responses to ambient illumination (see Chapter 11).

RETINAL SYNAPSES

Excitation and inhibition of ganglion cells depend on special properties of photoreceptors and bipolar cells. The presynaptic part of a photoreceptor leaks its transmitter continuously in darkness. The release of transmitter is suppressed by illumination. Thus, the activity of the receptor cell is suppressed by light. Bipolar cells do not conduct action potentials. Their neurites (and those of other retinal interneurons) are all called *dendrites*. Some bipolar cells respond to the transmitter from the photoreceptors with hyperpolarization of the cell membrane. Others respond to the same transmitter with partial depolarization. The quantity of transmitter released by the presynaptic neurites of a bipolar neuron varies with the magnitude of the partial depolarization of the cell.

The neurotransmitters in the retina are not yet certainly identified. Several candidate substances have been detected immunohistochemically in the human retina. These include glutamate, which is present in photoreceptors, many bipolar cells, and ganglion cells. Glutamate is known to be the excitatory transmitter at synapses in most other parts of the central nervous system (CNS).

ASSOCIATION NEURONS

Synaptic transmission in the retina is subject to modification by interneurons known as *association neurons* (see Fig. 20-1). **Horizontal cells** are located in the outer part of the zone occupied by the cell bodies of the bipolar cells. Their dendrites make contact with the synaptic terminals of the photoreceptors and with the dendrites of bipolar cells, which they inhibit. **Amacrine cells** are located in the inner part of the zone occupied by the cell bodies of the bipolar cells. The dendrites of an amacrine cell all emerge from the same side of the cell to ramify and then terminate in the synaptic complexes between bipolar and ganglion cells and on the interplexiform cells, which are described next. Amacrine cells contain many putative transmitters, and there are probably inhibitory and excitatory types. The **interplexiform cells** are interspersed among the cell bodies of the bipolar cells. They are postsynaptic to the amacrine cells and presynaptic to the horizontal and bipolar cells, thus providing a feedback loop through which neural information is passed back from the inner to the outer of the two layers of retinal synapses.

The retinal interneurons provide **lateral inhibition**, an arrangement that enhances central transmission from adjacent dark and illuminated regions of the retina. The signals sent to the brain are thus weighted in favor of the edges of images. (A simpler example of lateral inhibition is explained in Chapter 19.)

NEUROGLIAL CELLS

The innermost layers of the retina contain astrocytes similar to those in the gray matter of the brain. Large numbers of radial neuroglial cells, called **Müller cells**, are also present. These cells extend from the innermost layer of the retina to the junction of the inner segments of rods and cones with the rod and cone fibers. They have lateral processes that intervene between the neuronal elements of the retina and provide support equivalent to that of astrocytes (see Chapter 2) elsewhere in the CNS.

HISTOLOGICAL LAYERS

In sections stained with hemalum and eosin (a commonly used dye combination that colors cell nuclei blue purple and everything else pink), the retina is seen to consist of 10 layers. These are shown in Figure 20-5, which can be compared with the diagram of cells that constitute the retina in Figure 20-1.

BLOOD SUPPLY

The retina receives nourishment from two sources. The **central artery of the retina** enters the eye through the optic disk, and its branches spread out over the inner surface of the retina. Thin branches penetrate the retina and form a capillary network that extends to the outer border of the inner nuclear layer. The capillary bed drains into retinal veins that converge on the optic papilla to form the central vein of the retina. The other source of blood is the capillary layer of the **choroid**. Soluble nutrients, oxygen, and metabolites of small molecular size diffuse from the choroid into the outer part of the retina. The layers containing the pigment epithelium, the photoreceptor, and the bipolar neurons are devoid of capillaries.

Pathway to the Visual Cortex

There is a point-to-point projection from the retina to the dorsal nucleus of the lateral geniculate body of the thalamus and from this nucleus to the primary visual cortex of the occipital lobe. There is, therefore, a spatial pattern of cortical excitation according to the retinal image of the visual field. Before discussing the components of the visual pathway, it will be useful to establish certain general rules concerning the projection from the retina to the cortex.

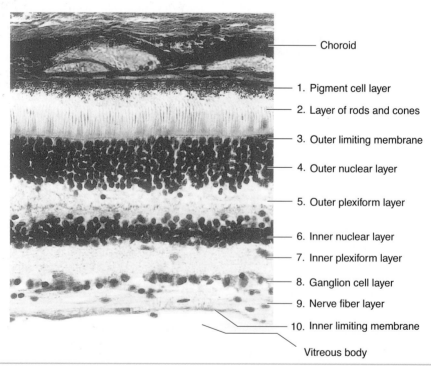

Choroid
1. Pigment cell layer
2. Layer of rods and cones
3. Outer limiting membrane
4. Outer nuclear layer
5. Outer plexiform layer
6. Inner nuclear layer
7. Inner plexiform layer
8. Ganglion cell layer
9. Nerve fiber layer
10. Inner limiting membrane
Vitreous body

FIGURE 20-5   Section of human retina showing the layers seen in a section stained with hemalum and eosin. (Compare with Fig. 20-1.)

Retinal Artery Occlusion

A small embolus, detached from a thrombus in the left atrium or a plaque of atheroma in a carotid artery, can obstruct the central artery of the retina at the optic disc, where the vessel is narrowed as it passes through the sclera. The eye immediately becomes blind. An even smaller embolus can block a branch of the central artery, causing a small visual field defect in one eye. Microscopic larvae of *Toxocara canis* and *T. cati* (nematodes commonly present in the intestines of dogs and cats) can enter the circulation of young children who eat dirt contaminated with the feces of pet animals. Visual field defects are produced when the larvae lodge in branches of retinal arteries. The parasitic embolus evokes a slow inflammatory response, generating a granular lesion that is easily seen with an ophthalmoscope.

RETINAL PROJECTIONS

For the purpose of describing the retinal projection, each retina is divided into nasal and temporal halves by a vertical line that passes through the fovea. A horizontal line, also passing through the fovea, divides each half of the retina into upper and lower quadrants. The macular area for central vision is represented separately from the remainder of the retina. Figure 20-6 illustrates the following rules with respect to the central projection of retinal areas:

1. Axons from the *right halves* of the two retinas terminate in the *right* lateral geniculate body, and the visual information is then relayed to the visual

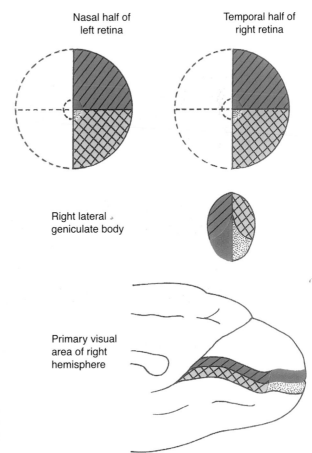

FIGURE 20-6 Topography of the projections from the retinas to the lateral geniculate body and primary visual cortex.

cortex of the right hemisphere. The converse holds true for the contralateral projection.

2. Axons from the *upper quadrants* peripheral to the macula end in the medial part of the lateral geniculate body, and impulses are relayed to the anterior two thirds of the visual cortex *above* the calcarine sulcus.

3. Axons from the *lower quadrants* peripheral to the macula end in the lateral portion of the lateral geniculate body, with a relay to the anterior two thirds of the visual cortex *below* the calcarine sulcus.

4. The *macula* projects to a relatively large posterior region of the lateral geniculate body, which, in turn, sends fibers to the *posterior* one third of the visual cortex in the region of the occipital pole. The macula is only 5 mm in diameter, but the proportions of the lateral geniculate body and visual cortex that receive fibers for macular vision are large because of the importance of central vision with maximal discrimination.

VISUAL FIELDS

Visual defects that result from interruption of the pathway at any point from the retina to the visual cortex are described in terms of the visual field rather than the retina. *The retinal image of an object in the visual field is inverted and reversed from right to left*, just as an image on the film in a camera is inverted and reversed. The following rules, therefore, apply to the nuclear and cortical representation of regions of the visual field.

1. The left visual field is represented in the right lateral geniculate body and in the visual cortex of the right hemisphere and vice versa.

2. The upper half of the visual field is represented in the lateral portion of the lateral geniculate body and in the visual cortex below the calcarine sulcus.

3. The lower half of the visual field is projected on the medial portion of the lateral geniculate body and on the visual cortex above the calcarine sulcus.

OPTIC NERVE, OPTIC CHIASMA, AND OPTIC TRACT

Each optic nerve contains about 1 million axons, all myelinated; this large number indicates the importance of human vision. The optic nerve is surrounded by extensions of the meninges (see also Chapter 26). The pia adheres to the nerve and is separated from the arachnoid by an extension of the subarachnoid space. The dura forms an outer sheath, and the meningeal extensions around the nerve fuse with the fibrous scleral coat of the eyeball. The central artery and central vein of the retina pierce the meningeal sheaths and are included in the anterior part of the optic nerve.

The **partial crossing** of optic nerve fibers in the optic chiasma is a requirement for binocular vision. Fibers from the nasal or medial half of each retina decussate in the chiasma and join uncrossed fibers from the temporal or lateral half of the retina to form the optic tract. Therefore, whereas impulses conducted to the right cerebral hemisphere by the right optic tract represent the left half of the field of vision, the right visual field is represented in the left hemisphere. Immediately after crossing in the chiasma, fibers from the nasal half of the retina loop forward for a short distance in the optic nerve. A lesion transecting the optic nerve close to the chiasma may, therefore, cause a temporal field defect in the opposite eye in addition to blindness in the eye whose optic nerve has been interrupted. The optic tract curves around the rostral end of the midbrain and ends in the lateral geniculate body of the thalamus.

Some of the fibers from the retina leave the optic chiasma and tract to proceed to sites other than the lateral geniculate body. These are described after a discussion of the pathway for conscious visual sensation.

LATERAL GENICULATE BODY, GENICULOCALCARINE TRACT, AND VISUAL CORTEX

The **lateral geniculate body** is a small swelling beneath the posterior projection of the pulvinar of the thalamus. The dorsal nucleus of the lateral geniculate body, in which the majority of the fibers of the optic tract terminate, consists of six layers of neurons. Within the general pattern

Papilledema

An increase in pressure of cerebrospinal fluid around the optic nerve impedes the return of venous blood. Edema or swelling of the optic disk (papilledema) results. This is visible with an ophthalmoscope and is a valuable indication of an in- crease in intracranial pressure. Part of the swelling is caused by enlargement of the axons in the disk, attributed to partial obstruction of anterograde axonal transport (see Chapter 2) within the optic nerve fibers.

shown in Figure 20-6 and described previously, crossed fibers of the optic tract end in layers 1, 4, and 6; uncrossed fibers end in layers 2, 3, and 5.

The **geniculocalcarine tract** originating in the lateral geniculate body first traverses the sublentiform and retrolentiform parts of the internal capsule. Its fibers then pass around the lateral ventricle, curving posteriorly toward the visual cortex (Fig. 20-7). Some of the geniculocalcarine fibers travel far forward over the temporal horn of the lateral ventricle. These fibers, which constitute the **temporal** or **Meyer's loop** of the geniculocalcarine tract, go to the visual cortex below the calcarine sulcus. It is evident from the retinal projection shown in Figure 20-6 that a temporal lobe lesion involving Meyer's loop causes a defect in the upper visual field on the side opposite the lesion. A lesion in the parietal lobe, on the other hand, may involve geniculocalcarine fibers that proceed to the visual cortex above the calcarine sulcus; the result is then a defect in the lower visual field on the side opposite the lesion.

The **primary visual cortex** occupies the upper and lower lips of the calcarine sulcus on the medial surface of the cerebral hemisphere. The

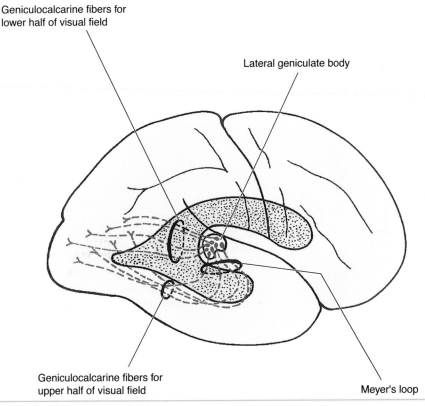

Geniculocalcarine fibers for lower half of visual field

Lateral geniculate body

Geniculocalcarine fibers for upper half of visual field

Meyer's loop

FIGURE 20-7   Geniculocalcarine projections.

area is much larger than suggested by cortical maps because of the depth of the calcarine sulcus. The primary visual cortex (area 17 of Brodmann) is marked by the line of Gennari (see Fig. 14-3) and is known alternatively as the **striate area**. There is a detailed point-to-point projection of the retina on the lateral geniculate body and on the visual cortex. The size of the retinal point is reduced to the diameter of a single cone for most acute vision in the central part of the fovea. Precise coordination of movements of the eyes ensures that the retinal patterns of activation correspond with one another, as required for binocular vision. The human **visual association cortex** is extensive, including the whole of

the occipital lobe, the adjacent posterior part of the parietal lobe, the posterior part of the lateral surface of the temporal lobe, and much of the inferior surface of the temporal lobe. This cortex is involved in recognition of objects and perception of color, depth, motion, and other aspects of vision that increase in complexity with distance from the calcarine sulcus. In general, the occipital and posterior parietal cortex examines the positions of objects in the visual fields, and the temporal cortex is concerned with their identification. Color recognition takes place in the cortex of the medial part of the inferior surfaces of the occipital and temporal lobes. The inferolateral surface of the temporal lobe, discussed

---

CLINICAL NOTE

Visual Defects Caused by Interruption of the Pathway

Certain general rules governing defects in the visual field as a result of lesions in the visual pathway are indicated by examples in Figure 20-8. *Example 1* is an obvious one: severe degenerative disease or injury involving an optic nerve results in blindness in the corresponding eye. Multiple sclerosis, in which central axons lose their myelin sheaths, can produce this effect. *Example 2* refers to interruption of decussating fibers in the optic chiasma, which causes **bitemporal hemianopia** if the full thickness of the chiasma is interrupted. (This name implies blindness in the lateral halves of the visual field, but each lateral half is still visible, with the unaffected half of the contralateral retina.) The medial halves of the visual fields have normal binocular vision, but there is only monocular vision in the lateral halves. The lesion that most commonly affects the optic chiasma is a pituitary tumor pressing on it from below. This first interrupts fibers from the inferior nasal quadrants of both retinas. The visual defect begins as a scotoma in each upper temporal quadrant of the visual field and spreads throughout the temporal fields as the chiasma is increasingly affected. Pressure on the lateral edge of the optic chiasma (*example 3*) happens rarely, but it may occur when there is an aneurysm of the internal carotid artery in this location. The field defect, in the case of pressure on the right

edge of the chiasma, is nasal hemianopia for the right eye. Interruption of the right optic tract (*example 4*) causes left **homonymous hemianopia.**

Example 5 is a large lesion that damages the geniculocalcarine tract or the primary visual cortex. An extensive right-sided lesion results in left homonymous hemianopia, except that central vision may remain intact (macular sparing). The cortex of the occipital lobe controls the involuntary eye movements that maintain fixation of the gaze on a target in the visual field. It is likely that a slight shifting of the patient's fixation or gaze during examination of the visual fields is responsible for the phenomenon known as *macular sparing* in patients with occipital cortical lesions. Destruction of only a part of the geniculocalcarine tract or the primary visual cortex causes field defects of lesser proportions than hemianopia. An example is provided by the upper quadrantic defect in the opposite visual field after interruption of fibers comprising Meyer's loop in the white matter of the temporal lobe (see Fig. 20-7).

It is important to remember that defects in the visual field can result from lesions of the eye as well as of the central pathways or cortex. For example, senile degeneration of the macula is a common condition that results in an area of blindness in the center of the field, often bilaterally. In chronic glaucoma, caused by increased intraocular pressure, atrophy of the peripheral parts of the retina occurs.

(continued)

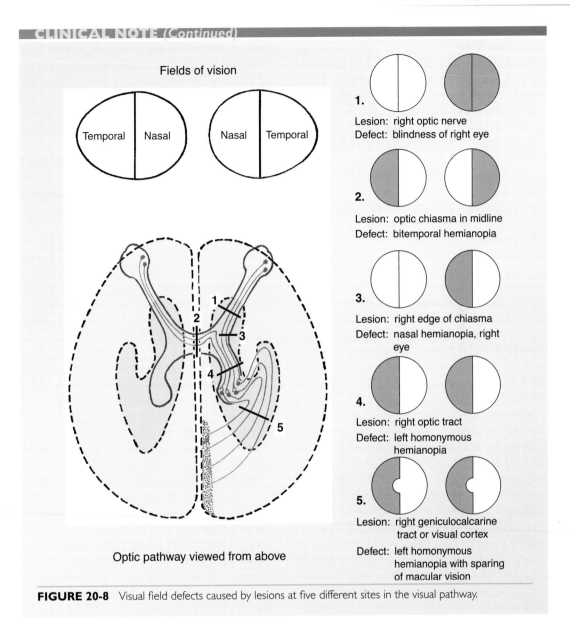

FIGURE 20-8   Visual field defects caused by lesions at five different sites in the visual pathway.

also in Chapters 15 and 18, is involved in interpreting, remembering, and recalling formed images. The organization of the visual cortex into columns of cells is briefly reviewed in Chapter 14. For disorders of the visual association cortex, see Chapter 15.

Visual Reflexes

A small bundle of axons from the optic tract bypasses the lateral geniculate body and enters the **superior brachium** (see Figs. 6-2 and 7-

15). These fibers, which participate in the afferent limbs of reflex arcs, go to the **superior colliculus** and to the **pretectal area**, which is a group of small nuclei immediately rostral to the superior colliculus.

The **pupillary light reflex** is tested in the routine neurological examination; the response consists of constriction of the pupil when light, as from a pen flashlight, is directed into the eye. Impulses from the retina stimulate neurons in the **olivary pretectal nucleus**, which is one of the nuclei of the pretectal area. Neurons in the pretectal area project to the Edinger-Westphal nucleus of the oculomotor complex, which, in turn, sends fibers to the ciliary ganglion in the orbit. This ganglion innervates the sphincter pupillae muscle of the iris (see Chapter 8 and Fig. 8-6). Both pupils constrict in response to light entering one eye because (1) each retina sends fibers into the optic tracts of both sides and (2) the pretectal area sends some fibers across the midline in the posterior commissure to the contralateral Edinger-Westphal nucleus.

Visual signals from the retina that reach the superior colliculus collaborate with input from the parietal and occipital cortex, frontal eye field, pallidum, and spinal cord, which are all sources of afferent fibers to the colliculus. The layered cytoarchitecture of the superior colliculus together with its diverse sources of afferent fibers indicate that considerable integrative activity occurs in the region. Efferent fibers go to the accessory oculomotor nuclei, paramedian pontine reticular formation, and pretectal area, and a few descend to the cervical segments of the spinal cord. This last pathway is known as the *tectospinal tract*.

The functions of the retinal afferents of the superior colliculus cannot be easily separated from the functions of the other afferents. The efferent fibers to the accessory oculomotor nuclei and to the paramedian pontine reticular formation are part of the pathway for control of both **voluntary and involuntary movement of the eyes**, as described in Chapter 8. An indirect connection to the Edinger-Westphal nucleus by way of the pretectal area controls the contractions of the ciliary and sphincter pupillae muscles in accommodation (see later). The small tectospinal tract is thought to influence movements of the head required for fixation of gaze.

When attention is directed to a near object, the **accommodation–convergence reaction** consists of three events: ocular convergence, pupillary constriction, and thickening of the lens. The reflex is tested by asking the subject to examine an object held about 30 cm in front of the eyes after looking into the distance and noting whether or not there is convergence and pupillary constriction. When attention is directed to a near object, the medial rectus muscles contract for convergence of the eyes. At the same time, contraction of the ciliary muscle allows the lens to thicken, increasing its refractive power, and pupillary constriction sharpens the image on the retina.

For accommodation to near objects, instructions from the visual association cortex reach the midbrain through fibers traversing the superior brachium and terminating in the superior colliculus. The subsequent connections to the nuclei of those cranial nerves that supply the extraocular muscles and to the Edinger-Westphal nucleus have already been described. *The frontal eye field, which is necessary for voluntary conjugate movements of the eyes, is not involved in convergence.* The pathways for constriction of the pupil in the light and accommodation reflexes are known to be different because they may be dissociated by disease.

Dilation of the pupils occurs in response to severe pain or strong emotional states. The pathway is presumed to begin with fibers from the amygdala and hypothalamus, which influence the intermediolateral cell column of the spinal cord. The pathway continues to the superior cervical ganglion of the sympathetic trunk, and it is completed by postganglionic fibers in the carotid plexus to the dilator pupillae muscle in the iris (see Chapter 24). At the same time, the parasympathetic supply to the sphincter pupillae muscle is inhibited.

CLINICAL NOTE

Argyll Robertson Pupil

Many patients with syphilis of the CNS (now a rare disease) have a loss of pupillary constriction in response to light but not to accommodation: the **Argyll Robertson pupil** or **light-near dissociation**. The lesion that typically causes dissociation of the responses is in the pretectal area, but cases have been described in which there was no abnormality in this part of the midbrain. The small size and slight irregularity of the Argyll Robertson pupil are probably caused by local disease of the iris.

Blindsight

The human condition known as **blindsight** is seen occasionally in patients with destructive lesions of the geniculostriate pathways. Despite the complete lack of conscious vision, behavioral tests can detect the perception of movements or of changes in illumination.

Other Optic Connections

Experimental investigations in animals have revealed that the axons of retinal ganglion cells end in several parts of the brain in addition to the lateral geniculate body, pretectal area, and superior colliculus.

Some retinal ganglion cells have axons that enter the **retinohypothalamic tract**, a small population of fibers that leave the dorsal surface of the optic chiasma and synapse with neurons in the **suprachiasmatic nucleus** of the hypothalamus. The visual input synchronizes the intrinsic circadian rhythm of the firing pattern of the neurons of the suprachiasmatic nucleus with the changes in ambient illumination. This is responsible for the influence of different levels of illumination on the secretion of pituitary gonadotrophins and the pineal hormone melatonin (see Chapter 11) in response to longer days and shorter nights. Retinohypothalamic projections may also influence sleep (see Chapter 9).

The **accessory optic tract** consists of small fascicles that pass from the optic tract to various small nuclei in the tegmentum of the midbrain. These nuclei project, directly and through synaptic relays in the inferior olivary nuclei, to the flocculonodular lobe of the cerebellum. (The principal input to this part of the cerebellum is from the vestibular system.) These connections implicate the accessory optic tract in coordination of movements of the eyes and head. Other fibers of the accessory optic tract turn rostrally, to terminate in the anterior perforated substance; they may be involved in integrated responses to visual and olfactory stimuli.

Some optic axons end in thalamic nuclei other than the lateral geniculate body. The main area of termination of such fibers is the **pulvinar**, which projects to the cortex of the occipital and parietal lobes, which include much of the visual association cortex. The function of this alternative pathway from the retina to the cerebral cortex is not yet understood, but evidence from animal studies indicates that this pathway may permit some residue of conscious vision after destruction of the lateral geniculate body or the primary visual cortex.

Suggested Reading

Barton JJS, Simpson T, Kiriakopoulos E, et al. Functional MRI of lateral occipitotemporal cortex during pursuit and motion perception. *Ann Neurol* 1996;40:387–398.

Berson DM. Strange vision: ganglion cells as circadian photoreceptors. *Trends Neurosci* 2003;26:314–320.

Borwein B. The retinal receptor: a description. In: Enoch JM ed. *Optics of Vertebrate Retinal Receptors*. Berlin: Springer-Verlag, 1982.

Cowey A, Stoerig P. The neurobiology of blindsight. *Trends Neurosci* 1991;14:140–145.

Dente C, Gurwood A. The Argyll Robertson pupil. *Optometry Today* 1999:23–25.

Elkington AR, Inman C, Steart PV, et al. The structure of the lamina cribrosa of the human eye: an immuno-histochemical and electron microscopical study. *Eye* 1990;4:42–57.

Grill-Spector K, Malach R. The human visual cortex. *Ann Rev Neurosci* 2003;27:649–677.

Hubel DH, Wiesel TN. Brain mechanisms of vision. *Sci Am* 1979;241:150–162.

Kawasaki A, Kardon AH. Intrinsically photosensitive retinal ganglion cells. *J Neuro-Ophthalmol* 2007;27:195–204.

Kolb H, Fernandez E, Nelson R. Webvision. The organization of the retina and visual system. Available online at http://retina.umh.es/Webvision/. Accessed April 11, 2008.

McKeefry DJ, Zeki S. The position and topography of the human colour centre as revealed by functional magnetic resonance imaging. *Brain* 1997;120:2229–2242.

Mick G, Cooper H, Magnin M. Retinal projection to the olfactory tubercle and basal telencephalon in primates. *J Comp Neurol* 1993;327:205–219.

Milner AD, Goodale MA. *The Visual Brain in Action*, 2nd ed. Oxford: Oxford University Press, 2006.

Moore RY, Speh JC, Card JP. The retinohypothalamic tract originates from a distinct subset of retinal ganglion cells. *J Comp Neurol* 1995;352:351–366.

Sakai K, Watanabe E, Onodera Y, et al. Functional mapping of the human colour centre with echo-planar magnetic resonance imaging. *Proc R Soc Lond Series B—Biological Sciences* 1995;261:89–98.

Sowka JW, Gurwood AS, Kabat AG. Toxocariasis (Ocular larva migrans). In: *Handbook of Ocular Disease Management*. New York: Obson Publishing LLC, 2001.

Szel A, Rohlich P, Caffe AR, et al. Distribution of cone photoreceptors in the mammalian retina. *Microsc Res Tech* 1996;35:445–462.

Tootell RBH, Dale AM, Sereno MI, et al. New images from human visual cortex. *Trends Neurosci* 1996;19:481–489.

Williams RW. The human retina has a cone enriched rim. *Vis Neurosci* 1991;6:403–406.

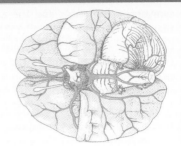

Chapter 21

AUDITORY SYSTEM

Important Facts

- The ossicles of the middle ear transfer vibrations from the air to the perilymph. Movement of the ossicles is restrained by the tensor tympani and stapedius muscles, innervated by cranial nerves V and VII, respectively.

- In the cochlea, the oscillations of the basilar membrane are detected by the inner and outer hair cells of the organ of Corti. The outer hair cells respond with movement, which is transmitted to the tectorial membrane and thence to the inner hair cells, increasing the sensitivity of the latter to sound. The inner hair cells respond by releasing their excitatory transmitter and stimulating the sensory terminals of the cochlear division of cranial nerve VIII.

- The primary sensory neurons have their somata in the spiral ganglion of the cochlea. Their axons end in the dorsal and ventral cochlear nuclei.

- Axons from the dorsal cochlear nucleus cross the midline, travel rostrally in the lateral lemniscus, and end in the inferior colliculus.

- Axons from the ventral cochlear nucleus end in the superior olivary nuclei of both sides. The convergence of signals from the left and right sides allows neurons in the superior olivary nucleus to respond to the different times of arrival of sound in the two ears, thus providing the ability to determine the direction of the source. The neurons in each superior olivary nucleus have axons that travel in the lateral lemniscus and end in the inferior colliculus.

- The inferior colliculus projects (through the inferior brachium) to the medial geniculate body, which projects to the primary auditory area of the cerebral cortex.

- The primary auditory cortex is located on the superior surface of the temporal lobe. It is connected with auditory association cortex of the superior temporal gyrus and nearby parts of the parietal lobe. In the left cerebral hemisphere (of most people), these regions are coextensive with the receptive language area.

- Descending pathways modify transmission in the central auditory system. The sensitivity of the organ of Corti is actively inhibited by efferent (olivocochlear) fibers in the cochlear nerve. These inhibit both the outer hair cells and the sensory terminals on the inner hair cells.

- Destructive lesions rostral to the cochlear nuclei do not cause unilateral deafness.

Hearing is second in importance among the special senses of humans, yielding first place only to sight. Their role in language accounts, to a large extent, for the reliance placed on these special senses. The auditory system consists of the external ear, middle ear, cochlea of the internal ear, cochlear nerve, and pathways in the central nervous system (CNS).

External and Middle Ear

The external ear consists of the auricle or pinna and the external acoustic meatus, with the latter being separated from the middle ear by the tympanic membrane. The function of the external ear is to collect sound waves, which cause vibration of the tympanic membrane. The vibration is transmitted across the middle ear by a chain of **ossicles** (little bones): the malleus, incus, and stapes. The **malleus** is attached to the tympanic membrane and articulates with the **incus**, which articulates in turn with the stirrup-shaped **stapes**. The footplate of the stapes occupies the **fenestra vestibuli** (oval window) in the wall between the middle and internal ears; the rim of the foot plate is attached to the margin of the fenestra vestibuli by the annular ligament, composed of elastic connective tissue. The ossicles constitute a bent lever with the longer of the two arms attached to the tympanic membrane, and the area of the foot plate of the stapes is considerably less than the area of the tympanic membrane. With this arrangement, the vibratory force of the tympanic membrane is magnified about 15 times at the fenestra vestibuli; the substantial increase in force is important because the sound waves are transferred from air to a liquid.

Protection against the effect of sudden, excessive noise is provided by reflex contraction of the tensor tympani and stapedius muscles, which are inserted on the malleus and stapes, respectively. The tensor tympani is innervated by the trigeminal nerve, and the stapedius is innervated by the facial nerve (see Chapter 8).

Inner Ear

The internal ear, which has two functions, consists of the **membranous labyrinth** encased in the **bony labyrinth**. Certain parts of the internal ear contain sensory areas for the vestibular system, which is discussed in Chapter 22. The cochlea is the part of the internal ear that contains the organ of Corti (spiral organ). This sense organ detects the sound waves produced in the fluid in the cochlea by vibration of the

stapes and sends action potentials centrally in the cochlear division of the vestibulocochlear nerve. A central pathway with several synaptic relays leads to the primary auditory area of the cerebral cortex. Other central connections in the brain stem cause reflex responses.

For more detailed descriptions of the cochlea and organ of Corti, see the CD-ROM that accompanies the printed book.

BONY AND MEMBRANOUS LABYRINTHS

The bony labyrinth (Fig. 21-1) is located in the petrous part of the temporal bone, which forms a prominent oblique ridge between the middle and posterior cranial fossae. The labyrinth is a system of tunnels within the bone. A preparation such as that represented in Figure 21-1 is made by chipping away the surrounding cancellous bone until only the walls of the tunnels (which are composed of compact bone) remain. The **fenestra vestibuli** or **oval window**, in which the foot plate of the stapes fits, is in the wall of the **vestibule**, the middle part of the bony labyrinth. The **fenestra cochleae** (**round window**) is located below the fenestra vestibuli; it is closed by a thin membrane that

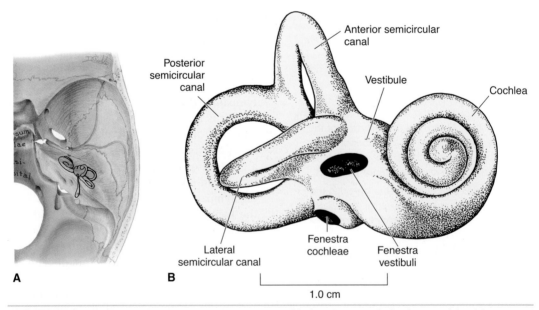

FIGURE 21-1 **(A)** Base of the skull showing the squamous (blue) and petrous (yellow) parts of the right temporal bone and the position of the labyrinth. (Reprinted with permission from Moore KL, Dalley AF. *Clinically Oriented Anatomy*, 5th ed. Philadelphia: Lippincott, Williams & Wilkins, 2006.) **(B)** Anterolateral view of the right bony labyrinth.

makes pressure waves possible in the fluid in the internal ear. The fluid would otherwise be completely enclosed in a rigid "box," except for the source of the waves at the fenestra vestibuli. Three **semicircular canals** extend posterolaterally from the vestibule, and the **cochlea** constitutes the anteromedial part of the bony labyrinth. The cochlea has the shape of a snail shell; its base abuts against the deep end of the internal acoustic meatus, which opens into the posterior cranial fossa.

The cochlear and vestibular divisions of the **vestibulocochlear nerve** leave the internal acoustic meatus and are attached to the lateral aspect of the brain stem at the junction of the medulla and pons. Within the internal meatus, the vestibulocochlear nerve is accompanied by the two divisions of the facial nerve (see Chapter 8) and the **labyrinthine artery** and vein (see Chapter 25).

The delicate membranous labyrinth conforms, for the most part, to the contours of the bony labyrinth (Fig. 21-2). There are, however, two dilations, the **utricle** and the **saccule**, in the vestibule of the bony labyrinth. Three **semicircular ducts** arise from the utricle. A patch of sensory epithelium is present on the inner surface of the utricle, the saccule, and each semicircular duct. The saccule is continuous with the **cochlear duct** through a narrow channel known as the **ductus reuniens**. The cochlear duct contains, along its entire length, the organ of Corti.

Whereas the lumen of the membranous labyrinth is filled with **endolymph**, the interval between the membranous and bony labyrinths is filled with **perilymph**. The vestibular part of the membranous labyrinth is suspended within the bony labyrinth by trabeculae of connective tissue. The cochlear duct is firmly attached along two sides to the bony wall of the cochlear canal.

COCHLEA

The **cochlear canal** makes 2.5 turns around a bony pillar or core, the **modiolus**, where channels for blood vessels and branches of the co-

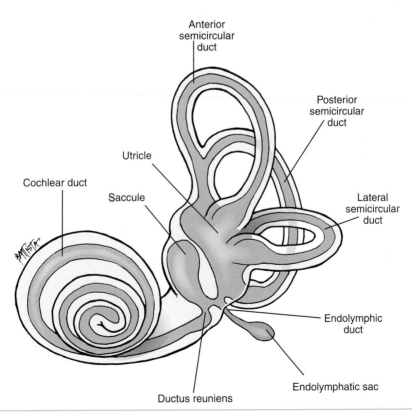

FIGURE 21-2 Anterolateral view of the right membranous labyrinth.

chlear nerve are present. The cochlea is most conveniently described as if it were resting on its base (Fig. 21-3), although its base actually faces posteromedially.

The cochlear canal, the cavity of this part of the bony labyrinth, is divided by two partitions into three spiral spaces. The middle of these is the **cochlear duct** (scala media), which contains endolymph. The cochlear duct is firmly fixed to the inner and outer walls of the cochlear canal. The remaining spiral spaces are the **scala vestibuli** and the **scala tympani**, which contain perilymph. The thin unspecialized wall of the cochlear duct apposing the scala vestibuli is called the **vestibular** or **Reissner's membrane**, and the thicker wall apposing the scala tympani constitutes the specialized **basilar membrane**, on which the organ of Corti rests.

The basilar membrane is of special importance in the physiology of hearing because it responds to vibration of the stapes in the following man-ner. As shown in Figure 21-4, vibration of the foot plate of the stapes produces corresponding waves in the perilymph, beginning with that of the vestibule. Sound waves propagate through the scala vestibuli, Reissner's membrane, the endolymph in the cochlear duct, and the basilar membrane to the scala tympani. These same waves create a vibration of the membrane closing the fenestra cochleae at the base of the scala tympani; this is essential to eliminate the damping of pressure waves that would otherwise occur in bone-encased fluid.

The perilymph filling the scala vestibuli and scala tympani is a watery fluid, similar in composition to cerebrospinal fluid. In fact, there is a communication, the tiny **cochlear canaliculus**, between the scala tympani and the subarachnoid space.

The **spiral ganglion** consists of cells in a spiral configuration at the periphery of the modiolus (see Fig. 21-3). The primary sensory neurons of both divisions of the vestibulocochlear nerve are bipo-

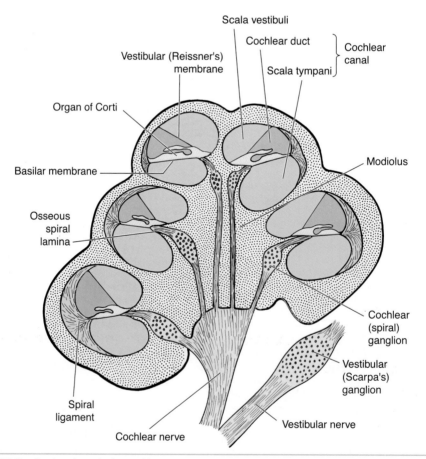

FIGURE 21-3 Section through the cochlea.

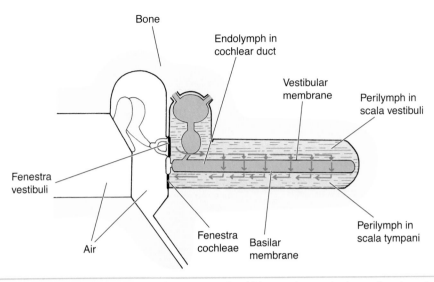

FIGURE 21-4 Schematic representation of the manner in which sound waves in the perilymph and endolymph cause vibration of the basilar membrane.

lar, rather than unipolar as in other cerebrospinal nerves, retaining this embryonic characteristic of primary sensory neurons. The two neurites, which are functionally both axons, are myelinated. The distal axons reach the organ of Corti by traversing openings in the osseous spiral lamina projecting from the modiolus, where myelin sheaths terminate. The central axons traverse channels in the modiolus, enter the internal acoustic meatus from the base of the cochlea, and continue in the cochlear nerve. Within the external acoustic meatus, a small anastomotic connection, the **Oort anastomosis**, carries efferent axons from the vestibular nerve into the cochlear nerve.

COCHLEAR DUCT

Vibration of the **basilar membrane** (Fig. 21-5) is essential in the transduction of mechanical stimuli (sound waves) to neural signals in the organ of Corti. The inner edge of the basilar membrane is attached to the **osseous spiral lamina**, which projects from the modiolus like the thread on a screw. The outer edge of the membrane is attached to the outer wall of the cochlear canal. The basilar membrane contains collagen and elastic fibers, mostly directed across the width of the membrane. The width of the basilar membrane steadily increases from the base to the apex of the cochlea; this is made possible by a progressive narrowing of the osseous spiral lamina. The width of the membrane at any point determines the pitch of sound to which it resonates maximally. *High tones, therefore, cause maximal vibration in the basal turn of the cochlea, and low tones cause maximal vibration near the apex.* The range of audible frequencies in the human ear is from 20 to 20,000 Hz. The range extends over 11 octaves, of which seven are used in musical instruments such as the piano. Ordinary conver-

High-Tone Deafness

Persistent exposure to loud sounds causes degenerative changes in the organ of Corti at the base of the cochlea, causing high-tone deafness. This is prone to occur in workers exposed to the sound of compression engines or jet engines and in those working for long hours on farm tractors. High-tone deafness was formerly encountered most frequently among workmen in boiler factories and is still sometimes called "boilermakers' disease."

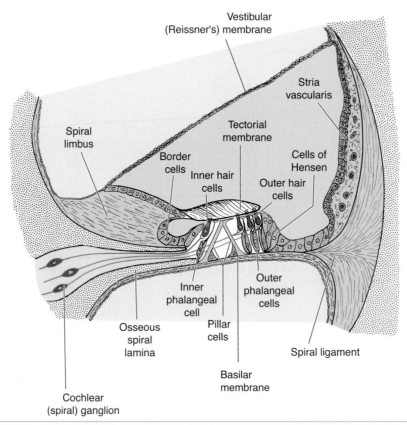

FIGURE 21-5   Structure of the cochlear duct and the spiral organ of Corti.

sation falls within the range of 300 to 3000 Hz. With advancing age, a gradual decrease in the perception of high frequencies takes place.

The **vestibular** or **Reissner's membrane** consists of two layers of simple squamous epithelium separated by a trace of connective tissue.

The outer wall of the cochlear duct is specialized as the **stria vascularis**, which consists of cuboidal epithelium overlying vascular connective tissue. The stria vascularis produces endolymph. This is similar to intracellular fluid in respect to its high concentration of potassium ions and low concentration of sodium ions. Endolymph fills the membranous labyrinth; absorption takes place into venules surrounding the **endolymphatic sac** in the dura mater on the posterior surface of the petrous part of the temporal bone. This sac is an expansion of the **endolymphatic duct**, which arises from the communication between the saccule and the utricle (see Fig. 21-2).

The epithelial lining of the membranous labyrinth, including the specialized sensory ar-

eas for the auditory and vestibular systems, is ectodermal in origin. The epithelium differentiates from the cells lining the **otic vesicle**. This is formed by an invagination of ectoderm at the level of the hindbrain of the early embryo.

ORGAN OF CORTI

The **organ of Corti** or **spiral organ** (see Fig. 21-5) consists of supporting cells and sensory cells. Supporting cells (**pillar cells** and **phalangeal cells**) form the sides and roof of the **tunnel of Corti**. The fluid in the tunnel of Corti has a chemical composition similar to that of perilymph rather than endolymph. The high concentration of potassium ions in endolymph would prevent impulse conduction by the neurites that cross the tunnel of Corti to reach the outer hair cells. Sensory hair cells are located on either side of the tunnel of Corti and are flanked by **border cells** on the inner aspect and by **cells of Hensen** at the outer edge of the basilar membrane.

The **tectorial membrane** is a ribbon-like structure of gelatinous consistency attached to the spiral limbus, a thickening of the periosteum on the osseous spiral lamina. The tectorial membrane extends over the organ of Corti, and the tips of the hairs of the outer hair cells are embedded in the membrane.

SUPPORTING CELLS OF THE ORGAN OF CORTI—MORE DETAILS

SENSORY CELLS

The sensory cells are called **hair cells** because of the hair-like projections from their free ends. There is a single row of about 7,000 inner hair cells; the 25,000 or so outer hair cells are arranged in three rows in the basal turn of the cochlea, increasing to five rows at the apex. The hairs are microvilli of an unusual type: they are rigid and of different lengths. Each hair has its tip joined by a linking protein molecule to an ion channel embedded in the cell membrane that forms the side of the adjacent hair. The mechanical stimulus of a vibration moves the whole bundle of hairs, which bend only at their points of attachment to the body of the cell; this applies tension to the link at the tip of each hair, which pulls on and opens the ion channel in the side of the adjacent hair. Entry of potassium and calcium ions from the endolymph depolarizes the cell membrane and initiates synaptic signaling to the innervating neurite.

The **inner hair cells** are the principal sensory elements. Each one synapses with the neurites of up to 10 rapidly conducting neurons whose myelinated axons make up at least 90% of the fibers of the cochlear nerve. No neuron is contacted by more than one inner hair cell. The **outer hair cells** synapse with branches of unmyelinated axons, which account for 5% to 10% of the fibers of the cochlear nerve. The zone of outer hair cells receives most of the efferent fibers of the cochlear nerve, which are described later. The outer hair cells are motile. Their microvilli move in response to transduced sound and produce corresponding vibrations of the tectorial membrane. This has the effect of lowering the threshold of excitation of the inner hair cells.

It is basic to the physiology of the cochlea that a particular region of the basilar membrane, depending on the pitch of sound, responds by maximal vibration. Bending of the hairs reduces the membrane potential of the hair cells, causing increased release of their chemical transmitter and initiation of action potentials in the sensory nerve endings. Regardless of the pitch of sound, vibration of the basilar membrane begins at the base of the cochlea and travels along the membrane with increasing magnitude to a point determined by the pitch. At this point, the vibration suddenly dies away, and impulses reaching the brain from the place of maximal stimulation of the organ of Corti are interpreted as a particular pitch of sound. An increase in the intensity of sound causes maximal vibration in a larger region of the basilar membrane, thereby activating more hair cells and neurons. Tonotopic localization is sharpened by lateral inhibition (see Chapter 19) in the nuclei of the ascending pathway to the auditory cortex and by various descending connections, including centrifugal fibers in the vestibulocochlear nerve.

Auditory Pathways

The **cochlear nerve** consists principally of axons of cells in the spiral ganglion, most of which are myelinated. It traverses the internal acoustic meatus in the petrous part of the temporal bone alongside the vestibular nerve, the two roots of the facial nerve (Chapter 8), and the labyrinthine artery (Chapter 25). On emerging from the internal meatus, the vestibulocochlear and facial nerves traverse the subarachnoid space in the **cerebellopontine angle**, a region between the middle and inferior cerebellar peduncles. The cochlear fibers enter the brain stem at this level and bifurcate, with one branch ending in the **dorsal cochlear nucleus** and the other branch in the **ventral cochlear nucleus** (Fig. 21-6). The cochlear nuclei are situated superficially in the rostral end of the medulla adjacent to the base of the inferior cerebellar peduncle (see Fig. 7-7). A tonotopic pattern of axonal endings has been demonstrated in both nuclei in laboratory animals and probably exists in humans. The dorsal and ventral cochlear nuclei differ in their contributions to the central pathways.

PATHWAY TO THE AUDITORY CORTEX

The pathway to the cerebral cortex is characterized by variable numbers of synaptic relays between the cochlear nuclei and the specific

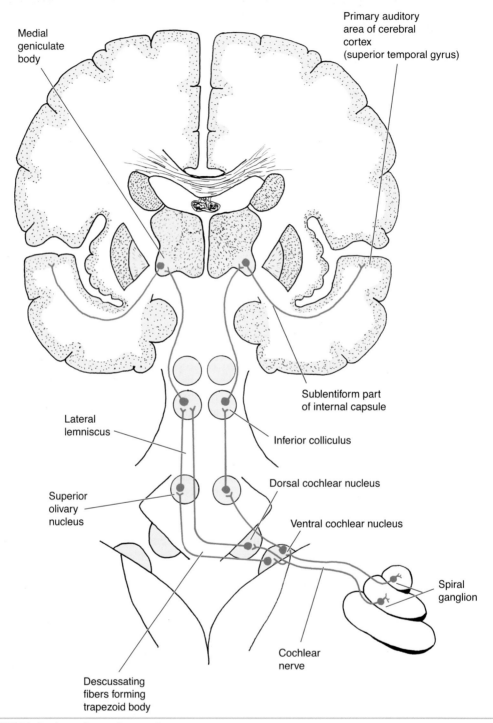

FIGURE 21-6   Ascending auditory pathway.

thalamic nucleus for hearing, the medial geniculate body (see Fig. 21-6). There is a relay in the inferior colliculus, and additional synaptic interruptions may occur in the superior olivary nucleus and in the nucleus of the lateral lemniscus. The pathway also includes a

Acoustic Neuroma

One of the more common types of intracranial neoplasm is a benign tumor derived from the neuroglial cells (Schwann cells) of the vestibular division of the eighth cranial nerve, within the internal auditory meatus. The correct name for the tumor is **vestibular schwannoma** (or neurilemmoma), but the older term *acoustic neuroma* is still in widespread use. Vertigo, the principal effect of damage to the vestibular system (see Chapter 22), occurs in some patients, but in most, the first symptom is slowly increasing hearing loss in the affected ear. This is due to pressure on the cochlear nerve, which is squeezed between the growing tumor and the bony wall of the meatus. In the early stages, there may also be tinnitus (a ringing or buzzing sound) due to abnormal stimulation of the sensory axons.

The tumor causes enlargement of the internal auditory meatus, a useful radiological sign, and expands into the subarachnoid space of the cerebellopontine angle. There, with further enlargement, the tumor presses upon and stretches the roots of nearby cranial nerves. The facial nerve, despite its close proximity to the vestibulocochlear, is surprisingly resistant to stretching, and the next symptom to develop is usually a tingling sensation in the face, with sensory impairment that can

be detected on examination. A decreased corneal reflex (Chapter 8) is often an early sign of involvement of the trigeminal nerve. With downward growth, the tumor impinges on glossopharyngeal rootlets, causing sensory impairment in the pharynx and posterior third of the tongue, with reduction or loss of the gag reflex. The clinical course of the disease is long (years) because of the slow growth of the tumor and the availability of a space—the cerebellopontine angle—that the tumor can occupy before it impinges on the brain stem. A large acoustic neuroma eventually presses on the medulla, obstructing the flow of cerebrospinal fluid through and out of the fourth ventricle, with resultant hydrocephalus (Chapter 26) and symptoms and signs of raised intracranial pressure (headache, vomiting, papilledema). Death ensues from loss of cardiovascular control and other vital functions of the medulla.

With early diagnosis, an acoustic neuroma can sometimes be removed without permanently damaging the cochlear nerve, but in most cases, the surgery is followed by permanent deafness. Severe vertigo is experienced postoperatively. Permanent facial paralysis and diminished function of the trigeminal and glossopharyngeal nerves frequently follow removal of larger tumors from the pontocerebellar angle.

significant ipsilateral projection to the cortex. The transmission of acoustic data to the cortex can best be described after certain components of the pathway in the brain stem have been identified.

The **superior olivary nucleus** is situated in the ventrolateral corner of the tegmentum of the pons at the level of the motor nucleus of the facial nerve (see Fig. 7-8). (Although considered here as a unit, the nucleus is a complex of four nuclei, whose connections differ in detail.) Auditory fibers that cross the pons in the ventral part of the tegmentum constitute the **trapezoid body** (see Fig. 7-8). The **lateral lemniscus**, the ascending auditory tract, extends from the region of the superior olivary nucleus, through the lateral part of the pontine tegmentum, and close to the surface of the brain stem in the isthmus region between the pons and midbrain (see Fig. 7-9).

The projection from the cochlear nuclei to the inferior colliculus and then to the medial

geniculate nucleus, through the components of the pathway just identified, is as follows (see Fig. 21-6). Axons from the **ventral cochlear nucleus** proceed to the region of the ipsilateral superior olivary nucleus, in which some of the fibers terminate. The majority of the axons continue across the pons, with a slight forward slope; these constitute the trapezoid body. On reaching the region of the superior olivary nucleus on the other side of the brain stem, the fibers either continue into the lateral lemniscus or terminate in the superior olivary nucleus, from which fibers are added to the lateral lemniscus. Fibers from the **dorsal cochlear nucleus** pass over the base of the inferior cerebellar peduncle, continue obliquely to the region of the contralateral superior olivary nucleus, and then turn rostrally in the lateral lemniscus. They end in the inferior colliculus.

Signals conveyed by the lateral lemniscus reach the **inferior colliculus** in the midbrain.

The complexity of neuronal organization in the inferior colliculus indicates integrative activity at this level. Ascending axons from the inferior colliculus traverse the inferior brachium (see Fig. 6-3) and end in the **medial geniculate body**.

The last link in the auditory pathway consists of the **auditory radiation** in the sublentiform part of the internal capsule, through which the medial geniculate body projects to the **primary auditory cortex** of the temporal lobe. This primary auditory area, corresponding to Brodmann's areas 41 and 42, is located in the floor of the lateral sulcus, extending only slightly onto the lateral surface of the hemisphere. A landmark is provided by the anterior transverse temporal gyri (Heschl's convolutions) on the dorsal surface of the superior temporal gyrus (see Fig. 15-3). The area receives afferent fibers from the tonotopically organized ventral part of the medial geniculate body. The tonotopic pattern in the auditory area is such that whereas fibers for low-frequency sounds end in the anterolateral part of the area, fibers for high-frequency sounds go to its posteromedial part. Some of the columns of neurons (see Chapter 14) within the primary auditory cortex occur in bands recognizable by virtue of their higher cytochrome oxidase activity. These columns may be involved in comprehension of speech.

Analysis of acoustic stimuli at a higher neural level, notably the recognition and interpretation of sounds on the basis of past experience, occurs in the **auditory association cortex** of the temporal lobe, which is located posteriorly to the primary auditory area. In addition to its afferents from the primary auditory area, the association cortex also receives projections from regions of the medial geniculate nucleus other than its tonotopically organized ventral part. In the cerebral hemisphere dominant for language (the left, in most people), the auditory association cortex is known as **Wernicke's area** (see Chapter 15), and along with the adjacent parietal lobe cortex, it is essential for the understanding of spoken and written language.

Above the level of the cochlear nuclei, the auditory pathway is both crossed and uncrossed because many axons ascend in the lateral lemniscus of the same side. In addition, the inferior colliculi of the two sides are connected by commissural fibers. Consequently, any loss of hearing that results from a unilateral corti-

cal lesion is so slight as to make detection difficult in audiometric testing. Most lesions in the vicinity of the auditory cortex also involve Wernicke's area and cause receptive aphasia when the dominant hemisphere for language is involved (see Chapter 15). The latter disability obscures any slight auditory deficiency.

The directions and distances of sources of sound are determined by the discrepancy in times of arrival of the stimulus in the left and right ears. Results obtained from investigations with animals indicate that the different inputs to the brain from the two cochleae are compared and analyzed in the superior olivary nuclei, although the auditory cortex is necessary if the coded information transmitted rostrally from the medulla is to have any meaning. The most severe loss of ability to judge the sources of sounds is that caused by unilateral deafness resulting from disease of the ear. The condition is equivalent to the loss of binocular vision that results from blindness in one eye.

TESTING IMPAIRED HEARING

DESCENDING PROJECTIONS IN THE AUDITORY PATHWAY

Parallel with the flow of information from the organ of Corti to the auditory cortex, some neurons with descending axons conduct in the reverse direction. The descending connections consist of the following: corticogeniculate fibers, which originate in the auditory and adjoining cortical areas and terminate in all parts of the medial geniculate body; corticocollicular fibers from the same cortical areas to the inferior colliculi of both sides; colliculo-olivary fibers from the inferior colliculus to the superior olivary nucleus; and colliculocochleonuclear fibers from the inferior colliculus to the dorsal and ventral cochlear nuclei. Except for the corticocollicular projection, which includes both crossed and uncrossed fibers, these descending pathways are ipsilateral.

As indicated earlier, control is exerted by the CNS over the initiation of auditory neural signals in the organ of Corti. Olivocochlear fibers, constituting the **olivocochlear bundle** of Rasmussen, are the axons of cholinergic neurons in the superior olivary nuclei. The axons leave the brain stem in the vestibular division of the vestibulocochlear nerve and then cross over into the cochlear division in a branch, the Oort anastomosis, located in the internal acoustic meatus.

The endings of the olivocochlear axons are applied to the outer hair cells (where their synaptic terminals outnumber those of afferent fibers) and to the preterminal parts of the sensory neurites that innervate the inner hair cells. The efferent axons are inhibitory to both the receptor cells and the sensory axons. Inhibition of the outer hair cells reduces the amplitude of the vibrations of the tectorial membrane, thereby raising the threshold of excitation of the inner hair cells. Thus, the efferent fibers of the cochlear nerve reduce the sensitivity of the ear.

The central transmission of data from the sensory hair cells is therefore far more than just a relay to the cortex. In the various cell stations of the pathway, a complex processing of acoustic data takes place that provides for refinement of such qualities as pitch, timbre, and volume of sound perception. In particular, feedback inhibition sharpens the perception of pitch, especially through the olivocochlear bundle. This is accomplished by inhibition in the organ of Corti except for the region in which the basilar membrane is responding by maximal vibration to a particular frequency of sound waves (auditory sharpening). Central inhibition probably suppresses background noise when attention is being concentrated on a particular sound.

AUDITORY REFLEXES

A few acoustic fibers from the inferior colliculus pass forward to the superior colliculus, which influences motor neurons of the cervical region of the spinal cord through the tectospinal tract. The superior colliculus also influences neurons of the oculomotor, trochlear, and abducens nuclei through indirect connections in the brain stem (see Chapter 8). These pathways provide for reflex turning of the head and eyes toward the source of a sudden loud sound.

Some axons from the superior olivary nucleus terminate in the motor nuclei of the trigeminal and facial nerves for reflex contraction of the tensor tympani and stapedius muscles, respectively.

Contraction of these muscles in response to loud sounds reduces the vibration of the tympanic membrane and the stapes, thereby protecting the delicate structures in the cochlea from mechanical damage.

Suggested Reading

Altschuler RA, Bobbin RD, Clopton BM, et al, eds. *Neurobiology of Hearing: The Central Auditory System*. New York: Raven Press, 1991.

Arnold W. Myelination of the human spiral ganglion. *Acta Otolaryngol (Stockh)* 1987;436:76–84.

Berry I, Demonet JF, Warach S, et al. Activation of association auditory cortex demonstrated with functional MRI. *NeuroImage* 1995;2:215–219.

Clarke S, Rivier F. Compartments within human primary auditory cortex: evidence from cytochrome oxidase and acetylcholinesterase staining. *Eur J Neurosci* 1998;10:741–745.

Clopton BM, Winfield JA, Flammino FJ. Tonotopic organization: review and analysis. *Brain Res* 1974;76:1–20.

García-Ánoveros J, Corey DP. The molecules of mechanosensation. *Annu Rev Neurosci* 1997;20:567–594.

Kelly JP. Hearing. In: Kandel ER, Schwartz JH, Jessell TM, eds. *Principles of Neural Science*, 3rd ed. New York: Elsevier-North Holland, 1991:258–268.

Liegeois-Chauvel C, Musolino A, Chauvel P. Localization of the primary auditory area in man. *Brain* 1991;114:139–145.

Lim DJ. Functional structure of the organ of Corti: a review. *Hearing Res* 1986;22:117–146.

Masterson RB. Neural mechanisms for sound localization. *Annu Rev Physiol* 1984;46:275–287.

Nadol JB. Synaptic morphology of inner and outer hair cells of the human organ of Corti. *J Electron Microsc Tech* 1990;15:187–196.

Roland PS. Skull base, acoustic neuroma (vestibular schwannoma), 2006. Available online at http://www.emedicine.com/ent/topic239.htm. Accessed November 2007.

Spoendlin H. The spiral ganglion and the innervation of the human organ of Corti. *Acta Otolaryngol (Stockholm)* 1988;105:403–410.

Webster DB. An overview of mammalian auditory pathways with an emphasis on humans. In: Webster DB, Popper AH, Fay RR, eds. *The Mammalian Auditory Pathway: Neuroanatomy*. New York: Springer-Verlag, 1992:1–22.

Yeomans JS, Frankland PW. The acoustic startle reflex: Neurons and connections. *Brain Res Rev* 1995;21:301–314.

Zatorre RJ, Ptito A, Villemure JG. Preserved auditory spatial localization following cerebral hemispherectomy. *Brain* 1995;118:879–889.

Zenner HP. Motile responses in outer hair cells. *Hearing Res* 1986;22:83–90.

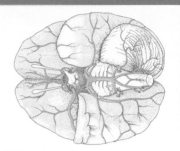

Chapter 22

VESTIBULAR SYSTEM

- The receptors in the saccule and utricle respond to the pull of gravity and to inertial movement caused by linear acceleration and deceleration.

- The receptors in the ampullae of the semicircular ducts respond to rotation of the head in any plane.

- The vestibular hair cells contact the distal neurites of bipolar neurons whose cell bodies are in the vestibular ganglion. Most of the central neurites (axons) of these neurons end in the vestibular nuclei, but a few go directly to the cerebellum.

- Neurons in the vestibular nuclei have axons that end in the vestibulocerebellum (fastigial nucleus and flocculonodular lobe); the nuclei of cranial nerves III, IV, and VI; and the spinal cord. There is also a pathway to the thalamus and cerebral cortex.

- Reflex movements of the eyes in response to stimulation of the kinetic labyrinth require the integrity of a reflex arc that includes fibers in the medial longitudinal fasciculus.

- Abnormal stimulation of any part of the vestibular system causes vertigo (dizziness), often associated with nausea or vomiting, and nystagmus (abnormal conjugate eye movements). Vertigo also follows unilateral loss of function of the kinetic labyrinth.

Three sources of sensory information are used by the nervous system in the maintenance of equilibrium. They are the eyes, proprioceptive endings throughout the body, and the vestibular apparatus of the internal ear. The role of the vestibular system, especially in relation to visual information, is illustrated by a person who has congenital atresia of the vestibular apparatus, usually accompanied by cochlear atresia and deaf–mutism. Such a person can orient himself satisfactorily by visual guidance but becomes disoriented in the dark or if submerged while swimming. In addition, vestibular impulses caused by motion of the head contribute to appropriate movements of the eyes to maintain fixation on an object in the visual field. These functions require a neural pathway from the vestibular labyrinth to motor neurons through pathways in the spinal cord, brain stem, and cerebellum, and there is also a projection to the cerebral cortex.

Whereas the static labyrinth, represented by the utricle and saccule, detects the position of the head with respect to gravity, the kinetic labyrinth represented by the semicircular ducts detects movement of the head. Both parts of the membranous labyrinth serve to maintain equilibrium, and the kinetic labyrinth has a special role in coordination of eye movement with rotation of the head.

Static Labyrinth

The **utricle** and **saccule** are endolymph-containing dilations of the membranous labyrinth, enclosed by the vestibule of the bony labyrinth (see Figs. 21-1 and 21-2). The utricle and saccule, which are derived from the otic vesicle of the embryo, are suspended from the wall of the vestibule by connective tissue trabeculae, and they are surrounded by space containing perilymph. Each dilatation includes a specialized area of sensory epithelium, the macula, about 2 by 3 mm in size. The **macula utriculi** is located in the floor of the utricle and parallel with the base of the skull, and the **macula sacculi** is vertically disposed on the anteromedial wall of the saccule. The two maculae are histologically identical (Fig. 22-1).

The columnar supporting cells of the maculae are continuous with the cuboidal epithelium

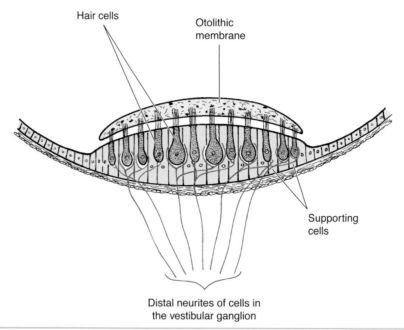

Hair cells

Otolithic membrane

Supporting cells

Distal neurites of cells in the vestibular ganglion

FIGURE 22-1 Structure of the macula utriculi.

that lines the utricle and saccule elsewhere. The sensory **hair cells**, of which two types have been identified in electron micrographs, are somewhat similar to hair cells in the organ of Corti (see Chapter 21). Type 1 hair cells are flask shaped, and type 2 hair cells are cylindrical. From 30 to 50 hairs project from each cell, together with a long cilium (the **kinocilium**) that arises from a centriole (see Fig. 22-2A). (Kinocilia are characteristic of vestibular hair cells. They do not occur in the organ of Corti.) The hairs, also called **stereocilia**, are large microvilli, 0.25 µm wide and up to 100 µm long. The lengths of the hairs increase toward the side of the bundle where the kinocilium emerges. The tips of the hairs and kinocilium are embedded in the gelatinous **otolithic membrane**, in which there are irregularly shaped concretions composed of protein and calcium carbonate. These are known as *otoliths*.

The otoliths give the otolithic membrane a higher specific gravity than the endolymph, thereby causing bending of the hairs in one direction or another, except when the macula is in a strictly horizontal plane. In each hair cell, the kinocilium is situated at one side of the tuft of hairs, and the position of the kinocilium at the periphery of the hairs differs from one region of the macula to another (see Fig. 22-2B). The

hair cells are excited when the hairs are bent in the direction of the kinocilium, and they are inhibited when the deflection is in the opposite direction (see Fig. 22-2A). The pattern of action potentials conducted by the axons of the vestibular nerve differs, therefore, according to the orientation of the macula to the direction of gravitational pull. The appropriate changes in muscle tone follow, as required to maintain equilibrium. The molecular mechanism of transduction of the mechanical stimulus by the stereocilia is the same as for the cochlear hair cells, described in Chapter 21.

Although the macula is predominantly a static organ, the higher specific gravity of the otolithic membrane with respect to the endolymph allows the macula to respond to linear acceleration and deceleration. Motion sickness is initiated by prolonged, fluctuating stimulation of the maculae.

The bipolar cell bodies of the primary sensory neurons are located in the **vestibular ganglion** (Scarpa's ganglion) at the lateral end of the internal acoustic meatus. The peripheral neurites enter the maculae and end on the hair cells (see Fig. 22-2A). In addition, efferent cholinergic axons in the vestibular nerve end as presynaptic terminals on the type 2 hair cells and on the sensory nerve endings that are postsynaptic to the type 1 cells. These axons, which are inhibi-

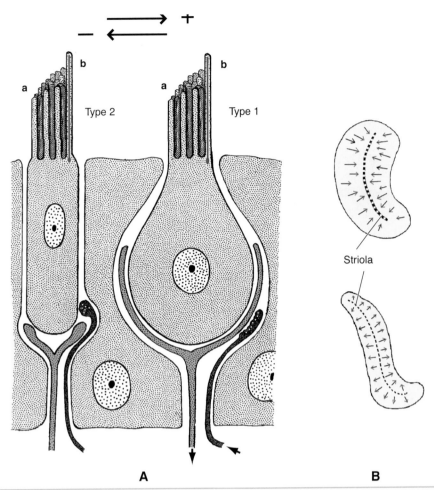

FIGURE 22-2   Vestibular hair cells, with their afferent and efferent innervation. **(A)** The two types of hair cells in a macula. Excitation occurs when the bundle of hairs or microvilli (a) bends in the direction of the kinocilium (b). Inhibition of the hair cell occurs when the hair bundle bends in the opposite direction. **(B)** Surfaces of the maculae of the utricle (above) and saccule (below), showing the positioning of the kinocilia *(heads of arrows)* relative to the tufts of hairs. Each arrow indicates the direction of gravitational pull for excitation of hair cells in that location. In the macula utriculi, the kinocilia of the hair cells face a central stripe, the striola. In the macula sacculi, the kinocilia face away from the striola. Hair cells are absent from the striola itself.

tory, originate from an unnamed group of neurons medial to the vestibular nuclei.

Kinetic Labyrinth

The three semicircular ducts are attached to the utricle and are enclosed in the semicircular canals of the bony labyrinth (see Figs. 21-1 and 21-2). The **anterior** and **posterior semicircular ducts** are in vertical planes; the former is transverse to and the latter is parallel with the long axis of the petrous part of the temporal bone. The **lateral semicircular duct** slopes downward and backward at an angle

of 30° to the horizontal plane. The sensory areas of the semicircular ducts respond only to movement, and the response is maximal when movement is in the plane of the duct.

Each semicircular duct has an expansion or **ampulla** at one end, in which the **crista ampullaris** or sensory epithelium is supported by a transverse septum of connective tissue projecting into the lumen (Fig. 22-3). Among the columnar supporting cells are the sensory **hair cells**, whose structural details and mode of innervation conform to those already described for hair cells of the static labyrinth. The hairs and kinocilium of each hair cell are embedded

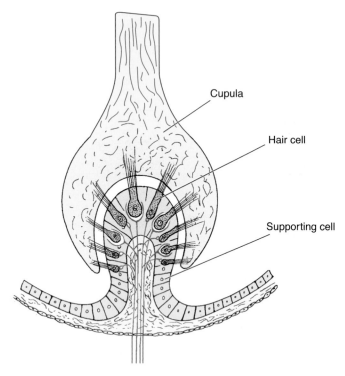

Cupula

Hair cell

Supporting cell

Distal neurites of cell in
the vestibular ganglion

FIGURE 22-3   Structure of a crista
ampullaris.

in gelatinous material that forms the **cupula**, in which otoliths are lacking. The cupula has the same specific gravity as the endolymph and is therefore not pulled on by gravity.

The cristae are sensors of rotary movement of the head, sometimes called *angular movement*, especially when accompanied by acceleration or deceleration. At the beginning of a movement in or near the plane of a semicircular duct, the endolymph lags because of inertia, and the cupula swings like a door in a direction opposite to that of the movement of the head. The momentum of the endolymph causes the cupula to swing momentarily in the opposite direction when the movement ceases. The hairs and kinocilia of the sensory cells bend accordingly. Depending on the direction of movement, this may reduce the membrane potentials of the hair cells, causing release of their chemical transmitter and the initiation of action potentials in the sensory nerve endings.

The kinocilium is consistently on the side of the tuft of hairs nearest the opening of the ampulla into the utricle. The excitation of hair cells occurs when the flow of endolymph is from the ampulla into the adjacent utricle; there is inhibition of the hair cells when the flow is in the opposite direction. The hair cells of the cristae, similar to those of the maculae, are supplied by primary sensory neurons whose bipolar cell bodies are situated in the vestibular ganglion.

Vestibular Pathways

On entering the brain stem at the junction of the medulla and pons, most of the vestibular nerve fibers bifurcate in the usual manner of afferent fibers and end in the vestibular nuclear complex. The remaining fibers go to the cerebellum through the inferior cerebellar peduncle.

VESTIBULAR NUCLEI

The vestibular nuclei are situated in the rostral medulla and caudal pons, partly beneath the lateral area of the floor of the fourth ventricle (see Figs. 6-3 and 22-4). Four vestibular nuclei are recognized on the basis of cytoarchitecture and the details of afferent and efferent connections. The **lateral ves-**

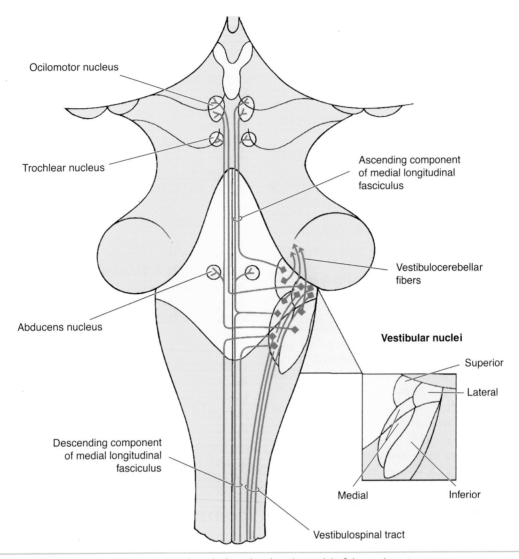

FIGURE 22-4 Vestibular pathways to the spinal cord and to the nuclei of the oculomotor nerves.

tibular nucleus, also known as **Deiters' nucleus**, consists mainly of large multipolar neurons with long axons. The **superior, medial,** and **inferior vestibular nuclei** consist of small- and medium-sized cells. The positions of the vestibular nuclei are described and illustrated in Chapter 7. The primary afferent vestibular neurons are excitatory to the neurons in the vestibular nuclei.

CONNECTIONS WITH THE CEREBELLUM

The **vestibulocerebellum**, consisting of the flocculonodular lobe, adjacent region of the inferior vermis and fastigial nuclei, receives its afferents from the superior, medial, and inferior vestibular nuclei in addition to a few axons directly from the vestibular nerve. In the reverse direction, efferent fibers of the vestibulocerebellum terminate throughout the vestibular nuclear complex (see Chapter 10 and Fig. 10-13). Some cerebellovestibular fibers are the axons of Purkinje cells (inhibitory); others are from the fastigial nucleus (excitatory). These afferent and efferent fibers of the vestibulocerebellum occupy the medial part of the inferior cerebellar peduncle. The role of the cerebellum in maintaining equilibrium is exerted mainly through pathways from the vestibular nuclei to the spinal cord.

CONNECTIONS WITH THE SPINAL CORD

The connection between the vestibular nuclei and the spinal cord is through descending fibers in the vestibulospinal tract and the medial longitudinal fasciculus. (Sometimes these tracts are called the *lateral* and *medial vestibulospinal tracts*, respectively.)

The **vestibulospinal tract**, which is uncrossed, originates exclusively in the lateral vestibular nucleus. The fibers descend in the medulla dorsal to the inferior olivary nucleus and continue into the ventral funiculus of the spinal cord. Vestibulospinal fibers terminate in the medial part of the ventral horn at all levels but most abundantly in the cervical and lumbosacral enlargements. A few vestibulospinal fibers synapse with medially located motor neurons that supply the axial musculature.

The vestibulospinal tract is of prime importance in regulating the tone of muscles involved in posture so that balance is maintained. Stimulation of the lateral vestibular nucleus causes excitation of motor neurons that supply extensor muscles of the ipsilateral lower limb. Flexors are inhibited, and the foot is pressed more firmly on the ground.

Axons from each medial vestibular nucleus project toward the midline and turn caudally in the descending component of the **medial longitudinal fasciculus** of both sides. This bundle of fibers is adjacent to the midline close to the floor of the fourth ventricle and ventral to the central canal of the medulla more caudally. The fibers continue into the medial part of the ventral funiculus of the spinal cord. They influence cervical motor neurons so that the head moves in a way that assists in maintaining equilibrium and fixation of gaze.

CONNECTIONS WITHIN THE BRAIN STEM

The ascending component of the **medial longitudinal fasciculus** is adjacent to the midline in the pons and midbrain, ventral to the floor of the fourth ventricle and the periaqueductal gray matter. The constituent axons connect the vestibular nuclei with the nuclei of the abducens, trochlear, and oculomotor nerves and with the accessory oculomotor nuclei of the midbrain.

Some of the ascending fibers are uncrossed; others cross the midline at the level of the vestibular nuclei. The medial longitudinal fasciculus provides for conjugate movement of the eyes, coordinated with movement of the head, to maintain visual fixation. Signals received by the vestibular nuclei from the cristae ampullares are responsible for the ocular adjustments to movement of the head. A small rotation of the head is accompanied by movement of the eyes through the same angle but in the opposite direction; this is called the **vestibulo-ocular reflex**.

The medial longitudinal fasciculus also contains the axons of internuclear neurons, which interconnect the nuclei of cranial nerves III, IV, and VI and fibers that originate in the paramedian pontine reticular formation. These connections and the effects of lesions of the medial longitudinal fasciculus are described in Chapter 8.

Excessive or prolonged stimulation of the vestibular system may cause nausea and vomiting. The connections responsible for these effects may be projections of vestibular nuclei to the solitary nucleus and the dorsal nucleus of the vagus nerve. Excessive input from the labyrinth to the vestibular nuclei is probably reduced to some extent by a feedback through the efferent inhibitory fibers in the vestibular nerve.

CORTICAL REPRESENTATION

The vestibular system acts mainly on the brain stem, cerebellum, and spinal cord, but a significant pathway to the cerebral cortex is also present. This provides for conscious awareness of position and movement of the head.

The ascending pathway from the vestibular nuclei is predominantly crossed and runs close to the medial lemniscus. The thalamic relay for the cortical projection is in the medial division of the ventral posterior nucleus (VPm), which also receives somatosensory fibers for the head. The vestibular cortical field is presumed to contribute information for use in higher motor regulation and for conscious spatial orientation. There is no known cortical area activated exclusively by vestibular stimulation.

Evoked potentials have been recorded in monkeys during electrical stimulation of the vestibular nerve. Two areas are thus identi-

■**CLINICAL NOTE**■

Caloric Testing and Doll's Eyes

The caloric test is used when there is a reason to suspect a tumor of the vestibulocochlear nerve or a lesion that interrupts the vestibular pathway in the brain stem. This procedure separately tests the pathway from each internal ear. The head is positioned so that the lateral semicircular duct is in a vertical plane, and the external acoustic meatus is irrigated with warm or cold water to induce convection currents in the endolymph. The ampulla of the duct is near the bone that is undergoing a change of temperature, and the endolymph "rises" or "falls," depending on whether it is warmed or cooled. In a *conscious* subject, the procedure causes nystagmus if the vestibular pathway for the side tested is intact. This nystagmus is a series of slow conjugate eye movements (driven by the vestibular nuclei), each followed by a rapid movement (driven by the cerebral cortex) to restore the original direction of gaze.

In a *comatose* patient with intact pathways in the brain stem, caloric stimulation with warm water makes the eyes deviate to the opposite side; cold water causes a conjugate deviation toward the cooled side. The deviation is the isolated slow component of a nystagmus. The fast component, which is a voluntary compensation, is prevented by the absence of consciousness.

The **doll's eyes phenomenon**, which is a vestibulo-ocular reflex uncomplicated by voluntary eye movements, is another clinical sign useful in the diagnosis of coma. If the vestibular apparatus, nuclei, and nerve; the medial longitudinal fasciculus; and the abducens and oculomotor nuclei are all intact, movement of the head will be accompanied by conjugate movement of the eyes in the opposite direction. Loss of caloric responses and of the doll's eyes reflex are two signs that can contribute to a diagnosis of **brain stem death**.

---

fied as receiving vestibular information: one is located in the posterior part of the insula, extending onto the parietal operculum, where it is coextensive with part of the second somatosensory area (see Chapter 15). The other area is located in the cortex that forms the anterior end of the intraparietal sulcus. Vertigo has been reported by human subjects after electrical stimulation at various sites in the parietal and temporal lobes. In positron emission tomography (PET) and functional nuclear magnetic resonance imaging (fMRI) studies, caloric stimulation of the human kinetic labyrinth has caused increased activation in various cortical areas. When the control subjects were patients whose vestibulocochlear nerves had been surgically removed (eliminating auditory as well as tactile and thermal sensations), significant cortical activation by caloric stimulation was detected only in the posterior insula and adjacent parietal operculum. The latter region is coextensive with the second somatosensory area (see Chapter 15).

Tracing experiments in monkeys reveal that neurons in various cortical regions (parts of the parietal lobe, insula, and premotor cortex of the

frontal lobe) have axons that end in the vestibular nuclei. These descending projections may suppress vestibular reflexes (i.e., movements of the eyes and neck) during the performance of voluntary movements.

Practical Aspects of the Vestibular System

ROTATION

The vestibular projections to nuclei that supply extraocular muscles and motor neurons in the spinal cord can be demonstrated by strong stimulation of the labyrinth. This may be done by rotating a subject around a vertical axis about 10 times in 20 seconds and then abruptly stopping the rotation. The responses are most pronounced if the head is bent forward 30 degrees to bring the lateral semicircular ducts in a horizontal plane. On stopping rotation, momentum acquired by the endolymph causes it to flow past (and deflect) the cupulae of the lateral semicircular ducts more suddenly and rapidly than for most movements.

Labyrinthine Disease

Labyrinthine irritation causes **vertigo** (an illusion of revolving motion), sometimes accompanied by nausea and vomiting, pallor, a cold sweat, and nystagmus. Paroxysms of labyrinthine irritation occur in **Ménière's disease,** a condition of obscure cause in which the endolymphatic pressure is abnormally high. Affected patients also have tinnitus (buzzing or ringing in the ears) and eventual deafness caused by degeneration of the receptor cells.

Benign paroxysmal positional vertigo is a common condition in which brief episodes of vertigo follow certain movements of the head. The condition is attributed to a particle of debris, such as a detached otolith, that has entered the endolymph of a semicircular duct. A sequence of head movements contrived to allow the particle to fall from the posterior semicircular duct into the utricle (the Dix-Hallpike maneuver) usually provides prolonged relief.

Sudden unilateral loss of vestibular function causes vertigo with considerable postural instability as well as a tendency to fall toward the abnormal side. This results from undue downward pressure on one foot, perhaps caused by excessive activity in the vestibulospinal tract of the normal side. The brain eventually accommodates to input from only one vestibular apparatus.

The responses of the hair cells in the cristae ampullares produce the following signs immediately after rotation ceases. Impulses conveyed by the ascending axons of the medial longitudinal fasciculus cause **nystagmus**, which is an oscillatory movement of the eyes consisting of fast and slow components.

1. The direction of nystagmus, right or left, is designated by that of the fast component, which is opposite to the direction of rotation. The slow component is driven by the vestibular nuclei; the fast component is a saccade (driven by the frontal eye field) to restore the direction of gaze.
2. The subject deviates in the direction of rotation if asked to walk in a straight line, and the finger deviates in the same direction when pointing to an object. These responses are caused by the effect of vestibulospinal projections on muscle tone.
3. There is a subjective feeling of turning in a direction opposite to that of rotation, for which both the cortical projection and the nystagmus are, presumably, responsible.
4. The spread of neuronal activity to nuclei of the vagus nerve may produce sweating and pallor as well as nausea in those who are susceptible to motion sickness.

Suggested Reading

Akbarian S, Grusser OJ, Guldin, WO. Corticofugal connections between the cerebral cortex and brainstem vestibular nuclei in the macaque monkey. *J Comp Neurol* 1994; 339:421–437.

Brandt T, Dieterich M. The vestibular cortex: its locations, functions and disorders. *Ann N Y Acad Sci* 1999;871: 293–312.

Carpenter MB, Chang L, Pereira AB, et al. Vestibular and cochlear efferent neurons in the monkey identified by immunocytochemical methods. *Brain Res* 1987;408: 275–280.

Donaldson JA, Lambert PM, Duckert LG, et al. *Surgical Anatomy of the Temporal Bone*, 4th ed. New York: Raven Press, 1992.

Emri M, Kisely, M, Lengyel Z, et al. Cortical projection of peripheral vestibular signaling. *J Neurophysiol* 2003;89: 2639–2646.

Gleeson MJ, Felix H, Johnsson LG. Ultrastructural aspects of the human peripheral vestibular system. *Acta Otolaryngol [Stockholm]* 1990;470(suppl):80–87.

Hawrylyshyn PA, Rubin AM, Tasker RR, et al. Vestibulothalamic projections in man: a sixth primary sensory pathway. *J Neurophysiol* 1978;41:394–401.

Highstein SM. The central nervous system efferent control of the organs of balance and equilibrium. *Neurosci Res* 1991;12:13–30.

Suarez C, Diaz C, Tolivia J, et al. Morphometric analysis of the human vestibular nuclei. *Anat Rec* 1997;247:271–288.

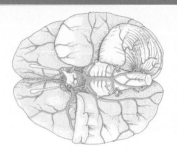

Chapter 23

MOTOR SYSTEMS

- A motor unit comprises a group of extrafusal muscle fibers and the alpha motor neuron that innervates them. Gamma motor neurons supply the intrafusal fibers of muscle spindles. The term *lower motor neuron* is applied collectively to motor neurons.

- A lower motor neuron lesion (e.g., destruction of cell bodies or transection of axons in a ventral root or peripheral nerve) causes flaccid paralysis, loss of the stretch reflex, and considerable atrophy.

- The stretch reflex is normally largely suppressed by the activity of descending pathways that end on motor neurons and nearby interneurons.

- The major descending pathways are the vestibulospinal, reticulospinal, and corticospinal (pyramidal) tracts. The first of these is largely concerned with postural adjustments, and the last is concerned with voluntary movements. Most corticospinal fibers decussate at the caudal end of the medulla.

- An upper motor neuron lesion (e.g., transection of corticospinal and corticoreticular fibers in the internal capsule) causes spastic paralysis, with exaggerated stretch reflexes and the abnormal Babinski reflex. Atrophy is not a prominent feature except when there is prolonged disuse.

- Corticobulbar and other descending axons end in the motor nuclei of cranial nerves, bilaterally in many cases. Transection of these fibers in the internal capsule causes contralateral weakness of muscles of the lower half of the face and of the tongue but not elsewhere in the head.

- The outputs of the cerebellum and the basal ganglia are channeled through the ventral lateral and ventral anterior nuclei of the thalamus to the four motor areas of the cerebral cortex. The connections of the cerebellum are ordered such that each cerebellar hemisphere is concerned with ipsilateral muscles.

- Disorders of the cerebellum cause inaccuracies in the rate, range, direction, and force of movements. Disorders of the basal ganglia cause dyskinesias or abnormalities of movement, including chorea, dystonia, hemiballismus, and parkinsonism.

Except for some visceral functions, overt expression of activity in the central nervous system (CNS) depends on the somatic or skeletal musculature. The muscles are supplied by the motor neurons in the ventral horns of the spinal cord and in the motor nuclei of cranial nerves, with these neurons constituting what Sherrington termed the "final common pathway" for determining muscle action. They are collectively known as the **lower motor neuron**, especially in clinical medicine. Another clinical expression is **upper motor neuron**, which embraces all the descending pathways of the brain and spinal cord involved in the volitional control of the musculature.

Components of the brain responsible for the execution of properly coordinated movements include the cerebral cortex, corpus striatum, thalamus, subthalamic nucleus, red nucleus, substantia nigra, reticular formation, vestibular nuclei, inferior olivary complex, and cerebellum. The connections of these structures have been described elsewhere in this book, but here they are reviewed with particular attention to their influence on the lower motor neuron. Although descending pathways can be traced from the motor areas of the cerebral cortex to the motor neurons, it is important to realize that the prefrontal cortex and the association areas of the parietal lobe are also importantly involved in the motivation and planning stages of the formulation of motor commands by the brain.

Lower Motor Neuron and Muscles

Skeletal muscles are supplied by motor neurons of two types, named alpha and gamma after the diameters of their axons. The large alpha motor neurons innervate the extrafusal fibers that constitute the main mass of the muscle, in which the axon of each neuron branches to supply the muscle fibers. The number supplied by a single neuron varies from fewer than 10 for small muscles whose contractions are precisely controlled to several hundred for large muscles that carry out strong but crude movements. An alpha motor neuron and the muscle fibers it supplies constitute a **motor unit**.

Different types of extrafusal muscle fiber are recognized on the basis of physiological and histochemical studies. The **type I fibers** contract slowly, are resistant to fatigue, and contain little stainable myofibrillar adenosine triphosphatase (ATPase). **Type II** fibers have faster contractions, are more rapidly fatigued than those of type I, and have high concentrations of ATPase in their myofibrils. Using other histochemical criteria, the type II muscle fibers are further divided into **types IIA and IIB**. All the muscle fibers in a motor unit are of the same type, and experimental evidence indicates that the type of fiber is determined by trophic influence of the innervating neuron. In addition to secreting acetylcholine to make the muscle fibers it supplies contract, a motor neuron provides trophic factors, which direct the differentiation of the muscle fibers and are necessary for their continued health. Proteins with myotrophic properties have been isolated from extracts of peripheral nerves.

The different types of muscle fiber respond differently to denervation: type IIB fibers atrophy most rapidly, and type I fibers atrophy most slowly.

Intrafusal muscle fibers supplied by gamma motor neurons control the length and tension

---

CLINICAL NOTE

Lower Motor Neuron Lesions

The syndrome of a lower motor neuron lesion occurs when a muscle is paralyzed or weakened as a result of disease or injury that affects the cell bodies or axons of the innervating neurons.

Typical causes include **poliomyelitis**, in which a virus selectively attacks ventral horn cells or equivalent neurons in the brain stem and **injuries** to peripheral nerves that transect some or all of the axons. The following clinical features are observed.

1. The muscle tone is reduced or absent (flaccid paresis or paralysis), owing to interruption of the efferent limb of the tonic stretch reflex.
2. The tendon-jerk reflexes are weak or absent. The cause is the same as that for flaccidity.
3. The muscles supplied by the affected neurons atrophy progressively. The atrophy is partly caused by loss of specific trophic factors normally provided by the motor nerve and partly to disuse.
4. Fibrillation potentials, caused by random contractions of individual denervated muscle fibers, can be detected by electromyog-

raphy. Fibrillation should not be confused with fasciculation, which is visible twitching that occurs at irregular intervals within a muscle. Although seen in partly denervated muscles, fasciculation is a rather unreliable diagnostic sign because it is quite common in some normal muscles.

5. In a partly denervated muscle, the intact nerve fibers sprout at the nodes of Ranvier and at motor end plates, with some of the new axonal branches innervating denervated muscle fibers. These changes can be seen in a suitably stained biopsy specimen, and the enlargement of the motor units can be detected by electromyography. Fasciculations in partly denervated muscles are contractions of enlarged motor units.

Signs similar to those of a lower motor neuron lesion occur in diseases of muscle in which synaptic transmission at the motor end plate is impaired (**myasthenia gravis**) or in which the contractile elements function inadequately (various forms of **dystrophy**, **myopathy**, and **myositis**). Biopsy and neurophysiological testing are used when a diagnosis cannot be made using clinical criteria.

of the neuromuscular spindles (see Chapter 3). The gamma motor neurons are much less numerous than the alpha motor neurons but are important because their patterns of firing determine the thresholds of the sensory nerve endings in the spindles. These endings are the receptors for the spinal stretch reflex, which is ordinarily suppressed as a result of activity in the descending tracts of the spinal cord. The muscle spindles are also receptors for the conscious awareness of position and movement.

Descending Pathways to the Spinal Cord

Motor neurons in the spinal cord are influenced by descending fibers from the cerebral cortex, central nuclei of the reticular formation, and lateral vestibular nucleus. Large tracts of fibers from these sites descend in the lateral and ventral funiculi of the spinal cord (see Fig. 5-9). Smaller contingents of descending fibers come from certain other nuclei in the brain stem.

CORTICOSPINAL TRACTS

The corticospinal tracts (Figs. 23-1 and 23-2) consist of the axons of cells in the frontal and parietal lobes. Motor corticospinal fibers arise in the primary motor, premotor, supplementary motor, and cingulate motor areas of the frontal lobe (see Chapter 15). Other corticospinal axons are from the first somatic sensory area in the parietal lobe; these probably do not have motor functions (see Chapter 15). The motor cortical areas have several other descending projections in addition to those to the spinal cord.

The organization of motor pathways (corticospinal and corticoreticulospinal) is both *parallel*, with axons descending from all the motor cortical areas, and *hierarchical*, with primary motor cortex receiving association fibers from the other motor areas, which, in turn, receive input from the prefrontal, parietal, and temporal association cortex. Thus, the motor output of the cerebral cortex is influenced by interpreted sensory input so that movements can be guided by touch, vision, and other senses as well as being dictated by those activities of the forebrain that constitute thinking.

The corticospinal fibers pass through the cerebral white matter, converging as they enter the posterior limb of the **internal capsule**, which is the band of white matter between the lentiform nucleus and thalamus (see Chapter 16). This part of the internal capsule also contains fibers that descend from the cortex to the red nucleus, reticular formation, pontine nuclei, and inferior olivary complex, together with many thalamocortical, corticothalamic, and corticostriate fibers. As will be seen, all these populations of axons are involved in the control of movement.

The internal capsule continues into the **basis pedunculi** of the midbrain. At this level, some of the corticospinal axons give off branches that terminate in the red nucleus. The corticospinal fibers occupy the middle three fifths of the basis pedunculi, flanked by and partly intermingled with corticopontine fibers. On reaching the ventral (basal) portion of the **pons**, the corticospinal tract breaks up into fasciculi that pass caudally with the bundles of corticopontine fibers (see Figs. 7-8 to 7-12). At this level, branches of some corticospinal axons enter and end in the central nuclei of the reticular formation.

At the caudal limit of the pons, the corticospinal axons reassemble to form, on the ventral surface of the medulla, the eminence known as the *pyramid*. The corticospinal fibers are therefore said to constitute the **pyramidal tract**. The term **pyramidal system** is applied to the corticospinal tracts together with the functionally equivalent **corticobulbar** (**corticonuclear**) **fibers**, which end in and near the motor nuclei of cranial nerves. At the caudal end of the medulla, in most people, about 85% of the corticospinal fibers cross the midline in the decussation of the pyramids (see Fig. 7-2) and enter the dorsal half of the lateral funiculus of the spinal cord, where they form the **lateral corticospinal tract**. The remaining 15% of the pyramidal fibers constitute the **ventral corticospinal tract**, which descends ipsilaterally in the medial part of the ventral funiculus. Most of the ventral corticospinal fibers decussate at segmental levels and end in the gray matter contralateral to their hemisphere of origin. (The relative sizes of the two corticospinal tracts are variable. In a few people, many of the fibers descend ipsilaterally in the ventral tract.)

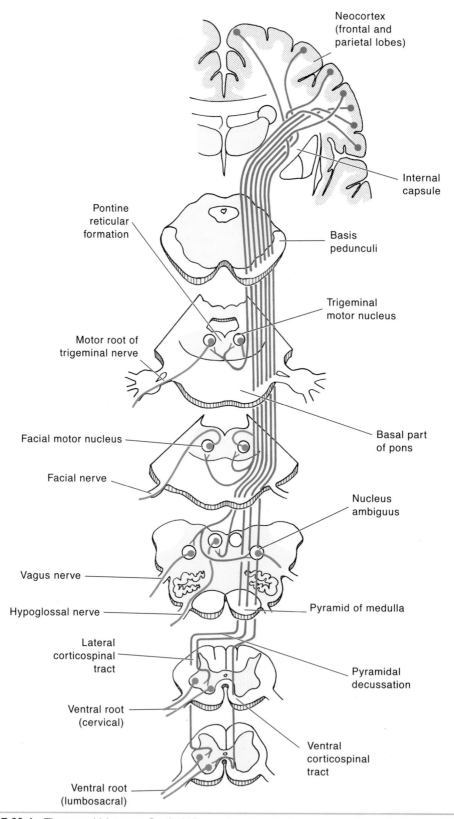

FIGURE 23-1 The pyramidal system. Corticobulbar and corticospinal neurons are shown in blue, and the motor neurons ("lower motor neuron") are shown in red.

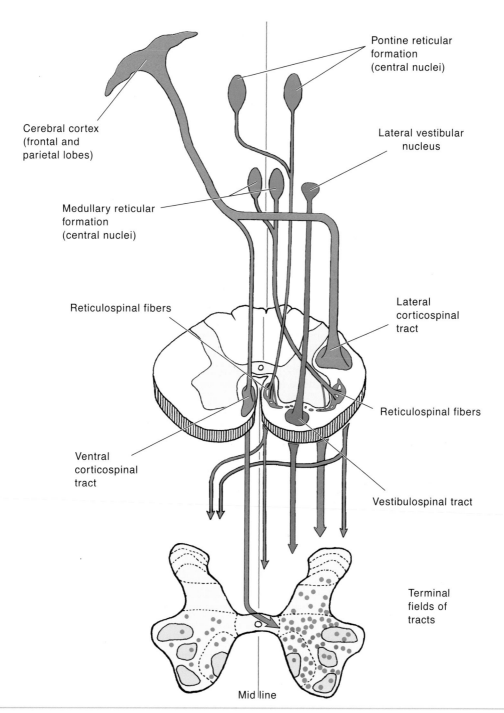

Pontine reticular
formation
(central nuclei)

Cerebral cortex
(frontal and
parietal lobes)

Lateral vestibular
nucleus

Medullary reticular
formation
(central nuclei)

Reticulospinal fibers

Lateral
corticospinal
tract

Reticulospinal fibers

Ventral
corticospinal
tract

Vestibulospinal tract

Terminal
fields of
tracts

Midline

FIGURE 23-2 Origins, courses, and terminal distributions of the major descending pathways concerned with the control of movement. The reticulospinal tracts indicated in green in the diagram represent a population of reticulospinal fibers present in the ventral and ventrolateral funiculi of the spinal white matter (see also Chapter 5). Corticospinal projections are red, and the vestibulospinal tract is blue. Columns of cell bodies of spinal motor neurons are indicated in yellow.

Selective Lesions of the Pyramidal Tract

There are about a dozen human case reports of medullary lesions confined to the pyramid. A contralateral flaccid hemiplegia was followed by recovery of most movements, with permanent clumsiness in movements of the fingers. The stretch reflexes were not abnormal. Neurosurgeons have cut through the middle part of the human basis pedunculi in attempts to relieve certain dyskinesias.

The effects of this lesion are similar to those of truly selective transection of the pyramid. These observations and comparable experimental studies in monkeys indicate that the most important function of the pyramidal tract is to control the precision and speed of skilled movements. The Babinski sign or response (described later in connection with upper motor neuron lesions) is probably due to transection of corticospinal fibers, but spasticity and other "upper motor neuron lesion" features are not so easily explained.

Within the **spinal gray matter**, most corticospinal axons terminate in the intermediate gray matter and the ventral horn. A minority synapse directly with the dendrites or cell bodies of motor neurons. Most corticospinal fibers are able to influence motor neurons only through the mediation of interneurons in the spinal gray matter. The corticospinal fibers that originate in the first somesthetic area of the parietal lobe end in the dorsal horn. These are not motor in function but instead modulate the transmission of data through the somesthetic pathways (see Chapter 19).

RETICULOSPINAL TRACTS

Reticulospinal fibers are present throughout the ventral funiculus and the ventral half of the lateral funiculus of the spinal white matter. Most are the axons of cells in the central group of nuclei of the reticular formation: the oral and caudal pontine reticular nuclei and the gigantocellular reticular nucleus of the medulla, mainly ipsilaterally. Many reticulospinal fibers shift from the ventral into the lateral funiculus as they descend. In humans, the fibers of pontine and medullary origin do not occupy separate zones of the white matter, as was once believed (see Chapter 5). Reticulospinal axons end bilaterally among spinal interneurons of the ventral horn, and a few enter the regions containing the cell bodies of motor neurons.

The central nuclei of the reticular formation receive afferents from all the sensory systems, from the premotor and supplementary motor areas of the cerebral cortex, from the fastigial nucleus of the vestibulocerebellum, and from other parts of the reticular formation (see Chapter 9). Afferents from the pedunculopontine nucleus provide a descending pathway through which the corpus striatum may indirectly modulate the activities of motor neurons.

Within the brain stem, the reticulospinal axons have short branches that synapse with other neurons of the reticular formation. Branching has been demonstrated also in the spinal cord, so that a single reticulospinal axon may have terminations in cervical, thoracic, and lumbar segments. This observation has led to the suggestion that the reticulospinal tracts control coordinated movements of muscles supplied from different segmental levels of the spinal cord, such as those of the upper and lower limbs in walking, running, and swimming. **Propriospinal (spinospinalis)** fibers may be equally important for synchronization of limb movements.

Most of what is known about the reticulospinal tracts is derived from research with animals. The tracts are present in a wide phylogenetic range of mammals, so it is likely to hold true also for humans. In view of what is known of other major descending pathways, it seems probable that the reticulospinal tracts mediate control over most movements that do not require dexterity or the maintenance of balance. Motor tracts from the human cerebral cortex can be studied by stimulating the motor areas electrically to evoke small movements. Normally, the delay between the stimulus and the beginning of the response is short enough to be attributable to direct (monosynaptic) activation of motor neurons by the corticospinal tract. The existence of a corticoreticulospinal pathway is supported by the finding of motor responses with longer delays in patients in whom the corticospinal fibers are known to have degenerated following infarction in the internal capsule.

From the foregoing paragraphs, it can be seen that the corticospinal and corticoreticulospinal pathways are influenced by the activities of several regions of the CNS that have connections with the cerebral cortex and the reticular formation. A greatly oversimplified scheme of these connections (Fig. 23-3) may help readers to envisage the overall organization of these major parts of the motor system.

VESTIBULOSPINAL TRACT

This tract (see Chapter 5 and Fig. 23-2), which arises ipsilaterally from the large cells of the lateral vestibular nucleus (Deiters' nucleus), is also known as the *lateral vestibulospinal tract*. It is composed of myelinated axons of large cali-

ber descending in the ventral funiculus of the spinal white matter. Most vestibulospinal fibers end in contact with interneurons in the medial part of the ventral horn of the spinal gray matter, but some synapse with the dendrites of motor neurons.

Electrical stimulation of the lateral vestibular nucleus in animals causes contraction of ipsilateral extensor muscles of the limbs and vertebral column, with relaxation of the flexors. These effects occur to a lesser extent contralaterally as well, probably because there are neurons in the medial part of the ventral horn with axons that cross the midline of the spinal cord. Transection of the brain stem above the vestibular nuclei causes a condition known as **decerebrate rigidity**, in which the extensor musculature of the whole body is in a continuous state of contraction. This condition is easily produced in laboratory animals and occasionally occurs in patients with large destructive lesions of the midbrain or pons. (The condition

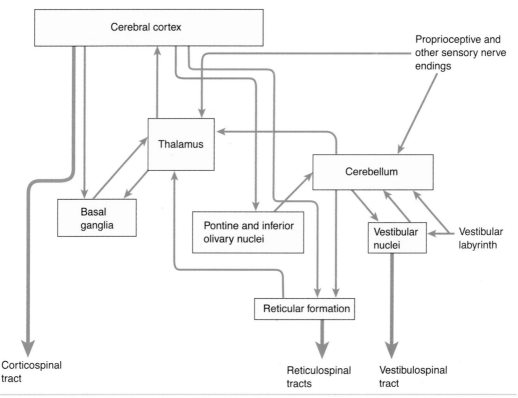

FIGURE 23-3   Diagram showing chains of command from sense organs and from the cerebral cortex to motor neurons, with sites at which the activities of corticospinal, reticulospinal, and vestibulospinal tracts can be modified by the basal ganglia and cerebellum. Descending motor pathways are red; other connections are blue. This simplified diagram omits many connections. For more details, see Figures 23-4 and 23-5.

can be caused by a large tumor or by thrombosis of the basilar artery.) The extensor spasm is abolished by destruction of the lateral vestibular nucleus, indicating that it is caused by the unopposed excessive activity of vestibulospinal neurons. The principal sources of afferent fibers to the lateral vestibular nucleus are the vestibular nerve, fastigial nucleus of the cerebellum, and vestibulocerebellar cortex.

The data summarized above support the view that the vestibulospinal tract is concerned with the maintenance of upright posture, which mainly results from the action of the extensor muscles in opposing gravity. Orderly functioning of the "antigravity" musculature is essential for balance, both at rest and during locomotion. Although the vestibulospinal tract does not mediate "voluntary" movements dictated by the cerebral cortex, it is essential for such highly skilled accomplishments of motor coordination as the feats of a gymnast or an acrobat. The learning of those aspects of skilled movement that involve posture and balance and that are effected through the vestibulospinal tract probably occurs in neuronal circuits that include the inferior olivary complex of nuclei and the cerebellum (see Chapter 10).

OTHER DESCENDING TRACTS

The parts of the brain that connect with the cells of origin of the corticospinal, reticulospinal, and vestibulospinal tracts are summarized in Figure 23-3. This diagram excludes some small descending tracts.

Two tracts in the medial part of the ventral funiculus terminate throughout the cervical segments of the spinal cord. These are the **tectospinal tract**, from the contralateral superior colliculus and the descending component of the **medial longitudinal fasciculus**. The former may be insignificantly small in humans. The latter, which is also called the *medial vestibulospinal tract*, arises from the medial vestibular nuclei of both sides but is mainly ipsilateral. Both tracts influence neurons that innervate the muscles of the neck, including those supplied by the accessory nerve, affecting movements of the head as required for fixation of gaze and maintaining equilibrium. The **rubrospinal tract** provides a motor pathway of some importance in most mammals, but in humans,

it is small and goes no further caudally than the second cervical segment.

Descending Pathways to Motor Nuclei of Cranial Nerves

Most of the muscles supplied by the cranial nerves participate in voluntarily initiated movements, and some of them are controlled with exquisite precision.

As described in Chapter 8, the oculomotor, trochlear, and abducens nuclei receive afferents through a complicated system of connections involving the cortex of the frontal, parietal and occipital lobes, superior colliculus, and various nuclei in the brain stem. It will be recalled that the cerebral cortex controls coordinated movements of the eyes. The frontal eye fields are necessary for changing the direction of gaze voluntarily. The posterior parietal cortex controls involuntary conjugate movements, as when tracking a moving object, and it also is necessary for convergence of the eyes to look at a near object.

Knowledge of the afferent connections of the other motor nuclei of cranial nerves is less complete. The nuclei concerned are the trigeminal and facial motor nuclei, nucleus ambiguus, and hypoglossal nucleus. Results of studies in animals indicate that **corticobulbar fibers** from the motor areas of the cortex end mainly in the reticular formation near the motor nuclei, with a few contacting the motor neurons directly. The motor nuclei also receive afferents from the reticular formation that are equivalent to the reticulospinal tracts. Therefore, upper motor neuron paralysis or paresis, caused by a lesion in the internal capsule, for example, is due to interruption of both corticobulbar and corticoreticular fibers.

With a unilateral lesion in the motor cortex or in the posterior limb of the internal capsule, the only paralyzed muscles in the head are those of the lower half of the face (moving the lips and cheeks) and of the tongue, contralaterally. The tongue paralysis is not permanent. The muscles supplied by the trigeminal motor nucleus, rostral portion of the facial motor nucleus, and nucleus

Upper Motor Neuron Lesions

The term *upper motor neuron* is unsatisfactory because it refers collectively to descending pathways that make different contributions to the voluntary control of muscle action. *Upper motor neuron lesion* is still useful in clinical medicine, however, because it is often necessary to determine whether a group of muscles is weakened or paralyzed as a result of denervation or as a consequence of some lesion in the CNS. Sudden development of paralysis due to a vascular lesion (hemorrhage, thrombosis, or embolism) in the brain constitutes a **stroke**. An infarction in the posterior limb of the internal capsule, for example, results in contralateral **hemiplegia** with the typical signs of an upper motor neuron lesion. Similar (although not identical) abnormalities occur below the level of a lesion that partly or completely transects the spinal cord. The clinical features of an upper motor neuron lesion are as follows.

1. Voluntary movements of the affected muscles are absent or weak.
2. Profound atrophy does not occur in the affected muscles, although there is slow wasting, and contractures may develop over several months if the condition does not improve. The muscles are not denervated, so the myotrophic effect of their motor innervation is preserved.
3. The tone of the muscles is increased. This phenomenon, known as **spasticity**, results from the continuous operation of the stretch reflex, which normally is suppressed by the activity of the descending tracts. The tendon jerks are exaggerated. When the examining physician attempts passive extension of a flexed joint, resistance is encountered because of operation of the stretch reflex. When greater force is applied, an inhibitory reflex is initiated by the Golgi tendon organs, which respond to tension rather than lengthening, and the muscles relax suddenly. This phenomenon is known as "clasp-knife rigidity." Alternating contractions and relaxations, known as **clonus**, may also occur when a tendon is stretched. A test for clonus is application of firm pressure to the ball of the foot, which dorsiflexes the ankle joint, pulls the tendo calcaneus (Achilles' tendon), and stretches the gastrocnemius and soleus muscles. Pushing the patella toward the foot can evoke clonus in the quadriceps muscles.
4. With a cerebral lesion, the extensor muscles of the paralyzed lower limb are stimulated by the intact vestibulospinal tract: the limb is extended and inwardly rotated. The upper limb is held in flexion at the elbow and wrist, perhaps as a result of activity in the reticulospinal tracts. A lesion in the spinal cord transects vestibulospinal fibers, and all the paralyzed limbs assume positions of flexion.
5. The **plantar reflex** is abnormal. Normally, there is plantar flexion of the big toe when the lateral margin of the sole is firmly stroked with a hard object. In the abnormal reflex, known as the **Babinski** sign or response, the toe is dorsiflexed. This movement is frequently associated with flexion at the knee and hip joints, although similar withdrawal is seen in normal people with sensitive soles. The descending tracts involved in the normal plantar reflex include the pyramidal tract. An extensor plantar response is normal in children under 1 year of age, and the response does not become unequivocally flexor until the 18th month. This maturation coincides with the myelination of most of the axons in the corticospinal tracts.
6. The **superficial reflexes** are suppressed or absent. These reflexes are the abdominal reflex (contraction of the anterior abdominal muscles when the overlying skin is firmly stroked) and the cremasteric reflex (withdrawal of the ipsilateral testis when the medial side of the thigh is stroked). The latter reflex is sluggish or absent in most men but is a useful clinical test in infants. These reflexes are presumed to be mediated by long tracts to and from the cerebral cortex, but their exact anatomical pathways are uncertain.
7. In the case of the facial muscles, only the lower half of the face is involved. For unknown reasons, muscle action expressing emotional changes is usually spared, and often there are abnormal emotional responses, such as laughter or crying on inappropriate occasions.
8. If the causative lesion in a cerebral hemisphere is small, there is gradual recovery of some function. Some patients develop "mirror movements," which occur symmetrically on attempting to use a single limb. Electrophysiological studies indicate that this is due to branches of corticospinal axons that pass from the intact to the disordered side of the spinal cord. These branches may be formed by axonal sprouting (see Chapter 2). Recovery from stroke is poorer in humans than in other animals with comparable lesions. This discrepancy has been attributed to the absence of a significant corticorubrospinal projection in the human CNS.

ambiguus are not affected on either side by a unilateral lesion in the cerebral hemisphere. It has been deduced that descending pathways are distributed bilaterally to all the motor nuclei of the brain stem except the caudal part of the facial motor nucleus, which receives only crossed descending afferents. Partial deafferentation of the bilaterally supplied nuclei is evidently compensated for by the intact connections from the ipsilateral hemisphere. The existence of these functional connections has been confirmed by more recent studies that involve stimulation of the normal human cerebral cortex.

The hypoglossal nucleus receives more crossed than uncrossed afferents, and if the former have been removed, the latter assume control after a few weeks. The accessory nucleus, in the upper cervical segments of the spinal cord, supplies the trapezius muscle, which elevates the shoulder and the sternocleidomastoid muscle, which turns the head to look to the contralateral side. After transection of descending motor fibers, there is paralysis of the contralateral trapezius and of the ipsilateral sternocleidomastoid. Evidently, the fibers descending to the sternocleidomastoid motor neurons do not cross the midline.

Systems That Control the Descending Pathways

The movements elicited by electrical stimulation of the motor cortical areas (see Chapter 15) are much simpler than those that ordinarily occur either in obedience to conscious thoughts or as part of involuntary or habitual patterns of activity. The physiological output of signals from the motor cortex must, therefore, be much more complex than its responses to simple, artificial electrical stimuli. The most numerous afferent connections of the motor areas are the association and commissural fibers from other cortical areas and projection fibers from the thalamus, especially the ventral anterior and ventral lateral nuclei. These thalamic nuclei receive projections from two other systems involved in the control of movement, the cerebellum and basal ganglia. (Connections and functions of the motor cortical areas are discussed at greater length in Chapter 15. For more about the cer-

ebellum and basal ganglia, see also Chapters 10 and 12.)

CEREBELLAR CIRCUITS

In connection with the motor systems, it is appropriate to review some of the connections of the cerebellum (Fig. 23-4). The cortex and central nuclei of the cerebellum receive input from extensive areas of the contralateral neocortex (by way of corticopontine and pontocerebellar projections); from ipsilateral proprioceptors in muscles, tendons, and joints (by way of the spinocerebellar and cuneocerebellar tracts); and from the vestibular apparatus. The inferior olivary complex, which receives most of its afferent fibers from the neocortical motor areas, red nucleus, and spinal cord, projects to the entire cerebellar cortex. In addition to these, the precerebellar reticular nuclei (see Chapter 10) relay information from the spinal cord, vestibular nuclei, and cerebral cortex. The cerebellar nuclei send their efferent fibers to the contralateral thalamus (ventral lateral nucleus) and red nucleus, as well as to the reticular formation bilaterally and to the ipsilateral vestibular nuclei.

Thus, the cerebellum receives information from the cerebral cortex, including motor areas, and it is also informed of changes in the lengths and tensions of muscles and of the position and angular movements of the head. These large contingents of afferent fibers are supplemented by smaller inputs that report on cutaneous, visual, and auditory sensations. The output of the cerebellar nuclei is brought to bear on the primary and supplementary motor areas through a relay in the posterior division of the ventral lateral thalamic nucleus (VLp). Other cerebellar efferents influence lower motor neurons through connections with the vestibular nuclei and the central group of nuclei of the reticular formation.

Electrophysiological investigations indicate that the cerebellum is informed through its olivary afferents of the program of neuronal instructions for any complex movement. The pontocerebellar afferents, which are active earlier than the primary motor area, are involved in the execution of movements. Cerebellar afferents activated by proprioceptive nerve endings enable a program of instructions to be modified in light of the changes in length and tension of muscles that are occurring.

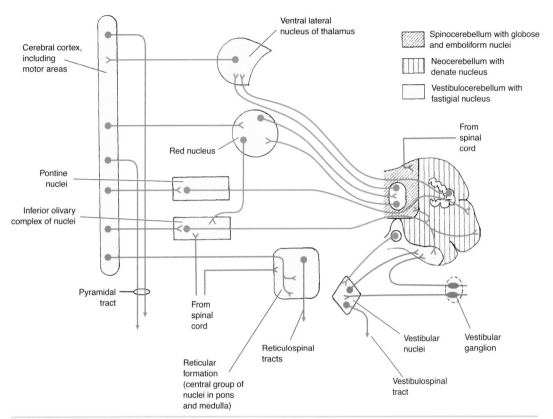

Cerebral cortex, including motor areas

Ventral lateral nucleus of thalamus

Spinocerebellum with globose and emboliform nuclei

Neocerebellum with denate nucleus

Vestibulocerebellum with fastigial nucleus

From spinal cord

Red nucleus

Pontine nuclei

Inferior olivary complex of nuclei

Pyramidal tract

From spinal cord

Reticular formation (central group of nuclei in pons and medulla)

Reticulospinal tracts

Vestibular nuclei

Vestibular ganglion

Vestibulospinal tract

FIGURE 23-4 Diagram of some neural connections involved in the control of movement, with emphasis on cerebellar circuitry (green neurons) and the major descending tracts (red neurons). Sensory inputs are represented by blue neurons. Other cerebellar connections are explained and illustrated in Chapter 10.

BASAL GANGLIA

The basal ganglia, which are not ganglia but nuclei, are the **corpus striatum** of the telencephalon, **subthalamic nucleus** of the diencephalon, and **substantia nigra** of the mesencephalon. The corpus striatum is functionally subdivided into the **striatum** and the external and internal divisions of the **pallidum**. (The unfortunate plethora of names associated with the basal ganglia and corpus striatum is explained in Chapter 12.) The putamen and caudate nucleus constitute the striatum. Its afferent fibers come from the whole neocortex, from the intralaminar thalamic nuclei, and from the substantia nigra (Fig. 23-5). The striatum projects to the pallidum, which influences the premotor and supplementary motor areas through inhibitory relays in the ventral anterior (VA) and the anterior division of the ventral lateral nucleus (VLa) of the thalamus. The activity of the striatum is modulated by a

two-way connection with the substantia nigra, and the activity of the pallidum is modulated by a two-way connection with the subthalamic nucleus. These connections are set out in more detail in Chapter 12.

A small contingent of pallidofugal fibers passes caudally and terminates in the **pedunculopontine nucleus** at the junction of the midbrain and pons (see Chapter 9). Among other projections, the pedunculopontine nucleus sends some fibers to the subthalamic nucleus, some to the pallidum, and some to the central group of nuclei of the reticular formation. A role in the timing of rhythmic activities, including locomotion and sleep, has been suggested for the pedunculopontine nucleus.

Clearly, the basal ganglia comprise a large mass of gray matter influenced by several parts of the CNS. The number and complexity of interconnections within the basal ganglia in-

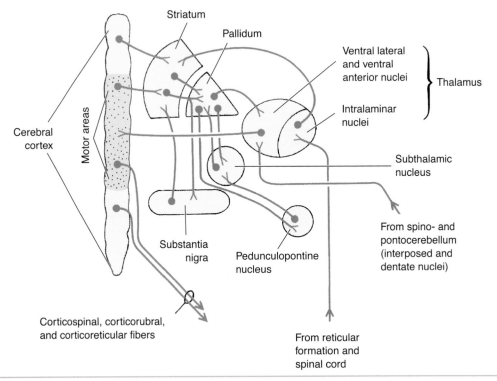

FIGURE 23-5   Diagram of some neural connections involved in the control of movement, with emphasis on the basal ganglia, thalamus, and motor cortex. Cortical projections are red; others are blue. For other circuitry of the basal ganglia, see Chapter 12.

dicate that much integrative activity must be occurring. Only part of the system is devoted to motor activities (see Chapter 12). Electrophysiological studies indicate that in the corpus striatum, as in the cerebellar nuclei, changes in activity precede and accompany movements. It is probable, therefore, that the motor circuitry of the basal ganglia is involved in the transfer of information from the whole of the neocortex to the motor areas, in particular the premotor and supplementary motor areas and that the corpus striatum serves as a repository of instructions for fragments of learned movements. The effects of disease also indicate a role in remembering encoded instructions for the initiation, control, and cessation of all the components of regularly made movements.

CONFUSING TERMINOLOGY

It was once erroneously thought that the pyramidal system controlled all deliberate move-ments and that there was a parallel "extrapyramidal" system largely concerned with the habitual or automatic activities of the muscles. Unfortunately, the term "extrapyramidal" has been applied not only to the reticulospinal and vestibulospinal tracts but also to pathways that include the corpus striatum, substantia nigra, and subthalamic nucleus because some of these structures were once thought to give rise to numerous descending fibers. From anatomical, physiologic, and clinical evidence, it is more appropriate to bracket the basal ganglia with the neocerebellum; the activity of both regions is directed through the thalamus to the motor areas of the cerebral cortex. Thus, the term "extrapyramidal system" does not represent any real entity and has caused much confusion. It is mentioned here because in clinical practice, dyskinesias (disorders in which abnormal spontaneous movements occur) are sometimes still called "extrapyramidal syndromes."

Disorders of Movement

Knowledge of the neurotransmitters and their excitatory or inhibitory actions within the motor circuitry might one day make it possible to provide tidy neuroanatomical explanations for different types of disordered movement comparable to those that account for some sensory deficits. Some progress in this direction has been made and is reviewed in Chapter 12. Conditions with well-defined clinical features are caused by circumscribed lesions in certain regions. The most straightforward is the lower motor neuron lesion, described earlier. Some others are now reviewed. Disordered movement is also discussed in Chapters 7, 11, and 12.

UPPER MOTOR NEURON AND CORTICAL LESIONS

The clinical signs comprising the upper motor neuron lesion were identified earlier in this chapter. The syndrome occurs in its most typical form after **infarction of the posterior limb of the internal capsule**, resulting in the severance of ascending and descending tracts, including corticospinal and corticobulbar fibers, together with corticopontine, cortico-olivary, corticoreticular, corticorubral, and thalamocortical projections. **Destruction of both the primary motor and the premotor cortex**, such as often follows occlusion of the middle cerebral artery, has similar consequences.

Lesions confined to the primary motor area cause a flaccid paralysis of the part of the body appropriate to the exact position of the destroyed cortex. As with other lesions in which only small cortical areas are damaged, recovery usually occurs as the functions are taken over by adjacent areas. **Destruction of the premotor area** causes contralateral weakness of the muscles that move the shoulder and hip joints. Locomotion is also impaired. The hand cannot be brought into a useful position for many ordinary tasks, and impairment of sequential actions of muscles and faulty execution of visually guided movement may also be present. (Sequences and logical ordering generally require the integrity of cortex rostral to the prefrontal area.) An ineffective movement may be repeated without improvement.

If the **supplementary motor area** is destroyed, the patient has a severe contralateral motor disability in which movements cannot be initiated. Bilateral lesions, especially if they involve the adjacent cingulate motor area, cause **akinetic mutism**. These symptoms are consonant with the normal involvement of the supplementary and cingulate motor areas in the initiation of movements (see Chapter 15), including those of the muscles used in speech. Akinetic mutism caused by bilateral medial cortical lesions must not be confused with the consequences of a destructive lesion in the upper pons in which the patient is apparently asleep with relaxed musculature. In the latter condition, also called *akinetic mutism*, the eyes open in response to loud sounds and follow moving objects, but other sensory stimuli are ineffective, and there is no other movement or speech.

A related condition, seen with a midpontine lesion, is the **locked-in syndrome,** in which the patient is awake but mute, with all muscles paralyzed except those that move the eyes. A lesion causing the locked-in syndrome transects the descending motor tracts but spares the somesthetic and special sensory pathways. A magazine editor, Jean-Dominique Bauby (1952–1997), became locked in after a brain stem stroke in 1995. He wrote a remarkable autobiographical book, dictated letter by letter with a code based on movements of his left eyelid. He also founded, in 1996, the *Association du Locked-in Syndrome*, based in Boulogne-Billancourt, France. The locked-in syndrome is extremely rare. Large pontine vascular lesions usually cause sudden death. Bauby wrote: "In the past . . . you simply died. But improved resuscitation techniques have now prolonged and refined the agony."

DYSKINESIAS

Dyskinesias are diseases in which unwanted superfluous movements occur. **Chorea** and various kinds of **dystonia**, which are thought to result from lesions of the corpora striata, are discussed in Chapter 12. **Ballism**, consisting of sudden flailing movements at the proximal joints of limbs, is usually caused by a vascular lesion in the contralateral subthalamic nucleus (see Chapters 11 and 12). The most frequently encountered dyskinesia is **Parkinson's disease**, which is characterized by muscular rigidity, tremor of distal muscles, and poverty of movement (bradykinesia). The primary lesion is loss of dopaminergic neurons in the pars compacta of the substantia nigra (see Chapters 7 and 12). Normally, such neurons are active at all times, irrespective of any movement being made, exerting a continuous modulating influence

(continued)

on the striatum and, indirectly, on the premotor and supplementary motor areas of the neocortex. The bradykinesia of parkinsonism has been attributed to withdrawal of an excitatory action of dopamine on some striatal neurons. This releases the pallidum from inhibition by the striatum, resulting in increased pallidal inhibition of the VLa nucleus of the thalamus. This thalamic nucleus is excitatory to the premotor cortex, so in Parkinson's disease, the cortical activity is reduced. (Refer to Fig. 12-6 to follow the logic of this argument, which, unfortunately, does not account for the tremors and rigidity.)

CEREBELLAR DYSFUNCTION

Finally, lesions of the cerebellum lead to a variety of motor disturbances, including a specific type of ataxia, hypotonia, and a characteristic intention tremor (see Chapter 10). Cerebellar lesions may be said to generally lead to errors in the rate, range, force, and direction of willed movements. **Unilateral damage** to a cerebellar hemisphere (vascular occlusion, a tumor, or demyelination of white matter in one or more cerebellar peduncles) results in symptoms that affect the same side of the body. Cerebellar dysfunction, which may be bilateral, is a common feature of multiple sclerosis (MS), an autoimmune disease in which plaques of demyelination develop in white matter throughout the brain and spinal cord. Cerebellothalamic fibers are often affected in MS. **Lesions in the midline** of the cerebellum affect the vestibular and spinal connections, so an ataxic gait is the most prominent abnormality.

Suggested Reading

Albin RL, Young AB, Penney JB. The functional anatomy of basal ganglia disorders. *Trends Neurosci* 1989;12:366–375.

Bauby JD. *The Diving Bell and the Butterfly* [translated by Leggatt J]. London: Fourth Estate, 1997.

Brouwer B, Ashby P. Corticospinal projections to upper and lower limb spinal motoneurons in man. *Electroenceph Clin Neurophysiol* 1990;76:509–519.

Bucy PC, Keplinger JE, Siqueira EB. Destruction of the "pyramidal tract" in man. *J Neurosurg* 1964;21:385–398.

Cangiano A, Buffelli M, Pasino E. Nerve-muscle trophic interaction. In: Gorio A, ed. *Neuroregeneration*. New York: Raven Press, 1993:145–167.

Cruccu G, Berardelli A, Inghilleri M, et al. Corticobulbar projections to upper and lower facial motoneurons: a study by magnetic transcranial stimulation in man. *Neurosci Lett* 1990;117:68–73.

Davidoff RA. The pyramidal tract. *Neurology* 1990;40:332–339.

Davis HL. Trophic effects of neurogenic substances on mature skeletal muscle in vivo. In: Fernandez HL, Donoso JA, eds. *Nerve-Muscle Cell Trophic Communication*. Boca Raton, FL: CRC Press, 1988:101–145.

Eyre JA, Miller S, Clowry GJ, et al. Functional corticospinal projections are established prenatally in the human foetus permitting involvement in the development of spinal motor centres. *Brain* 2000;123:51-64.

Freund H-J, Hummelsheim H. Lesions of premotor cortex in man. *Brain* 1985;108:697–733.

Fries W, Danek A, Witt TN. Motor responses after transcranial electrical stimulation of cerebral hemispheres with a degenerated pyramidal tract. *Ann Neurol* 1991;29:646–650.

Georgopoulos AP. Higher order motor control. *Annu Rev Neurosci* 1991;14:361–377.

Inglis WL, Winn P. The pedunculopontine tegmental nucleus: where the striatum meets the reticular formation. *Prog Neurobiol* 1995;47:1–29.

Nathan PH, Smith MC. The rubrospinal and central tegmental tracts in man. *Brain* 1982;105:223–269.

Nathan PN, Smith MC, Deacon P. Vestibulospinal, reticulospinal and descending propriospinal nerve fibers in man. *Brain* 1996;119:1809–1833.

Nudo RJ, Masterton RB. Descending pathways to the spinal cord, II. quantitative study of the tectospinal tract in 23 mammals. *J Comp Neurol* 1989;286:96–119.

O'Rahilly R, Muller F. *The Embryonic Human Brain. An Atlas of Developmental Stages*, 3rd ed. New York: Wiley-Liss, 2006.

Peterson BW. The reticulospinal system and its role in the control of movement. In: Barnes CD, ed. *Brainstem Control of Spinal Cord Function*. Orlando, FL: Academic Press, 1984:28–86.

Porter R, Lemon R. *Corticospinal Function and Voluntary Movement*. (Monographs of the Physiological Society, No. 45.) Oxford: Clarendon Press, 1993.

Rothwell JC. *Control of Human Voluntary Movement*, 2nd ed. London: Chapman & Hall, 1994.

Rouiller EM, Liang F, Babalian A, et al. Cerebellothalamocortical and pallidothalamocortical projections to the primary and supplementary motor cortical areas: a multiple tracing study in macaque monkeys. *J Comp Neurol* 1994;345:185–213.

Wise SP, Soussadoud D, Johnson PB, et al. Premotor and parietal cortex: corticocortical connectivity and combinatorial computations. *Annu Rev Neurosci* 1997;20:25–42.

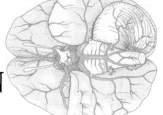

VISCERAL INNERVATION

Important Facts

- The control of smooth muscle, cardiac muscle, and secretory tissues by the central nervous system always involves a chain of at least two neurons, preganglionic and postganglionic, with the cell body of the latter being in an autonomic ganglion.

- Whereas parasympathetic ganglia are near the organs they innervate, most sympathetic ganglia are paravertebral or preaortic. The enteric ganglia are located in the myenteric and submucous plexuses of the alimentary canal.

- Preganglionic parasympathetic neurons are present in certain nuclei of cranial nerves III, VII, IX, and X and in the intermediolateral cell columns of spinal segments S2, S3, and S4.

- Parasympathetic ganglia supply the sphincter pupillae and ciliary muscles, the lacrimal and salivary glands, thoracic and abdominal viscera (including the heart), the urinary bladder and other pelvic organs, and the erectile tissue of the genitalia.

- Preganglionic sympathetic neurons are located in the intermediolateral cell column of spinal segments T1 to L2. Their axons pass through the ventral roots and the white communicating rami into the sympathetic trunk. They reach paravertebral ganglia by way of the sympathetic trunk or preaortic ganglia by way of splanchnic nerves.

- Gray communicating rami carry postganglionic sympathetic axons into mixed nerves to supply blood vessels, sweat glands, and piloarrector muscles. Postganglionic fibers to the head travel along the carotid arteries and their branches. Cardiac sympathetic nerves arising in the cervical ganglia supply the heart. Mesenteric and similar nerve plexuses carry postganglionic sympathetic fibers from preaortic ganglia to abdominal organs. The adrenal medulla is a modified sympathetic ganglion with neurons that release their transmitters directly into the blood.

- The enteric nervous system can work independently, but its activities are modulated by preganglionic parasympathetic and postganglionic sympathetic axons. The enteric plexuses contain sensory neurons, interneurons, and cells that provide excitatory and inhibitory innervation to the gut.

- Acetylcholine is the principal neurotransmitter of all preganglionic neurons and all parasympathetic postganglionic neurons. Noradrenaline is the principal transmitter of all postganglionic sympathetic neurons except those that supply sweat glands, which are cholinergic. Several peptides also occur in autonomic neurons.

- The activities of the autonomic nervous system are subject to control by descending central pathways from the medial prefrontal cortex, amygdala, septal area, hypothalamus, and reticular formation. The descending pathway mediating sympathetic effects in the eye and face passes ipsilaterally through the lateral part of the medulla and then in the medial part of the lateral funiculus of the spinal cord.

- Fibers for visceral pain have cell bodies in dorsal root ganglia and axons that accompany the preganglionic and postganglionic sympathetic fibers. Pain is often referred to somatic structures supplied by the same spinal segments as the affected organ. The central pathway to the cerebral cortex is the spinothalamic system.

- Most sensory neurons for visceral reflexes (and for conscious sensation of fullness) have cell bodies in the inferior ganglion of the vagus nerve and axons that accompany the preganglionic parasympathetic fibers. The sensory neurons project centrally to the solitary nucleus, which is connected with preganglionic autonomic neurons, the hypothalamus, various regions of the reticular formation, and the amygdala. There are indirect projections to the mediodorsal thalamic nucleus and to the insular and medial prefrontal cortex.

Chapter 24

In neurobiology, the adjective *visceral* is applied to innervated smooth and cardiac muscle and secretory cells in all parts of the body. The primary role of visceral innervation is to maintain optimal homeostasis. This end is attained through regulation of the organs and structures concerned with digestion, circulation, respiration, maintenance of normal body temperature, excretion, and reproduction. In addition to the regulating role of visceral reflexes, the activities of smooth muscles, glandular elements, and cardiac muscle can be altered by influences from the highest levels of the brain, especially in response to emotion and to the external environment.

Afferent signals of visceral origin reach the central nervous system (CNS) through primary sensory neurons similar to those for general sensation. Under normal conditions, these impulses elicit reflex responses in viscera and feelings of fullness of hollow organs such as the stomach, large intestine, and urinary bladder. Visceral sensation also contributes to feelings of well-being or malaise. In the presence of abnormal function and disease, visceral afferents transmit impulses for pain. The painful sensation often is referred to a part of the body wall or a limb supplied by the same segmental nerves as the affected organ.

The motor or efferent supply of smooth muscle cells (SMC), cardiac muscle, and gland cells differs from that of voluntary muscles in that the connection between the CNS, and the viscus consists of a succession of at least two neurons rather than a single motor neuron (see Fig. 3-2). The cell body of the first neuron is in the brain stem or the spinal cord; its axon terminates on a neuron in an autonomic ganglion, and the axon of the latter neuron ends either on effector cells or on a third neuron. The first and second neurons are called **preganglionic** and **postganglionic** neurons, respectively. The third neuron, when present, is part of the plexuses within the wall of the alimentary canal. In 1898, J.N. Langley assigned the term **autonomic nervous system** to the visceral efferents. He later (1921) subdivided the autonomic system into the **parasympathetic**, **sympathetic**, and **enteric** divisions, and this classification is still in use.

Visceral Efferent or Autonomic System

The SMCs, secretory cells of viscera, and also cardiac muscle come under the dual influence of the sympathetic and parasympathetic divisions of the autonomic nervous system. In some organs, these are functionally antagonistic, and a delicate balance between the two systems maintains a more or less constant level of visceral activity. Autonomic innervation extends beyond the organs in the major body cavities to include the muscles of the iris and ciliary body in the eye, smooth muscles in the orbit, the lacrimal and salivary glands, sweat glands and arrector pili muscles of the skin, and blood vessels everywhere. In addition, the alimentary canal contains its own intrinsic nerve supply, the enteric nervous system, which is able to control at least the simpler forms of gastrointestinal (GI) motility.

AUTONOMIC GANGLIA

An autonomic ganglion receives thin, myelinated (group B) afferent fibers from the brain stem or spinal cord. Its efferent fibers, which supply visceral structures, are the axons of the principal cells of the ganglion. They are unmyelinated (group C) and are more numerous than the preganglionic fibers. Thus, the synapses in the ganglion provide for divergence in the efferent pathway so that relatively small numbers of neurons in the CNS control large numbers of smooth muscle and gland cells in the periphery. The divergence is enhanced by preterminal branching of the postganglionic fibers and, in the alimentary canal, by further synapses with the neurons of the enteric nervous system.

Divergence cannot be the sole reason for the existence of autonomic ganglia; the same effect could be more simply achieved by further branching of axons. Evidence for integration and comparison of neural inputs is seen in the synaptic organization of the ganglion (Fig. 24-1). Each principal cell is inhibited at the dendrodendritic synapses with nearby principal cells and from the small intrinsic neurons of the ganglion. These interneurons, whose only cytoplasmic processes are short dendrites, are ex-

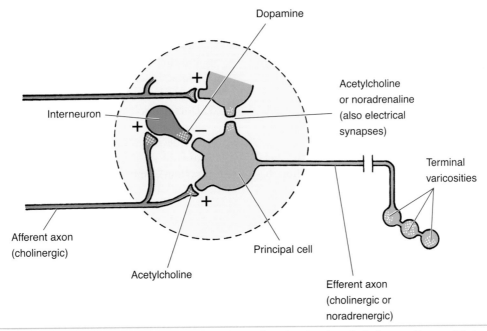

FIGURE 24-1 Synaptic organization of an autonomic ganglion, showing the principal transmitters and their excitatory (**1**) or inhibitory (**2**) actions.

cited by branches of the preganglionic axons. In at least some autonomic ganglia, sensory fibers that are passing through give off branches that synapse with the principal cells. This arrangement may provide for reflexes that do not involve the CNS.

NEUROTRANSMITTERS

The preganglionic neurons are invariably cholinergic. The principal cells are all cholinergic in parasympathetic ganglia, but only a small proportion of them are cholinergic in sympathetic ganglia. Most of the principal cells of sympathetic ganglia are noradrenergic at their peripheral synapses. The intrinsic neurons of the ganglia contain dopamine, which they are believed to use as a transmitter. All the neurons in autonomic ganglia also contain two or more peptides, which may serve as additional neurotransmitters or as neuromodulators. Several clinically valuable drugs selectively enhance or inhibit both the synthesis and the metabolism of acetylcholine, dopamine, and noradrenaline. Other drugs imitate or block the actions of these transmitters at postsynaptic sites. Information about synaptic connections in autonomic gan-

glia is therefore valuable in understanding some of the physiological effects of these drugs.

PARASYMPATHETIC DIVISION

The actions of the parasympathetic system include a decrease in the rate and force of the heart beat, augmentation of the activity of the digestive system (promoting propulsion and secretion), emptying of the urinary bladder, and tumescence of the genital erectile tissue. As previously stated, acetylcholine is the chemical mediator at the synapses between preganglionic and postganglionic neurons and at the contacts between postganglionic terminals and effector cells, with various peptides also being released. The parasympathetic system is therefore **cholinergic**. It acts in localized and discrete regions rather than causing effects throughout the body. The discrete nature of the response is a result of the fact that there is less divergence than there is in the sympathetic system. Acetylcholine is rapidly inactivated by acetylcholinesterase; each parasympathetic discharge is, consequently, of short duration.

Preganglionic parasympathetic neurons, which have long axons, are located in the brain stem and in the middle three sacral segments (S2–S4) of the spinal cord (Fig. 24-2). The preganglionic parasympathetic nuclei and the sites of the corresponding postganglionic neurons are as follows:

1. **Edinger-Westphal nucleus** of the oculomotor complex and the **ciliary ganglion** behind the eyeball
2. **Superior salivatory nucleus** of the facial nerve and **submandibular ganglion** beneath the floor of the mouth
3. **Lacrimal nucleus** of the facial nerve and **pterygopalatine ganglion** beneath the base of the skull
4. **Inferior salivatory nucleus** of the glossopharyngeal nerve and **otic ganglion** beneath the base of the skull
5. **Dorsal nucleus of the vagus nerve** and ganglia in the pulmonary plexus, cells in the myenteric and submucosal plexuses of the GI tract (the enteric nervous system), and postganglionic neurons at other sites

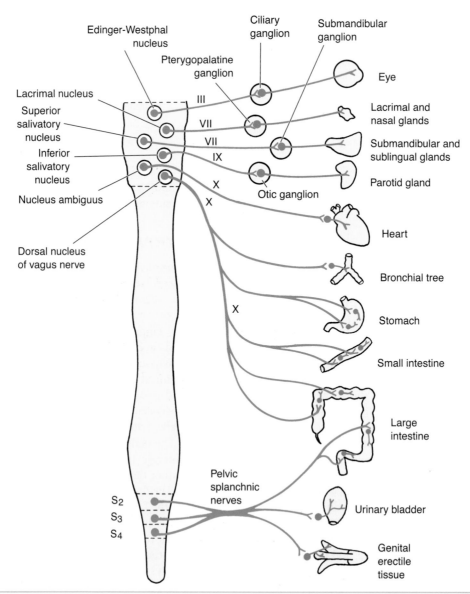

FIGURE 24-2 Plan of the parasympathetic nervous system. Preganglionic neurons are red, and postganglionic neurons are blue.

6. **Nucleus ambiguus** and **cardiac ganglia**. The cardiac parasympathetic ganglia are most numerous in the atria, around the entering great veins. Ganglionated plexuses are formed by numerous slender nerves that interconnect the ganglia.

7. **Sacral parasympathetic nucleus** and postganglionic neurons in and near the pelvic viscera.

The locations of the cranial nerve nuclei are described and illustrated in Chapters 7 and 8, and the sacral parasympathetic nucleus is described in Chapter 5.

SYMPATHETIC DIVISION

Paravertebral ganglia are associated with all the spinal nerves, although at the cervical levels, eight segments share three ganglia. The sympathetic outflow originates in the **inter-** **mediolateral cell column** (lateral horn) of all thoracic spinal segments and the upper two or three lumbar segments (Figs. 24-3 and 24-4). The axons of preganglionic neurons reach the **sympathetic trunk** by way of the corresponding ventral roots and **white communicating rami** (see Fig. 24-3). With respect to the sympathetic supply of structures in the head and thorax, the preganglionic fibers terminate in the ganglia of the sympathetic trunk. For smooth muscles and glands in the head, the synapses between preganglionic and postganglionic neurons are mainly located in the superior cervical ganglion of the sympathetic trunk, and the postganglionic axons are located in the **carotid plexus**, which accompanies the carotid artery and its branches. In the case of thoracic viscera, the synapses are located in the three cervical sympathetic ganglia (superior, middle, and inferior) and the upper five ganglia of the thoracic portion of the sympathetic trunk.

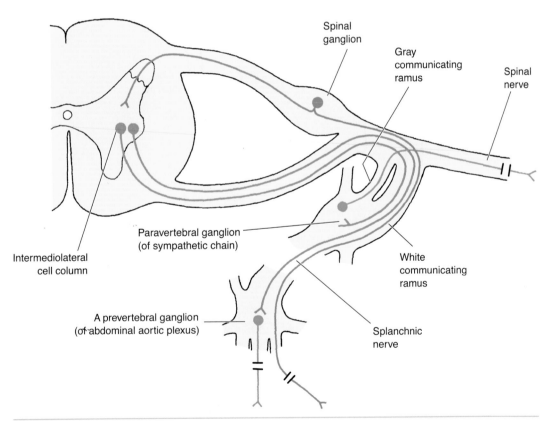

FIGURE 24-3 Visceral efferent and afferent neurons associated with a thoracic segment of the spinal cord. Preganglionic neurons are red, and postganglionic neurons are green. A sensory (pain) neuron supplying an internal organ of the abdomen is shown in blue. Visceral sensory axons pass through autonomic ganglia, but their cell bodies are located in dorsal root ganglia.

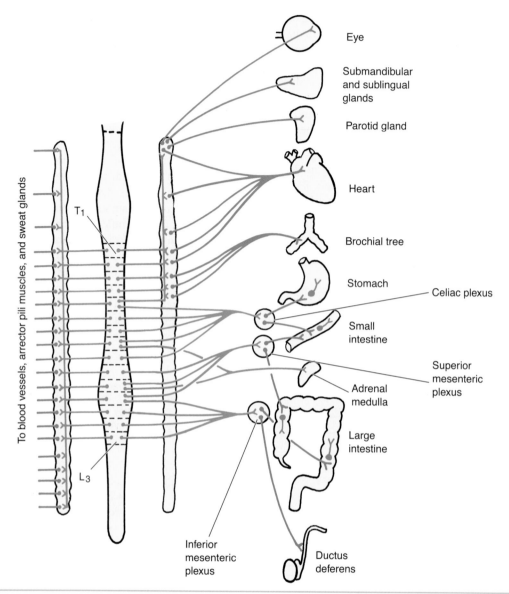

FIGURE 24-4   Plan of the sympathetic nervous system. Preganglionic neurons are red, postganglionic neurons are blue, and enteric neurons are green.

Preganglionic fibers for abdominal and pelvic viscera proceed without interruption through the sympathetic trunk and into the **splanchnic nerves**. The axons terminate on postganglionic neurons located in **preaortic ganglia** (also known as *collateral ganglia*), which are situated in the plexuses that surround the main branches of the abdominal aorta. The largest are the **celiac plexus** and the superior and inferior **mesenteric plexuses**. The sympathetic supply to the **adrenal medulla** is

exceptional. The secretory cells of the medulla, which are derived from the neural crest, are postganglionic sympathetic neurons that lack axons or dendrites. The adrenal medulla is, consequently, supplied directly by preganglionic sympathetic neurons. The alimentary canal is chiefly supplied by the ganglia in the celiac and mesenteric plexuses; the postganglionic fibers do not terminate directly on SMCs and gland cells but on neurons of the enteric nervous system.

For the body wall and the limbs, preganglionic fibers terminate in all ganglia of the sympathetic trunk, from which postganglionic fibers are distributed by way of **gray communicating rami** (see Fig. 24-3) and spinal nerves to blood vessels, arrector pili muscles, and sweat glands. Gray communicating rami are gray because the postganglionic axons are unmyelinated (group C) fibers; white rami contain thin (group B) myelinated axons.

The sympathetic system stimulates activities that are accompanied by an expenditure of energy. These include acceleration of the heart and increase in force of the heartbeat, increase in arterial pressure, and direction of blood flow to skeletal muscles at the expense of visceral and cutaneous circulation. Sympathetic responses are most dramatically expressed during stress and emergency situations (the fight-or-flight reaction). The neurotransmitter substance between preganglionic and postganglionic neurons is acetylcholine, as in the parasympathetic system. In the case of the sympathetic system, **noradrenaline** (also known as **norepinephrine**) is the transmitter released by most postganglionic axons. The sympathetic system is therefore said to be **noradrenergic**. The sympathetic supply to sweat glands is cholinergic, constituting an exception to the general rule. Cutaneous areas lack parasympathetic fibers; the cholinergic sudomotor neurons are anatomically sympathetic but are functionally similar to those of parasympathetic ganglia.

Noradrenaline has different actions in different tissues, according to the type of receptor molecule on the responding cells. **Alpha receptors** occur on the surfaces of smooth muscle cells in the dilator pupillae muscle and in the blood vessels of the skin and internal organs. These cells contract when noradrenaline is bound by their alpha receptors, with consequent pupillary dilatation and cutaneous and visceral vasoconstriction. The enteric neurons that cause closure of sphincters also bear alpha receptors. The **beta receptors** occur on cardiac muscle cells in the atrial pacemaker tissue and in the ventricles, on smooth muscle cells in the bronchioles, in blood vessels of skeletal muscle, and on enteric neurons that inhibit propulsive movements of the alimentary tract. SMCs with beta receptors relax in response to noradrenaline so dilatation of the bronchioles and vasodilation in skeletal muscles

take place. The rate and force of contraction of the heart are increased, and propulsion along the gut is inhibited. Several clinically important drugs act by stimulating or blocking the alpha or beta receptors.

Strong sympathetic stimulation produces diffuse effects because of the following factors, which are the converse of those present in the parasympathetic system. Each sympathetic preganglionic neuron synapses with many postganglionic neurons, and each of the latter supplies numerous effector cells or enteric neurons. Hence, there is much divergence. Noradrenaline liberated at postganglionic terminals is deactivated by being taken up into the axonal terminals from which it was released, and this is a slower process than the enzyme-catalyzed hydrolysis of acetylcholine.

ENTERIC NERVOUS SYSTEM

From the esophagus to the rectum, the walls of the human alimentary canal contain some 10^8 neurons, a population comparable to the number of neurons in the spinal cord. The cell bodies occur in two zones. The **myenteric plexus** (Auerbach's plexus) lies between the longitudinal and circular muscle layers, and the **submucosal plexus** (of Meissner) lies in the connective tissue between the circular muscle layer and the muscularis mucosae. Each plexus consists of small enteric ganglia, joined to one another by thin nerves in which all the axons are unmyelinated. Similar nerves connect the two plexuses across the circular muscle layer and carry branches from the plexuses into the smooth muscle layers and the lamina propria of the mucosa. Most of the neurons are multipolar, but there are also many bipolar and unipolar ones, especially in the submucous plexus. In addition to neurons, the enteric nervous system contains neuroglial cells, which ensheath the neurons and their processes. The nervous tissue is avascular and receives its nutrients by diffusion from capillary vessels outside the glial sheath.

The synaptic organization of the enteric nervous system (Fig. 24-5) is not simple. Several types of neuron are found in the plexuses. The bipolar and unipolar cells are presumed to have sensory functions, especially in initiating the peristaltic reflex. Neurons of two types have

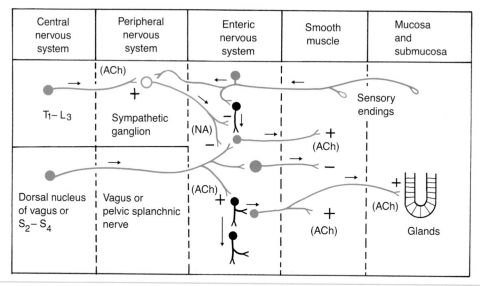

FIGURE 24-5   Organization of the enteric nervous system. For simplification, the myenteric and submucosal plexuses have been combined. The sites of some known transmitters are shown, as are sites of excitation (+) and inhibition (−). The inhibitory transmitter to smooth muscle may be adenosine triphosphate or nitric oxide or both of these compounds. Arrows indicate directions of axonal conduction. Cholinergic neurons are red, the noradrenergic neuron is green, the sensory enteric neuron is blue, the neuron inhibitory to smooth muscle is magenta, and intrinsic enteric neurons (interneurons) are black. ACh, acetylcholine; NA, noradrenaline.

axons that end on smooth muscle and gland cells; the excitatory neurons are cholinergic. The nonadrenergic, noncholinergic inhibitory neurons may use a peptide, a nucleotide, or nitric oxide. Some enteric neurons send axons centripetally in the nerves that accompany the mesenteric and other abdominal arteries to the celiac and mesenteric sympathetic ganglia.

Enteric neurons have been shown to contain many different peptides with pharmacologically demonstrable actions on the gut, and it is considered probable that at least some of these substances serve as neurotransmitters.

The fibers afferent to the enteric nervous system are of two types. Cholinergic axons of preganglionic parasympathetic neurons

Hirschsprung's Disease

In about one in 5,000 infants, 80% of them male, cells of the neural crest fail to migrate into the most caudal part of the large intestine. Intrinsic enteric neurons are absent from the distal rectum and for a variable distance rostrally, often to the sigmoid colon. In the absence of intrinsic neurons, there is no peristalsis, and the circular smooth muscle is tonically contracted, creating a functional obstruction to the movement of feces. The proximal parts of the colon, which have normal innervation, become greatly distended, giving the condition its alternative name of **congenital megacolon**. Preganglionic cholinergic nerve fibers are present in abnormally high numbers in

the rectum. The presence of these fibers in biopsies of the rectal mucosa confirms the diagnosis of Hirschsprung's disease. The condition is treated by surgical removal of the aganglionic segment.

Acquired megacolon in adults can have a variety of causes—disease such as diabetes mellitus, scleroderma, or amyloidosis that can interfere with smooth muscle and its innervation. **Chagas' disease** (South American trypanosomiasis) is a parasitic infection in which enteric neurons are destroyed by an autoimmune mechanism. This occasionally results in megacolon, but more frequently, the aganglionic region is above the junction of the esophagus with the stomach, and the esophagus becomes greatly distended.

terminate on the dendrites and cell bodies of interneurons and of neurons that supply smooth muscle and secretory cells and glands. The noradrenergic axons of sympathetic neurons terminate in axoaxonal synapses on both parasympathetic and intrinsic fibers. They are believed to mediate presynaptic inhibition of the cholinergic neurons that stimulate contraction of the musculature and glandular secretion.

Central Control of the Autonomic Nervous System

The hypothalamus has a diverse afferent input, and its efferent connections include projections to neurons that constitute the autonomic outflow. It is therefore an important controlling and integrating center for the autonomic system.

Through afferent connections described in Chapter 11, the hypothalamus is influenced by the neocortex, hippocampal formation, amygdala and septal area, and olfactory areas. Ascending pathways from the spinal cord and brain stem convey information of visceral and gustatory origin. In addition, hypothalamic neurons respond directly to changes in the temperature, osmolarity, and concentrations of various substances (including hormones) in the circulating blood. Depending on specific sensitivities, these neurons are related either to the autonomic system or to the pituitary gland.

Signals that originate in the hypothalamus reach autonomic nuclei in the brain stem and spinal cord directly and through relays in the reticular formation. Direct projections from the amygdala and septal area to preganglionic autonomic neurons have also been described. The autonomic neurons are also influenced by visceral "centers" and by visceral afferent nuclei, notably the solitary nucleus, in the medulla. The autonomic outflow therefore comes under a wide range of influences: visceral (including taste and smell), emotional (both basic drives and moods), and even mental processes at the neocortical level. Cortical areas that are functionally active at the same time as the sympathetic nervous system include the medial

prefrontal cortex and the anterior parts of the insula and cingulate gyrus.

CENTRAL SYMPATHETIC PATHWAY FOR THE EYE AND FACE

Central pathways that control the sympathetic innervation of the head can be interrupted by lesions in the brain stem. Horner's syndrome (see Chapter 7) and loss of thermoregulatory sweating of facial skin can occur after the development of ipsilateral lesions in the medulla, dorsal to the inferior olivary nucleus. The sympathetic dysfunction is part of Wallenberg's syndrome, and the position of the lesion (see Fig. 7-17) indicates that nuclei or descending fibers essential for pupillary dilation and facial vasomotor control descend through the lateral part of the medullary reticular formation. Lateral medullary lesions prevent thermally induced but not emotionally induced facial sweating, indicating the existence of more than one descending pathway to the preganglionic sympathetic neurons. In the human spinal cord, descending fibers that originate in or pass through the lateral medulla are deeply located in the lateral funiculus of the spinal white matter just lateral to the ventral horn.

Visceral Afferents

The unipolar cell bodies of general visceral afferent neurons are situated in the inferior ganglia of the glossopharyngeal and vagus nerves and in the ganglia of spinal nerves. The peripheral processes of visceral afferent neurons traverse autonomic ganglia and plexuses without interruption to reach the organs they supply. These neurons are functionally of two kinds: physiological afferents and afferents for pain. Most physiological afferents accompany fibers of the parasympathetic division of the autonomic nervous system. The afferents for pain accompany the fibers of the sympathetic division (see Fig. 24-3).

PHYSIOLOGICAL AFFERENTS

Visceral afferents of special physiological importance are associated with the parasympathetic division of the autonomic system. The following examples illustrate the reflex arcs of which they form the afferent limbs.

Cardiovascular System

Terminals of sensory fibers in the aortic arch and carotid sinus (at the bifurcation of the common carotid artery) serve as **baroreceptors**, signaling changes in arterial blood pressure (BP). Whereas the cell bodies of neurons supplying the aortic arch are located in the inferior (nodose) ganglion of the vagus nerve, those for the carotid sinus are in the inferior ganglion of the glossopharyngeal nerve. The central processes terminate in the solitary nucleus in the medulla, from which fibers pass to regions of the reticular formation commonly called **cardiovascular "centers."** Axons from the solitary nucleus and the reticular formation project to the nucleus ambiguus and intermediolateral cell column of the spinal cord. Through the reflex pathways thereby established, a rapid increase in arterial pressure causes a decrease in heart rate (vagus nerve) and vasodilation through inhibition of the vasoconstrictor action of the sympathetic outflow. A decrease in arterial pressure, such as occurs after hemorrhage, initiates reflex responses that are the reverse of those caused by an increase in arterial pressure. Visceral afferents in the glossopharyngeal and vagus nerves therefore participate in the maintenance of normal arterial BP.

The cardiac output is also regulated by the **Bainbridge reflex**, which is triggered by vagally innervated receptors in the right atrium; these monitor the central venous pressure. The central connections provide for stimulation of the sympathetic nervous system and inhibition of the vagal slowing of the heart. Thus, the cardiac output is increased as the volume of the venous return increases.

Respiratory System

Three **respiratory "centers"** are present in the brain stem for automatic control of respiratory movements. Two such regions are situated in the reticular formation of the medulla: an **inspiratory center** medially and an **expiratory center** laterally. In addition, a **pneumotaxic center** in the parabrachial area, at the level of the pontine isthmus, regulates the rhythmicity of inspiration and expiration. The inspiratory

and expiratory "centers," as well as those for the cardiovascular system, are probably fields within the network of long dendrites in the reticular formation rather than compact collections of cell bodies. Inspiration is initiated by stimulation of neurons in the inspiratory center by carbon dioxide of the circulating blood. The chemosensory neurons, by means of reticulospinal connections, stimulate the motor neurons that supply the diaphragm and intercostal muscles.

Respiratory movements are also influenced by signals conducted centrally from the carotid bodies situated near the bifurcation of each common carotid artery and from small aortic bodies adjacent to the aortic arch. These bodies serve as **chemoreceptors** that respond to decreased oxygen concentration in the blood. The resulting signals are sent to the solitary nucleus through neurons with cell bodies in the inferior ganglia of the glossopharyngeal and vagus nerves. Further connections with respiratory "centers" in the brain stem bring about increased rate and depth of respiratory movements. This reflex operates in vigorous exercise, when a person is exposed to a lowered oxygen tension (as at high altitudes), or in any circumstances that produce asphyxia.

Sensory neurons in the vagus nerve constitute the afferent limb of the **Hering-Breuer reflex**, through which expiration is initiated. Sensory endings in the bronchial tree, especially the smaller branches, discharge at an increasing rate as the lungs are inflated. These signals reach the expiratory center through a relay in the solitary nucleus. Neurons in the expiratory center then inhibit those of the inspiratory center. Expiration ensues as a passive (elastic) process when the inspiratory muscles relax.

Other Systems

Sensory axons in the vagus nerve are distributed to the GI tract at least as far as the junction of the transverse and descending parts of the colon (the splenic flexure). The nerve terminals are stimulated by distention of the stomach and intestine, contraction of the smooth musculature, and irritation of the mucosa. Although motility and secretion are not dependent on the extrinsic nerves, they are modified by reflex action involving vagal afferent and efferent neurons. The distal colon, rectum, and urinary bladder are supplied by splanchnic branches of the second, third, and fourth sacral nerves. Reflexes in these segments of the spinal cord and the sacral component of the parasympathetic system stimulate emptying of the large bowel and urinary bladder, subject to voluntary control.

ASCENDING PATHWAYS FOR FULLNESS

Some ascending visceral pathways are distinct from those for pain (described in the next section). One such pathway originates in the solitary nucleus in the medulla, which receives general visceral afferents from the vagus nerve predominantly. A second pathway originates in segments T1 to L2 and S2 to S4 of the spinal cord. These ascending fibers are included in the spinoreticular and spinothalamic tracts. Through the pathways from the medulla and spinal cord, signals of visceral origin reach the reticular formation of the brain stem, hypothalamus, and the lateral division of the ventral posterior nucleus (VPl) of the thalamus. A thalamocortical projection provides for a conscious feeling of fullness when the stomach is distended and a feeling of hunger when the stomach is empty. Feelings of fullness in the distal colon and urinary bladder are also mediated by these spinoreticular and spinothalamic connections.

CLINICAL NOTE

Pain From Internal Organs

The **heart** is supplied with pain fibers by the middle and inferior cervical cardiac nerves and by the thoracic cardiac branches of the left sympathetic trunk. Central processes of the primary sensory neurons enter segments T1 to T5. Pain of cardiac origin is therefore referred to the center of the chest and the inner aspect of the left arm. Deviations from this zone of reference are common and are probably attributable to variations in the laterality and segmental levels of the cardiac innervation.

Pain from the **gallbladder** or **bile ducts** passes centrally in the right greater splanchnic nerve, entering the spinal cord through dorsal roots T7 and T8. The pain is referred to the upper quadrant of the abdomen and the infrascapular region on the right side. Disease of the liver or gallbladder may irritate the peritoneum covering the **diaphragm**. The resulting pain is referred to the top of the shoulder because the diaphragm is supplied with sensory (as well as motor) fibers by the phrenic nerve, which originates from segments C3, C4, and C5.

Pain of gastric origin is felt in the epigastrium because the **stomach** is supplied with pain afferents that reach segments T7 and T8 by way of the left and right greater splanchnic nerves. Pain from the **duodenum**, as in duodenal ulcer, is referred to the anterior abdominal wall just above the umbilicus, with both this area and the duodenum being supplied by nerves T9 and T10. Afferent fibers from the **appendix** are included in the lesser splanchnic nerve, which contains axons from the T10 dorsal root ganglion. The pain of appendicitis is initially referred to the region of the umbilicus, which lies in the T10 dermatome. The pain shifts to the lower right quadrant of the abdomen when the parietal peritoneum becomes involved in the inflammatory process. (The parietal peritoneum and pleura are supplied by segmental somatic nerves in a distribution similar to that of the skin of the trunk.) Pain fibers from the **renal pelvis** and **ureter** are included in the least splanchnic nerve; they enter segments L1 and L2 of the spinal cord, and the pain is referred to the loin and the groin.

There is no entirely satisfactory explanation for the referral of pain. An early proposal was that afferent fibers for visceral and somatic pain synapse with the same tract cells in the spinal cord, with these cells being excited by subliminal somatic stimuli when receiving impulses of visceral origin. A more recent hypothesis is that both visceral and somatic pain from regions served by a specific segment of the spinal cord are relayed to the same group of cells in the ventral posterior nucleus of the thalamus. The topographic representation of the body in the thalamus and cerebral cortex allows recognition of the sources of ordinary somatic sensations. Localization may be in error when pain originates internally, perhaps because pain of somatic origin is a more common experience than pain caused by visceral malfunction or disease. It is of interest that more than 230 years ago, John Hunter called referred pain a "delusion of the mind."

PAIN AFFERENTS

The sensory endings for pain arising in internal organs are stimulated in various ways in the presence of abnormal function or disease. The pain is most commonly caused by distention of a hollow viscus such as the intestine. This may occur proximal to localized and forcible contraction of the smooth muscle. Similarly, distention of a bile duct or a ureter occurs when the lumen is obstructed by a stone. Visceral pain also results from rapid stretching of the capsule of a solid organ, such as the liver or spleen. Peritoneal or pleural irritation contributes to the pain of inflammatory disease. In the case of angina and the pain of myocardial infarction, the effective stimulus is anoxia of cardiac muscle.

The sensory neurons for pain arising in thoracic and abdominal organs are associated only with the sympathetic nervous system. The cell bodies of the primary sensory neurons are located in the dorsal root ganglia of the thoracic and upper lumbar nerves (see Fig. 24-4). The peripheral processes of these neurons reach the sympathetic trunk by way of white communicating rami (see Fig. 24-3); they run in the sympathetic trunk for variable distances and then continue to the viscera by way of the cardiac, pulmonary, and splanchnic nerves. The corresponding dorsal root fibers probably enter the dorsolateral tract of Lissauer along with somatic pain fibers and end similarly in the dorsal horn of the spinal cord. The ascending pathway for visceral pain corresponds, in part, with the pathway for somatic pain (see Chapter 19), through crossed fibers in the spinothalamic tract. There are also bilateral spinoreticular fibers and relays in the reticular formation, as in the pathway for pain from somatic structures.

REFERRED PAIN

Visceral pain has characteristics that distinguish it from pain arising in somatic structures, notably diffuse localization and radiation to somatic areas (i.e., referred pain). The zone of reference of the pain from an internal organ coincides with the part of the body served by somatic sensory neurons associated with the same segments of the spinal cord. The principle of referred pain is illustrated by the examples in the Clinical Note on page 363. The reader should compare the areas of reference with the distribution of segmental innervation of the skin (see Fig. 5-13).

Suggested Reading

Armour JA, Murphy DA, Yuan BX, et al. Gross and microscopic anatomy of the human intrinsic cardiac nervous system. *Anat Rec* 1997;247:289–298.

Brading A. *The Autonomic Nervous System and its Effectors.* Oxford: Blackwell, 1999.

Bruce EN, Cherniak NS. Central chemoreceptors. *J Appl Physiol* 1987;62:389–402.

Critchley HD, Elliott R, Mathias CJ, et al. Neural activity relating to generation and representation of galvanic skin conductance responses: a functional magnetic resonance imaging study. *J Neurosci* 2000;20:3033–3040.

Critchley HD, Mathias CJ, Josephs O, et al. Human cingulate cortex and autonomic control: converging neuroimaging and clinical evidence. *Brain* 2003;126:2139–2152.

Elfvin L-G, Lindh B, Hokfelt T. The chemical neuroanatomy of sympathetic ganglia. *Annu Rev Neurosci* 1993;16:471–507.

Gai WP, Blessing WW. Human brainstem preganglionic parasympathetic neurons localized by markers for nitric oxide synthesis. *Brain* 1996;119:1145–1152.

Grundy D. *Gastrointestinal Motility.* Lancaster & Boston: MTP Press, 1985.

Hainsworth R. Reflexes from the heart. *Physiol Rev* 1991; 71:617–658.

Karczmar AG, Koketsu K, Nishi S, eds. *Autonomic and Enteric Ganglia.* New York: Plenum Press, 1986.

Kincaid JC. The autonomic nervous system. In: Rhoades RA, Tanner GA, eds. *Medical Physiology*, 2nd ed. Philadelphia: Lippincott, Williams & Wilkins, 2003:108–118.

Nathan PW, Smith MC. The location of descending fibres to sympathetic neurons supplying the eye and sudomotor neurons supplying the head and neck. *J Neurol Neurosurg Psychiatry* 1986;49:187–194.

Parker TL, Kesse WK, Mohamed AA, et al. The innervation of the mammalian adrenal gland. *J Anat* 1993;183:265–276.

Pauza D, Skripka V, Pauziene N, et al. Morphology, distribution and variability of the epicardiac neural ganglionated subplexuses in the human heart. *Anat Rec* 2000; 259:353–382.

Rowell LB. *Human Cardiovascular Control.* New York: Oxford University Press, 1993.

Sanders KM, Ward SM. Nitric oxide as a mediator of nonadrenergic noncholinergic neurotransmission. *Am J Physiol* 1992;262:G379–G392.

Smith OA, DeVito JL. Central neural integration for the control of autonomic responses associated with emotion. *Annu Rev Neurosci* 1984;7:43–65.

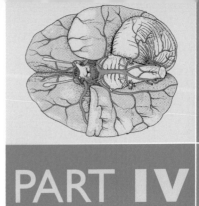

PART IV

Blood Supply
and the Meninges

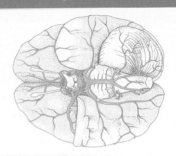

Chapter 25

BLOOD SUPPLY OF THE CENTRAL NERVOUS SYSTEM

Important Facts

- Blood flow through arteries in the central nervous system is kept constant by a process known as *autoregulation*.

- Exchange through the capillaries of the central nervous system is regulated by endothelial transport mechanisms. These vessels are impermeable to large molecules, except in a few small regions that have no blood–brain barrier.

- The anterior choroidal artery supplies the optic tract and parts of the internal capsule.

- The anterior cerebral artery gives rise to the recurrent artery of Heubner, which supplies parts of the corpus striatum and internal capsule and to the anterior communicating artery. It then continues and supplies the medial and superior surfaces of the frontal and parietal lobes.

- The middle cerebral artery supplies the lateral surface of the frontal, parietal, and temporal lobes, including the motor and somesthetic areas for the face, trunk, upper limbs, and (on the left side) the language areas. The geniculocalcarine tract is also supplied by this vessel.

- The spinal cord is supplied by branches of the vertebral and radicular arteries.

- The largest branch of the vertebral artery is the posterior inferior cerebellar artery, which supplies the lateral part of the medulla and much of the cerebellum.

- The anterior inferior and the superior cerebellar arteries are branches of the basilar artery, which also has smaller branches that supply the pons and the labyrinth of the inner ear.

- The posterior cerebral artery gives rise to the posterior choroidal artery, connects with the posterior communicating artery, and then supplies the occipital lobe, the inferior surface of the temporal lobe, and parts of the hippocampal formation.

- Internal structures of the cerebral hemisphere and diencephalon are supplied by central arteries, which are proximal branches of the three cerebral arteries.

- Aneurysms at sites of arterial bifurcation in and near the circle of Willis are common sources of subarachnoid hemorrhage.

- Superior cerebral veins drain into the superior sagittal sinus. Blood from the inferior surfaces of the cortex and from the interior of the brain is eventually collected by the great cerebral vein, which empties into the straight sinus.

The blood supply of the central nervous system (CNS) is of special interest because of the metabolic demands of nervous tissue. The brain depends on aerobic metabolism of glucose and is one of the most metabolically active organs of the body. Although composing only 2% of body weight, the brain receives about 17% of the cardiac output and consumes about 20% of the oxygen used by the entire body. Unconsciousness occurs after cessation of cerebral circulation in about 10 seconds. Lesions of vascular origin are responsible for more neurological disorders than any other category of disease process.

Arterial Supply of the Brain

The brain is supplied by the paired internal carotid and vertebral arteries through an extensive system of branches. Descriptions of the arteries follow, with some notes on their clinical significance. Later in this chapter, summaries are provided of cortical areas and deeper parts of the brain, indicating the arteries by which they are supplied.

INTERNAL CAROTID SYSTEM

The **internal carotid artery**, a terminal branch of the common carotid artery, traverses the carotid canal in the base of the skull and enters

Cerebrovascular Disease

Arterial occlusion by an embolus or a thrombus is usually followed by infarction of a portion of the region supplied. Anastomotic channels are present between branches of the major arteries on the surface of the brain. There are also communications at the arteriolar level, and the capillary bed is continuous throughout the brain. These anastomoses, however, are usually insufficient to sustain the circulation in the region normally supplied by a major artery. The size of an infarction depends on the caliber of the occluded artery, existing anastomoses, and the time elapsing before complete obstruction. In addition to intracranial occlusions, impairment of the cerebral circulation is often caused by stenosis of a carotid or vertebral artery in the neck.

The slender, thin-walled arteries that penetrate the ventral surface of the brain to supply the internal capsule and adjacent gray masses are especially prone to rupture. Hypertension and degenerative changes in these arteries are major factors that lead to **cerebral hemorrhage**. An **aneurysm** usually occurs at the site of branching of one of the larger arteries at the base of the brain. An aneurysm may leak or rupture, and there is bleeding into the subarachnoid space. In some cases, adhesion of the aneurysmal sac to adjacent structures can give rise to hemorrhage that is intracerebral or into a cranial nerve.

the middle cranial fossa beside the dorsum sellae of the sphenoid bone. Beyond this point, the artery undergoes the following sequence of bends that constitute the **carotid siphon** in a cerebral angiogram (Fig. 25-1). The internal carotid artery first runs forward in the cavernous venous sinus and then turns upward on the medial side of the anterior clinoid process. At this point, the artery enters the subarachnoid space by piercing the dura mater and arachnoid, courses backward below the optic nerve, and finally turns upward immediately lateral to the optic chiasma. This brings the artery under the anterior perforated substance, where it divides into the middle and anterior cerebral arteries (Fig. 25-2).

Collateral Branches

The following branches arise from the internal carotid artery before its terminal bifurcation.

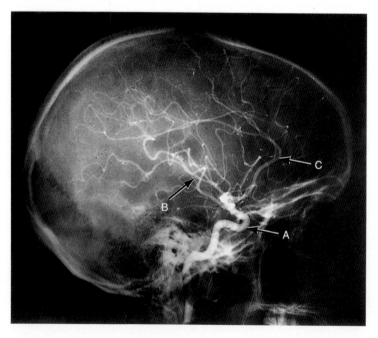

FIGURE 25-1 Carotid angiogram (lateral view). A, carotid siphon; B, branches of the middle cerebral artery; C, anterior cerebral artery. (Courtesy of Dr. J. M. Allcock.)

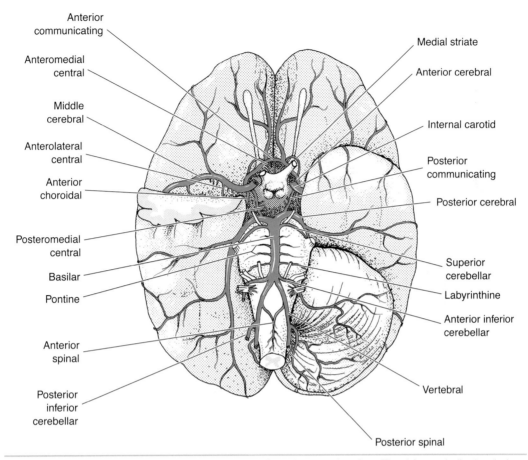

FIGURE 25-2   Arteries that supply the brain, as seen from the ventral surface. The right cerebellar hemisphere and the tip of the right temporal lobe have been removed.

Hypophysial Arteries

The posterior hypophysial arteries supply the neural (posterior) lobe of the pituitary gland, and the anterior hypophysial arteries enter the median eminence of the hypothalamus. The latter blood vessels break up into capillary loops, into which hypothalamic releasing factors gain access, and the capillary loops drain through small **hypophysial portal veins** into the capillaries of the anterior lobe. This constitutes the system through which the hypothalamus controls the output of anterior pituitary hormones (see also Chapter 11).

Ophthalmic Artery

This branch comes off immediately after the internal carotid artery enters the subarachnoid space. The ophthalmic artery passes through the optic foramen into the orbit, supplying the eye and other orbital contents, frontal area of the scalp, frontal and ethmoid paranasal sinuses, and parts of the nose.

Posterior Communicating Artery

This slender artery arises from the internal carotid artery close to its terminal bifurcation and runs backward to join the proximal part of the posterior cerebral artery, thereby forming part of the arterial circle (circle of Willis). Some of the posteromedial central arteries, described later, are branches of the posterior communicating artery.

Anterior Choroidal Artery

This branch has a wider distribution than its name suggests. The artery passes back along the optic tract and the choroid fissure at the medial edge of the temporal lobe. The anterior choroidal artery sends branches to the optic

Internal Carotid Occlusion

Occlusion of the internal carotid artery has serious consequences. Blindness of the ipsilateral eye (supplied by the ophthalmic artery) and the contralateral half of the visual field of the other eye (from infarction of the optic tract and lateral geniculate body, supplied by the anterior choroidal artery) are added to the effects of occlusion of the middle and anterior cerebral arteries (principally a contralateral hemiplegia and hemianopsia, with global apha-sia if the affected hemisphere is the dominant one for language).

Occlusion of the **anterior choroidal artery** alone can be asymptomatic, or it may have a variety of effects, depending on the site of the obstruction and the efficiency of the anastomoses with the posterior choroidal artery. Symptoms can include contralateral hemiplegia and sensory abnormalities (internal capsule) and contralateral homonymous hemianopia (optic tract and lateral geniculate body).

tract, uncus, amygdala, hippocampus, globus pallidus, lateral geniculate body, and ventral part of the internal capsule. Branching is variable, and this artery sometimes supplies the subthalamus, ventral parts of the thalamus, and the rostral part of the midbrain. The terminal branches of the anterior choroidal artery supply the choroid plexus in the temporal horn of the lateral ventricle and anastomose there with branches of the posterior choroidal artery.

Middle Cerebral Artery

Of the terminal branches of the internal carotid artery, the middle cerebral artery is the larger and more direct continuation of the parent vessel (see Fig. 25-2). This artery runs deep in the lateral sulcus between the frontal and temporal lobes. Central arteries arise from the proximal part of the middle cerebral artery, lateral to the optic chiasma. They enter the base of the hemisphere and supply internal structures, including the internal capsule. **Frontal, parietal,** and **temporal branches** emerge from the lateral sulcus of the cerebral hemisphere (Fig. 25-3) to supply a large area of cortex and subcortical white matter in the three corresponding lobes of the cerebrum.

The territory of distribution of the middle cerebral artery includes most of the primary motor and premotor cortex, the frontal eye field, and the primary somatosensory area. The motor and sensory cortex for the lower limb and the perineum are excluded (compare Figs.

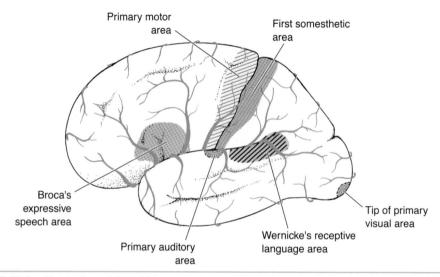

FIGURE 25-3   Distribution of the middle cerebral artery on the lateral surface of the left cerebral hemisphere. Terminal branches of the anterior and posterior cerebral arteries are also visible.

Middle Cerebral Artery Occlusion

Loss of function of the cortical areas supplied by the middle cerebral artery results in contralateral paralysis most noticeable in the lower part of the face and in the arm, together with general somatic sensory deficits of the cortical type. Involvement of the geniculocalcarine tract results in hemianopia of the contralateral visual fields of both eyes (see Chapter 20). The auditory cortex is included in the area of distribution, but a unilateral lesion causes no demonstrable impairment of hearing because of the bilateral cortical projection from the organ of Corti (see Chapter 21). Occlusion of the middle cerebral artery of the hemisphere dominant for language causes global aphasia (see Chapter 15).

Fragments of the complete syndrome, such as monoplegia or receptive aphasia, are seen when individual cortical branches of the artery are blocked. Obstruction of the central branches can cause hemiplegia attributable to infarction of motor fibers in the internal capsule. A lesion in the internal capsule does not cause aphasia because the connections of the language areas with the contralateral hemisphere are intact.

15-3 and 25-3). The left middle cerebral artery (in most people) supplies all the cortical areas concerned with language. These are the receptive language areas in the temporal and parietal lobes and Broca's expressive speech area in the inferior frontal gyrus (see Fig. 25-3 and Chapter 15). The white matter underlying the parietal cortex contains the geniculocalcarine tract.

Anterior Cerebral Artery

The smaller terminal branch of the internal carotid artery is the anterior cerebral artery, which is first directed medially above the optic nerve (see Fig. 25-2). The two anterior cerebral arteries almost meet at the midline where they are joined together by the **anterior communicating artery**. A special branch of the anterior cerebral artery is given off just proximal to the anterior communicating artery. This is the **medial striate artery** (also called *recurrent artery of Heubner*), which penetrates the anterior perforated substance to supply the ventral part of the head of the caudate nucleus, the adjacent part of the putamen, and the anterior limb and genu of the internal capsule.

The anterior cerebral artery ascends in the longitudinal fissure and bends backward around the genu of the corpus callosum (Fig. 25-4). Branches given off just distal to the anterior communicating artery supply the medial part of the orbital surface of the frontal lobe, including the olfactory bulb and olfactory tract. The artery continues along the upper surface of the corpus callosum as the **pericallosal artery**, and a large branch, the **callosomarginal artery**, follows the cingulate sulcus. The anterior cerebral artery supplies the medial surfaces of the frontal and parietal lobes and the corpus callosum. In addition, branches extend over the dorsomedial border of the hemisphere and supply a strip on the lateral surface (see Fig. 25-3). The supplementary and cingulate motor areas and the dorsal parts of the primary motor and primary somatosensory areas are included in its territory.

VERTEBROBASILAR SYSTEM

The **vertebral artery**, a branch of the subclavian artery, ascends in the foramina of the transverse processes of the upper six cervical vertebrae. On reaching the base of the skull, the artery winds around the lateral mass of the atlas, pierces the posterior atlanto-occipital membrane, and enters the subarachnoid space at the level of the foramen magnum by piercing the dura and arachnoid. The artery then runs forward with a medial inclination, giving off small branches that deeply penetrate the medial parts of the medulla. The left and right vertebral arteries join at the caudal border of the pons to form the **basilar artery**. The latter vessel runs rostrally in the midline of the pons and divides into the **posterior cerebral arteries** (see Fig. 25-2).

Branches of the Vertebral Artery

Spinal Arteries

The rostral segments of the cervical cord receive blood through spinal branches of the vertebral arteries. A single **anterior spinal artery** is formed by a contribution from each vertebral artery. A **posterior spinal artery** arises on each side as a branch

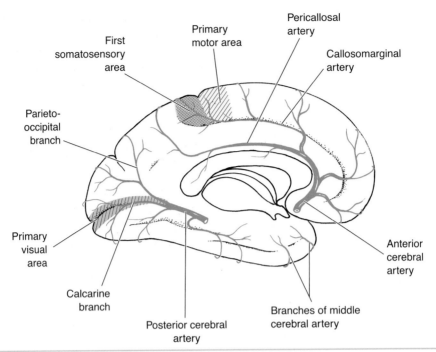

First somatosensory area
Primary motor area
Pericallosal artery
Callosomarginal artery
Parieto-occipital branch
Primary visual area
Calcarine branch
Posterior cerebral artery
Branches of middle cerebral artery
Anterior cerebral artery

FIGURE 25-4 Distribution of the anterior and posterior cerebral arteries on the medial surface of the left cerebral hemisphere.

of either the vertebral or the posterior inferior cerebellar artery (see Fig. 25-2). The anterior and posterior spinal arteries continue throughout the length of the spinal cord. These are small vessels, however, and most of their blood comes from reinforcements by the anterior and posterior radicular arteries, which are described later.

Posterior Inferior Cerebellar Artery

The posterior inferior cerebellar artery (PICA) is the largest branch of the vertebral artery. It pursues an irregular course between the medulla and cerebellum. Branches are distributed to the posterior part of the cerebellar hemisphere, inferior vermis, central nuclei of the cerebellum, and choroid plexus of the fourth ventricle. There are also important **medullary branches** to the dorsolateral region of the medulla.

Branches of the Basilar Artery

The basilar artery gives off the following branches before dividing into the posterior cerebral arteries at the rostral border of the pons.

Anterior Cerebral Artery Occlusion

Occlusion of the anterior cerebral artery causes paralysis and sensory deficits in the contralateral leg and perineum. Commonly, affected patients have urinary incontinence caused by inadequate perineal sensation and defective cortical control of the pelvic floor musculature. If the obstruction is in the proximal part of the vessel, blocking the medial striate artery, patients also have contralateral upper motor neuron weakness of the face, tongue, and upper limb because of corticofugal motor fibers that are in or near the genu of the internal capsule before they pass into its posterior limb (see Chapter 16). A proximal occlusion may also cause ipsilateral anosmia attributable to infarction of the olfactory bulb and tract.

Anterior cerebral artery syndromes often are associated with mental confusion and dysphasia, perhaps attributable to loss of functions of the prefrontal cortex, the cingulate gyrus, and the supplementary motor area.

Anterior Inferior Cerebellar Artery

Arising from the caudal end of the basilar artery, the anterior inferior cerebellar artery (AICA) supplies the cortex of the inferior surface of the cerebellum anteriorly and the underlying white matter; it assists in the supply of the central cerebellar nuclei. In addition, slender twigs from the artery penetrate the upper medulla and the tegmentum of the lower pons.

Labyrinthine Artery

This vessel is a branch of the basilar artery (see Fig. 25-2) or, more frequently, the AICA. The labyrinthine artery traverses the internal acoustic meatus and ramifies throughout the membranous labyrinth of the internal ear.

Pontine Arteries

These are slender branches of variable length that arise from the basilar artery along its length. The short **paramedian pontine arteries** supply the basal part of the pons, including most of the bundles of corticospinal fibers, pontine nuclei, and transverse (pontocerebellar) fibers. These paramedian vessels extend dorsally to the floor of the fourth ventricle, supplying the medial parts of the pontine tegmentum. Longer **circumferential pontine arteries** pierce and supply the lateral parts of the pons and middle cerebellar peduncle and then turn medially to supply the lateral part of the tegmentum.

Superior Cerebellar Artery

This branch arises close to the terminal bifurcation of the basilar artery, ramifies over the dorsal surface of the cerebellum, and supplies the cortex, white matter, and central nuclei. Branches from the proximal part of the superior cerebellar artery are distributed to the rostral pontine tegmentum, superior cerebellar peduncle, and inferior colliculus of the midbrain.

CLINICAL NOTE

Vascular Lesions That Affect the Brain Stem

A substantial hemorrhage within the pons is instantly fatal. Thrombosis of the whole basilar artery causes coma and decerebrate rigidity (see Chapter 23), soon followed by death attributable to failure of the central control of respiration.

An embolus that passes through a vertebral artery typically lodges at the bifurcation of the basilar artery, bilaterally occluding the superior cerebellar and the posteromedial central arteries. The latter are the first branches of the posterior cerebral arteries. Infarction in the reticular formation of the rostral pons and caudal midbrain causes coma, and the associated destruction of the fibers of both oculomotor nerves results in bilateral divergence of the eyes with fixed, dilated pupils (see Chapter 8). This syndrome can resemble the end stage of compression of the oculomotor nerves and midbrain caused by herniation through the tentorial incisura (see Chapter 26), but the effects of an embolus are sudden, not gradual. A small embolus that lodges in one of the posteromedial central arteries can cause a small infarct in the midbrain, such as the lesion responsible for Weber's syndrome (see Chapter 7).

Many syndromes have been described as resulting from small infarcts caused by occlusion of individual branches of the vertebral and basilar arteries. The positions and levels of the lesions can be deduced from the effects of transection of tracts and destruction of nuclei or fibers of cranial nerves. A few examples are cited in Chapter 7. Of these, the most common is the **lateral medullary** (**Wallenberg's**) **syndrome**, typically caused by obstruction of the PICA. This syndrome may also occur after thrombosis of the vertebral artery.

Although a rare occurrence, occlusion of the **labyrinthine artery** (or of its usual parent vessel, the AICA) results in the expected deafness in the corresponding ear and vestibular dysfunction (vertigo, with a tendency to fall toward the side of the lesion).

Infarction of the ventral part of the **pons** transects motor tracts. This causes paralysis of all voluntary movement except that of the eyes (because the medial longitudinal fasciculus is spared). The general and special sensory pathways and the reticular formation are spared, and the patient is conscious but can communicate only by means of eye movements. This condition is called the **locked-in syndrome**. More dorsally located lesions in the rostral pons or caudal midbrain cause one of the two forms of **akinetic mutism** (see Chapter 23). In this form, consciousness is severely impaired.

Posterior Cerebral Artery

The **posteromedial central arteries** arise at and near the bifurcation of the basilar artery. Each posterior cerebral artery then curves around the midbrain, above the tentorium, and reaches the medial surface of the cerebral hemisphere beneath the splenium of the corpus callosum (see Fig. 25-4). The artery gives off **temporal branches**, which ramify over the inferior surface of the temporal lobe and **calcarine** and **parieto-occipital branches**, which run along the corresponding sulci. All these arteries send branches around the border of the cerebral hemisphere to supply a peripheral strip on the lateral surface (see Fig. 25-3). The calcarine branch is of special significance because it supplies all the primary and some of the association cortex for vision. Much of the parahippocampal gyrus is supplied by the temporal branches, along with parts of the hippocampus.

The **posterior choroidal artery** (not seen in Fig. 25-4) comes off the posterior cerebral artery in the region of the splenium and runs forward in the transverse fissure beneath the corpus callosum. The posterior choroidal artery supplies the choroid plexus of the central part of the lateral ventricle, the choroid plexus of the third ventricle, the posterior part of the thalamus, the fornix, and the tectum of the midbrain. Its terminal branches anastomose with those of the anterior choroidal artery within the choroid plexus of the lateral ventricle.

ANASTOMOSES BETWEEN CORTICAL ARTERIES

Anastomoses between branches of the anterior, middle, and posterior cerebral arteries are concealed in the sulci. The caliber of an anastomotic vessel may be sufficient to sustain part of the territory of another artery if the latter is occluded. The cerebral arteries are also interconnected through an arteriolar network in the pia mater. Whereas short cortical branches from the pial plexus supply the rich capillary network of the cortex, longer branches of arteries in the subarachnoid space penetrate into the white matter and form a less profuse capillary network.

ARTERIAL CIRCLE (CIRCLE OF WILLIS)

The major arteries that supply the cerebrum are joined to one another at the base of the brain in the circle of Willis (see Fig. 25-2). Starting from the midline in front, the circle consists of the anterior communicating, an-

---

CLINICAL NOTE

Posterior Cerebral Artery Occlusion

Infarction of the cortical areas and subcortical white matter supplied by the posterior cerebral artery causes blindness in the contralateral fields of vision of both eyes (homonymous hemianopia; see Chapter 20). Ischemia of the hippocampal formation can result in a disturbance of memory after the arterial occlusion, but patients recover from this because lesions in the limbic system must be bilateral to cause lasting disability. If the infarct is located in the hemisphere dominant for language (usually the left) and extends into the splenium of the corpus callosum, the contralateral (intact) visual cortex is disconnected from the language areas of the dominant hemisphere. This causes alexia (see Chapter 15) in addition to the homonymous hemianopia.

Herniation of the uncus and midbrain through the tentorial incisura, caused by an expanding space-occupying lesion in the supratentorial compartment of the cranial cavity, can stretch and compress one or both posterior cerebral arteries over the rigid anterior edge of the tentorium (see Chapter 26). Even if the cause is treated surgically, necrosis of the areas supplied by the compressed arteries may develop. Cortical blindness results, and the patient may also have permanent impairment of the ability to form new memories (see Chapter 18) because of bilateral hippocampal involvement. Intracranial hemorrhage caused by head injury can lead to these consequences of bilateral ischemia in the territory of the posterior cerebral artery.

Intracranial Aneurysms

Aneurysms often develop at sites of branching of arteries in and near the arterial circle, and they can rupture or leak, causing **subarachnoid hemorrhage**. The most common sites for such aneurysms are the terminal part of the internal carotid artery, the anterior communicating artery, the proximal part of the middle cerebral artery, and the posterior communicating artery. A subarachnoid hemorrhage causes a severe headache of sudden onset, with a stiff neck and other signs of meningeal irritation.

terior cerebral, internal carotid (a short segment), posterior communicating, and posterior cerebral arteries; then it continues to the starting point in reverse order. Normally, little exchange of blood takes place between the main arteries through the slender communicating vessels. The arterial circle provides alternative routes, however, when one of the major arteries leading into it is occluded. Frequently, these anastomoses are inadequate, especially in elderly people in whom the large vessels and communicating arteries may be narrowed by atheroma.

Many variants of the conventional configuration of the arterial circle exist. Each posterior cerebral artery starts out as a branch of the internal carotid artery. In later embryonic development, the posterior cerebral arteries become the terminal branches of the basilar arteries, leaving the left and right posterior communicating arteries as vestiges of the earlier condition. About one in three people has one posterior cerebral artery as a major branch of the internal carotid artery. This type of connection of the posterior cerebral artery seldom occurs bilaterally. Often one anterior cerebral artery is unusually small in the first part of its course, in which case the anterior communicating artery has a larger-than-usual caliber, and one carotid artery provides blood for the medial surfaces of both cerebral hemispheres.

Central Arteries

Numerous central arteries arise from the region of the arterial circle as four groups (see Fig. 25-2). These slender, thin-walled blood vessels, also known as *ganglionic, nuclear, striate,* or *thalamic perforating arteries,* supply parts of the corpus striatum, internal capsule, diencephalon, and midbrain. The medial striate artery (recurrent artery of Heubner) is similar to the central arteries with respect to its distribution, as are the anterior and posterior choroidal arteries with respect to parts of their distributions. Table 25-1 summarizes the origins and distributions of the groups of central arteries.

DISTRIBUTION OF CENTRAL ARTERIES

Table 25-2 identifies the blood supply of structures within the regions of the brain that are supplied by the central arteries.

Cerebral Hemorrhage

Branches of striate arteries in the claustrum and external capsule are the most common site of cerebral hemorrhage caused by hypertension. The escaping blood destroys the surrounding brain tissue and may eventually occupy a substantial proportion of the volume of the cerebral hemisphere. Blood also commonly enters the ventricular system of the brain. A large hemorrhage of this kind causes contralateral hemiplegia, which is likely to be followed by coma and death.

Some hypertensive cerebral hemorrhages originate in **Charcot-Bouchard aneurysms**, which are dilatations of arterioles attributed to degenerative changes in the vessel wall. These microaneurysms probably develop much less frequently than was formerly believed, however, even in hypertensive individuals.

TABLE 25-1 **Origin and Distribution of Central Arteries of the Brain**

Central Arteries	Origin (Site of Entry Into Brain)	Structures Supplied
Anteromedial group	Anterior cerebral and anterior communicating arteries (anterior perforated substance)	Anterior hypothalamus and preoptic area
Anterolateral group (lateral striate arteries)	Middle cerebral artery (anterior perforated substance)	Head of caudate nucleus, putamen, lateral part of pallidum, internal capsule (anterior limb, genu and part of posterior limb), external capsule, claustrum, lateral hypothalamus
Posteromedial group	Posterior cerebral and posterior communicating arteries (posterior perforated substance)	Thalamus (anterior and medial parts), subthalamus, hypothalamus (middle and posterior parts), midbrain (medial part of cerebral peduncle)
Posterolateral group	Posterior cerebral artery lateral to midbrain (thalamus and midbrain)	Thalamus (posterior parts, including geniculate bodies), midbrain (tectum and lateral part of cerebral peduncle)

TABLE 25-2 **Structures Supplied by Central Arteries**

Structure	Arteries
Amygdala, uncus, and hippocampal formation	Anterior choroidal artery, temporal branches of posterior cerebral artery
Cerebral peduncle (basis pedunculi, substantia nigra, and midbrain tegmentum)	Posteromedial and posterolateral central arteries, anterior choroidal artery
External capsule and claustrum	Anterolateral central arteries
Hypothalamus	Anteromedial, posteromedial, and anterolateral central arteries
Internal capsule	Anterolateral and posterolateral central arteries, anterior choroidal artery, medial striate artery
Pallidum (globus pallidus)	Anterolateral central arteries, anterior choroidal artery
Pineal gland	Posterolateral central arteries
Striatum (head of caudate nucleus and putamen)	Anterolateral central arteries, medial striate artery
Tectum (colliculi of midbrain)	Posterolateral central arteries, posterior choroidal artery, superior cerebellar artery
Thalamus	Posteromedial and posterolateral central arteries, anterior and posterior choroidal arteries
Subthalamus	Posteromedial central arteries, anterior choroidal artery

Vasomotor Control

The calibers of small arteries in the brain are controlled by **autoregulation**, which means that their muscular walls contract if the pressure inside increases and relax if the pressure decreases, so that a constant rate of flow tends to be maintained. The increased blood flow in active areas of gray matter is probably caused by vasodilator metabolites, notably carbon dioxide. Noradrenergic axons (from the sympathetic system and from the locus coeruleus) are present in the walls of many cerebral blood vessels, but their functional importance has not yet been ascertained.

Cerebral Blood Flow and Intracranial Pressure

Venous Drainage of the Brain

The brain stem and cerebellum are drained by unnamed veins that empty into the dural venous sinuses adjacent to the posterior cranial fossa. The cerebrum has an external and an internal venous system. Whereas the external cerebral veins lie in the subarachnoid space on all surfaces of the hemispheres, the central core of the cerebrum is drained by internal cerebral veins situated beneath the corpus callosum in the transverse fissure (which is described in Chapter 13). Both sets of cerebral veins empty into dural venous sinuses, which are described in Chapter 26.

EXTERNAL CEREBRAL VEINS

The **superior cerebral veins**, of which there are eight to 12 in number, course upward over the lateral surface of the hemisphere. On nearing the midline, they pierce the arachnoid, run between the arachnoid and the dura mater for 1 to 2 cm, and empty into the superior sagittal sinus or into venous lacunae adjacent to the sinus.

The **superficial middle cerebral vein** runs downward and forward along the lateral sulcus and empties into the cavernous sinus. Anastomotic channels allow for drainage in other directions (Fig. 25-5A). These are the superior anastomotic vein (vein of Trolard), which opens into the superior sagittal sinus and the inferior anastomotic vein (vein of Labbé), which opens into the transverse sinus.

The **deep middle cerebral vein** runs downward and forward in the depths of the lateral sulcus to the ventral surface of the brain. The **anterior cerebral vein** accompanies the anterior cerebral artery. These veins unite in the region of the anterior perforated substance to form the **basal vein** (vein of Rosenthal), which runs backward at the base of the brain, curves around the midbrain, and empties into the great cerebral vein (Fig. 25-5B; see also the section "Internal Cerebral Veins" in this chapter). The basal vein receives tributaries from the optic tract, hypothalamus, temporal lobe, and midbrain.

In addition to the veins just noted, numerous small vessels drain limited areas. These have no consistent pattern and empty into adjacent dural sinuses.

INTERNAL CEREBRAL VEINS

The internal venous system forms adjacent to each lateral ventricle and continues through the transverse cerebral fissure beneath the corpus callosum (see Chapter 13 and Fig. 25-5C). The **thalamostriate vein** (vena terminalis) begins in the region of the amygdaloid body in

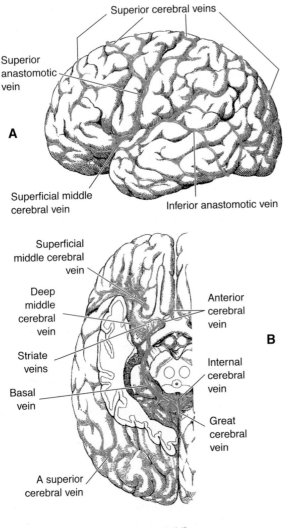

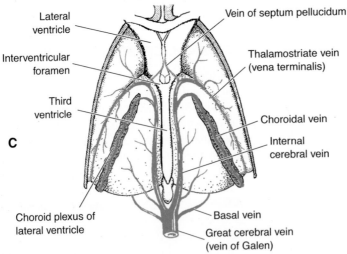

FIGURE 25-5 Internal cerebral system of veins, as seen from above after removal of the corpus callosum and fornix. Veins of the cerebrum. **(A)** Veins on the lateral aspect of the left hemisphere. **(B)** Veins of the right hemisphere, viewed from below. Part of the temporal lobe has been cut away, revealing the choroid plexus of the lateral ventricle. **(C)** Internal system of veins, as seen from above after removal of the corpus callosum and fornix.

the temporal lobe and follows the curve of the tail of the caudate nucleus on its medial side, receiving tributaries from the corpus striatum, internal capsule, thalamus, fornix, and septum pellucidum. The tortuous **choroidal vein** runs along the choroid plexus of the lateral ventricle. In addition to draining the choroid plexus, this vein receives tributaries from the hippocampus, fornix, and corpus callosum. The thalamostriate vein and choroidal vein unite immediately behind the interventricular foramen to form the **internal cerebral vein**. The paired internal cerebral veins run posteriorly in the transverse fissure, uniting beneath the splenium of the corpus callosum to form the **great cerebral vein** (vein of Galen). The latter vein, which is no more than 2 cm long, also receives the basal veins and tributaries from the cerebellum. The great cerebral vein empties into the straight sinus, which is in the midline of the tentorium cerebelli.

Blood Supply of the Spinal Cord

SPINAL ARTERIES

The median **anterior spinal artery** and the paired **posterior spinal arteries** run longitudinally throughout the length of the spinal cord. The anterior spinal artery originates in a Y-shaped configuration from the vertebral arteries, as already described, and runs caudally along the ventral median fissure. Each posterior spinal artery is a branch of either the vertebral or the PICA and consists of multiple anastomosing channels along the line of attachment of the dorsal roots of the spinal nerves.

The blood received by the spinal arteries from the vertebral arteries is sufficient for only the upper cervical segments of the spinal cord. The arteries are therefore reinforced at intervals in the following manner. The vertebral artery in the cervical region, the posterior intercostal branches of the thoracic aorta, and the lumbar branches of the abdominal aorta give off segmental **spinal arteries**, which enter the vertebral canal through the intervertebral foramina. In addition to supplying the vertebrae, these segmental spinal arteries give rise to **anterior** and **posterior radicular arteries**,

which run along the ventral and dorsal roots of the spinal nerves. Most of the radicular arteries are of small caliber, sufficient only to supply the nerve roots and contribute to a vascular plexus in the pia mater covering the spinal cord. A variable number of anterior radicular arteries of substantial size, about 12 including both sides, join the anterior spinal artery. Similarly, a variable number of posterior radicular arteries, about 14 including both sides, join the posterior spinal arteries. These larger radicular arteries are in the lower cervical, lower thoracic, and upper lumbar regions; the largest, an anterior radicular artery known as the **spinal artery of Adamkiewicz**, is usually situated in the upper lumbar region. The spinal cord is vulnerable to circulatory impairment if the important contribution by a major radicular artery is compromised by injury or by the placing of a surgical ligature.

Sulcal branches arise in succession from the anterior spinal artery and enter the right and left sides of the spinal cord alternately from the ventral median fissure. The sulcal arteries are least frequent in the thoracic part of the spinal cord. The anterior spinal artery supplies the ventral gray horns, part of the dorsal gray horns, and the ventral and lateral white funiculi. Penetrating branches from the posterior spinal arteries supply the remainder of the dorsal gray horns and the dorsal funiculi of white matter. A fine plexus (the **vasocorona**) derived from the spinal arteries is present in the pia mater on the lateral and ventral surfaces of the cord. Penetrating branches from the vasocorona supply a narrow zone of white matter beneath the pia mater.

SPINAL VEINS

Although the pattern of spinal veins is irregular, there are essentially six of them. **Anterior spinal veins** run along the midline and along the line of ventral rootlets. **Posterior spinal veins** are situated in the midline and along the line of dorsal rootlets. The spinal veins are drained at intervals by up to 12 **anterior radicular veins** and by a similar number of **posterior radicular veins**. The radicular veins empty into an epidural venous plexus, which, in turn, drains into an external vertebral plexus through channels in the intervertebral foramina. Blood from the external vertebral plexus empties into the vertebral, intercostal, and lumbar veins.

Imaging Cerebral Blood Vessels

In 1927, de Egas Moniz introduced the technique of **cerebral angiography**, which developed into a valuable diagnostic aid in the hands of neuroradiologists. The method consists of injecting a radiopaque solution into the artery, followed by serial radiographic photography at about 1-second intervals. The radiographs show the contrast medium in progressive stages of its passage through the arterial tree and the venous return. Injection into the common carotid artery or the internal carotid artery shows the distribution of the middle and anterior cerebral arteries (see Figs. 25-1 and 25-6). Similarly, injection of the vertebral artery permits visualization of the vertebral, basilar, and posterior cerebral arteries together with their branches (Fig. 25-7) The cerebral veins are seen in later pictures of a series.

(The internal carotid and vertebral arteries are approached with a long catheter passed through a femoral artery and the aorta.)

The technique of cerebral angiography is especially useful in identifying vascular malformations and aneurysms. The method often provides valuable information concerning occlusive vascular disease and space-occupying lesions that displace blood vessels.

The larger cerebral vessels can be demonstrated by **computed tomography** after intravenous injection of a contrast medium and by **nuclear magnetic resonance imaging** (see Chapter 4). **Ultrasound** can provide information about the anatomy and blood flow in the carotid arteries. These less invasive techniques do not display the vascular anatomy in as much detail as angiography.

Blood–Brain Barrier

Certain substances fail to pass from capillary blood into the CNS, although the same sub-

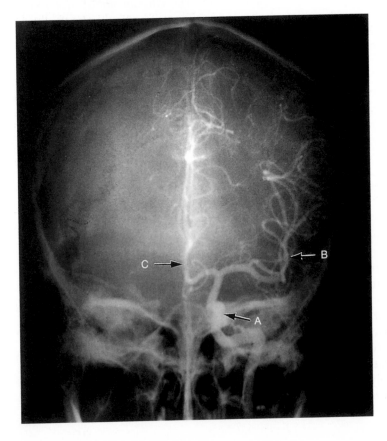

FIGURE 25-6 Carotid angiogram (anteroposterior view). A, carotid siphon; B, branches of the middle cerebral artery; C, anterior cerebral artery. (Courtesy of Dr. J. M. Allcock.)

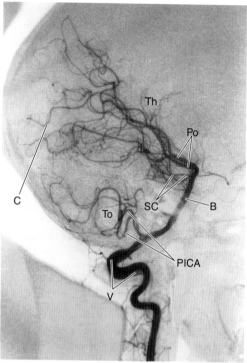

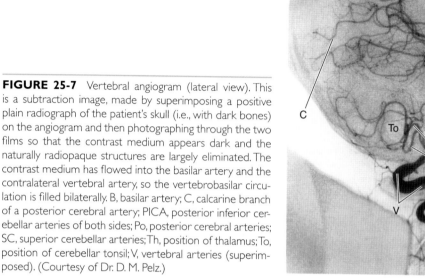

FIGURE 25-7 Vertebral angiogram (lateral view). This is a subtraction image, made by superimposing a positive plain radiograph of the patient's skull (i.e., with dark bones) on the angiogram and then photographing through the two films so that the contrast medium appears dark and the naturally radiopaque structures are largely eliminated. The contrast medium has flowed into the basilar artery and the contralateral vertebral artery, so the vertebrobasilar circulation is filled bilaterally. B, basilar artery; C, calcarine branch of a posterior cerebral artery; PICA, posterior inferior cerebellar arteries of both sides; Po, posterior cerebral arteries; SC, superior cerebellar arteries; Th, position of thalamus; To, position of cerebellar tonsil; V, vertebral arteries (superimposed). (Courtesy of Dr. D. M. Pelz.)

stances gain access to non-nervous tissues. They include dyes used in animal experimentation and some antibiotics and other drugs that would otherwise be of therapeutic value. In the blood, these substances are bound to plasma protein molecules, which are unable to leave normal cerebral blood vessels. The lumen of a capillary and the parenchyma of the brain and spinal cord are separated by endothelium, a basal lamina, and perivascular end feet of astrocytic processes. In mammals, the blood–brain barrier to proteins is formed by the internal plasma membranes of the endothelial cells and the tight junctions between them. The barrier properties of the endothelium are induced by the adjacent cells, principally astrocytes, of the CNS tissue. Small hydrophobic molecules, including oxygen, carbon dioxide, and ethanol, can diffuse through endothelial cell membranes and cytoplasm and are not excluded by the brain.

Tight junctions between cells of the choroid epithelium and arachnoid prevent diffusion of plasma proteins into the CSF from the extracellular spaces of the choroid plexus and dura mater, respectively. Molecules of all sizes can diffuse freely between the CSF and the extracellular spaces of the CNS.

The entry of small molecules into the brain is restricted by carrier mechanisms within the endothelial cells of the cerebral blood vessels. These regulate the transport of glucose (the GLUT-1 transporter), amino acids (the L-1 transporter), and other substances from the blood to the neurons and neuroglia. An efflux transporter (P-glycoprotein) returns unwanted hydrophobic substances from the endothelial cytoplasm to the blood. The composition of CSF is similarly controlled by the choroid epithelial cells.

In a few small regions known as **circumventricular organs** (e.g., the area postrema in the medulla, the subfornical organ, and the neurohypophysis), the blood–brain barrier is lacking. Sensory and autonomic ganglia are permeated by plasma proteins and so are spinal nerve roots. The capillaries within the endoneurium of a peripheral nerve are partly permeable to proteins, and the innermost layer of the perineurium (see Chapter 3) restricts diffusion of proteins from the epineurium, which has fully permeable blood vessels.

The blood–brain barrier is defective for 2 to 3 weeks after injury, and it also fails in various pathological states, such as inflammatory and neoplastic diseases. It is possible to make images of sites of abnormal vascular permeability by administering an appropriate radioactive tracer and scanning the head for the emitted radiation. Other tracers (gadolinium compounds) make permeable regions visible in images produced by nuclear magnetic resonance imaging.

Suggested Reading

Abbott NJ. Astrocyte-endothelial interactions and blood-brain barrier permeability. *J Anat* 2002;200:629–638.

Blumenfeld H. *Neuroanatomy through Clinical Cases.* Sunderland, MA: Sinauer, 2002.

Challa VR, Moody DM, Bell MA. The Charcot-Bouchard aneurysm controversy: impact of a new histologic technique. *J Neuropath Exp Neurol* 1992;51:264–271.

Davson H. History of the blood-brain barrier concept. In: Neuwelt EA, ed. *Implications of the Blood-Brain Barrier and Its Manipulation,* vol 1. New York: Plenum Press, 1989:27–52.

Gross PM. Morphology and physiology of capillary systems in subregions of the subfornical organ and area postrema. *Can J Physiol Pharmacol* 1991;69:1010–1025.

Haines DE, ed. *Fundamental Neuroscience,* 3rd ed. New York: Churchill-Livingstone, 2006.

Kiernan JA. Vascular permeability in the peripheral autonomic and somatic nervous systems: controversial aspects and comparisons with the blood-brain barrier. *Microsc Res Tech* 1996;35:122–136.

Lee DH, Gao FQ, Rankin RN, et al. Duplex and color Doppler flow sonography of occlusion and near occlusion of the carotid artery. *Am J Neuroradiol* 1996;17:1267–1274.

Montemurro DG, Bruni JE. *The Human Brain in Dissection,* 2nd ed. Philadelphia: WB Saunders, 1988.

Nonaka H, Akima M, Nagayama T, et al. The microvasculature of the cerebral white matter: arteries of the subcortical white matter. *J Neuropathol Exp Neurol* 2003;62: 154–161.

Pardridge WM, ed. *The Blood-Brain Barrier. Cellular and Molecular Biology.* New York: Raven Press, 1993.

Pullicino PM. The courses and territories of cerebral small arteries. *Adv Neurol* 1993;62:11–39.

Pullicino PM. Diagrams of perforating artery territories in axial, coronal and sagittal planes. *Adv Neurol* 1993;62: 41–72.

Rowell LB. *Human Cardiovascular Control.* New York: Oxford University Press, 1993.

Salamon G. *Atlas de la Vascularization Artérielle du Cerveau chez l'Homme,* 2nd ed. Paris: Sandoz Editions, 1973.

Thron AK, Rossberg C, Mironov A. *Vascular Anatomy of the Spinal Cord. Neuroradial Investigations and Clinical Syndromes.* Vienna: Springer-Verlag, 1988.

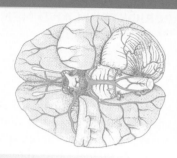

Chapter 26

MENINGES AND CEREBROSPINAL FLUID

- The cranial dura mater adheres to the skull, but an extradural hemorrhage from the middle meningeal artery can compress the brain. The spinal epidural space contains fat, nerve roots, and veins.

- The sensory innervation of most of the cranial dura is from branches of the trigeminal nerve. The vagus nerve innervates the dura of the posterior fossa.

- The largest dural reflections are the falx cerebri and the tentorium cerebelli.

- Pressure on a cerebral hemisphere can lead to transtentorial herniation. This causes compression of the ipsilateral oculomotor nerve and uncus, either cerebral peduncle, and sometimes the posterior cerebral arteries.

- Veins leaving the cerebral cortex traverse the subarachnoid and subdural spaces before entering the superior sagittal sinus. A head injury can tear these veins, which then bleed into the subdural space.

- Most other cerebral veins empty into the straight sinus. All the venous blood from the brain eventually passes through the sigmoid sinuses into the internal jugular veins.

- The epithelium of the arachnoid has occluding tight junctions that form a barrier between the cerebrospinal fluid (CSF) and the dura. There is free exchange across the pia mater between the CSF and the extracellular spaces of the central nervous system.

- The width of the subarachnoid space varies because the arachnoid adheres to the dura and the pia to the external glial-limiting membrane. The widest spaces are the subarachnoid cisterns, of which the lumbar and cerebellomedullary are the largest.

- The subarachnoid space accompanies the optic nerve as far as the optic disc. Raised intracranial pressure causes swelling of the disc (papilledema).

- CSF is secreted by the choroid plexuses; circulates through the ventricles, the apertures of the fourth ventricle, and the subarachnoid space; and is absorbed into the dural sinuses by way of the arachnoid villi.

- Hydrocephalus can be caused by obstruction of the flow of CSF through the ventricular system or subarachnoid space or to obstruction of the arachnoid villi. The sites of accumulation of fluid are appropriate to the position of the blockage.

In addition to the protection provided by the skull and the vertebral column and its ligaments, the soft, gelatinous central nervous system (CNS) receives physical support from the meninges. These are the thick **dura mater** externally, the delicate **arachnoid** lining the dura, and the thin **pia mater** adhering to the brain and spinal cord. The latter two layers bound the subarachnoid space, which is filled with cerebrospinal fluid (CSF). The main support and protection provided by the meninges come from the dura mater and the cushion of CSF in the subarachnoid space.

Dura Mater and Associated Structures

The internal surfaces of the cranial bones are clothed by periosteum, which is continuous with the periosteum on the external surface at the margins of the foramen magnum and of smaller foramina for nerves and blood vessels. The cranial dura mater is intimately attached to the periosteum, which is sometimes incorrectly called the "external layer" of the dura mater.

PERIOSTEUM AND MENINGEAL BLOOD VESSELS

The periosteum consists of collagenous connective tissue and contains arteries, somewhat inappropriately called *meningeal arteries*, which mainly supply the adjoining bone. Of these, the largest is the **middle meningeal artery**, a branch of the maxillary artery that enters the cranial cavity through the foramen spinosum in the floor of the middle cranial fossa. Its branches extend over the lateral interior surface of the cranium, producing grooves on the bones. Smaller meningeal arteries are branches of the ophthalmic, occipital, and vertebral arteries.

The meningeal arteries are accompanied by **meningeal veins**, which are also subject to tearing in fractures of the skull. The largest meningeal veins accompany the middle meningeal artery, leave the cranial cavity through the foramen spinosum or the foramen ovale, and drain into the pterygoid venous plexus. **Diploic veins**, within the cancellous bone of the vault of the skull, drain into the veins of the scalp and into the dural venous sinuses described below.

DURA MATER

The dura mater, or **pachymeninx**, is a dense, firm layer of collagenous connective tissue. The **spinal dura mater** takes the form of a tube, pierced by the roots of spinal nerves, that extends from the foramen magnum to the second segment of the sacrum. The spinal dura mater is separated from the wall of the spinal canal by an **epidural (extradural) space** that contains adipose tissue and a venous plexus. The **cranial dura mater** is firmly attached to the periosteum, as previously described, from which it

receives small blood vessels. The outer layer of the dura consists largely of collagen and elastic fibers, and the smooth inner surface of the dura is a simple squamous epithelium. A microscopically narrow film of fluid occupies the **subdural space** between the dura and outer layer of cells of the arachnoid. The cranial dura mater has several features of importance, notably the dural reflections and dural venous sinuses.

DURAL REFLECTIONS

The dura is reflected along certain lines to form the dural reflections or septa. The intervals between the periosteum and dura along the lines of attachment of the septa accommodate dural venous sinuses (Fig. 26-1). The largest septa, the falx cerebri, and the tentorium cerebelli form incomplete partitions that divide the cranial cavity into three compartments (Fig. 26-2).

The **falx cerebri** is a vertical partition in the longitudinal fissure between the cerebral hemispheres. This dural reflection is attached to the crista galli of the ethmoid bone in front, to the midline of the vault as far back as the internal occipital protuberance, and to the tentorium cerebelli. The anterior end of the falx cerebri is often fenestrated.

The **tentorium cerebelli** intervenes between the occipital lobes and the cerebellum. The attachment of the falx cerebri along the midline draws the tentorium upward, giving it a shallow, tent-like shape. The peripheral border of the tentorium is attached to the upper edges of the petrous parts of both temporal bones and to the occipital bone at the margins of the sulci for the transverse sinuses. The free anterior border bounds the **incisura of the tentorium** (tentorial notch), which accommodates the midbrain.

CLINICAL NOTE

Extradural Hemorrhage

A fracture in the temporal region of the skull may tear a branch of the middle meningeal artery. The extravasated blood accumulates between the bone and the periosteum. As in the case of any space-occupying lesion in the nonexpansile cranial cavity, intracranial pressure increases, and prompt surgical intervention

is necessary. The effects of the expanding lesion are similar to those of a subdural hemorrhage (see Chapter 25) and are discussed in this chapter under the heading "Transtentorial and Other Herniations." With arterial blood escaping at high pressure, the deterioration is typically faster than with venous bleeding into the subdural space.

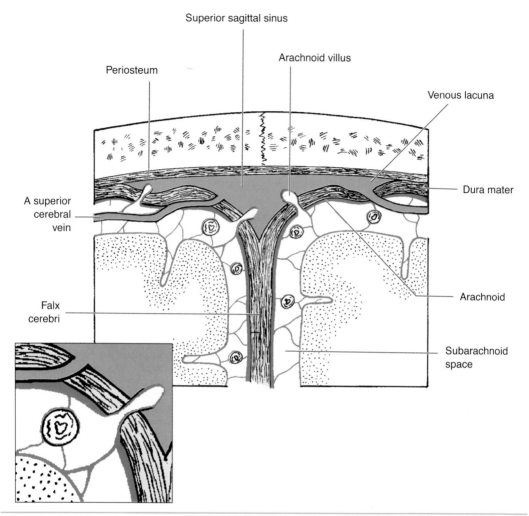

FIGURE 26-1   Coronal section at the vertex of the skull, including the superior sagittal sinus (venous blood is blue) and the attachment of the falx cerebri. The dura mater is yellow, and the pia-arachnoid is green.

The **falx cerebelli** is a small dural fold in the posterior cranial fossa, extending vertically for a short distance between the cerebellar hemispheres. The **diaphragma sellae** roofs over the pituitary fossa or sella turcica of the sphenoid bone and has a hole in its middle for passage of the pituitary stalk.

NERVE SUPPLY OF THE DURA MATER

The dura mater is innervated by nerves that travel alongside the arteries and veins. The cranial dura has a plentiful sensory supply, mainly from branches of all three divisions of the trigeminal nerve. The sensory fibers terminate as unencapsulated endings in the outer, fibroelastic layer of the dura, and they are of significance in certain types of headache. Sympathetic axons also accompany the dural blood vessels.

The dura lining the anterior and middle cranial fossae is supplied by branches from all three divisions of the trigeminal nerve. The dura lining the floor of the posterior cranial fossa is supplied by a meningeal branch from the superior ganglion of the vagus nerve and also by sensory twigs from spinal nerves C1 to C3, which enter the posterior fossa through the hypoglossal canal. (Nerve C1 lacks a sensory component in about half of individuals.)

Recurrent branches of all spinal nerves enter the vertebral canal through the intervertebral

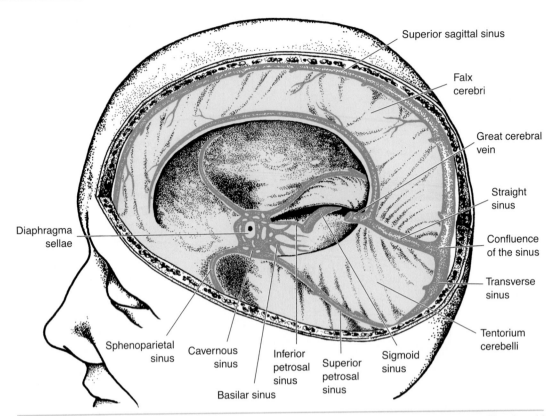

FIGURE 26-2   Dural reflections (yellow) and dural venous sinuses (blue) after removal of the brain. The sigmoid sinus of the right side is seen through the tentorial incisura.

foramina and give off meningeal branches to the spinal dura mater.

DURAL VENOUS SINUSES

As described in Chapter 25, the veins draining the brain empty into the venous sinuses of the dura mater, from which blood flows into the internal jugular veins. The walls of the sinuses consist of dura mater (and periosteum) lined by endothelium. The locations of most of the dural venous sinuses are shown in Figure 26-2.

The **superior sagittal sinus** lies along the attached border of the falx cerebri. It begins in front of the crista galli of the ethmoid bone, where there may be a narrow communication with nasal veins. **Venous lacunae**, which are shallow, blood-filled spaces within the dura, lie alongside the superior sagittal sinus and open into it. The superior cerebral veins drain into the sinus or into the lacunae. The superior sagittal sinus is usually continuous with the right transverse sinus.

The small **inferior sagittal sinus** runs along the free border of the falx cerebri, receiving veins from the medial aspects of the cerebral hemispheres. The inferior sagittal sinus opens into the **straight sinus**, which lies in the attachment of the falx cerebri to the tentorium cerebelli. The straight sinus also receives the great cerebral vein (see Fig. 25-4). The straight sinus is usually continuous with the left transverse sinus. Venous channels connect the transverse sinuses at the internal occipital protuberance; the configuration of venous channels in this location is called the **confluence of the sinuses** or **torcular Herophili**. It also receives the small **occipital sinus**, which is in the attached margin of the falx cerebelli.

Each **transverse sinus** lies in a groove on the occipital bone along the attached margin of the tentorium cerebelli. On reaching the petrous part of the temporal bone, the transverse sinus continues as the **sigmoid sinus**. The latter follows a curved course in the posterior fossa and becomes continuous with the internal jugular vein at the jugular foramen.

Transtentorial and Other Herniations

The narrow interval between the midbrain and the boundary of the tentorial incisura is the only communication between the subtentorial and supratentorial compartments of the cranial cavity. An expanding lesion in the supratentorial compartment, such as a subdural hematoma or a tumor in a cerebral hemisphere, may push the medial part of the temporal lobe (the uncus) down into the incisura of the tentorium. An uncal herniation presses on the ipsilateral oculomotor nerve. The first clinical sign of this event is impairment of the pupillary light reflex (see Chapter 8) because the preganglionic parasympathetic fibers for constriction of the pupil are superficially located in the nerve.

Further herniation can damage descending motor fibers in one or both cerebral peduncles, causing weakness, spasticity, and exaggerated tendon reflexes on either side or bilaterally. When the midbrain is displaced toward the opposite side, the pressure of the rigid edge of the tentorium on the basis pedunculi may result in the unusual finding of upper motor neuron paresis on the same side of the body as the cerebral le-

sion. Sometimes the downward displacement of the brain occludes one or both posterior cerebral arteries by stretching these vessels over the free edge of the tentorium, with consequences that are explained in Chapter 25. In the later stages of transtentorial herniation, the contralateral oculomotor nerve may be affected. The pupil that dilates first is the most reliable lateralizing sign for the causative lesion.

There are other abnormal movements of parts of the brain from one dural compartment to another. A **subfalcial herniation** occurs when a space-occupying lesion pushes the cingulate gyrus of one hemisphere across the midline beneath the anterior part of the free edge of the falx cerebri. In an **upward transtentorial herniation**, the brain stem and cerebellum are displaced into the supratentorial compartment by a mass in the posterior fossa. Such a mass may also cause **medullary coning**, when the brain stem and part of the cerebellum descend through the foramen magnum into the spinal canal. Medullary coning can occur after withdrawal of CSF from the lumbar subarachnoid space in a patient with raised intracranial pressure. The tonsils of the cerebellum compress the medulla, and the condition can be quickly fatal.

The **cavernous sinus** is an extradural compartment filled with very thin-walled veins and traversed by the internal carotid artery and various nerves, present on each side of the body of the sphenoid bone and connected by venous channels in the anterior and posterior margins of the diaphragma sellae. A more correct but seldom-used name is **lateral sellar** (or **parasellar**) **compartment**. Each cavernous sinus receives the ophthalmic vein and the superficial middle cerebral vein

Thrombosis in Venous Sinuses

Thrombosis in the **superior sagittal sinus** can occur after a fracture that damages the dura. If the posterior part of the sinus is obstructed, blood cannot escape from much of the cerebral cortex, and areas of infarction form in the frontal and parietal lobes.

Sometimes, infective particles can become dislodged from a facial lesion (e.g., a carbuncle of the upper lip) and pass through the veins of the orbit and the ophthalmic vein into the **cavernous sinus**. The effects of septic thrombosis of the cavernous sinus include compression of the oculomotor, trochlear, abducens, and maxillary

nerves, which are located in the walls of the sinus (see Chapter 8), together with swelling and protrusion of the conjunctiva and systemic signs of a serious infection. A congenital weakness in the wall of the internal carotid artery may cause a split that leaks into the cavernous sinus. Similar to a septic thrombosis, this **arteriovenous fistula** compresses the nerves that pass through the sinus and causes considerable venous congestion of the eye. The eyeball protrudes and pulsates, and a loud pulsating sound is heard by the patient and by anyone applying a stethoscope to the head.

and drains into the transverse sinus through the **superior petrosal sinus**, which runs along the attachment of the tentorium cerebelli to the petrous part of the temporal bone. The **inferior petrosal sinus** lies in the groove between the petrous part of the temporal bone and the basilar part of the occipital bone, providing a communication between the cavernous sinus and the internal jugular vein. The sinuses at the base of the cranium receive veins from adjacent parts of the brain.

Within the orbit, the ophthalmic vein has anastomotic communications with the superficial veins of the middle part of the face. Some blood from the facial skin can therefore enter the cavernous sinus and pass into the internal jugular vein. **Emissary veins** connect dural venous sinuses with veins outside the cranial cavity. Blood may flow in either direction, depending on venous pressures. The parietal and mastoid emissary veins are the largest of these connecting channels. The parietal emissary vein joins the superior sagittal sinus with tributaries of the occipital veins. The mastoid emissary vein joins the sigmoid sinus with the occipital and posterior auricular veins.

Pia-Arachnoid

The **pia mater** and the **arachnoid** together constitute the **leptomeninges** (thin membranes). They develop initially as a single layer from the mesoderm surrounding the embryonic brain and spinal cord. Fluid-filled spaces form within the layer and coalesce to become the subarachnoid space. The origin from a single membrane is reflected in the numerous trabeculae passing between the two layers (Fig. 26-3). The arach-

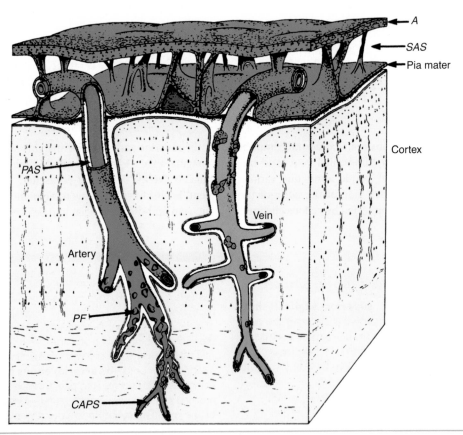

FIGURE 26-3 Perivascular spaces in the brain. The subarachnoid space (SAS) separates the arachnoid (A) from the pia mater. The pia splits to ensheath the artery but not the vein. The periarterial space (PAS) has subpial and intrapial compartments, which become continuous as the pial periarterial sheath becomes perforated (PF). Capillaries (CAPS) have no pial ensheathment. (With permission from Zhang ET, Inman CBE, Weller RO. Interrelationships of the pia mater and the perivascular [Virchow-Robin] spaces of the human cerebrum. J Anat 1990;170:111–123.)

noid is closely applied to the inside of the dura mater, so the **subdural space** normally contains only a film of extracellular fluid. The pia mater adheres to the external glial-limiting membrane of the CNS (see Chapter 2).

The arachnoid is thick enough to be manipulated with fingers or forceps. In contrast, the pia mater is barely visible to the unaided eye, although it imparts a shiny appearance to the surface of the brain. Both surfaces of the arachnoid and the external surface of the pia are covered by simple squamous epithelium. The trabeculae crossing the subarachnoid space are delicate strands of connective tissue with squamous epithelial cells on their surfaces. Tight junctions (zonulae occludentes) connect adjacent arachnoid epithelial cells, preventing exchange of large molecules between the blood in the dural vasculature and the CSF. No tight junctions exist between the pial cells, so there can be free exchange of macromolecules between the CSF and the CNS tissue.

The avascular arachnoid is separated from the dura mater by a film of fluid. The pia mater, which contains a network of fine blood vessels, adheres to the surface of the brain and spinal cord, following all their contours. The collagen fibers in the spinal pia-arachnoid run mostly in a longitudinal direction. This is accentuated along the ventromedian line of the spinal cord, where a thickened strand of fibers, the **linea splendens**, lies superficial to the anterior spinal artery. The **denticulate ligament**, described in Chapter 5, is also derived from the pia-arachnoid.

PERIVASCULAR SPACES

It was formerly thought that the subarachnoid space continued around arteries and veins entering and leaving the CNS tissue. Electron microscopy of surgically removed human cerebral cortex, however, reveals that where an artery enters the substance of the brain, the pia mater splits, and one leaflet forms a cellular sheath that constitutes the adventitia of the vessel. A **periarterial subpial space** separates the pia-adventitia from the external glial-limiting membrane of the brain. An **intrapial periarterial space** is also present between the smooth muscle of the artery and the pia. The latter space is a continuation of the space that separates an artery from its leptomeningeal covering as it crosses the subarachnoid space (see Fig. 26-3). Veins do not have pial extensions, so the **perivenular spaces** within the brain are equivalent to the intrapial periarterial spaces. The subarachnoid space is continuous, through fenestrations in the pia, with all three types of perivascular space.

The old term **Virchow-Robin spaces** applies to all perivascular spaces seen in sections prepared for light microscopy. Capillary blood vessels in the CNS are surrounded by single basal laminae, against which abut the foot processes of astrocytes (see Chapter 2). Spaces are often seen around capillaries in material conventionally prepared for light microscopy, but these are artifacts caused by differential shrinkage, as are the spaces commonly seen around the cell bodies of neurons.

SUBARACHNOID CISTERNS

The width of the subarachnoid space varies because whereas the arachnoid rests on the dura mater, the pia mater adheres to the irregular contours of the brain. The space is narrow over the summits of gyri, wider in the regions of major sulci, and wider yet at the base of the brain and in the lumbosacral region of the spinal canal. Regions of the subarachnoid space that contain more substantial amounts of CSF are called **subarachnoid cisterns** (Fig. 26-4).

The **cerebellomedullary cistern** (**cisterna magna**) occupies the interval between the cerebellum and medulla and receives CSF through the median aperture of the fourth ventricle. The basal cisterns beneath the brain stem and diencephalon include the **pontine** and **interpeduncular cisterns** and the **cistern of the optic chiasma**. The cistern of the optic chiasma is continuous with the **cistern of the lamina terminalis**, which, in turn, continues into the **cistern of the corpus callosum** above this commissure. The subarachnoid space dorsal to the midbrain is called the **superior cistern** or, alternatively, the **cistern of the great cerebral vein**. This cistern and subarachnoid space on the sides of the midbrain constitute the **cisterna ambiens** or perimesencephalic cistern (not seen in Fig. 26-4). The **cistern of the lateral sulcus** corresponds with that sulcus. The **lumbar cistern** of the spinal subarachnoid space

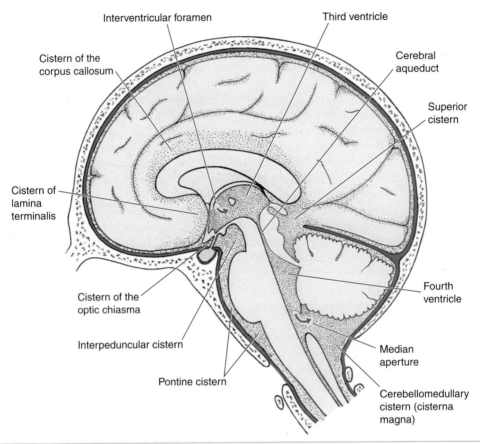

FIGURE 26-4   Subarachnoid cisterns of the head, in and near the median plane. Red arrows show the flow of cerebrospinal fluid from the lateral to the third ventricle through the right interventricular foramen and from the fourth ventricle, through the median aperture, into the cerebellomedullary cistern. Regions occupied by cerebrospinal fluid are light blue, and the dura is green. The cisterna ambiens (extending laterally from the superior and interpeduncular cisterns) and the cistern of the lateral sulcus (see text) are not shown because they are outside the median plane.

is especially large, extending from the second lumbar vertebra to the second segment of the sacrum. It contains the cauda equina, formed by lumbosacral spinal nerve roots.

The meningeal layers and subarachnoid space extend around cranial nerves and spinal nerve roots for a distance approximately to the level of sensory ganglia when these are present. For example, the trigeminal cave (Meckel's cave) is an extension of the subarachnoid space, enclosed by dura mater, around the proximal part of the trigeminal

---

CLINICAL NOTE

Papilledema

The meningeal extension of greatest clinical importance surrounds the optic nerve to its attachment to the eyeball. The central artery and central vein of the retina run within the anterior part of the optic nerve and cross the extension of the subarachnoid space to join the ophthalmic artery and ophthalmic vein. An increase of CSF pressure slows the return of venous blood, causing edema of the retina. This is most apparent on ophthalmoscopic examination as swelling of the optic papilla or disc **(papilledema)**. Dilatation of the axons of the optic nerve, caused by impairment of the slow component of anterograde axoplasmic transport, also contributes to the swelling. Inspection of the ocular fundi is an important part of every physical examination of a patient.

ganglion at the tip of the petrous part of the temporal bone.

Cerebrospinal Fluid

PRODUCTION

The CSF is produced mainly by the choroid plexuses of the lateral, third, and fourth ventricles, with those in the lateral ventricles being the largest and most important.

The **choroid plexus** of each lateral ventricle is formed by an invagination of vascular pia mater (the **tela choroidea**) on the medial surface of the cerebral hemisphere. The vascular connective tissue picks up a covering layer of epithelium from the ependymal lining of the ventricle. The choroid plexuses of the third and fourth ventricles are similarly formed by invaginations of the tela choroidea attached to the roofs of these ventricles. Each choroid plexus, which has a minutely folded surface, consists of a core of connective tissue containing many wide capillaries and a surface layer of cuboidal or low columnar epithelium (the choroid epithelium; Fig. 26-5). The surface area of the choroid plexuses of the two lateral ventricles combined is about 40 cm².

Several features of the choroid epithelium as seen in electron micrographs are of functional interest (Fig. 26-6). The large nucleus, abundant cytoplasm, and many mitochondria indicate that production of CSF is an active process that requires expenditure of energy on the part of these cells. The plasma membrane at the free surface is greatly increased in area by irregular microvilli. A basement membrane separates the epithelium from the subjacent stroma with its rich vascular network. The capillaries, unlike those generally supplying nervous tissue, have endothelial fenestrations and are permeable to large molecules. The blood–CSF barrier to macromolecules is formed by the cells of the choroid epithelium and the tight junctions (zonulae occludentes) between adjacent cells.

Production of CSF is a complex process. Some components of the blood plasma, notably water, enter and leave the CSF by diffusion. Others reach the fluid with the assistance of metabolic activity on the part of the choroid

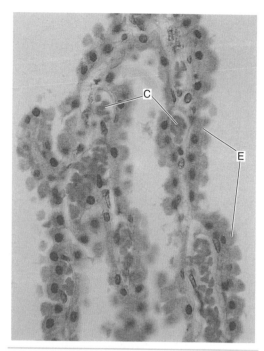

FIGURE 26-5   Fragment of choroid plexus, showing large capillaries *(C)* and the choroid epithelium *(E)*. Stained with hemalum and eosin.

epithelial cells. An important factor is active transport of certain ions (notably sodium) through the epithelial cells, followed by passive movement of water to maintain osmotic equilibrium. Transporter proteins in the choroid epithelial cells allow controlled movement of glucose and amino acids into the CSF.

CIRCULATION

CSF flows from the lateral ventricles into the third ventricle through the interventricular foramina and then into the fourth ventricle by way of the cerebral aqueduct. CSF leaves the ventricular system through the median and lateral apertures of the fourth ventricle, with the former opening into the cerebellomedullary cistern and the latter into the pontine cistern (see Figs. 6-4 and 6-5). From these sites, fluid moves sluggishly through the spinal subarachnoid space, determined partly by movements of the vertebral column. More importantly, the CSF flows slowly forward through the basal cisterns and then upward over the medial and lateral surfaces of the cerebral hemispheres. Movement of CSF is assisted by the pulsation

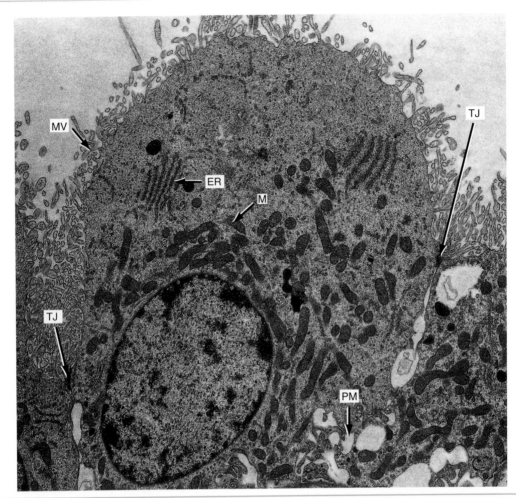

FIGURE 26-6 Electron micrograph of a choroid epithelial cell. ER, endoplasmic reticulum; M, mitochondria; MV, microvilli; N, nucleus; PM, folds of plasma membrane; TJ, tight junction (zonula occludens) (×8,000; courtesy of Dr. D. H. Dickson).

of arteries, especially in the subarachnoid space around the spinal cord.

ABSORPTION

The main site of absorption of the CSF into venous blood is through the **arachnoid villi** projecting into dural venous sinuses, especially the superior sagittal sinus and its adjacent lacunae (see Fig. 26-1). Each arachnoid villus consists of a thin cellular layer, derived from the endothelium of the sinus, which encloses an extension of the subarachnoid space containing arachnoid cells and collagenous trabeculae (Fig. 26-7). The absorptive mechanism depends on the hydrostatic pressure of the CSF being higher than

that of the venous blood in the dural sinuses. An increase in venous pressure collapses the extracellular channels of the villus, preventing the reflux of blood into the subarachnoid space. The final stage of absorption is the movement of fluid in large vesicles that form in the cytoplasm of the endothelial cells. Arachnoid villi become hypertrophied with age, becoming visible to the unaided eye. They are then called **arachnoid granulations** or **pacchionian bodies**; some are sufficiently large to produce erosion or pitting of the parietal bones.

Some CSF is absorbed into arachnoid villi that protrude into veins that pass alongside the spinal and cranial nerve roots before emptying into the epidural venous plexus.

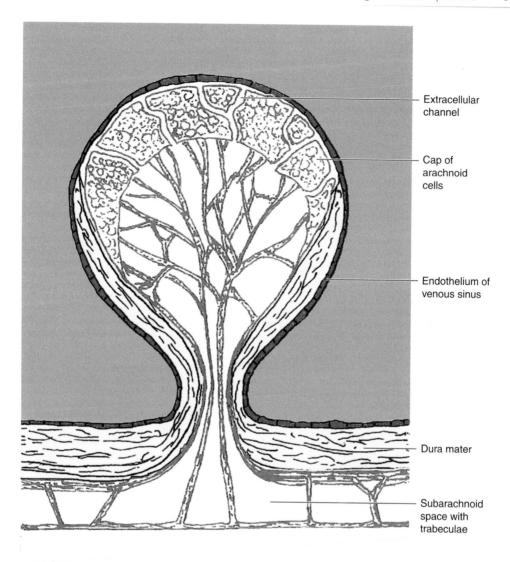

FIGURE 26-7   Structure of an arachnoid granulation. The venous blood in the sinus is blue. Pia-arachnoid tissue is green, the endothelium of the sinus is red, the dura is yellow, and the cerebral cortex (stippled) is gray. Cerebrospinal fluid occupies the white areas in the subarachnoid space, between collagenous trabeculae within the granulation and between the cap of arachnoid epithelial cells and the endothelium.

PRESSURE AND PROPERTIES

The volume of the CSF varies from 80 to 150 mL; these figures include the fluid in the ventricles and the subarachnoid space. The ventricular system alone contains from 15 to 40 mL of fluid. The rate of production is sufficient to effect a total replacement several times daily. The pressure of CSF is from 80 to 180 cm H_2O when a subject is recumbent; the pressure in the lumbar cistern is about twice as high when measured in a sitting position. Venous congestion in the closed space of the cranial cavity and the spinal canal, as produced by straining or coughing, is reflected in a prompt increase of CSF pressure.

CSF is clear and colorless, with a density of 1.003 to 1.008 g/cm³. The few cells present are mainly lymphocytes. These vary in number from one to eight in each cubic millimeter; a count of more than 10 cells indicates disease. The glucose level is about one-half that of blood, and the protein content is very low (15 to 45 mg/dL).

Hydrocephalus

When there is an excess of CSF, the condition is known as *hydrocephalus*, of which there are several types. **External hydrocephalus**, in which the excess fluid is mainly located in the subarachnoid space, is found in senile atrophy of the brain. **Internal hydrocephalus** refers to dilatation of the ventricles. All the ventricles are enlarged if the apertures of the fourth ventricle are occluded. The third and lateral ventricles enlarge if the obstruction is located in the cerebral aqueduct. In the rare occurrence of occlusion of an interventricular foramen, the hydrocephalus is confined to the ipsilateral lateral ventricle.

The term **communicating hydrocephalus** refers to a combination of internal and external hydrocephalus. The most common cause is obstruction of the arachnoid villi by blood after a subarachnoid hemorrhage. Communicating hydrocephalus can also occur in bacterial meningitis, with pus as the obstructing material. If the flow of CSF through the incisura of the tentorium around the midbrain is obstructed, the excess fluid accumulates in the ventricles and in the part of the subarachnoid space below the tentorium.

Suggested Reading

Baumbach GL, Cancilla PA, Hayreh MS, et al. Experimental injury of the optic nerve with optic disc swelling. *Lab Invest* 1978;39:50–60.

Boulton M, Young A, Hay J, et al. Drainage of CSF through lymphatic pathways and arachnoid villi in sheep: measurement of I-125-albumin clearance. *Neuropathol Appl Neurobiol* 1996;22:325–333.

Dandy WE. Experimental hydrocephalus. *Trans Am Surg Assoc* 1919;37:397–428.

Davson H, Segal MB. *Physiology of the CSF and Blood-Brain Barriers.* Boca Raton, FL: CRC Press, 1996.

Greitz D, Wirestam R, Franck A, et al. Pulsatile brain movement and associated hydrodynamics studied by magnetic resonance phase imaging: the Monro-Kellie doctrine revisited. *Neuroradiology* 1992;34:370–380.

Lowhagen P, Johansson BB, Nordborg C. The nasal route of cerebrospinal fluid drainage in man: a light-microscope study. *Neuropathol Appl Neurobiol* 1994;20:543–550.

Parkinson D. Human spinal arachnoid septa, trabeculae, and rogue strands. *Am J Anat* 1991;192:498–509.

Parkinson D. Lateral sellar compartment OT (cavernous sinus): history, anatomy, terminology. Anat Rec 1998; 251:486–490.

Strazielle N, Ghersiegea JF. Choroid plexus in the central nervous system: biology and physiopathology. *J Neuropathol Exp Neurol* 2000;59:561–574.

Vandenabeele F, Creemers J, Lambrichts I. Ultrastructure of the human spinal arachnoid mater and dura mater. *J Anat* 1996;189:417–430.

Weller RO, Kida S, Zhang ET. Pathways of fluid drainage from the brain: morphological aspects and immunological significance in rat and man. *Brain Pathol* 1992;2: 277–284.

Weninger WJ, Pramhas D. Compartments of the adult parasellar region. *J Anat* 2000;197:681–686.

Zhang ET, Inman CBE, Weller RO. Interrelationships of the pia mater and the perivascular (Virchow-Robin) spaces of the human cerebrum. *J Anat* 1990;170:111–123.

Glossary of Neuroanatomical and Related Terms

In this text, the standard Latin forms of anatomical names are anglicized wherever this is possible without loss of euphony. Most anatomical terms have Latin origins, and most names related to diseases are derived from Greek words. Many words are defined and explained (without etymology) in the text. If you cannot find a word in this glossary, try the Index. For eponyms (names of people, applied to structures, syndromes, or diseases) consult the CD-ROM that accompanies the printed book.

Abbreviations

Eng., *English*; Fr., *French*; Ger., *German*; Gr., *Greek*; L., *Latin*; O.E., *Old English*

A

Abducens. L. *ab*, from + *ducens*, leading. Abducens (or abducent) nerve supplies the muscle that moves the direction of gaze away from the midline.

Abulia. Gr. *a*, without + *boule*, will. A loss of willpower. (Also spelled **aboulia**.)

Accumbens. L. reclining. The nucleus accumbens is the ventral part of the head of the caudate nucleus, anterior and ventral to the anterior limb of the internal capsule.

Adenohypophysis. Gr. *aden*, gland + *hypophysis* (which see). The part of the pituitary gland derived from the pharyngeal endoderm (Rathke's pouch). Its largest part is the anterior lobe of the pituitary gland.

Adiadochokinesia. *a*, neg. + Gr. *diadochos*, succeeding + *kinesis*, movement. Inability to perform rapidly alternating movements. Also called dysdiadochokinesia.

Ageusia. Gr. *a*, without + *geuein*, to taste. Loss of the sense of taste.

Agnosia. *a*, neg. + Gr. *gnosis*, knowledge. Lack of ability to recognize the significance of sensory stimuli (auditory, visual, tactile, etc., agnosia).

Agraphia. *a*, neg. + Gr. *graphein*, to write. Inability to express thoughts in writing owing to a central lesion.

Akinesia. *a*, neg. + Gr. *kinesis*, movement. Loss of movement (adjective, **akinetic**). Often used to mean severe bradykinesia, a feature of advanced Parkinson's disease.

Ala cinerea. L. wing + *cinereus*, ashen-hued. Vagal triangle in floor of fourth ventricle.

Alexia. *a*, neg. + Gr. *lexis*, word. Loss of the power to grasp the meaning of written or printed words and sentences.

Alimentary. L. *alimentarius*, about food. The alimentary canal or tract is the passage extending from the mouth to the anus.

Allocortex. Gr. *allos*, other + L. *cortex*, bark. Phylogenetically older cerebral cortex, usually consisting of three layers. Includes paleocortex and archicortex.

Allodynia. Gr. *allos*, other + *dynamis*, power or force. A condition in which the nervous system misinterprets a sensory stimulus. The word is usually used when a harmless sensation such as touch is consciously felt as pain, which may be excruciating.

Alveus. L. trough. Thin layer of white matter covering the ventricular surface of the hippocampus. (The name seems quite inappropriate but has become an accepted part of anatomical terminology.)

Amacrine. *a*, neg. + Gr. *makros*, long + *inos*, fiber. Amacrine nerve cell of the retina.

Ambiguus. L. changeable or doubtful. Nucleus ambiguus (Chs. 7 and 8) occupies an atypically ventral position for a cranial nerve nucleus, and its limits are somewhat indistinct.

Ammon's horn. Hippocampus, which has an outline in cross section suggestive of a ram's horn. Also known as the cornu Ammonis. Ammon was an Egyptian deity with a ram's head.

Amoeboid. Gr. *amoibe*, change. Relating to a cell that continuously changes its shape and looks like an amoeba.

Ampulla. L. *ampla*, full + *bulla*, vase. A bulge in a tubular structure.

Amygdala. L. *amygdalum*, from Gr. *amygdale*, almond. Amygdala or amygdaloid body in the temporal lobe of the cerebral hemisphere.

Aneurysm. Gr. *aneurysma*, dilation or widening. An abnormal widening of an artery. It can compress nearby structures and may burst.

Anlage. Ger. arrangement, layout (among other meanings). The grouping of cells in an embryo that is the beginning of an anatomical structure (Plural: **anlagen**).

Anopia. (also **Anopsia**). *an*, neg. + Gr. *opsis*, vision. Defect of vision.

Ansa hypoglossi. L. *ansa*, handle + Gr. *hypo*, under + Gr. *glossa*, tongue. Loop of nerves containing axons of the first three cervical roots that encircles the common carotid artery and internal jugular vein in the neck. The fibers from C1 pass within the trunk of the hypoglossal nerve before joining the ansa. Also called the **ansa cervicalis**.

Anterior. L. *anterior* (from *ante*), before. Nearer to the front or head. In human anatomy, synonymous with ventral. In animals that do not walk upright, anterior and ventral are different directions.

Antidromic. Gr. *anti*, against + *dromos*, racecourse. Of impulses traveling in the opposite direction to what is usual in an axon.

Aphasia. *a*, neg. + Gr. *phasis*, speech. Defect of the power of expression by speech or of comprehending spoken or written language.

Apraxia. *a*, neg. + Gr. *prassein*, to do. Inability to carry out purposeful movements in the absence of paralysis.

Arachnoid. Gr. *arachne*, spider's web + *eidos*, resemblance. Meningeal layer that forms the outer boundary of the subarachnoid space.

Archicerebellum. Gr. *arche*, beginning + diminutive of cerebrum. Phylogenetically old part of the cerebellum, functioning in the maintenance of equilibrium. Also spelled archeocerebellum.

Archicortex. Gr. *arche*, beginning + L. *cortex*, bark. Three-layered cortex included in the limbic system; located mainly in the hippocampus and dentate gyrus of the temporal lobe. Also spelled archeocortex.

Area postrema. Area in the caudal part of the floor of the fourth ventricle.

Arrector pili. L. *arrectus*, upright + *pilus*, hair. A cutaneous muscle that moves a hair.

Astereognosis. *a*, neg. + *stereos*, solid + *gnosis*, knowledge. Loss of ability to recognize objects or to appreciate their form by touching or feeling them.

Astrocyte. Gr. *astron*, star + *kytos*, hollow (cell). Type of neuroglial cell.

Asynergy. *a*, neg. + Gr. *syn*, with + *ergon*, work. Disturbance of the proper association in the contraction of muscles that ensures that the different components of an act follow in proper sequence, at the proper moment, and of the proper degree, so that the act is executed accurately.

Ataxia. *a*, neg. + Gr. *taxis*, order. Loss of power of muscle coordination, with irregularity of muscle action.

Atheroma. Gr. *athere*, porridge. Thickening of the lining of an artery caused by deposition of lipid material.

Athetosis. Gr. *athetos*, without position or place. Affliction of the nervous system caused by degenerative changes in the corpus striatum and cerebral cortex and characterized by bizarre, writhing movements of the fingers and toes, especially.

Atlas. Gr. *atlao*, I sustain. The first cervical vertebra.

Atresia. *a*, neg. + Gr. *tresis*, perforation. Absence of a passage caused by an error in development.

Atrophy. *a*, neg. + Gr. *trophe*, nourishment. Diminution of size and functional activity; wasting; emaciation.

Autoimmunity. Gr. *auto*, self + *im*, not + *munis*, serving. A condition in which antibodies or cells of the immune system attack a part of their own body.

Autonomic. Gr. *autos*, self + *nomos*, law. Autonomic system; the efferent or motor innervation of viscera.

Autoradiography. Gr. *autos*, self + L. *radius*, ray + Gr. *graphein*, to write. Technique that uses a photographic emulsion to detect the location of radioactive isotopes in tissue sections. Also called radioautography.

Axolemma. Gr. *axon*, axis + *lemma*, husk. Plasma membrane of an axon.

Axon. Gr. *axon*, axis. Efferent process of a neuron that conducts impulses to other neurons or to muscle fibers (striated and smooth) and gland cells.

Axon hillock. Region of the nerve cell body from which the axon arises; it contains no Nissl material.

Axon reaction. Changes in the cell body of a neuron after damage to its axon.

Axoplasm. Gr. *axon*, axis + *plasm*, anything formed or molded. Cytoplasm of the axon.

B

Ballism. See hemiballismus.

Baroreceptor. Gr. *baros*, weight + *receptor*, receiver. Sensory nerve terminal that is stimulated by changes in pressure, as in the carotid sinus and aortic arch.

Basis pedunculi. Ventral part of the cerebral peduncle of the midbrain on each side, separated from the dorsal part by the substantia nigra. Also called the crus cerebri.

Brachium. L. from Gr. *brachion*, arm. As used in the central nervous system, denotes a large bundle of fibers that connects one part with another (e.g., brachia associated with the colliculi of the midbrain).

Bradykinesia. Gr. *brady*, slow + *kinesis*, movement. Abnormal slowness of movements; one of the three major abnormalities resulting from Parkinson's disease.

Brain stem. In the mature human brain, denotes the medulla, pons, and midbrain. In descriptions of the embryonic brain, the diencephalon is included as well.

Bulb. Referred at one time to the medulla oblongata, but in the context of "corticobulbar tract," refers to the brain stem, in which motor nuclei of cranial nerves are located.

Bulbospongiosus muscle. L. *bulbus*, bulb or onion + *spongia*, sponge. Muscle surrounding the corpus spongiosus, the body of erectile tissue surrounding the urethra at the base of the penis.

C

Calamus scriptorius. L. *calamus*, a reed, therefore a reed pen. Refers to an area in the caudal part of the floor of the fourth ventricle that is shaped somewhat like a pen point.

Calcaneus. L. *calcaneum*, the heel. Relating to the calcaneum, which is the bone in the heel of the foot. The tendo calcaneus (Achilles' tendon) inserts into the superior surface of the posterior end of the calcaneum.

Calcar. L. spur, used to denote any spur-shaped structure. Calcar avis, an elevation on the medial aspects of the lateral ventricles at the junction of occipital and temporal horns. Also calcarine sulcus of occipital lobe, which is responsible for the calcar avis.

Cauda equina. L. horse's tail. Lumbar and sacral spinal nerve roots in the lower part of the spinal canal.

Caudal. L. *cauda*, tail. Along the axis of the central nervous system, toward the tail. In human anatomy, approximately equivalent in the brain stem and spinal cord to "inferior" and in the forebrain to "posterior." Opposite of rostral.

Caudate nucleus. Part of the corpus striatum, so named because it has a long extension or tail.

Cerebellum. L. diminutive of *cerebrum*, brain. Large part of the brain with motor functions situated in the posterior cranial fossa.

Cerebrum. L. brain. Principal portion of the brain, including the diencephalon and cerebral hemispheres but not the brain stem and cerebellum.

Channel. A protein molecule in a cell membrane that allows the passage of a particular ion, such as sodium, calcium, potassium or chloride, into or out of the cell, following a concentration gradient. Channels typically are gated, meaning that they open and close in response to neurotransmitters or local changes in membrane potential.

Cholinergic. Using acetylcholine as a neurotransmitter.

Chordotomy. Gr. *chorde*, cord + *tome*, a cutting. Division of the spinothalamic and spinoreticular tracts for intractable pain (tractotomy). Also spelled cordotomy.

Chorea. L. from Gr. *choros*, a dance. Disorder characterized by irregular, spasmodic, involuntary movements of the limbs or facial muscles. Attributed to degenerative changes in the neostriatum.

Choroid. Gr. *chorion*, a delicate membrane + *eidos*, form. Choroid or vascular coat of the eye; choroid plexuses in the ventricles of the brain. Also spelled chorioid.

Chromatolysis. Gr. *chroma*, color + *lysis*, dissolution. Dispersal of the Nissl material of neurons after axon section or in viral infections of the nervous system.

Cinereum. L. *cinereum*, ashen-hued, from *cinis*, ash. Refers to gray matter, but limited in usage. Tuber cinereum (ventral portion of the hypothalamus, from which the neurohypophysis arises); tuberculum cinereum (slight elevation on medulla formed by spinal tract and nucleus of trigeminal nerve); ala cinerea (vagal triangle in floor of fourth ventricle).

Cingulum. L. girdle. Bundle of association fibers in the white matter of the cingulate gyrus on the medial surface of the cerebral hemisphere.

Circumventricular organs. Small regions composed of atypical brain tissue in the walls of the third (see Ch. 11) and fourth (see Ch. 9) ventricles. These structures lack a blood-brain barrier and have chemoreceptor or neurosecretory functions.

Claustrum. L. a barrier. Thin sheet of gray matter of unknown function situated between the lentiform nucleus and the insula.

Clinoid processes. Gr. *kline*, bed + *oides*, shape. The anterior and posterior clinoid processes are four bony points at the corners of the diaphragma sellae (*q.v.*), named from a fancied resemblance to a four-poster bed.

Clivus. L. slope. The sloping bone between the pituitary fossa and the foramen magnum, formed from the fused sphenoid and occipital bones.

Cochlea. L. *coclea* and Gr. *kocklias*, snail. The spiral cavity of the inner ear and its contents.

Colliculus. L. Small elevation or mound. Superior and inferior colliculi composing the tectum of the midbrain; facial colliculus in the floor of the fourth ventricle.

Commissure. L. a joining together. Bundle of nerve fibers that passes from one side to the other in the brain or spinal cord. Strictly, this term should be applied to tracts that connect symmetrical structures (cf. **decussation**).

Conjugate. L. *con-*, together + *jugum*, a yoke. Relating to coordinated movements of both eyes in the same direction.

Contracture. Persistent shortening, as in a muscle paralyzed for a long time.

Contralateral. L. *contra*, opposite + *lateris* of a side. Of the other (left or right) side of the body. Opposite of "ipsilateral."

Cornu. L. horn. See **Ammon's horn**. Horns of the lateral ventricle and of the spinal gray matter are also formally named as cornua.

Corona. L. *corona* (or Gr. *korone*), a crown. Corona radiata (fibers radiating from the internal capsule to various parts of the cerebral cortex).

Coronal. Gr. *korone* or L. *corona*, a crown. The coronal suture traverses the top of the head, separating the frontal bone from the parietal bones. A coronal section is one cut in or parallel to the plane of the coronal suture; these planes are sometimes called frontal.

Corpus callosum. L. body + hard. L. *callum* can also mean a beam or rafter. Main neocortical commissure of the cerebral hemispheres. (In the second century AD, Galen called this structure a beam or rafter. It has a tougher consistency than the cerebral cortex.)

Corpus luteum. L. body + *luteum*, yellow. Progesterone-secreting endocrine tissue that forms in the ovary after ovulation.

Corpus striatum. L. body + *striatus*, furrowed or striped. Mass of gray matter with motor functions at the base of each cerebral hemisphere.

Cortex. L. bark. Outer layer of gray matter of the cerebral hemispheres and cerebellum.

Cortical. L. *corticis*, of bark. Of or relating to a cortex.

Corticofugal. L. *cortico*, from bark + *fugere*. to flee from. Describes efferent axons of neurons in a region of a cortex that terminate somewhere else: in a remote cortical area or in a subcortical nucleus of the cerebrum or cerebellum.

Corticopetal. L. *cortico*, to bark + *petere*, to seek. Describes axons afferent to a cortex.

Cribriform. L. *cribrum*, sieve + *formare*, to shape. Perforated by numerous holes. The cribriform plate of the ethmoid bone has about 20 small foramina on each side, accommodating the olfactory nerves.

Crista. L. crest. Used in anatomy for various ridge-like structures, including the cristae ampullares of the kinetic labyrinth. The crista galli (L. *galli*, of a cockerel) is an upward projection of the ethmoid bone in the midline of the anterior cranial fossa.

Crus. L. leg. Crus cerebri is the ventral part of the cerebral peduncle of the midbrain on each side, separated from the dorsal part by the substantia nigra. Also called the basis pedunculi. Crus of the fornix.

Cuneus. L. wedge. Gyrus on the medial surface of the cerebral hemisphere. Fasciculus cuneatus in the spinal cord and medulla; nucleus cuneatus in the medulla.

Cupula. L. diminutive of *cupa*, tub. A small concave structure. The gelatinous cap of the crista ampullaris. Also applied to the apex of the cochlea.

Cytosol. Gr. *kytos*, a hollow vessel + solution. Soluble portion of the cytoplasm, excluding all membranous and particulate components.

D

Decussation. L. *decussatio*, from *decussis*, the numeral X. Point of crossing of paired tracts. Decussations of the pyramids, medial lemnisci, and superior cerebellar peduncles are examples. A decussation connects asymmetrical parts of the nervous system.

Dendrite. Gr. *dendrites*, related to a tree. Process of a nerve cell on which axons of other neurons terminate. Sometimes also used for the peripheral process of a primary sensory neuron, although this has the histological and physiological properties of an axon.

Denervation. Loss of innervation due to transection of axons or death of the somata of the innervating neurons.

Dentate. L. *dentatus*, toothed. Dentate nucleus of the cerebellum; dentate gyrus in the temporal lobe.

Diabetes. Gr. *diabetes*, a syphon. Disease with excessive production of urine. In **diabetes mellitus** (L. *mellitus*, sweet), the urine contains sugar, whereas in **diabetes insipidus** (L. *in*, not + *sapor*, flavor), the urine is watery and quite tasteless.

Diaphragma sellae. Gr. *dia*, across + *phragma*, wall + L. *sellae*, of a saddle. The membrane of dura mater that covers the sella turcica and is pierced by the pituitary stalk.

Diencephalon. Gr. *dia*, through + *enkephalos*, brain. Part of the cerebrum, consisting of the thalamus, epithalamus, subthalamus, and hypothalamus; the more caudal and medial part of the prosencephalon of the developing embryo.

Diplopia. Gr. *diploos*, double + *ops*, eye. Double vision.

Dorsal. L. *dorsum*, the back. Toward the back; the direction opposite to ventral. In human anatomy, dorsal is synonymous with posterior when applied to structures in the head and trunk.

Dorsiflexion. From dorsal and flexor. Movement at the ankle that raises the toes and depresses the heel.

Dorsum sellae. L. *dorsum*, the back + *sellae*, of a saddle. The part of the ethmoid bone that forms the posterior wall of the sella turcica or pituitary fossa in the base of the skull.

Dura. L. *dura*, hard. Dura mater (the thick external layer of the meninges).

Dyskinesia. Gr. *dys*, difficult or disordered + *kinesis*, movement. Abnormality of motor function characterized by involuntary, purposeless movements.

Dysmetria. Gr. *dys*, difficult or disordered + *metron*, measure. Disturbance of the power to control the range of movement in muscle action.

E

Ectoderm. Gr. *ektos*, outside + *derma*, skin. Most dorsal layer of cells of the early embryo, which gives rise to the epidermis, neural tube, neural crest, etc.

Edema (oedema). Gr. *oidema*, swelling. Abnormal accumulation of fluid in a tissue.

Emboliform. Gr. *embolos*, plug + L. *forma*, form. Emboliform nucleus of the cerebellum.

Embolus. Gr. *embolos*, plug. Fragment of a thrombus that breaks loose and eventually obstructs an artery.

Endomysium. Gr. *endo*, within + *myos* (*mys*), muscle. The delicate connective tissue that surrounds and separates individual contractile fibers of a muscle.

Endoneurium. Gr. *endon*, within + *neuron*, nerve. Delicate connective tissue sheath surrounding an individual nerve fiber of a peripheral nerve. Also called the sheath of Henle.

Endoplasmic reticulum. Gr. *endo*, within + *a molded form* (cytoplasm) + L. *reticulum*, small net. An array of membranes within a cell. Rough endoplasmic reticulum is associated with ribosomes, where protein molecules are assembled.

Engram. Gr. *en*, in + *gramma*, mark. Used in psychology to mean the lasting trace left in the brain by previous experience; a latent memory picture.

Entorhinal. Gr. *entos*, within + *rhis* (*rhin*-), nose. The entorhinal area is the anterior part of the parahippocampal gyrus of the temporal lobe adjacent to the uncus. It is included in the lateral olfactory area.

Eosin Y. Gr. *eos*, dawn + in (suffix that denotes an organic compound that is not a base) + Y (for yellowish, in contrast to eosin B which has a bluish cast). A red anionic dye of the xanthene series, used as a microscopical stain. It colors cytoplasm and connective tissue components various shades of orange, pink, and red.

Ependyma. Gr. *ependyma*, an upper garment. Lining epithelium of the ventricles of the brain and central canal of the spinal cord.

Epineurium. Gr. *epi*, upon + *neuron*, nerve. Connective tissue sheath surrounding a peripheral nerve.

Epithalamus. Gr. *epi*, upon + *thalamos*, inner chamber. Region of the diencephalon above the thalamus; includes the pineal gland.

Epithelium. Gr. *epi*, upon + *thele*, nipple. A layer (or multiple layers) of cells covering any external or internal surface. Originally (1700) this word meant thin skin covering the nipples or lips; later, it was applied to all skin. By the 1870s, the term was being used in its present sense.

Estrogen (oestrogen). L. *oestrus*, gadfly or frenzy + *generator*, producer. Steroid hormones (estradiol, estrone, estriol) secreted by the ovary that stimulate the secondary sex organs, especially before ovulation.

Ethmoid. Gr. *ethmos*, sieve + *oides*, shape. A bone of the skull that forms the medial part of the floor of the anterior cranial fossa and the upper part of the skeleton of the nasal cavities. The bone includes the cribriform plate.

Euphony. Gr. *eu*, well + *phone*, sound. Agreeable sound or easy pronunciation.

Exteroceptor. L. *exterus*, external + *receptor*, receiver. Sensory receptor that serves to acquaint the individual with his or her environment (exteroception).

Extrafusal. L. *extra*, outside + *fusus*, spindle. Relates to the great majority of contractile fibers of a skeletal muscle, which are outside the sensory receptor organs known as neuromuscular spindles.

Extrapyramidal system. Vague and confusing term applied to motor parts of the central nervous system other than the pyramidal motor system.

F

Falx. L. sickle. Two of the dural partitions in the cranial cavity are the falx cerebri and the small falx cerebelli.

Fasciculus. L. diminutive of *fascis*, bundle. Bundle of nerve fibers.

Fastigial. L. *fastigium*, the top of a gabled roof. Fastigial nucleus of the cerebellum.

Fenestra. L. window. A hole. Fenestra rotunda (round) and fenestra ovale (oval) are between the middle and inner ear. Capillary blood vessels are fenestrated when their endothelial cells have pores, each closed by a diaphragm that does not prevent the egress of large molecules. Such vessels typically occur in endocrine organs.

Fimbria. L. *fimbriae*, fringe. Band of nerve fibers along the medial edge of the hippocampus, continuing as the fornix.

Fistula. L. pipe. Abnormal communication between two cavities or between a cavity and the surface of the body.

In an arteriovenous fistula, blood is shunted directly from an artery into a vein or venous sinus.

Flexor. L. *flexus*, bent; *flectere*, to bend. A muscle that bends a joint.

Foramen (plural, **foramina**). L. *forare*, to pierce. A hole.

Forceps. L. a pair of tongs. Used for the U-shaped configuration of fibers that constitute the anterior and posterior portions of the corpus callosum (forceps frontalis and forceps occipitalis).

Fornix. L. arch. Efferent tract of the hippocampal formation, arching over the thalamus and terminating mainly in the mamillary body of the hypothalamus.

Fossa. L. hole, ditch or grave. An indentation.

Fovea. L. a pit or depression. Fovea centralis (depression in the center of the macula lutea of the retina).

Frontal. L. *frons*, forehead. The frontal bone forms the anterior part of the cranium, including the roofs of the orbits, containing the frontal lobes of the cerebral hemispheres.

Fundus. L. bottom. Rounded interior of a hollow organ. The ocular fundus is lined by the retina, with its blood vessels, the optic disc, and other landmarks visible through an ophthalmoscope.

Funiculus. L. diminutive of *funis*, cord. Area of white matter that may consist of several functionally different fasciculi, as in the lateral funiculus of white matter of the spinal cord.

Fusiform. L. *fusus*, spindle + *forma*, shape. Widest in the middle and tapering at both ends. The fusiform gyrus is on the inferior surface of the temporal lobe, lateral to the parahippocampal gyrus.

G

GABAergic. Describes a neuron that uses gamma-aminobutyrate (GABA) as its principal synaptic transmitter.

Ganglion. Gr. knot or subcutaneous tumor. Swelling composed of nerve cells, as in cerebrospinal and sympathetic ganglia. Also used inappropriately for certain regions of gray matter in the brain (e.g., basal ganglia of the cerebral hemisphere).

Gastrocnemius. Gr. *gaster*, belly + *kneme*, leg. The muscle largely responsible for the bulging contour of the calf of the human leg.

Gemmule. L. *gemmula*, diminutive of *gemma*, bud. Minute projections on dendrites of certain neurons, especially pyramidal cells and Purkinje cells, for synaptic contact with other neurons.

Genu. L. *genu*, knee. Anterior end of corpus callosum; genu of facial nerve. Also geniculate ganglion of facial nerve and geniculate bodies of thalamus.

Glia. Gr. glue. Neuroglia, the interstitial or accessory cells of the central nervous system.

Glioblast. Gr. *glia*, glue + *blastos*, germ. Embryonic neuroglial cell.

Gliosomes. Gr. *glia*, glue + *soma*, body. Granules seen by light microscopy in neuroglial cells, especially astrocytes. They are probably mitochondria.

Globus pallidus. L. ball + pale. Medial part of lentiform nucleus of corpus striatum. Also globose nuclei of cerebellum.

Glomerulus. Diminutive of L. *glomus*, ball of yarn. Synaptic glomeruli of the olfactory bulb and cerebellum.

Glomus. L. ball of yarn. Applied to various small organs, including the carotid and aortic bodies, and to one of their characteristic cell types.

Glycocalyx. Gr. *glycyx*, sweet + *kalyx*, cup. Outer coating of carbohydrate molecules on the surface of cells.

Golgi apparatus. An array of membranous compartments within the cytoplasm, where proteins combine with carbohydrates to form glycoproteins.

Gonadotrophic (also **gonadotropic**). Gr. *gone*, generation + *trephein*, to feed (*trophe*, food), or *trepein*, to turn (*tropos*, a turning). Gonadotrophic hormones are secreted by the anterior lobe of the pituitary gland and in pregnancy by the placenta. They act upon the gonads (ovary or testis) and are essential for the functions of these organs.

Gracilis. L. slender. Fasciculus gracilis of the spinal cord and medulla; nucleus gracilis and gracile tubercle of the medulla.

Granule. L. *granulum*, diminutive of *granum*, grain. Used to denote small neurons, such as granule cells of cerebellar cortex and stellate cells of cerebral cortex. Hence granular cell layers of both cortices.

H

Habenula. L. diminutive of *habena*, strap or rein. Small swelling in the epithalamus adjacent to the posterior end of the roof of the third ventricle.

Haarscheibe. Ger. *haar*, hair + *scheibe*, disk. Small elevated area of skin that develops in association with specialized hair follicles and serves as a receptor for tactile stimuli.

Helicotrema. Gr. *helix*, snail or coil + *trema*, hole. The communication between the scala tympani and scala vestibuli at the apex of the cochlea.

Hemalum. From Eng. hematein + alum. A solution containing hematein and aluminum ions, used to stain the nuclei of cells blue. (Hematein is a yellow dye made by oxidation of hematoxylin, which is a colorless compound extracted from the wood of the logwood tree, *Hematoxylon campechianum*.) Hemalum is frequently used with eosin Y, a dye that colors tissue components other than nuclei pink. The combination ("H & E") is the most frequently used staining method in pathology laboratories.

Hemianopia. Gr. *hemi*, half + *an*, neg. + *opsis*, vision. Loss of half of a field of vision. Also called hemianopsia.

Hemiballismus. Gr. *hemi*, half + *ballismos*, jumping. Violent form of motor restlessness that involves one side of the body, caused by a destructive lesion involving the subthalamic nucleus.

Hemiplegia. Gr. *hemi*, half + *plege*, a blow or stroke. Paralysis of one side of the body.

Herpes zoster Gr. *herpein*, to creep + *zoster*, waist-belt. Virus infection of neurons in a sensory ganglion, causing painful inflammation with small blisters in the corresponding area of skin. (Also called *shingles*; systemic invection with the same virus causes chicken pox.)

Hippocampus. Gr. *hippos*, horse + *kampos*, sea monster; also the zoological name for a genus of small fishes known as sea horses. Rather inappropriate name given to a gyrus that constitutes an important part of the limbic system; produces an elevation on the floor of the temporal horn of the lateral ventricle.

Homeostasis. Gr. *homois*, like + *stasis*, standing. Tendency toward stability in the internal environment of the organism.

Homonymous. Gr. *homonymos* and L. *homonymus*, having the same name. Applied to defects in the same part (left or right) of the visual field of both eyes, in consequence of transection of the visual pathway posterior to the optic chiasma.

Hormone. Gr. *hormaein*, to stir up. A compound secreted into the blood, which exercises a specific physiological function elsewhere in the body.

Hydrocephalus. Gr. *hydror*, water + *kephale*, head. Excessive accumulation of cerebrospinal fluid.

Hyperacusis. Gr. *hyper*, over + *acacias*, a hearing. Abnormal loudness of perceived sounds.

Hypertension. Gr. *hyper*, above measure + L. *tension*, I stretch. (Before 1700, the word tension was incorrectly used as a synonym for pressure.) Abnormally high arterial blood pressure.

Hypophysis. Gr. from *hypo*, under + *phytin*, to grow. The pituitary gland (considered as an attachment underneath the brain).

Hypothalamus. Gr. *hypo*, under + *thalamus*, inner chamber. Region of the diencephalon that serves as the main controlling center of the autonomic nervous system.

I

Induction. L. *inducere*, to bring in. In embryology, action of one population of cells on the development of another population nearby.

Indusium. L. a garment, from *induo*, to put on. Indusium griseum, thin layer of gray matter on the dorsal surface of the corpus callosum (gray tunic).

Inferior. L. comparative of *inferus* (from *infra*), lower or below. In human anatomy, nearer to the soles of the feet. In animals that are not bipedal, the equivalent term is posterior.

Infarction. L. *infarcire*, to stuff or fill in. Regional death of tissue caused by loss of blood supply. The resulting piece of nonfunctional material is called an **infarct**. In the central nervous system, an infarct replaces axons and/or cell bodies of neurons.

Infundibulum. L. funnel. Infundibular stem of the neurohypophysis.

Innervation. The normal condition in which axons and their presynaptic endings make functional contact with other cells. The associated verb is **innervate**.

Insula. L. island. Cerebral cortex concealed from surface view and lying at the bottom of the lateral sulcus. Also called the island of Reil.

Interoceptor. L. *inter*, between + *receptor*, receiver. One of the sensory end organs within viscera.

Interstitial. L. *inter*, between + *statum*, placed. Within spaces. Interstitial cells of the testis are in the spaces between the seminiferous tubules.

Intrafusal. L. *intra*, within + *fusus*, spindle. Relates to the contractile muscle fibers within the capsule of a neuromuscular spindle.

Ipsilateral. L. *ipse*, itself + *lateris* of a side. Of the same side (left or right) of the body. Opposite of "contralateral."

Ischemia. Gr. *ischein*, to check + *haimos*, blood. Condition of tissue that is not adequately perfused with oxygenated blood.

Ischiocavernosus muscle. Gr. *ischion*, hip joint + L. *caverna*, cave or hollow. Paired muscle associated with the bodies of erectile tissue on either side of the base of the penis.

Isocortex. Gr. *isos*, equal + L. *cortex*, bark. Cerebral cortex having six layers (neocortex).

J

Juxtarestiform body. L. *juxta*, next door to + *restis*, rope + *forma*, shape. Vestibulocerebellar fibers, which lie along the medial surface of the restiform body (*q.v.*).

K

Kinesthesia. Gr. *kinesis*, movement + *aisthesis*, sensation. Sense of perception of movement.

Koniocortex. Gr. *konis*, dust + L. *cortex*, bark. Areas of cerebral cortex that contain large numbers of small neurons; typical of sensory areas.

L

Labyrinth. Gr *labyrinthos*, building with intricate passages. The cavities and canals of the inner ear within the petrous part of the temporal bone.

Lamella. Diminutive of L. *lamina*, plate or leaf. A thin layer or membrane.

Lamina propria. L. *lamina*, plate or leaf + *propria*, characteristic, one's own. Connective tissue layer underlying an epithelium.

Lateral. L. *latus*, side or flank. Away from the midline.

Lemniscus. Gr. *lemniskos*, fillet (a ribbon or band). Used to designate a bundle of nerve fibers in the central nervous system (e.g., medial lemniscus and lateral lemniscus).

Lentiform. L. *lens* (*lent*-), a lentil (lens) + *forma*, shape. Lens-shaped. Lentiform nucleus, a component of the corpus striatum. Also called lenticular nucleus.

Leptomeninges. Gr. *leptos*, slender + *meninx*, membrane. Arachnoid and pia mater.

Lesion. L. *laesum*, hurt or wounded. Applied to any abnormality. In the nervous system, a lesion may be destructive (such as an infarct, injury, hemorrhage, or tumor), or it may stimulate neurons (as in epilepsy).

Limbus. L. a hem or border. Limbic lobe: C-shaped configuration of cortex on the medial surface of the cerebral hemisphere that consists of the septal area and the cingulate and parahippocampal gyri. Limbic system: limbic lobe, hippocampal formation, and portions of the diencephalon, especially the mamillary body and anterior thalamic nuclei.

Limen. L. threshold. Limen insulae: ventral part of the insula; included in the lateral olfactory area.

Locus coeruleus. L. place + *caeruleus*, dark blue. Small dark spot on each side of the floor of the fourth ventricle; marks the position of a group of nerve cells that contain melanin pigment.

M

Macroglia. Gr. *makros*, large + *glia*, glue. Larger types of neuroglial cells: astrocytes, oligodendrocytes, and ependymal cells.

Macrophage. Gr. *makros*, great + *phagein*, to eat. A type of white blood cell (monocyte) that has entered connective tissue and assumed phagocytic properties.

Macrosmatic. Gr. *makros*, large + *osme*, smell. Having the sense of smell strongly or acutely developed.

Macula. L. a spot. Macula lutea: spot at the posterior pole of the eye that has a yellow color when viewed with red-free light. Maculae sacculi and utriculi: sensory areas in the vestibular portion of the membranous labyrinth.

Mamillary. L. *mammilla*, diminutive of *mamma*, breast (shaped like a nipple). Mamillary bodies: swellings on the ventral surface of the hypothalamus. Also spelled mammillary.

Massa intermedia. Bridge of gray matter that connects the thalami of the two sides across the third ventricle; present in 70% of human brains. Also called the interthalamic adhesion.

Mastoid. Gr. *mastos*, breast + *oeides*, shape. The mastoid process is the downwardly projecting part of the temporal bone behind the ear.

Meatus. L. passage. The internal acoustic meatus is the bony canal that contains the eighth cranial nerves and the labyrinthine vessels as they pass within the petrous part of the temporal bone.

Medial. L. *medius*, middle. Toward the midline (a relative term).

Median. L. *medianus*, in the middle. Located in the midline.

Medulla. L. marrow, from *medius*, middle. Medulla spinalis: spinal cord. Medulla oblongata: caudal portion of the brain stem. In current usage, "medulla" means the medulla oblongata.

Medulloblastoma. Malignant tumor of young children, usually in the midline of the cerebellum, enlarging into the fourth ventricle and spreading by way of the subarachnoid space to other parts of the central nervous system.

Mesencephalon. Gr. *mesos*, middle + *enkephalos*, brain. The midbrain; also its embryonic precursor, the part of the neural tube interposed between the forebrain and hindbrain.

Mesoderm. Gr. *mesos*, middle + *derma*, skin. Middle layer of cells of the early embryo, which gives rise to connective tissues, muscle, etc.

Metathalamus. Gr. *meta*, after + *thalamus*, inner chamber. Medial and lateral geniculate bodies (nuclei).

Metencephalon. Gr. *meta*, after + *enkephalos*, brain. Pons and cerebellum; the more rostral of the two divisions of the rhombencephalon or hindbrain.

Microglia. Gr. *mikros*, small + *glia*, glue. Type of neuroglial cell.

Microsmatic. Gr. *mikros*, small + *osme*, smell. Having a sense of smell, but of relatively poor development.

Microvillus. Gr. *mikros*, small + L. *villus*, hair. Hair-like projections of a cell, typically presenting a striated appearance in light microscopy but individually resolved by the electron microscope and seen to be cytoplasmic protrusions.

Mimetic. Gr. *mimetikos*, imitative. Muscles of expression supplied by the facial nerve; sometimes referred to as mimetic muscles.

Miotic. Gr. *meiosis*, diminution. A drug causing constriction of the pupil of the eye.

Mitochondrion. Gr. *mitos*, thread + *chondros*, granule. A cytoplasmic organelle with distinctive ultrastructure, containing respiratory enzymes.

Mitral. L. *mitra*, a turban; later the tall, cleft hat (miter) of a bishop. Mitral cells of the olfactory bulb.

Mnemonic. Gr. *mneme*, memory. Pertaining to memory.

Molecular. L. *molecula*, diminutive of *moles*, mass. Used in neurohistology to denote tissue that contains large numbers of fine nerve fibers and that, therefore, has a punctate appearance in silver-stained sections. Molecular layers of cerebral and cerebellar cortices.

Mucosa or **mucous membrane.** From L. mucus. The moist lining of a cavity or hollow organ, consisting of an epithelium with glands that secrete mucus, the underlying lamina propria, and (in the alimentary tract) the muscularis mucosae.

Muscularis mucosae. L. muscle + of mucosa. A thin layer of smooth muscle tissue beneath (external to) the lamina propria in the mucosa of the alimentary tract.

Mutism. L. *mutus*, silent or dumb. Inability to speak.

Myasthenia gravis. Gr. *myos*, muscle + *a*, without + *sthenos*, strength + L. *gravis*, heavy (severe). Disease in which there is failure of neuromuscular transmission (see Ch. 3).

Myelencephalon. Gr. *myelos*, marrow + *enkephalos*, brain. Medulla oblongata; the more caudal of the two divisions of the rhombencephalon or hindbrain.

Myelin. Gr. *myelos*, marrow. Layers of lipid and protein substances that form a sheath around axons.

Myenteric. Gr. *myos*, muscle + *enteron*, intestine. The myenteric plexus lies between the longitudinal (outer) and circular layers of smooth muscle of the intestine and other parts of the alimentary tract.

Mydriatic. Gr. *mydriasis*, enlargement of the pupil. A drug causing dilation of the pupil of the eye.

Myoepithelial cell. Gr. *myos*, muscle + *epi*, upon + *thele*, nipple. Contractile cell that embraces a secretory unit (acinus or alveolus) of a gland and propels the contents into a duct.

Myotrophic. Gr. *myos*, muscle + *trephein*, to nourish. Responsible for maintaining the structural and functional integrity of muscle (principally by chemical agents from motor neurons, hence the earlier but ambiguous term "neurotrophic").

N

Neocerebellum. Gr. *neos*, new + diminutive of cerebrum. Phylogenetically newest part of the cerebellum present in mammals and especially well developed in humans. Ensures smooth muscle action in the finer voluntary movements.

Neocortex. Gr. *neos*, new + L. *cortex*, bark. Six-layered cortex, characteristic of mammals and constituting most of the cerebral cortex in humans.

Neostriatum. Gr. *neos*, new + L. *striatus*, striped or grooved. Phylogenetically newer part of the corpus striatum that consists of the caudate nucleus and putamen; the striatum.

Neuralgia. Gr. *neuron*, nerve + *algein*, to suffer. Pain attributed to abnormal stimulation of sensory fibers in the peripheral nervous system.

Neurite. Gr. *neurites*, of a nerve. Cytoplasmic processes of neurons. The term embraces both axons and dendrites.

Neurobiotaxis. Gr. *neuron*, nerve + *bios*, life + *taxis*, arrangement. Tendency of nerve cells to move during embryological development toward the area from which they receive the most stimuli.

Neuroblast. Gr. *neuron*, a nerve + *blastos*, germ. Embryonic nerve cell.

Neurofibril. Gr. *neuron*, nerve + L. *fibrilla*, diminutive of *fibra*, fiber. Filaments in the cytoplasm of neurons (see Ch. 2).

Neuroglia. Gr. *neuron*, nerve + *glia*, glue. Accessory or interstitial cells of the nervous system; includes astrocytes, oligodendrocytes, microglial cells, ependymal cells, satellite cells, and Schwann cells.

Neurohypophysis. Gr. *neuron*, nerve + *hypophysis*. An endocrine organ that is a ventral protuberance of the hypothalamus, comprising the median eminence of the tuber cinereum, the infundibular stem (which is the nervous tissue of the pituitary stalk) and the neural lobe or infundibular process, which is the major part of the posterior lobe of the pituitary gland.

Neurokeratin. Gr. *neuron*, nerve + *keras* (*kerat-*), horn. Fibrillar material consisting of proteins that remain after lipids have been dissolved from myelin sheaths.

Neurolemma. Gr. *neuron*, nerve + *lemma*, husk. Delicate sheath surrounding a peripheral nerve fiber consisting of a series of neurolemma cells or Schwann cells. Also spelled neurilemma.

Neuroma. Gr. *neuron*, nerve + *-oma*, indicating a tumor. Swelling of a severed or otherwise injured nerve, containing a profusion of axonal sprouts that have failed to regrow usefully.

Neuron. Gr. a nerve. Morphological unit of the nervous system consisting of the nerve cell body and its processes (dendrites and axon).

Neuropil. Gr. *neuron*, nerve + *pilos*, felt. Complex net of nerve cell processes that occupies the intervals between cell bodies in gray matter.

Neurosecretion. The activity of a cell that has the signaling properties of a neuron and the secretory properties of an endocrine cell: a neuron that releases a hormone into the blood.

Nociceptive. L. *noceo*, I injure + *capio*, I take. Responsive to injurious stimuli.

Nucleolus. Diminutive of *nucleus* (see below). An inclusion within the nucleus of a cell, composed of protein and RNA.

Nucleus. L. nut, kernel. (1) Body in a cell that contains, in the DNA of its chromosomes, the genetic information that encodes the amino acid sequences of proteins. (2) Collection of neuronal cell bodies, which may be large (like the caudate nucleus) or microscopic (like many nuclei in the brain stem).

Nystagmus. Gr. *nystagmos*, a nodding, from *nystazein*, to be sleepy. Involuntary oscillation of the eyes.

O

Obex. L. bar, bolt, or barrier. Small transverse fold overhanging the opening of the fourth ventricle into the central canal of the closed portion of the medulla.

Occipital. L. *occipitium*, back of the head. Pertaining to the back of the head, which can be called the occiput. Occipital bone and occipital lobes of the cerebral hemisphere.

Oligodendrocyte. Gr. *oligos*, few + *dendron*, tree + *kytos*, hollow (cell). Type of neuroglial cell. Forms the myelin

sheath in the central nervous system in the same manner as the Schwann cell in peripheral nerves.

Olive. L. *oliva*. Oval bulging of the lateral area of the medulla. Inferior, accessory, and superior olivary nuclei.

Ontogeny. Gr. *ontos*, being + *genesis*, generation. Development of an individual. The adjective **ontogenetic**, which means much the same as "embryological" or "developmental," is used in contrast to "phylogenetic" (which see).

Operculum. L. a cover or lid, from L. *opertum*, covered. Frontal, parietal, and temporal opercula bound the lateral sulcus of the cerebral hemisphere and conceal the insula.

Osseous. L. *ossis*, of bone. Composed of bone: osseous spiral lamina of the cochlea.

Otic. Gr. *otos*, of the ear. The otic vesicle is the anlage of the inner ear. The otic ganglion is near the middle ear.

Otolith. Gr. *otos*, of the ear + *lithos*, stone. One of the particles of calcium carbonate associated with the hair cells of the utricle and saccule (otolithic organs) of the inner ear.

Oxytocin. Gr. *oxys*, sharp + *tokos*, birth. An octapeptide hormone of the neurohypophysis that stimulates the smooth muscle of the uterus and the myoepithelial cells of the mammary glands.

P

Pachymeninx. Gr. *pachys*, thick + *meninx*, membrane. Dura mater.

Paleocerebellum. Gr. *palaios*, old + diminutive of cerebrum. Phylogenetically old part of the cerebellum that functions in postural changes and locomotion.

Paleocortex. Gr. *palaios*, old + L. *cortex*, bark. Olfactory cortex consisting of three to five layers.

Paleostriatum. Gr. *palaios*, old + L. *striatum*, striped or grooved. Phylogenetically older and efferent part of the corpus striatum; the globus pallidus or pallidum.

Pallidofugal. Pallidum (see below) + L. *fugere*, to flee from. Describes the axons of neurons in the globus pallidus that conduct impulses to other parts of the brain.

Pallidum. L. *pallidus*, (*-um*), pale. Globus pallidus of the corpus striatum; medial portion of the lentiform nucleus comprising the paleostriatum.

Pallium. L. cloak. Cerebral cortex with subjacent white matter but usually used synonymously with cortex.

Paralysis. Gr. *paralysis*, secret undoing; from *para*, beside + *lyein*, to loosen. Loss of the power of motion.

Paraplegia. Gr. *para*, beside or beyond + *plege*, a stroke or blow. Paralysis of both legs and lower part of trunk.

Paramedian. Gr. *para*, beside + L. *medianus*, in the middle. In a plane parallel to the median or midsagittal plane.

Parasagittal. Gr. *para*, beside + L. *sagitta*, arrow. A word sometimes used instead of sagittal for a sagittal plane or section that is parallel to but not in the midline.

Parenchyma. Gr. *parenchein*, to pour in beside. Essential and distinctive tissue of an organ. (The name is from an early notion that internal organs contained material poured in by their blood vessels.)

Paresis. Gr. *parienai*, to relax. Partial paralysis.

Parietal. L. *parietalis*, pertaining to walls. The parietal lobes are beneath the parietal bones, which form much of the wall of the top of the cranium.

Patella. Diminutive of L. *patina*, a pan. The kneecap bone embedded in the tendon of the quadriceps group of muscles, which are extensors of the knee joint.

Pathway. Eng. Route within the central nervous system consisting of interconnected populations of neurons that serve a common function. A pathway often contains one or more tracts.

Perikaryon. Gr. *peri*, around + *karyon*, nut, kernel. Cytoplasm surrounding the nucleus. Sometimes refers to the cell body of a neuron.

Perineum. Gr. *perinaion*. Region consisting of the genitalia, the anus, and the immediately surrounding and intervening region.

Perineurium. Gr. *peri*, around + *neuron*, nerve. Cellular and connective tissue sheath surrounding a bundle of nerve fibers in a peripheral nerve.

Pernicious anemia. L. *per*, through + *necis*, of murder + Gr. *an*, negative + *haimos*, blood. Disease caused by failure to absorb vitamin B_{12} (cyanocobalamin). The vitamin deficiency results in defective production of red blood cells and degeneration in the central nervous system, including subacute combined degeneration in the spinal cord (see Ch. 5).

Pes. L. foot. Pes hippocampi: anterior thickened end of the hippocampus that slightly resembles a cat's paw.

Petrous. L. *petrosus*, rocky. The petrous part of the temporal bone, containing the inner ear, has a craggy appearance.

Phagocyte. Gr. *phagein*, to eat + *kytos*, vessel (cell). A cell that can engulf and internalize smaller objects such as bacteria and fragments of dead cells.

Phalangeal. Gr. *phalanx*, a formation of soldiers. Phalangeal cells are in lines alongside the sensory cells of the organ of Corti.

Phylogeny. Gr. *phylon*, race + *genesis*, origin. Evolutionary history, typically as deduced from comparative anatomy.

Pia mater. L. tender mother. Thin innermost layer of the meninges attached to the surface of the brain and spinal cord; forms the inner boundary of the subarachnoid space.

Pineal. L. *pineus*, relating to the pine. Shaped like a pine cone (pertaining to the pineal gland).

Plantar. From L. *planta*, plant; also applied to the foot. An adjective that relates to the sole of the foot (which often treads on small plants). The **plantaris** muscle is a small calf muscle that pulls on the sole of the foot. It is very small in the human leg but larger in the legs of quadrupeds. **Plantar flexion** is bending the ankle so that the toes point downward.

Plexus. L. plaited, interwoven. Arrangement of interwoven and intercommunicating nerve trunks or fibers or of blood vessels.

Pneumoencephalography. Gr. *pneuma*, air + *enkephalos*, brain + *graphe*, a writing. Replacement of cerebrospinal fluid by air followed by x-ray examination (pneumoencephalogram); permits visualization of the ventricles and subarachnoid space. This technique has been replaced by computed tomography (CT scan).

Pons. L. bridge. Part of the brain stem that lies between the medulla and the midbrain; appears to constitute a bridge between the right and left halves of the cerebellum.

Portal. L. *porta*, gate. A portal vein drains a capillary bed, but instead of joining larger veins that lead to the heart, it ends by branching into capillaries elsewhere.

Positron. (From *positive electron*.) Subatomic particle with the same mass as an electron and equal but opposite charge. Positrons emitted by radioactive elements combine with electrons, with elimination of matter and emission of x-rays. Detection of the latter forms the basis of positron emission tomography (PET).

Posterior. L. comparative of *post*, after. Nearer to the back or tail. In human anatomy, synonymous with dorsal when applied to structures in the head and trunk.

Postpartum. L *post*, after + *parturire*, to bring forth. Describes the condition of a mother who has recently given birth.

Progesterone. Steroid hormone secreted by the corpus luteum and the placenta.

Projection. L. *proiectus*, thrown forward. Applied to the axons of a population of neurons and their sites of termination. Often used when the axons do not constitute a circumscribed tract.

Proprioceptor. L. *proprius*, one's own + *capere*, to take (or *receptor*, receiver). One of the sensory endings in muscles, tendons, and joints; provides information concerning movement and position of parts of the body (proprioception).

Prosencephalon. Gr. *pros*, before + *enkephalos*, brain. Forebrain, consisting of the telencephalon (cerebral hemispheres) and diencephalon (thalamus and nearby structures).

Prosopagnosia. Gr. *prosopon*, person or face + agnosia (*q.v.*). Inability to recognize previously familiar faces.

Psalterium. Gr. *psalterion*, an ancient stringed instrument like a zither. The name is sometimes given to the posterior part of the body of the fornix, including the hippocampal commissure.

Ptosis. Gr. *ptosis*, a falling. Drooping of the upper eyelid.

Pulvinar. L. a cushioned seat. Posterior projection of the thalamus above the medial and lateral geniculate bodies.

Pump. A molecular channel in a cell membrane associated with enzymes that enable it to move ions in or out of the cell against a concentration gradient, with expenditure of energy.

Punctate. L. *punctum*, pricked. Apparently composed of dots, as when many axons or dendrites are seen in transverse section.

Putamen. L. shell, husk. Larger and lateral part of the lentiform nucleus of the corpus striatum.

Pyramidal system. Corticospinal and corticobulbar tracts. So-called because the corticospinal tracts occupy the fancifully pyramid-shaped area on the ventral surface of the medulla. The term pyramidal tract refers specifically to the corticospinal tract.

Pyriform. L. *pyrum*, pear + *forma*, form. Pyriform area is a region of olfactory cortex consisting of the uncus, limen insulae, and entorhinal area; has a pear-shaped outline in animals with a well-developed olfactory system.

Q

Quadriplegia. L. *quadri*, four + Gr. *plege*, stroke. Paralysis that affects the four limbs. Also called tetraplegia.

R

Ramus. L. branch. One of the first branches (*dorsal, ventral*) of a spinal nerve, or a communicating branch going to (*white*) or from (*gray*) a sympathetic ganglion. Some branches of cerebral sulci are named as rami.

Raphe. Gr. seam. Anatomical structure in the midline. In the brain, several raphe nuclei are in the midline of the medulla, pons, and midbrain. Their names are partly Latinized, as in nucleus raphes magnus (great nucleus of the raphe), etc.

Receptor. L. *receptus*, received. Word used in two ways in neurobiology: (1) Structure of any size or complexity that collects and usually also edits information about conditions inside or outside the body. Examples are the eye, the muscle spindle, and the free ending of the peripheral neurite of a sensory neuron. (2) Protein molecule embedded in the surface of a cell (or sometimes inside the cell) that specifically binds the molecules of hormones, neurotransmitters, drugs, or other substances that can change the activity of the cell.

Restiform. L. *restis*, rope + *forma*, shape. Restiform body is an old name for the inferior cerebellar peduncle.

Reticular. L. *reticularis*, pertaining to or resembling a net. Reticular formation of the brain stem.

Rhinal. Gr. *rhis*, nose, therefore related to the nose. Rhinal sulcus in the temporal lobe indicates the margin of the lateral olfactory area.

Rhinencephalon. Gr. *rhis* (rhin-), nose + *enkephalos*, brain. Obsolete term that referred to components of the olfactory system. In comparative neurology, structures incorporated in the limbic system (especially the hippocampus and dentate gyrus) were included.

Rhombencephalon. Gr. *rhombos*, a lozenge-shaped figure + *enkephalos*, brain. Pons and cerebellum (metencephalon) and medulla (myelencephalon).

Roentgenogram. After Wilhelm Konrad Roentgen (1845–1923), who discovered x-rays, + Gr. *gramma*, a letter or record. Picture made with x-rays; more often called an x-ray or a radiograph.

Rostral. Adjective from L. *rostrum*, beak, snout. Along the axis of the central nervous system, toward the nose. In human anatomy, approximately equivalent in the brain stem and spinal cord to "superior" and in the forebrain to "anterior." Opposite of caudal.

Rostrum. L. beak. Recurved portion of the corpus callosum, passing backward from the genu to the lamina terminalis.

Rubro-. L. *ruber*, red. Pertaining to the red nucleus (nucleus ruber), as in rubrospinal and corticorubral.

S

Saccadic. Fr. *saccader*, to jerk. Saccadic or quick movements of the eyes in altering direction of gaze.

Sagittal. L. *sagitta*, arrow. The sagittal suture is in the midline of the cranial vault, between the parietal bones. A sagittal section is one cut in or parallel to the median plane.

Satellite. L. *satteles*, attendant. Satellite cells: flattened cells of ectodermal origin that encapsulate nerve cell bodies in ganglia. Also satellite oligodendrocytes adjacent to nerve cell bodies in the central nervous system.

Scala. L. flight of steps. The scalae tympani, media and vestibuli mount up to the apex of the cochlea, but they do not include any steps.

Scotoma. Gr. *skotos*, darkness. A blind area in the field of vision, due to damage in the retina or central nervous system.

Sella turcica. L. Turkish saddle. The pituitary (hypophysial) fossa, a depression in the midline of the sphenoid bone that contains the pituitary gland.

Septal area. Area ventral to the genu and rostrum of the corpus callosum on the medial aspect of the frontal lobe that is the site of the septal nuclei.

Septum pellucidum. L. partition + transparent. Triangular double membrane between the frontal horns of the lateral ventricles; it fills in the interval between the corpus callosum and the fornix.

Sinus. L. word applied to various curved, folded, or hollowed-out shapes. Anatomical uses of the word include air cavities in some cranial bones and the large venous channels of the dura mater.

Sinusoid. L. *sinus* (q.v.) + Gr. *oeides*, shape. A component of a network of thin-walled blood vessels with wider diameter than ordinary capillaries, in the liver, spleen, and some endocrine organs such as the anterior lobe of the pituitary gland.

Soleus. From L. *solea*, sole of a foot or sandal, or the flat fish called sole in English. A muscle in the calf of the leg, deep to the gastrocnemius. Its action presses the sole onto the ground.

Somatic. Gr. *somatikos*, bodily. Denoting the body, exclusive of the viscera (as in somatic efferent neurons that supply the skeletal musculature).

Somatosensory. Having to do with somatic sensation. Synonymous with **somesthetic**.

Somatotopic. Gr. *soma*, body + *topos*, place. Representation of parts of the body in corresponding parts of the brain.

Somesthetic. Gr. *soma*, body + *aisthesis*, perception. Consciousness of having a body. Somesthetic senses are those of pain, temperature, touch, pressure, position, movement, and vibration. Also spelled somaesthetic.

Sphenoid. Gr. *sphen*, wedge + *oeides*, shape. A bone of complex form that extends across the base of the skull. It is interposed ("wedged") between the cranial vault and the bones of the facial skeleton.

Splenium. Gr. *splenion*, bandage. Thickened posterior extremity of the corpus callosum.

Squint. From Middle English *asquint*, with the eyes askew. See also **strabismus**.

Stellate. L. *stella*, star. Stellate neuron has many short dendrites that radiate in all directions.

Stenosis. Gr. *stenos*, narrow. Abnormal narrowing of a tube or passage.

Stereotaxic. Gr. *stereos*, solid + *taxis*, arrangement. Relating to a surgical procedure for introducing the tip of an electrode or other instrument into a predetermined position within the brain. The position is calculated from three-dimensional coordinates based on bony landmarks and supplemented by images obtained by CT or MRI.

Strabismus. Gr. *strabismos*, a squinting. Constant lack of parallelism of the visual axes of the eyes. Also known as a **squint**. (This is the only correct usage of the word squint.)

Stria terminalis. L. a furrow, groove + boundary, limit. Slender strand of fibers running along the medial side of the tail of the caudate nucleus. Originating in the amygdaloid body, most of the fibers end in the septal area and hypothalamus.

Striatum. L. *striatus*, furrowed. Phylogenetically more recent part of the corpus striatum (neostriatum) consisting of the caudate nucleus and the putamen or lateral portion of the lentiform nucleus. In comparative anatomy, striatum refers to a region of the brain in fishes, amphibians, and reptiles that is comparable to the corpus striatum of mammals.

Subiculum. L. *subicere*, to bring under or near. An underlying structure. The subiculum hippocampi is the transitional cortex between that of the parahippocampal gyrus and the hippocampus. In a coronal section of the human temporal lobe, the subiculum is beneath the hippocampus.

Submucosal. L. *sub*, under + mucosal (from mucus). In the wall of a hollow organ, the layer that separates mucosa from the external muscular layers; it consists of vascular connective tissue with much collagen and also contains the submucosal (Meissner's) plexus.

Substantia gelatinosa. Column of small neurons at the apex of the dorsal gray horn throughout the spinal cord.

Substantia nigra. L. black substance. Large nucleus with motor functions in the midbrain; many of the constituent cells contain melanin.

Subthalamus. L. under + Gr. *thalamus*, inner chamber. Region of the diencephalon beneath the thalamus, containing fiber tracts and the subthalamic nucleus.

Sudomotor. L. *sudor*, sweat + *motor*, mover. Applies to sympathetic neurons that stimulate secretion from sweat glands.

Superior. L. comparative of *superus* (from *super*), above. In human anatomy, nearer to the top of the head. In animals that are not bipedal, the equivalent term is anterior.

Synapse. Gr. *synapsis*, junction. Word introduced by Sherrington in 1897 for the site at which one neuron is excited or inhibited by another neuron.

Syndrome. Gr. *syndrome*, the act of running together or combining. Collection of concurring clinical symptoms and signs. A syndrome usually is due to a single cause. The word is often used incorrectly as a synonym for "disease."

Syringomyelia. Gr. *syrinx*, pipe, tube + *myelos*, marrow. Condition characterized by central cavitation of the spinal cord and gliosis around the cavity.

T

Tangential. L. *tangens*, touching. In the direction of a line or plane that touches a curved surface. Used in anatomy for a plane of section approximately parallel to the surface of an organ.

Tanycyte. Gr. *tanyo*, stretch + *kytos*, hollow (cell). Specialized type of elongated ependymal cell present in the floor of the third ventricle.

Tapetum. L. *tapete*, a carpet. Fibers of the corpus callosum sweeping over the lateral ventricle and forming the lateral wall of its temporal horn.

Tectum. L. roof. Roof of the midbrain consisting of the paired superior and inferior colliculi.

Tegmentum. L. *tegmentum*, a covering. Dorsal portion of the pons; also the major portion of the cerebral peduncle of the midbrain, lying between the substantia nigra and the tectum.

Tela choroidea. L. a web + Gr. *chorioeides*, like a membrane. Vascular connective tissue continuous with that of the pia mater that continues into the core of the choroid plexuses.

Telencephalon. Gr. *telos*, end + *enkephalos*, brain. Cerebral hemispheres; the more lateral and rostral of the two divisions of the prosencephalon or forebrain.

Telodendria. Gr. *telos*, end + *dendrion*, tree. Terminal branches of axons.

Temporal. L. *tempus*, time. The temporal lobe is named after the overlying temporal bone of the skull. The bone is named for the overlying skin (the temple), where the hair first goes gray with the ravages of time.

Tendon. L. *tendo*. A cord, band, or sheet of collagen fibers (sinew) that attaches a muscle to a bone or other structure. The **tendo calcaneus** is shared by the calf muscles (gastrocnemius, plantaris, and soleus), which all insert onto the calcaneus or heel bone to mediate plantar flexion at the ankle joint.

Tentorium. L. tent. Tentorium cerebelli is a dural partition between the occipital lobes of the cerebral hemispheres and the cerebellum.

Tetraplegia. Gr. *tetra-*, four + *plege*, a blow or stroke. Paralysis that affects the four limbs. Also called quadriplegia.

Thalamus. Gr. *thalamus*, an inner chamber; also meant a bridal couch, so that the pulvinar (*q.v.*) was its cushion or pillow. Galen made up the word thalamus, and Willis was probably the first to use the word in its modern sense.

Threshold. O.E. *therscwald*, a house's door sill or point of entry. In physiology, the point at which a stimulus brings about a response.

Thrombus. Gr. *thrombos*, clot. Clotted blood in a living blood vessel. Thrombosis occurs at sites of irregularity, typically due to atheroma in arteries.

Tomography. Gr. *tomos*, cutting + *graphein*, to write. Production of images of sections through a part of the body. Computed tomography with x-rays and nuclear magnetic resonance imaging are valuable diagnostic techniques.

Tone, tonus. Gr. *tonos*, pitch (sound), or tension. The normal state of firmness and elasticity of muscles caused by partial contraction of some of their fibers.

Tonofibril. Gr. *tonos*, or tension + L. *fibra*, thread. An intracellular filament that contributes to maintaining the shape and position of a cell.

Torcular. L. wine press, from *torquere*, to twist. Confluence of the dural venous sinuses at the internal occipital protuberance was formerly known as the torcular Herophili.

Trabecula. Diminutive of L. *traba* or Gr. *trapes*, a wooden beam. A component of a net-like arrangement of fibrous, muscular or bony structures, such as the connective tissue filaments that bridge the subarachnoid space, or the spicules and lamellae of cancellous bone.

Tract. L. *tractus*, a region or district. Region of the central nervous system largely occupied by a population of axons that all have the same origin and destination (which often form the name, as in "spinothalamic tract").

Transducer. L. *transducere*, to lead across. Structure or mechanism for converting one form of energy into another; applied to sensory receptors.

Trapezoid body. Transverse fibers of the auditory pathway situated at the junction of the dorsal and ventral portions of the pons.

Trigeminal. L. born three at a time. Trigeminal nerve has three large branches or divisions.

Trochlear. L. *trochlea*, a pulley. Trochlear nerve supplies the superior oblique muscle, whose tendon passes through a fibrous ring, the trochlea. This ring changes the direction in which the muscle pulls.

Trophic. Gr. *trephein*, to feed; *trophe*, food or nourishment; *trophos*, a feeder. Relating to nutrition. The term is extended to chemically mediated beneficial interactions among cells and organs. Frequently part of a word, as in thyrotrophic hormone, which stimulates the thyroid gland.

Tropism. Gr. *tropos*, a turning. An influence that changes or controls the direction in which a molecule, a cell or an organ moves. Usually encountered as the suffix **-tropic** or **-tropism**. Tropisms are important in the embryonic development of the nervous system. As a suffix, **-tropic** is sometimes interchangeable with **-trophic** (*q.v.*). For example, the name thyrotropic hormone signifies that this pituitary hormone passes from the blood into the thyroid gland. The name thyrotrophic hormone indicates its action on the gland.

U

Uncinate. L. hook-shaped. Uncinate fasciculus: association fibers connecting cortex of the ventral surface of the frontal lobe with that of the temporal pole. Also a bundle of fastigiobulbar fibers (uncinate fasciculus of Russell) that curves over the superior cerebellar peduncle in its passage to the inferior cerebellar peduncle.

Uncus. L. a hook. Hooked-back portion of the rostral end of the parahippocampal gyrus of the temporal lobe, constituting a landmark for the lateral olfactory area.

Uvula. L. little grape. A part of the inferior vermis of the cerebellum.

V

Vagus. L. wandering. Tenth cranial nerve is so named on account of the wide distribution of its branches in the thorax and abdomen.

Vallecula. L. diminutive of *vallis*, valley. Midline depression on the inferior aspect of the cerebellum.

Varicosity. L. *varix*, a varicose vein. In the nervous system, one of many dilations along the course of a neurite.

Vasopressin. L. vessel + pressure. An octapeptide hormone of the neurohypophysis. Large doses increase blood pressure by constricting small arteries. The alternative name of *antidiuretic hormone* describes its physiological action on the kidney.

Velate. L. *velum*, sail, curtain, veil. Velate or protoplasmic astrocytes have flattened processes.

Velum. L. sail, curtain, veil. Membranous structure. Superior and inferior medullary vela forming the roof of the fourth ventricle.

Ventral. L. *venter*, belly. Opposite of dorsal. In human anatomy, synonymous with anterior when applied to structures in the head and trunk. In animals that do not stand upright, ventral and anterior are different directions.

Ventricle. L. *ventriculus*, diminutive of *venter*, belly. Lateral, third, and fourth ventricles of the brain.

Vergence. L. *vergere*, to bend or incline. Relating to coordinated movements of both eyes in opposite directions, either medially (*convergence*) or laterally (*divergence*).

Vermis. L. worm. Midline portion of the cerebellum. Its ventral surface looks a little like a folded earthworm.

Vertigo. L. whirling, from *vertere*, to turn. A false sensation of rotation, either of self or surroundings.

Vestibular. L. *vestibulum*, forecourt or entrance hall. Relating to the equilibratory sense organs of the inner ear, which are connected with a common cavity, the vestibule of the labyrinth.

Z

Zona incerta. L. *zona*, belt + uncertain. Gray matter in the subthalamus representing a rostral extension of the reticular formation of the brain stem.

Zonula occludens. L. diminutive of *zona*, belt + occluding. Also known as a tight junction. Form of continuous close apposition of the membranes of neighboring cells, impermeable to macromolecules.

Suggested Reading

Dobson J. *Anatomical Eponyms*, 2nd ed. London: Livingstone, 1962.

Field EJ, Harrison RJ. *Anatomical Terms. Their Origin and Derivation*, 3rd ed. Cambridge: Heffer, 1968.

Index

Page numbers in *italic* denote figures and page numbers followed by t denote tables.